SURGERY
FOR
RHEUMATOID ARTHRITIS

A Comprehensive Team Approach

SURGERY FOR RHEUMATOID ARTHRITIS

A Comprehensive Team Approach

Edited by

Mack L. Clayton, M.D.

Clinical Professor of Orthopaedic Surgery
Department of Orthopaedics
Clinical Professor of Surgery (Hand)
Department of Surgery
University of Colorado Health Sciences Center
Assistant Chief, Division of Orthopedic Surgery
Veterans Administration Medical Center
Orthopedic Surgeon (retired) and Founder
Denver Orthopedic Clinic
Denver, Colorado
Senior Clinical Lecturer
Division of Orthopedics, Department of Surgery
University of Arizona College of Medicine
Tucson, Arizona

Charley J. Smyth, M.D., M.S.(Path), Sc.D.(hon)

Clinical Professor
Division of Rheumatic Diseases
Department of Medicine
University of Colorado Health Sciences Center
Rheumatologist (retired)
Denver Orthopedic Clinic
Denver, Colorado

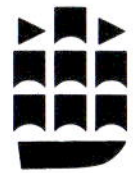

Churchill Livingstone
New York, Edinburgh, London, Melbourne, Tokyo

Library of Congress Cataloging-in-Publication Data

Surgery for rheumatoid arthritis : a comprehensive team approach /
    edited by Mack L. Clayton, Charley J. Smith.
        p.   cm.
    Includes bibliographical references and index.
    ISBN 0-443-08217-0
    1. Rheumatoid arthritis—Surgery. 2. Rheumatoid arthritis-
-Treatment. 3. Health care teams.
    [DNLM: 1. Arthritis, Rheumatoid—surgery. 2. Patient Care Team.
3. Surgery, Operative—methods.   WE 346 S9585]
RD686.S85 1992
617.4'72—dc20
DNLM/DLC
for Library of Congress   92-9503
                                                                   CIP

Distributed in the United Kingdom by Churchill Livingstone, Robert Stevenson House, 1–3 Baxter's Place, Leith Walk, Edinburgh EH1 3AF, and by associated companies, branches, and representatives throughout the world.

Accurate indications, adverse reactions, and dosage schedules for drugs are provided in this book, but it is possible that they may change. The reader is urged to review the package information data of the manufacturers of the medications mentioned.

The Publishers have made every effort to trace the copyright holders for borrowed material. If they have inadvertently overlooked any, they will be pleased to make the necessary arrangements at the first opportunity.

Copy Editor: *Donna C. Balopole*
Production Designer: *Jill Little*
Production Supervisor: *Sharon Tuder*
Cover Design: *Paul Moran*
Production services provided by Bermedica Productions, Ltd.

Printed in the United States of America

First published in 1992   7 6 5 4 3 2 1

This book is dedicated to Charley J. Smyth, M.D., a giant in the field of rheumatology. He started the arthritis service at the University of Colorado School of Medicine in 1948 and has trained many rheumatologists. He was one of the original founders of The Arthritis Foundation (national) and its Michigan and Rocky Mountain chapters. He is a Past President of the American Rheumatism Association (now the American College of Rheumatology) and was recently honored with a "Master" in the College. There is now a Charley J. Smyth Rheumatology Professorship at the University of Colorado, with endowment by his many patients and friends.

I became associated with Charley in 1954 at the University of Colorado, where we set up a combined Orthopaedic-Rheumatology Clinic to emphasize a "team approach" to this crippling disease, and we have continued to work as a team during the ensuing years. He practiced at the Denver Orthopedic Clinic from 1978 until his retirement in 1991.

Charley Smyth has strongly supported the team approach between rheumatology and orthopedics on which this book is based. He is my mentor, consultant, associate, and friend. He is, indeed, a "friend to man."

Mack L. Clayton, M.D.

Contributors

Mack L. Clayton, M.D.
Clinical Professor of Orthopaedic Surgery, Department of Orthopaedics, and Clinical Professor of Surgery (Hand), Department of Surgery, University of Colorado Health Sciences Center; Assistant Chief, Division of Orthopedic Surgery, Veterans Administration Medical Center; Orthopedic Surgeon (retired) and Founder, Denver Orthopedic Clinic, Denver, Colorado; Senior Clinical Lecturer, Division of Orthopedics, Department of Surgery, University of Arizona College of Medicine, Tucson, Arizona

Douglas A. Dennis, M.D.
Assistant Clinical Professor, Department of Orthopaedics, University of Colorado Health Sciences Center; Orthopedic Surgeon, Denver Orthopedic Clinic, Denver, Colorado

Donald C. Ferlic, M.D.
Associate Clinical Professor, Department of Orthopaedics, University of Colorado Health Sciences Center; Orthopedic Surgeon, Denver Orthopedic Clinic, Denver, Colorado

Alan E. Heilman, M.D.
Clinical Assistant Professor, Department of Orthopedic Surgery, Baylor College of Medicine; Orthopedic Surgeon, Fondren Orthopedic Group, Inc., Houston, Texas. Formerly, Orthopedic Surgeon, Denver Orthopedic Clinic, Denver, Colorado

Charley J. Smyth, M.D., M.S.(Path), Sc.D.(hon)
Clinical Professor, Division of Rheumatic Diseases, Department of Medicine, University of Colorado Health Sciences Center; Rheumatologist (retired), Denver Orthopedic Clinic, Denver, Colorado

Morris H. Susman, M.D.
Orthopedic Surgeon, Denver Orthopedic Clinic, Denver, Colorado

David A. Wong, M.D., M.Sc., F.R.C.S.(C)
Assistant Clinical Professor, Department of Orthopaedics, University of Colorado Health Sciences Center; Orthopedic Surgeon, Denver Orthopedic Clinic, Denver, Colorado

Strengthen the weak hands,
and make firm the feeble knees.
Say to those who are of a fearful heart,
Be strong, fear not!

Isaiah 35:3

Preface

Rheumatoid arthritis is one of the most common and widespread forms of nonfatal chronic polyarthritis in the United States. Its prevalence approaches 1 percent of all adults (age 18 and older) and occurs between two and three times more frequently in women than in men. In people 65 years and older, the prevalence ranges from 2 percent in men to 5 percent in women. The impact of rheumatoid arthritis, in terms of human suffering and financial burden, is monumental. About one-third of all patients with this disease become disabled within 10 years after diagnosis, largely from joint destruction.

The primary focus of *Surgery for Rheumatoid Arthritis: A Comprehensive Team Approach* is the orthopaedic management of joints damaged by rheumatoid inflammation. Patients disabled by rheumatoid arthritis have been surgically treated for almost a century, but developments in reconstructive surgery have been made rapidly over the past few decades. The contributions of orthopaedic surgery to the restoration of function and the reduction of pain in these patients mark some of the most significant advances in the management of this disease.

An additional contribution to disease management has been the remarkable progress in the overall understanding of rheumatoid arthritis. This has resulted from the contributions of multiple basic science and clinical disciplines, including major advances in the understanding of the mechanism of joint inflammation, application of newer diagnostic methods, and development of more effective drugs and rehabilitation procedures. The introductory chapters of this book are designed to provide a concise analysis of the current knowledge in each of these areas.

In the mid-1950s, we adopted a team approach to the comprehensive management of the rheumatoid arthritic patient. It became evident that maximum benefit could be accomplished only by combining the talents of physicians with those of skilled nurses, physical and occupational therapists, social workers, and family members, all working with an informed and motivated patient. The education of all team members has been essential in the success of the team approach. The efforts of The Arthritis Foundation in educating the general public have played a key role in making these advances known and available to a larger number of patients.

This book is based upon our experiences during the past 35 years, and is primarily a record of personal opinions. A number of key references are included, but this is not intended to constitute a survey of the literature. The book is aimed toward all comprehensive-minded orthopaedic surgeons, physiatrists, clinical rheumatologists, orthopaedic and rheumatology trainees, and general physicians who are treating arthritis patients, with a special emphasis upon the current status of reconstructive surgery in rheumatoid arthritis and the value of the team approach. The book should also prove valuable for use in training programs for the entire treatment team.

There has been a great interest and growth in surgery of the hand and of the entire upper extremity relating to the crippled arthritic patient. These advances are reviewed here, including the development of total joint arthroplasty and tendon and other soft tissue reconstructive procedures.

A critical analysis is made of the current status of lower extremity reconstruction through hip and knee replacements in the rheumatoid patient. The successes following total hip replacement have been so outstanding that many patients as well as rheumatologists have come to expect too much from other reconstructive procedures; however, the total knee replacement is now as successful as the total hip replacement. Forefoot arthroplasty has been successful for over 35 years, longer than any other widely used procedure for the leg. A number of individual case reports are included to illustrate the priorities and timing when multiple procedures are necessary.

Spinal problems related to rheumatoid arthritis are discussed, including ankylosing spondylitis, which is also an "inflammatory" arthritis. The surgical procedures employed in rheumatoid patients are not significantly different from those used in other patients who require a similar operation. However, the bony erosions, osteopenia, and synovial and capsular changes of the rheumatoid patient require that the operation be tailored to accommodate these changes in each patient. Synovectomy is an important part of rheumatoid surgery; the history, subsequent improvements in technique, and current role of this procedure are presented here.

Reconstructive surgery in the patient with generalized rheumatoid disease is only one step in a comprehensive plan of treatment; it is often a dramatic event indeed. In order for it to be successful, the patient and each team member must be active contributors. The coordination and timing of drug therapy, physical therapy, and patient education—before and after each surgical procedure—will give the best opportunity for maximum benefit. It is this entire process of preoperative and postoperative care, provided through either physical means or adequate drugs, that is of critical importance to the success of any surgical intervention. Included in these decisions are the status of the patient's overall health and social and family situations, the degree of active disease in all joints, and the presence of any co-existing disease. It is essential that the surgeon be aware of the prior course of the patient's illness before introducing the new factor of surgical intervention.

Despite the advances in surgical techniques and prosthetic designs for those afflicted with rheumatoid arthritis, the key to optimum results remains prudent medical-surgical judgment in patient selection combined with careful preoperative planning and appropriate operative technique.

Mack L. Clayton, M.D.
Charley J. Smyth, M.D.

Acknowledgments

This book is a product of the Denver Orthopedic Clinic. A decade-long labor of love, it has entailed the efforts of many obliging hands along the way. All contributors are or have been associated with the Clinic, which has resulted in the book's unified approach.

The administrative staff of Bruce McKinnon and Paul Sauer have been an unfailing source of support and encouragement during this endeavor. Research Coordinator Anne Szymanski, with her background in English and library research, was invaluable in coordinating the many details of revision, bibliographic verification, and illustrations for each author. Medical Research Consultant Elizabeth Stringer assisted in the preparation of clinical reports. Secretaries Donna Erickson and Jana Gleason spent long hours typing and retyping my (M.L.C.) manuscripts, as did the secretaries of the other authors for them. The majority of fine illustrations in this book have been precisely executed by my son, James Clayton.

As a group, the 33 orthopaedic-rheumatology fellows that have trained at the Denver Orthopedic Clinic have made significant contributions in service, fresh ideas, and clinical research. In addition, the University of Colorado residents have provided stimulation and made life more pleasant. Drs. William Winter (Chief of Orthopedics at the Denver Veterans Administration Medical Center) and Jerome Wiedel (Professor and Chief of Orthopaedics, University of Colorado School of Medicine) have encouraged us to "get the book finished after all these years." Our team approach never would have succeeded without the endorsement of the referring physicians and all members of the team, including nurses, physical and occupational therapists, social workers, and the patients themselves.

Last but not least, Sally Clayton and Laura Smyth have constituted the major support group for this book. Without their love and encouragement, it never would have happened.

Mack L. Clayton, M.D.
Charley J. Smyth, M.D.

Contents

MEDICAL CONSIDERATIONS

I

Medical Perspectives of Surgery for Rheumatoid Arthritis

Charley J. Smyth

The terms *arthritis* and *rheumatism* cover more than 100 types of joint and connective tissues diseases. An estimated 35 million Americans, or one in seven, suffer from these disorders, making arthritis and related diseases this nation's most common cause of pain, disability, and disfigurement.[18] Because most of these illnesses are chronic and frequently require lifelong medical care, the annual cost of hospitalization, professional services, drugs, and loss of productivity is estimated to be a staggering $18.6 billion annually.

Today there is general agreement that rheumatoid arthritis is one of the most frequently occurring types of these rheumatic diseases. Its etiology remains unknown. The diagnosis of this type is established by the manner in which it involves multiple joints and its tendency to progressively destroy articular tissues, resulting in characteristic deformities. Also, it is now generally recognized that rheumatoid arthritis is a multisystem disease with frequent extra-articular lesions (e.g., granulomatous nodules in the skin, lungs, bursae, and tendons), arteritis, episcleritis, pericarditis, lymphadenopathy, splenomegaly, and occasionally amyloid deposits in the kidneys. Although the articular tendon synovium bears the brunt of the destructive changes typical of this disease, many other organs are involved; hence it is more aptly termed *rheumatoid disease*. It is generally regarded as the prototype of autoimmune connective tissue disease. Some helpful but unspecific laboratory diagnostic tests include serum antibodies to certain immunoglobulins (rheumatoid arthritis factor, IgM, IgG), immune complexes, and elevated erythrocyte sedimentation rates. Other laboratory tests have shown an association between certain histocompatible antigens: HLA-D4, HLA-DR4, MT3, and rheumatoid arthritis. Roentgenographic joint changes frequently provide assistance in establishing the diagnosis of rheumatoid arthritis.

The ability to distinguish this disease from other chronic types of arthritis today contrasts sharply from the situation that existed when the term "rheumatoid arthritis" was first used in England in 1859 by Garrod.[6] At that time and throughout the last half of the nineteenth century there was considerable controversy about the existence of this chronic polyarthritis as a separate clinical disease. During these years the views of the famous German pathologist Rudolph Virchow[19] prevailed and gained universal acceptance in both Europe and America. In 1869, when he introduced the term "arthritis deformans," he did not differentiate degenerative joint disease (osteoarthritis) from rheumatoid arthritis but considered them together as one form of progressive chronic polyarthritis.

It was not until the last decade of the nineteenth century and early in the twentieth century that the results of the American studies, each using roentgenograms of affected joints in patients with chronic rheumatic diseases, showed clear-cut differences between rheumatoid arthritis and osteoarthritis. Three studies (Goldthwait,[7]

Painter,[13] and Nichols and Richardson[12]) clearly distinguished rheumatoid arthritis as a single entity.

RHEUMATOLOGIC SURGERY

One of the rewarding and successful developments in the management of the rheumatic diseases has been the liaison between primary physicians and orthopaedic surgeons. Before rheumatology had been developed as a specialty within internal medicine, patients with arthritis first consulted an orthopaedist, and many still do. Today, with advances in the knowledge and effectiveness of total hip replacement, synovectomies, tendon repair, osteotomies, and other arthritis reconstructive procedures, and the reduction of complications of sepsis, loosening, and fractures, there has been a growing respect between these two specialties dealing with disorders of the locomotor system.

PREVALENCE

Among the more than 100 types of arthritis currently recognized, rheumatoid arthritis ranks second in prevalence only to degenerative joint disease or osteoarthritis. In a survey of 14 worldwide epidemiologic studies, including a National Health Examination survey in the United States, the prevalence rate varied from 0.3 to 1.5 percent of the population.[20] This wide range can be attributed in part to the various criteria that were used to gather these data and to the lack of agreement among epidemiologists regarding the best method for conducting such studies. Other difficulties in the ascertainment of a more exact prevalence results from the uncertainty when detecting early cases. During the first several months of rheumatoid arthritis it is often impossible to be certain about the diagnosis, and it may be confused with a different disease altogether. Uncertainty may also be caused by the insidious onset. Another factor is the re-

mitting nature of the illness, especially during the first 2 years.

Still other variables include the frequency of rheumatoid arthritis among certain subgroups of the population. For example, it is two to three times more common in women than in men, although this female predominance disappears when only patients with positive serologic tests for rheumatoid factor and erosive changes on roentgenograms are considered. The prevalence of rheumatoid arthritis also varies among ethnic groups. For instance, Yakima Indian women have a much higher incidence than women in the general population (3.4 percent versus 1.4 percent).[1] In urban South African blacks, the prevalence is 3.3 percent compared with 0.87 percent in rural blacks in the same country. American Blacks may have a lower prevalence than whites.[3] The annual incidence rates for persons age 15 and older have been estimated at 67/100,000 for the sexes combined.[10] Other studies have clearly shown an increased incidence with age: 0.3 percent incidence in adults under 35 years of age, with an increase during subsequent decades to exceed 10 percent in persons 65 years and older.

There is now general agreement that hereditary factors exert major influences in the susceptibility to rheumatoid arthritis.[21] Major advances in knowledge of familial aggregation and studies of identical (monozygotic) twins indicate that the association with rheumatoid arthritis is more than 30 times the expected rate. Additional support for the concept for a major role in the development of rheumatoid arthritis has been the demonstration of the specificity of DR-4 in the immune response genes of HLA-DR locus in population studies of rheumatoid arthritis patients. This genetic factor has been demonstrated in up to 60 percent of patients with this disease.

COURSE AND PROGNOSIS

Surprisingly little is known about the clinical course of this common disease if it is untreated. It is not known how often patients with minimal symptoms and little or no functional loss tolerate these changes by taking simple analgesics and not seeking medical attention. It appears that this practice is a frequent occurrence, and so these individuals are not incorporated into any study designed to determine the long-term course of this disease. As a result, it is not possible to know the number or the course of patients with rheumatoid arthritis that goes unrecognized. Although controlled studies are lacking, it can be estimated that approximately one-third of all patients who develop rheumatoid arthritis undergo, with or without treatment of any kind, a complete and permanent remission within 2 years after the onset of their illness. This self-limited clinical course has been called course I (Fig. 1-1). It is important to keep this group of patients in mind whenever any type of high-risk drug management program "preventive" orthopaedic procedure is being considered. The marked and unpredictable variability is not limited to the early stage of the disease but occurs throughout its clinical course, making evaluation of any form of therapy difficult.

In contrast to the above relatively benign or self-limited course (course I), a far greater number of patients who develop rheumatoid arthritis follow a slowly progressive course, with moderate activity interspersed with short episodes of acute arthritis. The periods of acute activity are more likely to occur early and become more sustained with the passage of time. Patients in this second group (course II) may have only minimally active disease and experience long periods of apparent inactivity. There is another subset of a few patients within this course II group who are characterized by recurrent episodes of severe synovitis of short duration (a few hours to a few days) with complete recovery and no residual deformity. These patients are said to have a "palindromic type" of onset of rheumatoid arthritis.

There remains a third major group of rheumatoid arthritis patients who experience a more unrelenting, progressive, and destructive form of the disease, with deformities, disfigurement, and occasionally even death (course III). Fortunately, this more progressive or malignant type is seen in only 10 to 15 percent of patients with this illness.

In a given patient it is not possible at the onset of the disease to predict its future course. If subcutaneous nodules occur, a high titer of rheumatoid factor develops, and erosive roentgenographic changes are demonstrated after the disease is established, there is a strong probability that rapid progression and marked destructive changes are inevitable.

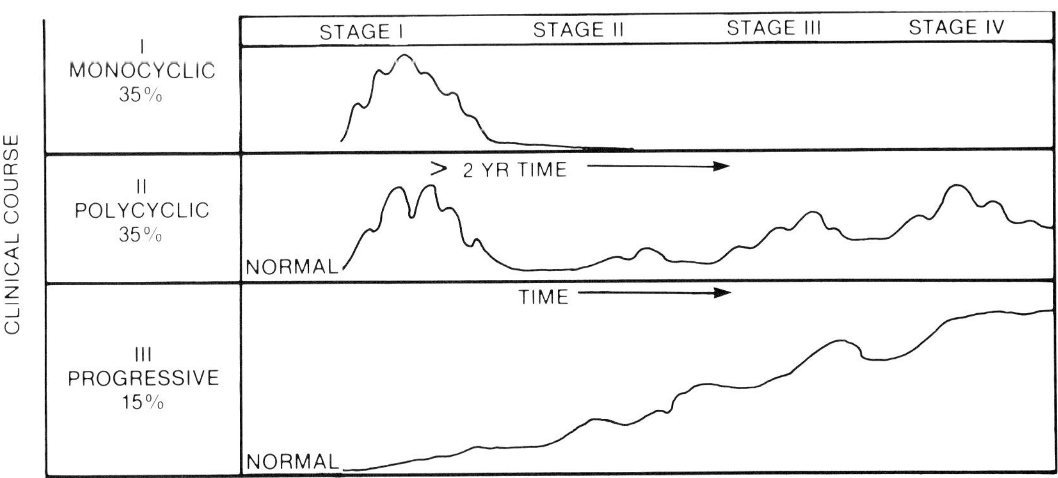

Fig. 1-1. Three characteristic clinical courses of rheumatoid arthritis showing approximate percentages of patients who follow each pattern and the relation to the stage of the disease and time.

PROGRESS IN MANAGEMENT

Rapid and major advancements in the control of rheumatoid arthritis has been made during the twentieth century. This progress has paralleled, and in some respects surpassed, the significant progress made in the care of other types of arthritis and allied disorders. These therapeutic achievements were possible only because of the remarkable contributions made by fundamental research. Investigation using advanced biotechnology has resulted in improved methods for controlling infections, understanding inflammatory mechanisms and its biochemical mediators, and providing new knowledge regarding immunoregulation and immunogenetics. In addition, valuable new information has been added about the ultrastructure of cartilage and connective tissue and the biomechanics of joints. From the pharmacology laboratories have come drugs that effectively alter the action of the mediators and reduce inflammation and cellular proliferation.

The application of this new knowledge to the clinical management of rheumatoid arthritis patients by primary physicians, rheumatologists, and orthopaedists has accomplished remarkable benefits. The rapid strides made during the past 50 years far exceeds those of any previous period in history.

EARLY YEARS

During the first quarter of the twentieth century there was little interest in arthritis by the medical profession. The limited treatment available consisted in salicylates, liniments, hot baths, the use of splints, and a few operative procedures. Synovectomy was one of the first operations performed for rheumatoid arthritis in the United States, when it was brought into rather general use in 1923 by Swett[17] in the hope of curing the disease. It enjoyed moderate popularity for some 15 years, then fell out of use only to be reinstated during the 1960s. Subsequently, the treatment was almost exclusively in the hands of the primary physicians, internists, and physiatrists. It

was during the first quarter of the twentieth century that a wide variety of methods were tried to control the disease: drugs, vaccines, vitamins, and physiotherapy. Most of these nonsurgical measures proved ineffective or, if any benefit was derived it was accompanied by adverse side effects. It was not until the 1930s that there were any significant advances in drug therapy for rheumatoid arthritis.

Among the prominent therapeutic methods tried was removal of focal infections followed by administration of polyvalent vaccines and gold injections. The concept that rheumatoid arthritis was caused by foci of infection was introduced in 1912 by Billings[2] of Chicago. There was almost universal acceptance of the idea, and this practice held full sway into the 1930s. The number of innocent teeth and tonsils and even gallbladders removed because of this erroneous therapy is incalculable. Hand in hand with the removal of suspected foci was the use of vaccines. Finally, controlled clinical trials of polyvalent vaccines proved their lack of value, and this sad period in the treatment of rheumatoid arthritis gradually came to an end.

It was not until 1876, with the discovery of salicylates, that any effective drugs for the relief of pain and inflammation of rheumatoid arthritis were known. In the English-speaking world, MacLagan[11] of England is usually credited with the use of salicin extracted from the bark of the willow. That same year, two German observers, Reiss[14] and Stricker,[16] reported the use of salicylic acid. The year 1876 therefore marked a turning point with three independent therapeutic trials of salicylate.

It was more than a half-century later before another effective agent was advocated for the treatment of this disease. Based on the belief that tuberculosis and rheumatoid arthritis had a common (infectious) etiology, Forestier[5] in France applied gold-thiopropanol sodium sulfanate (allodrysine) for the treatment of rheumatoid arthritis. His favorable experiences with more than 550 cases, in which improvement was noted in 70 to 80 percent, were published in 1935. Numerous others have subsequently confirmed these observations, including those reporting double-blind studies.[4,8,15] Gold is still highly regarded and frequently used as an effective remission-inducing agent.

CORTISONE INITIATING A NEW DRUG ERA

With the introduction of cortisone by Hench et al.[9] in 1949 came a productive period of drug-related research in the rheumatic disease field. Since then, rapid advances have been made in the development of a great number of beneficial and relatively safe nonsteroidal anti-inflammatory drugs (NSAIDs) as well as agents that have strong remission-inducing capabilities. These drugs include gold, D-penicillamine, cyclophosphamide, azathioprine, methotrexate, sulfasalazine, and hydroxychloroquine. They have been designated disease-modifying antirheumatic drugs (DMARDs), or second line agents.

ADVANCES IN ORTHOPAEDIC MANAGEMENT

The greatest contributions to the care of patients with established rheumatoid arthritis during the last quarter-century have been made in orthopaedic surgery. The prolonged pain relief and the restoration to normal or near-normal function resulting from reconstructive surgical procedures in disabled rheumatoid arthritis patients is a remarkable therapeutic advance. Numerous long term studies confirm the usefulness, lasting benefits, and safety of total joint replacement of hips, knees, shoulders, elbows, wrists, and small joints of the hand and toes.

These results have come through the combined efforts of material scientists, bioengineers, orthopaedic and hand surgeons, rheumatologists, and both medical and paramedical rehabilitation specialists. Additional factors contributing to the success of the operative management of the rheumatoid arthritis patient have been the availability and use of effective antibiotic agents, refinements in aseptic techniques, use of modern anesthesia methods, and blood and fluid replacement.

TEAM APPROACH

As these advances in preventive and reconstructive care have occurred over the past few decades, several significant changes have taken place. They include increased participation by orthopaedists in the total management of the rheumatoid arthritis patient and a growing awareness of the importance of effective rehabilitative services to gain maximum improvement from reconstructive procedures. During this same period, primary physicians, rheumatologists, allied health professionals, and all other health care providers have become increasingly aware of the benefits that can be achieved in overcoming disability and correcting deformities. It is now clear that it is no longer possible to provide adequate care to rheumatoid arthritis patients without these services.

The delivery of this type of comprehensive care demands a close working relationship between members of the various health professions involved. This team includes the primary physician, rheumatologist, orthopaedist, physiatrist, physical and occupational therapists, nurse, social worker, dietitian, and occupational counselor. This interdisciplinary approach has proved effective for providing total patient services and for recording and evaluating the end results of the various procedures carried out.

ARTHRITIS CENTERS

Within all branches of the medical profession and the allied health professionals as well as the general public, there is a growing recognition of the significant progress being made to improve the care of many patients with arthritis. With this recognition has come a general increased demand for improvement in the delivery of the latest treatment. Physicians with particular interest in the management of victims of these crippling diseases, rheumatologists, and orthopaedists have joined with hospital administrators and government agencies in a search for more efficient ways to meet the special needs of this group of patients. In Great Britain and on the continent of

Europe, special clinics, hospitals, or designated areas within hospitals have existed for several decades, providing the opportunity for the medical staff to work closely with other members of the rehabilitation team. In such units the entire professional staff responsible for the patient's care are able to confer frequently about all aspects of the problems presented by any individual patient, and thus each member of the team has a clear understanding of his or her responsibility in carrying out the treatment regimen.

The development of these comprehensive interdepartmental treatment facilities in Europe preceded by several decades such units in the United States. Few specialized arthritis treatment centers were established here until the 1930s. Since then the number has increased rapidly, serving many regions throughout the nation. Experience gained since the 1950s by bringing the programs and personnel involved with every phase of arthritis research, training, and patient care into one area has made it clear that such a team approach adds greatly to more efficient delivery of total patient care. It is important to stress that the overall responsibility of individual patients admitted to an arthritis center rests with a single physician. In most hospitals it is the primary physician, usually a rheumatologist, physiatrist, or orthopaedist, who will coordinate all phases of the diagnosis and treatment.

REFERENCES

1. Beasley RP, Willkens RF, Bennett PA: High prevalence of rheumatoid arthritis in Yakima Indians. Arthritis Rheum 16:143, 1973
2. Billings FL: Chronic focal infections and their etiologic relation to arthritis and nephritis. Arch Intern Med 9:484, 1912
3. Cunningham LS, Kelsey JL: Epidemiology of musculoskeletal impairments and associated disabilities. Am J Public Health 74:574, 1984
4. Empire Rheumatism Council: Gold therapy in rheumatoid arthritis; final report of a multicentre controlled trial. Am Rheum Dis 20:1315, 1961
5. Forestier J: Rheumatoid arthritis and its treatment by gold salts. J Lab Clin Med 10:827, 1935
6. Garrod AB: Treatise on Gout and Rheumatic Gout. Griffin, London, 1859
7. Goldthwait JE: Treatment of disabled joints resulting from the so-called rheumatic diseases. Boston Med Surg J 136:79, 1897
8. Hartfall SJ, Garland HG, Goldie W: Gold treatment of arthritis; a review of 900 cases. Lancet 233:838, 1937
9. Hench PS, Kendall AC, Slocumb CH et al: Effects of a hormone of the adrenal cortex (17-hydroxy-11-dehydrocorticosterone: compound E) and of pituitary adrenocorticotrophic hormone on rheumatoid arthritis. Proc Staff Meet Mayo Clin 24:181, 1949
10. Hochberg MC: Adult and juvenile rheumatoid arthritis; current epidemiologic concepts. Epidemiol Rev 3:27, 1981
11. MacLagan T: The treatment of acute rheumatism by salicin. Lancet 1:342, 1876
12. Nichols EH, Richardson FL: Arthritis deformans. J Med Res 16:149, 1909
13. Painter CF: Pathological lesions in rheumatoid arthritis. Boston Med Surg J 145:593, 1901
14. Reiss I: Uber die innerliehen anwendung der salicylsaure insbesonders bei dem acutem gelenkrheumatismus. Berlin Klin Wochenschr 13:86, 1876
15. Sigler JW, Bluhm GB, Duncan H et al: Gold salts in the treatment of rheumatoid arthritis: a double-blind study. Ann Intern Med 80:21, 1974
16. Stricker W: Uber die resultate der behandlung der polyarthritis rheumatica mit salicylsaure. Berlin Klin Wochenschr 1:15, 1876
17. Swett PP: A review of synovectomy. J Bone Joint Surg 20:68, 1938
18. US Department of Health and Human Services: Initiatives for Arthritis: Progress and Future Directions; a Report of the National Arthritis Advisory Board. NIH Publ. 84-2678, 1984
19. Virchow R: Knochen vom hohlenbaren mut krankaften veranderungen. Litschr Ethnol Ber 17:706, 1859
20. Wolfe AM: The epidemiology of rheumatoid arthritis: a review. Bull Rheum Dis 19:518, 1968
21. Wordsworth MB: The immunogenetics of rheumatoid arthritis. Curr Opin Rheum 2:423, 1990

2

Rheumatoid Arthritis: A Major Rheumatic Disease

Charley J. Smyth

Rheumatoid arthritis occurs worldwide and involves all racial, ethnic, and income groups. Several studies have shown that there is no basis for the belief that it is a disease of temperate climates, occurring infrequently in the tropics and subpolar regions. Additional predisposing factors have been considered, including heavy manual work and other work exposures, specific nutritional deficiencies, nervous dysfunctions, and personality disorders, but none of these factors led to increased risk of development of the disease.

EPIDEMIOLOGY

Prevalence

In an extensive analysis of data from population studies of rheumatoid arthritis in the United States defined by the American Rheumatism Association criteria for classic/definite disease, the rate of occurrence is consistently between 1 and 2 percent of the adult populations in every part of the world.[22] A few subpopulation studies have shown a high predisposition to the development of rheumatoid arthritis. Frequencies of 3.4 and 5.3 percent were found in Yakima and Chippewa Indians, respectively, compared with a prevalence of 1.4 percent in the general population.[3,10] A study in South Africa found a striking increase in the disease among those living in urban areas (3.3 percent) compared with those in rural areas (0.87 percent).[30]

There is general agreement that prevalence increases with age for both sexes. The U.S. National Health Examination Survey found a prevalence of 0.3 percent in adults under 35 years of age that increased steadily during subsequent decades, exceeding 10 percent in persons 65 years and older.[24]

Incidence

The number of new cases of rheumatoid arthritis that appears within a definite period of time varies with the criteria used; it is reported to range from a high of 2.9 to a low of 0.097 per 1,000 population for both men and women.[22] The only study to look at incidence longitudinally is that of Linos et al.,[21] which is based on hospital and physician records at the Mayo Clinic and other institutions in Rochester, Minnesota. Attendees between 1950 and 1974 showed an overall rate of 2.9 per 10,000 population over this period for men and women combined. In the United States in 1988 it was estimated that there were between four million and six million cases, with 100,000 to 200,000 new cases each year.

Hormonal and Reproductive Factors

A large number of clinical and experimental studies provide clear evidence of a linkage between sex hormones and rheumatoid arthritis. Population surveys from many parts of the world have found that there is a 2.5 : 1.0 female/male predominance in the prevalence of this disease. This ratio is less when only those with positive serology tests for rheumatoid factor and erosive bony changes are considered.

In 1938 Hench, of the Mayo Clinic, noted marked improvement in 22 women with active rheumatoid arthritis during 33 pregnancies,[11] and since then many investigators have confirmed his observations. Relapse postpartum is an almost universal finding and usually occurs within the first month after delivery. In a series of 56 pregnancies in rheumatoid arthritis patients, more than 90 percent had symptomatic relief during pregnancy but had exacerbations within 8 weeks postpartum.[25]

One report presented data indicating a decrease in the numbers of two subsets of T lymphocytes (OKT3[+] and OKT4[+]) during gestation in 84 women and offered it as a possible explanation for the long recognized reduction of rheumatoid activity associated with pregnancy.[33]

The 10-year population study by Linos et al.[21] observed a dramatic decline in the incidence of rheumatoid arthritis in the female population compared with the relatively stable rate in the male population. They attributed this decrease to the use of oral contraceptives and postmenopausal estrogens. Another study in England reported that the incidence of rheumatoid arthritis among women who had used contraceptives was about 50 percent less than in nonusers.[36]

Studies focused on the androgenic status of male rheumatoid patients following confirmed reports that these individuals have low serum testosterone concentrations. Further convincing data relating to the immunosuppressive effects associated with rheumatoid arthritis are the beneficial results in a trial involving seven male rheumatoid patients who received oral testosterone undeconate. All showed marked clinical improvement measured by a significant reduction in the number of affected joints as well as favorable laboratory changes. There was a rise in serum testosterone levels, a rise in the CD8[+] lymphocytes, and a decrease in the CD4[+]/CD8[+] lymphocyte ratio.[4] Other studies confirmed that a decrease in this ratio is a reliable index of reduc-

tion in the activity and severity of rheumatoid arthritis.

Hereditary Factors

Several types of investigation have established a genetic predisposition to rheumatoid arthritis. Occasionally, several cases of rheumatoid arthritis occur in the same family. This observation has led to a large number of population studies to determine the degree of aggregation or concentration of this disease. An analysis of ten such investigations by Mitchell failed to reveal evidence of familial aggregation.[22] Major advances relating to the role of heredity in the development of this disease have come from studies of twins with one parent known to have arthritis. In an extensive study in Great Britain involving 428 twins, there was a striking association in identical (monozygotic) twins, with 30 percent developing seropositive arthritis; of the fraternal (dizygotic) twins, 6 percent had seropositive arthritis.[20]

There is broad agreement that the concordance rates for rheumatoid arthritis are four to five times greater among monozygotic twins than dizygotic twins. A study of three monozygotic twin pairs from a rheumatoid arthritis family noted that there may be a marked delay before both twins develop the disease. This finding indicates that the concordance rate may be much higher and thus increases the relative importance of genetic factors.

Additional support for the importance of hereditary susceptibility to rheumatoid arthritis is the high incidence of affected first degree relatives with this disease. Familial aggregation of rheumatoid arthritis is well described, and one study showed that at least 11 percent of the patients with rheumatoid arthritis in this population study had one or more affected relatives.[37]

These highly significant immunogenetic investigations have clearly established a sound basis for the genetic contributions to rheumatoid arthritis and allied autoimmune rheumatic diseases. Extensive studies using a wide range of intricate techniques (e.g., serology, cellular typing, monoclonal antibodies, DNA amino acid sequencing) have shown that there is a strong association with the genes located in chromosome 6 in the major histocompatibility complex (MHC), alternately termed the human lymphocyte antigen (HLA) system. It is now established that the genes in this region govern the immune responses and act as risk factors for a variety of autoimmune diseases, including ankylosing spondylitis, systemic lupus erythematosus (SLE), and rheumatoid arthritis. These advances began after the observation that certain immunoglobulins of the IgG class were present in rheumatoid factor (RF) in the blood of rheumatoid arthritis patients.[28]

The genes in this region of chromosome 6 were first detected using HLA. Subsequently, four major subregions—A, B, C, D—were identified; and in the D or DR region, further subdivisions having specific autoimmune disease associations have been established. The strongest rheumatic disease association is between HLA-B27 and ankylosing spondylitis. Also, there is now agreement that the association of rheumatoid arthritis with a subunit of the DR locus (HLA-Dw4 and HLA-DRw4) is highly significant. Many believe that these two antigens are identical (Fig. 2-1).

Patients who have these HLA-DR4 antigens were first reported in 1978 by Statsny,[31] and an analysis of the results was published confirming these observations.[6] There is agreement that the specificity of this locus for rheumatoid arthritis is by no means as strong as the HLA-B27 marker for ankylosing spondylitis[9]; and there is general agreement that in the presence of this antigen the

relative risk of developing the disease is about fourfold.[38]

The identification of the precise marker in the immune response has greatly clarified our understanding of the immunogenic aspects of rheumatoid arthritis. This major advance may lead to detection of individuals predisposed to rheumatoid arthritis, thus aiding in early detection and therapeutic potential.

PATHOLOGY

Stage I: Early Events

The earliest events in rheumatoid arthritis occur in synovial tissues, with involvement of the microvasculature and resulting in endothelial cell injury and edema (Fig. 2-2). These early changes suggest that the responsible triggering factor is carried to the synovium by the circulation. Three specific types of vascular abnormality are recognized: The most common is *arteritis*, which involves the digital arteris. Noninflammatory, with internal proliferation and obliterative endoarteritis, it causes splinter infarcts in the nail beds and paronychial regions as well as peripheral neuritis. *Leukoblastic vasculitis* is the second type, with fibrinoid necrosis and polymorphonuclear (PMN) and mononuclear inflammatory infiltrates that produce papules or urticaria often involving the lower legs. The third type is *necrotizing arteritis*, which involves both small and medium-sized arteries and all layers of the vessel wall with an intense inflammatory reac-

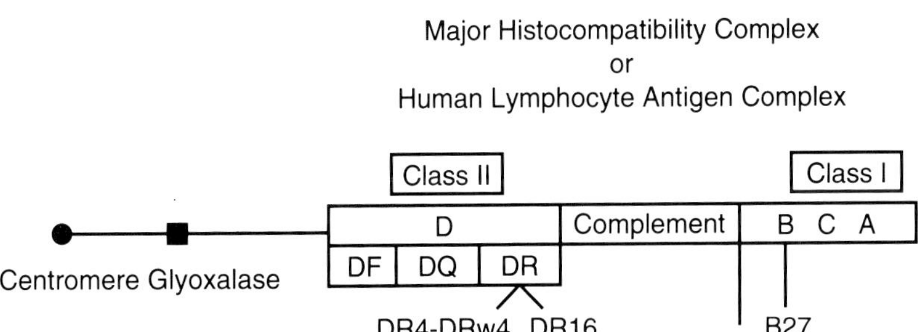

Fig. 2-1. Chromosome 6, showing the locations of HLA antigens responsible for the predisposition to the development of rheumatoid arthritis (DR-4, DRw4, and DR-16) and ankylosing spondylitis (B-27).

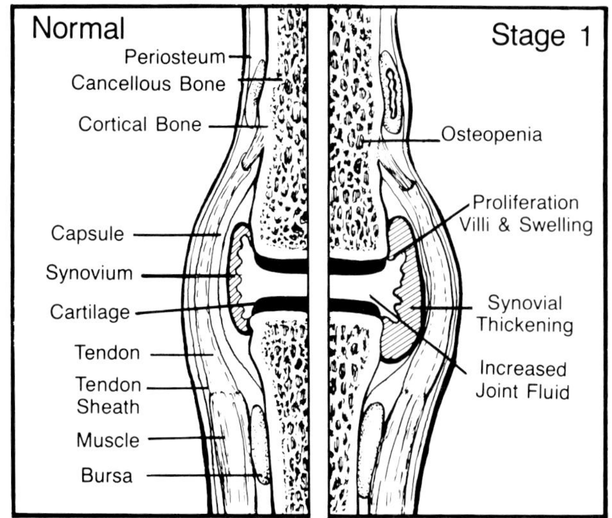

Fig. 2-2. Diarthrodial joint showing normal structures and the early pathologic changes of rheumatoid arthritis (stage I).

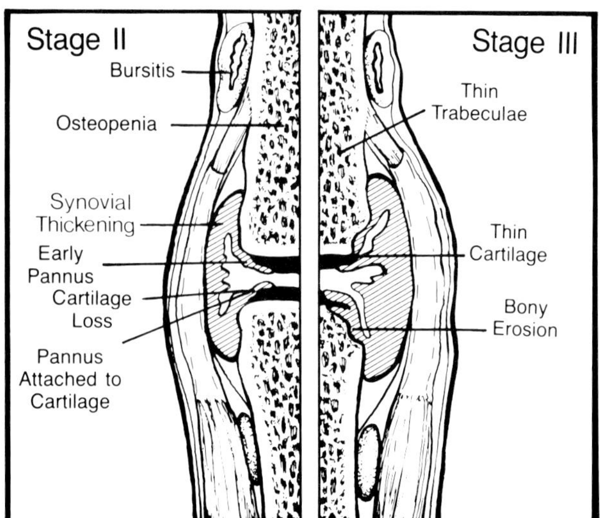

Fig. 2-3. **(A)** Stage II: moderately advanced with early pannus and beginning cartilage loss. **(B)** Stage III: late absorptive changes in cartilage with bony erosions.

tion, fibrinoid necrosis, and thrombosis. Fortunately, this type occurs infrequently, but when it does it leads to serious illness.

Stage II

At about the same time as the events in late Stage I are taking place, proliferation of the synovial lining cells occurs with hyperplasia and hypertrophy, resulting in an increase from the normal 1- to 3-cell surface layer to a depth of 6 to 10 cells (Fig. 2-3A). In the superficial synovium, the small blood vessels become surrounded by collections of monocytes, including macrophages and small lymphocytes that are often arranged in nodular aggregates; tiny thrombi are often seen as well. The subsynovial layer in the normal state is acellular but becomes packed with inflammatory cells that collect in the perivascular area. Small lymphocytes usually predominate in these collections; and monocytes/macrophages, plasma cells, and mast cells are also usual findings. Studies have shown that most of the lymphocytes in the synovial membrane are T cells of the helper subclass, but there are also large numbers of immunoglobulin-producing B lympho-

cytes. PMNs are infrequently seen even in clinically active joints, although they are commonly found in the synovial fluid. Rarely are germinal centers found in these synovial aggregates.

Stage III: Established Disease

With established rheumatoid arthritis, the synovium develops slender villous projections that appear as edematous finger-like protrusions into the joint cavity. As the inflammation proceeds, these tongues of inflamed synovium become adherent to the adjacent margins of the articular cartilage (Fig. 2-3B), and this adherent inflammatory tissue invades the cartilage as it creeps progressively over the cartilage. At the articular margins, the pannus also replaces bone, and in this position the loss of bone gives rise to the radiologically visible erosions characteristic of this disease. Pannus may also extend through the subchondral bone and destroy trabeculae, producing cysts or geodes.

Active synovitis is accompanied by an increase in the amount of synovial fluid. Characteristically, this effusion is an exudate. The total white blood cell (WBC) count ranges from 5,000 to

20,000/cu mm, although values in excess of 50,000/cu mm are encountered.[27] Mononuclear cells usually predominate early in the disease, but in established stages about two-thirds of the cells are PMNs. Many of these cells contain small intracytoplasmic granules of phagocytosed RFs and are called rheumatoid arthritis cells, or *ragocytes*.[13] The synovial fluid is cloudy and of low viscosity, and it forms a loose friable clot with the addition of dilute acetic acid (mucin clot test). The protein content, normally less than 2 g%, often exceeds 3.5 g%. Hemolytic complement levels are usually less than one-third of the serum values; C4 and C2 levels are profoundly depressed, and glucose values may be low or normal.

The subcutaneous nodule is the characteristic pathologic finding and is present at some time in approximately 20 to 25 percent of patients with established rheumatoid arthritis. They are almost invariably associated with RF-positive disease and usually with a more severe, destructive arthritis. These diagnostic lesions are firm, rounded masses that occur in the subcutaneous tissue and vary in size from 0.5 to 2.0 cm in diameter. They are most often found in periarticular structures and areas that are frequently subjected to mechanical pressure. Common sites include the olecranon bursae, the extensor surface of the forearms, and the Achilles tendon. These granulomatous lesions also occur in lungs and pleura, meninges, ears, along the tendon sheaths of the writs, and in the flexor tendons of the palms, where they commonly cause "triggering." Histologically, these nodules are composed of a central zone of fibrinoid necrosis surrounded by

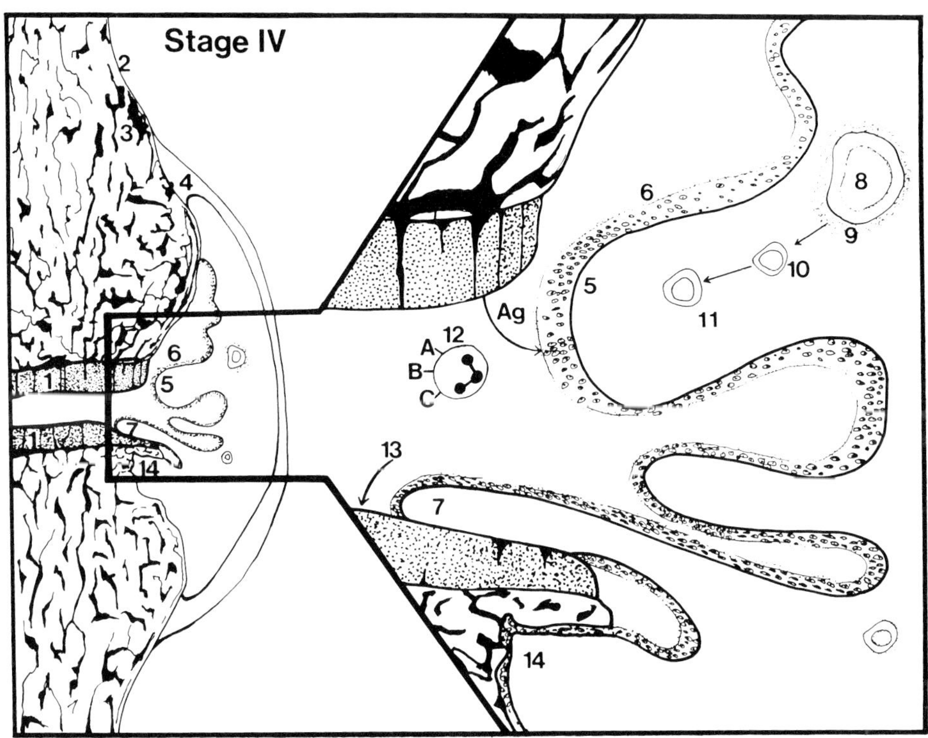

Fig. 2-4. Stage IV: advanced joint destruction with marked or complete loss of cartilage. There is atrophy of cortical and trabecular bone with erosions leading to subluxation and fibrous or bony union (or both) across joint space. 1, articular cartilage; 2, cortex of bone; 3, trabeculae of bone; 4, capsule; 5, hypertrophied villus; 6, proliferating synovial lining cells; 7, pannus; 8, blood vessel; 9, monocytes/macrophages; 10, T lymphocytes; 11, B lymphocytes; 12,A, chemotoxis; 12,B, complement activation; 12,C, lysosomes; 13, immune complex deposits; 14, bone erosion.

elongated connective tissue cells radically arranged in a palisade fashion around the central necrotic zone. A third, or outer, zone of mature granulation tissue contains chronic inflammatory cells and a few giant cells.

Periarticular tissue (tendon sheaths, bursae, joint capsules, ligaments, muscles, and nerves) share in the inflammatory changes that are continuing within the joint. Arteritis involving small and medium-sized vessels often accompanies rheumatoid arthritis. Intimal proliferation commonly affects the digital and mesenteric vessels of the lower extremities in the area of the malleoli, resulting in chronic skin ulcers. Rarely an acute "rheumatoid arteritis" occurs with widespread multisystem lesions, including sensory motor neuropathy, digital and intestinal infarction, episcleritis, pleuritis, myocarditis, or pericarditis. The fulminant form of vasculitis may be complicated by malnutrition, infection, or congestive heart failure, and it may be a fatal illness.

Stage IV: Advanced Changes

If the condition progresses, the articular cartilage becomes extensively destroyed by the lytic enzymes in the synovial fluid and is replaced by pannus. The opposing bone surfaces are in direct opposition of the two articular surfaces and become increasingly bound together by the relatively acellular mature fibrous tissue transformed from the pannus. The resulting scar-like tissues serve to restrict the movement of the affected joint and may cause fibrous or even bony ankylosis (Fig. 2-4).

At this late stage of rheumatoid arthritis with extensive cartilage and bone damage, the changes of secondary degenerative joint disease (osteoarthritis) are frequently superimposed. At this stage it may be difficult to distinguish the effects of this degenerative process from those of the underlying inflammatory disease.

During the late stages of the disease, as a result of cartilage loss, erosion of bone, and direct involvement of the capsule and accessory ligaments, the joints become unstable and permit subluxation and dislocation. Direct involvement of the muscles and capsule adds to this instability. Another cause of fixed contractures and dislo-

cations is tenosynovitis, and direct invasion of the tendons by granulation tissue may lead to their rupture.

PATHOGENESIS

Although the etiology of rheumatoid arthritis remains unknown, progress in recent years has greatly advanced our understanding of its pathogenesis. The foregoing description of the distinctive histopathologic changes in this disease may serve as a guide for identifying and interpreting the pathways of activation and perpetuation of this aggressive inflammatory disease. Knowledge from many fields of study, including molecular and cellular biology, immunology, biochemistry, and genetics, has provided insight into the production of the articular and systemic manifestations of this disease. There is general agreement that the resulting inflammatory response becomes chronic, and the persistence of this immune reaction and its tendency to be localized within joints and tendon synovium distinguishes rheumatoid arthritis from other forms of inflammation. When considering the complex series of events that occurs in diarthrodial joints with rheumatoid arthritis, it is important to note that each structural component (synovium, synovial fluid, cartilage, and subchondral bone) are functionally and metabolically interdependent. The vascular nature of the synovium allows relatively free transfer of nutrients and cell products in the synovium to move into the synovial fluid and bathe the avascular cartilage.

Although the joint tissues bear the brunt of the destructive changes typical of this disorder, many organs may become involved. Inflammation is not always clinically apparent but affects a wide variety of visceral and peripheral organs, e.g., heart, lungs, eyes, peripheral nerves, and vessels, providing compelling evidence for considering rheumatoid arthritis a systemic disease. In view of this multisystem involvement, it is more aptly termed "rheumatoid disease" and is regarded as a prototype of autoimmune-related connective tissue disease.

A limited review of the advances in knowledge of the mechanisms of rheumatoid arthritis induced inflammation and tissue destruction requires an understanding of the terminology of the intricate biochemical immunologic and genetic methods and substances. In the following discussion the sequence of events that leads to the production of joint and systemic damage in rheumatoid arthritis patients is presented in four segments, or steps (Fig. 2-5).

Step I: Etiology

The initiating events of rheumatoid arthritis occur as an immune response involving the vasculature and adjacent synovium resulting from an unknown stimulus or antigen in a genetically susceptible individual. Despite our ignorance of the precise course of rheumatoid arthritis, there is strong evidence that two host factors are major determinants in its development, the most dominant of which is immune susceptibility; the other is gender.

Based on the similarity of joint and extra-articular manifestations and the histopathology of the synovium among these patients, rheumatoid arthritis is considered to be a single disease. There is evidence, however, that it may be a heterogeneous group of connective tissue diseases. This view comes from the dissimilar clinical findings in individual patients, the variable course out-

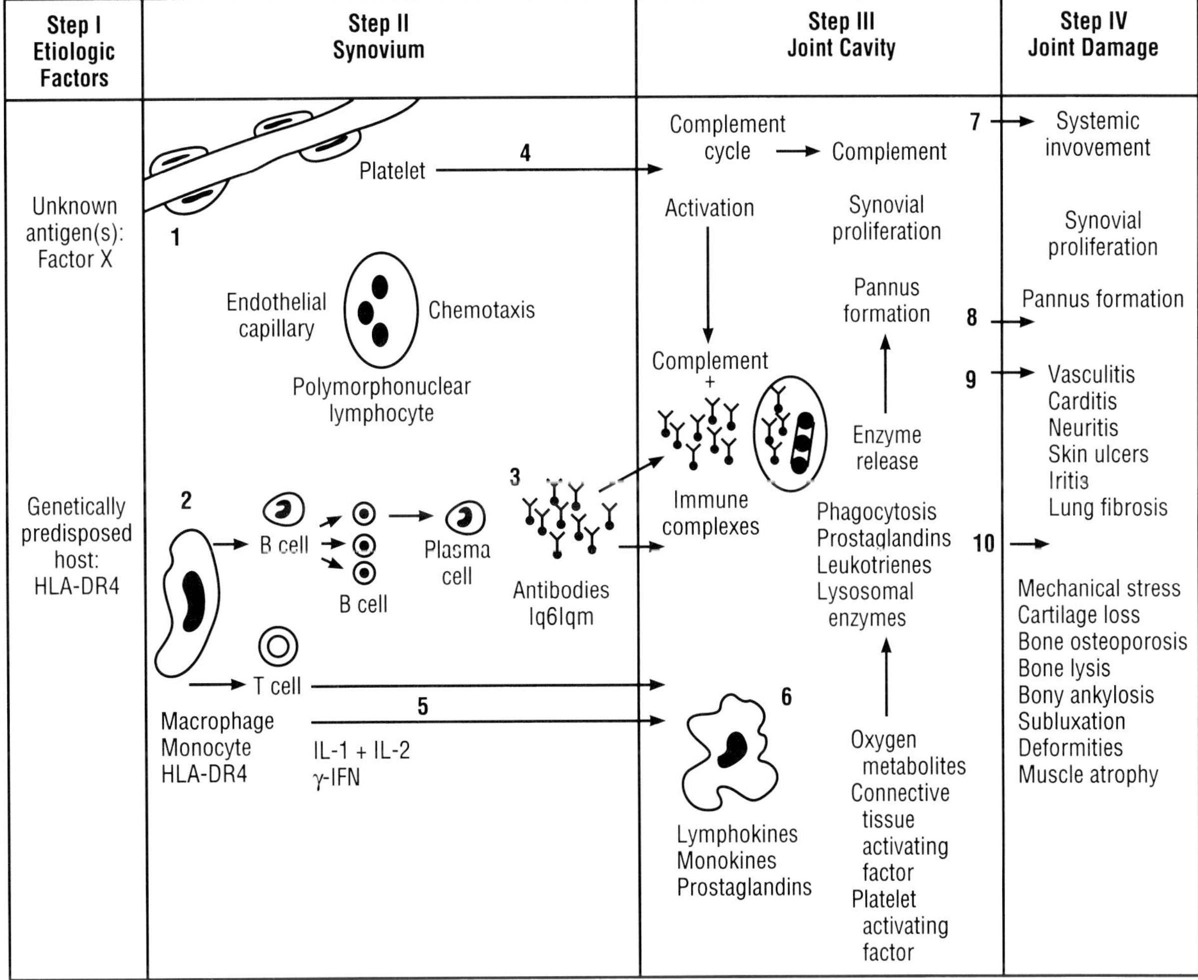

Fig. 2-5. Pathogenesis of rheumatoid arthritis (a complex sequence of self-perpetuating events).

comes, the presence or absence of serum rheumatoid factors, and the marked differences in genetic markers of those affected.

Initiating Factors

Despite many years of intensive search, the exact causative agent or triggering substance acting as an antigen is not yet known. Many approaches have been tried, including studies of metabolic, endocrinologic, infectious, and nutritional factors. The two leading potential sources of initiating factors or antigens are either exogenous (i.e., outside the host) or endogenous (i.e., originating from normal body tissues).

Potential Exogenous Factors. Among those outside agents that have been implicated are bacteria or bacterial debris, mycoplasma, or viral agents. Studies have demonstrated an anti-rheumatoid arthritis nuclear antigen (RANA) and the Epstein-Barr virus nuclear antigen (EBNA). Antibodies to these antigens are found in more patients with rheumatoid arthritis than in those who do not have the disease; however, the antibody is not specific for this disease. Many persons have been infected with this virus, which causes infectious mononucleosis, and have developed antibodies to components of this agent, but they do not develop rheumatoid arthritis.

Other viruses have been implicated in rheumatoid etiopathology, including cytomegaloviruses, parvoviruses, and viruses of the adenovirus type I group. Each has been reported to have been isolated from synovial cells or synovial fluid of patients with rheumatoid arthritis.

Potential Endogenous Factors. One of the agents within the body that is being considered and intensively investigated as the cause of rheumatoid arthritis is collagen. Rats and mice injected with collagen develop an antibody-mediated chronic arthritis. There are convincing data to document an association of both humoral and cellular immunity against collagen in patients with rheumatoid arthritis. This reaction is related primarily to type II collagen.[34]

Another possible endogenous agent to initiate rheumatoid arthritis is immunoglobulin. There is a definite increase in morbidity and mortality in patients with rheumatoid factor, and deposits of immune complexes containing IgG and IgM in

blood vessel walls show evidence of vasculitis. It has been established that rheumatoid arthritis synovial cells produce predominantly IgG, a substance that has been shown to associate or unite with other immunoglobulin molecules and become phagocytosed, leading to an inflammatory response within the joint space.[12] The union of IgG and another immunoglobulin, IgE, may cause mast cell degranulation and contribute to acute synovitis. There is rapidly accumulating evidence that rheumatoid arthritis develops upon interaction between one or more of these potential triggering agents and genetic factors in a susceptible host.

Step II: Synovium

The next series of events in the pathogenesis of rheumatoid arthritis involves a number of vascular and cellular reactions that take place within the synovium of affected joints. Evidence that ties immunologic events to the pathogenesis of rheumatoid arthritis has mounted steadily since it was first noted that the disease was associated with the presence of anti-gamma globulins (rheumatoid arthritis factors).[29] At that time there was a lack of understanding of the normal immune mechanisms in most diseases, and these observations were by and large regarded as incidental findings. Another cause for the delay of investigations into immune factors was the discovery of adrenocorticoids and the dramatic clinical response to these agents. After their introduction there was a flurry of research aimed at uncovering a metabolic cause. It was not until these efforts proved futile that investigators returned to the relatively unexplored area of possible immunopathogenesis of rheumatoid arthritis. Another major reason for clinical interest resulted from developments relating to organ transplantation immunity and hypersensitivity reactions associated with rejection of homografts.

Since the late 1970s numerous reports have appeared involving patients with rheumatoid arthritis and related connective tissue disease, especially systemic lupus erythematosus, and studies have established beyond doubt that immunologic reactions contribute greatly to the tissue injury that characterizes these diseases. They are now generally regarded as autoimmune disorders.

It is basic to an understanding of the role played by immunologic responses in the pathogenesis of rheumatoid arthritis to consider the cells found in the synovial tissues of joints, tendons, bursae, cartilage, and bone that have been shown to participate in the immune mechanisms leading to tissue destruction. The key cells that play a role are capillary endothelia, monocyte/macrophages, lymphocytes of the T and B types, PMNs, platelets, chondrocytes, and osteoblasts.

Patients with rheumatoid arthritis exhibit abnormalities of the humoral and cellular components of their immune systems that may be important to the pathogenesis of this disorder. Based on available evidence, the first impact of the as yet unidentified agent (antigen) occurs as an injury to the capillary endothelial cells. This injury to the vessel walls permits transfer of blood cells into the loose perivascular synovial tissues, causing accumulation of lymphocytes, macrophages, plasma cells, mast cells, and PMNs, often in nodular aggregates. Using monoclonal antibodies and immunochemical staining techniques, the cells in this synovium have been further identified. Most of the small lymphocytes are of the T or B cell type.

1. *T-Lymphocyte function.* T lymphocytes have on their cell membranes antigens associated with either helper/inducer function (CD4) or suppressor cytotoxic-associated antigens (CD8).[16] These nodular aggregates are rich cells that have HLA-DR genetic markers on their surfaces.[30] These monocyte/macrophage cells have been found in close cell-to-cell contact with the T lymphocyte designated a helper or inducer cell. It has also been shown that the activated monocytes produce an angiogenetic factor (perhaps interleukin-1, or IL-1), which stimulates endothelial proliferation and development of new capillaries. With the formation of new blood vessels, growth of synovial villae is sustained.

In this initial immune reaction between macrophages with HLA-DR genetic markers and IL-1, T lymphocytes proliferate and B lymphocytes secrete immunoglobulins and a variety of mediators (lymphokines). The synovial monocytes/macrophages also produce a number of cell mediators (monokines) that include IL-1, mononuclear cell activator, fibroblastic activator factor, plasminogen activator, collagenase, prostaglandins, and lysosomal enzymes. These lymphokines and monokines, in addition to regulating the expansion and function of other inflammatory cells, stimulate the growth of synovial living cells and fibroblasts.

These same synovial cell interactions are involved in the formation and function of pannus. It is this membrane, composed of proliferating fibroblasts, small blood vessels, collagen, and inflammatory cells, that contributes to excess levels of collagenase and prostaglandins, leading to the destruction of cartilage and the erosion of subchondral bone and other structures adjacent to these cells.

2. *B-Lymphocyte function.* The primary role of B lymphocytes in the pathogenesis of rheumatoid arthritis lies in proliferation and differentiation into plasma cells and antibody production. They migrate from the circulation and are activated by monocyte (macrophages) antigen-presenting cells that express major histocompatibility complex class II molecules on their surface. A number of regulatory molecules, including IL-1 and other lymphokines plus γ-interferon (γ-IFN), enhance the proliferation of B cells and their differentiation into immunoglobulin and antibody-forming cells. These mature cells, once stimulated, synthesize all four classes of immunoglobulins (IgG, IgM, IgA, IgE). The resulting autoantibodies are determined by the genetic material transferred during activation of these cells.

A variety of methods are available for detecting the antiglobulins (RFs) produced by the synovial membrane, including agglutination with latex or bentonite particles and sheep red blood cells, precipitation, complement fixation, radioimmunoassays, and immunosolvent assay (ELISA). These systems detect anti-γ-globulins (RFs) in all classes, with IgM and IgG occurring most frequently. Using the standard latex agglutination method, approximately 75 percent of patients with rheumatoid arthritis are positive depending on the criteria used for the diagnosis. Patients with rheumatoid arthritis and titers that fall below the normal range are considered seronegative. These patients usually have milder synovitis than seropositive rheumatoid arthritis patients, and they seldom develop extra-articular manifestations.

The detection of RF is not specific for rheumatoid arthritis because this test is found to be positive in low titer in the sera of a variety of patients with acute and chronic inflammatory diseases, including other rheumatic diseases, viral infections, and neoplastic diseases. The finding of RF in the serum or synovial fluid is frequently used to confirm the diagnosis of suspected rheumatoid arthritis. It has been shown to contribute to the amplification and perpetuation of rheumatoid synovitis through activation of complement and in the synovial fluid to form immune complexes that are phagocytosed by PMNs. It has not been established that RFs are directly involved in the etiology of rheumatoid arthritis by being linked to the genes of the DR4 of the class II antigens that predispose to this disease. A number of studies have, however, shown a strong association between the histocompatibility antigen DR4 and seropositive rheumatoid arthritis patients but no significant association with seronegative patients.

It is through the application of the powerful tools of molecular biology with monoclonal antibody technology that rapid progress has led to an understanding of the function of the various cells of the rheumatoid synovium and their products. These developments have promise in directing future investigations in therapy toward ameliorating definite abnormalities and intercellular reactions that characterize rheumatoid inflammation.

Step III: Joint Cavity

At step III a complex succession of biochemical, immunologic, and hematologic events involving numerous cells and soluble mediators of inflammation occur in the synovial cavity. T and B lymphocytes, macrophages, and PMNs and their products originating in the synovium move into the joint space; and the rheumatoid pannus, containing these same cells and fibroblasts, migrates medially and becomes attached to the hyaline articular cartilage. The synovial cavity becomes a mixing bowl of cells, chemotactic factors, enzymes, and inflammatory mediators.

Immune Complexes

An initiating and perpetuating event is the union of immunoglobulins, predominantly IgM, with unknown factor(s) (antigen) being joined by complement to form immune complexes.[32] Large numbers of PMNs—10,000 to 15,000/cu mm—are attracted; they phagocytize the immune complexes and release a variety of proteolytic substances, including lysosomal enzymes, oxygen-free radicals, prostaglandins (PGE_2), platelet activating factor, connective tissue activating factor, thromboxanes, and proteases. Each of these substances is capable of producing and sustaining the inflammatory response.

Cytokines

Some studies have identified the function of additional biologically active mediator substances called cytokines from the synovial fluid of rheumatoid arthritis patients.[1,5,14] Those that play an important role in inflammation and joint destruction include interleukins (IL-1, IL-2, IL-6, tumor necrosis factor-α (TNF-α), and γ-IFN. These agents are primarily the products of macrophages and activated T and B lymphocytes, and they function as stimulants or agonists in cell-to-cell interactions in rheumatoid joints. It has been shown that IL-1 and TNF-α stimulate fibroblasts in pannus and chondrocytes in cartilage to secrete PGE_2, collagenase, and other neutral proteases, resulting in the destruction of cartilage, bone, and periarticular structures. Other responses of IL-1 include chemotaxis of PMNs, fibroblast proliferation, collagen production, and stimulation of T and B lymphocytes. Specific IL-1 and TNF-α inhibitors have been identified that act as a controlling mechanism by preventing these cytokines from interacting with target cells. Thus it is possible that inadequate synthesis of these inhibitors would allow their continued proinflammatory effects in rheumatoid synovitis.

Each of these chemical mediators released into or formed in the synovial fluid bathe the articular cartilage and act as a chemoattractant for pannus to move into the joint cavity and attach to the cartilage and bone.[36] They are capable of acting to release and sustain the inflammatory response: They cause the fibroblasts of the pannus and chondroctyes to produce PGE_2 and collagenase, leading to the destruction of joint tissues.[37]

High levels of yet another cytokine, IL-6, are present in inflammatory synovial fluids from rheumatoid arthritis patients. These levels exceed those of IL-1 and TNF-α in the same fluids and are correlated with systemic disease activity, elevated erythrocyte sedimentation rate (ESR), and increased levels of acute phase reactants.[1] Unconfirmed reports indicate that the role of IL-6 in rheumatoid arthritis may be to modify the proinflammatory effects of other cytokines by inducing the synthesis of acute phase proteins and stimulating RF production locally.[1,15]

Step IV: Joint Damage

The end result of chronic rheumatoid synovitis is permanent damage to the involved joints and periarticular structures, with dislocation, deformities, and loss of function. As active joint manifestations continue, leading to destructive local changes, evidence shows that rheumatoid arthritis is not simply a disease of joints. During the early weeks and months, constitutional symptoms such as fatigue, low-grade fever, malaise, generalized muscle weakness, and weight loss suggest a diffuse disease. Inflammatory lesions are not always apparent early in the illness and involve a variety of visceral and peripheral organs such as skin, lungs, heart, and nerves, providing further evidence that rheumatoid arthritis is a systemic illness. Additional evidence comes from laboratory studies. Within weeks after the onset of joint symptoms, anemia, leukocytosis, elevated ESR, and C-reactive proteins are common. Also, after several months immunologic abnormalities involving antibodies may be demonstrated using the RF assay, immune complex level, and low complement levels in the serum and synovial fluid.

Cartilage Loss

The first process leading to cartilage destruction results from the interaction of antigens and antibodies forming IgG, IgM, and collagen II immune complexes. Other components that are found in these complexes include fibrinogen, collagen fiber fragments, cell membranes, and soluble nucleoproteins. These complexes are trapped in the rheumatoid cartilage and play an important role in cartilage damage.[18] These observations provide a mechanism to explain the self-perpetuating and chronic nature of cartilage degradation in rheumatoid arthritis. The site of major collagen and proteoglycon dissolution is in the region immediately adjacent to mononuclear cells at the junction between the granulation tissue of the pannus and cartilage.

Another key source of soluble substances responsible for cartilage destruction is the large numbers of PMNs that are attracted by complement-derived chemotactic factors into the joint space. During the process of phagocytosis of immune complexes they die and release hydrolytic lysosomal enzymes, including neutral proteases, elastoses, collagenases, cathepsins, and polysaccharidases, each of which is capable of destroying cartilage fibers.[35]

Another soluble mediator contained in rheumatoid arthritis joint effusions is plasminogen activator, which is produced by the synovial membrane. Upon entering the inflamed joint it is converted to plasmin, which activates latent collagenase bound to collagen fibers.[38] Collagenase in turn rapidly destroys the collagen II fiber of articular cartilage. Plasmin also degrades proteoglycan. The activities of these destructive proteinases in the joint fluid are controlled by naturally occurring enzyme inhibitors. Among these are α_2-macroglobulins and tissue inhibitor metalloproteinase, which coexist with the active proteinases.[2] Through this mechanism the numerous patent proteolytic enzymes are maintained in balance by inhibitor enzymes.

Jasin and Dingle demonstrated that articular chondrocytes can be influenced by a substance from synovial cells called catabolin, which has been found to be identical with IL-1. It is capable of releasing the proteinases that break down the surrounding cartilage matrix.[17] Chondrocytes have also been shown to produce immune mediators identified as metalloproteinase, capable of destroying proteoglycans. This loss destroys the ability of cartilage to rebound from a deforming loan and renders the cartilage biologically and mechanically ineffective.[8]

Bone Resorption

Rheumatoid arthritis is characterized by both juxta-articular and systemic osteoporosis. An early radiographic finding is the reduced bone density limited to bone adjacent to joints with active synovitis. The generalized loss of bone substance occurs insidiously and is recognized only later in the disease.

Local Bone Loss

The reduced bone density is due to the narrow spaces being invaded by inflammatory tissue that is histologically similar to the synovial membrane. It is continuous with the synovium and enters the bone through defects in the cortex or through bare areas over the end of bones denuded of cartilage.

A comprehensive review of osteoporosis associated with rheumatoid arthritis indicates that the cause of the bone loss results from multifactorial processes, summarizing the research that is focused primarily on the products of the various cells in the inflamed rheumatoid synovium and pannus.[19] There is substantial evidence that the cytokines, IL-1, tumor necrosis factor, and γ-IFN, which originates from lymphocytes and macrophages, are the major mediators of localized osteoporosis. Also, IL-1 activates chondrocytes to secrete collagenases, proteoglycanases, and neutral proteases. Thus stimulation of synovial cells, osteoblasts, and chondrocytes, and these cytokines and inhibitors, which have been demonstrated to be elevated in the synovial fluid of rheumatoid patients, are potent stimulators of bone resorption.

Prostaglandin E_2 is the most potent stimulator of bone resorption of the prostaglandins. It is synthesized in large amounts by synovial cells, macrophages, and chondrocytes within the inflamed tissue and secreted by PMNs into joint fluid. It is considered to be another key mediator that acts either directly or indirectly in bone destruction. Another substance, osteoclast-activating factor,

has been identified as a product of activated T lymphocytes and is dependent on PGE_2. Mast cells are present in increased numbers in the synovium and synovial effusion of active rheumatoid arthritis. Products of these cells can stimulate the production of PGE_2 by synovial cells.[7] Monocytes have also been shown to resorb bone directly but probably act by releasing PGE_2 and collagenases.[23]

Generalized Osteoporosis

The etiology of generalized osteoporosis has been difficult to elucidate. Multiple factors are known to affect the systemic loss of bone including the duration of disease, its severity, sex hormone status, physical activity, drug therapy (corticosteroids, cyclosporine, methotrexate), and systemic elevated cytokines. Studies of bone density in patients with rheumatoid arthritis using dual energy radiographic photon absorption to be decreased by 1 to 2 percent per year. Total bone mass correlated significantly with disease duration and parameters of disease activity.[26]

Adhesions, Dislocation, Deformities

After the phase of cartilage destruction and resorption of bone in areas adjacent to the involved joints, the granulation tissue is transformed into fibrous adhesions and scar tissue. The opposing bone surfaces become adherent through this cicatrix. The weakened capsule and adjacent bursae, tendons, and tendon sheaths frequently become entrapped in fibrotic adhesions. These fibrous bands associated with muscle shortenings dislocate the opposing ends of bones. The sum of these pathologic changes, in conjunction with mechanical forces of weight-bearing and muscle pull, produce the characteristic deformities of rheumatoid arthritis. With long-standing disease, metaplasia of the scar tissue may result in cartilaginous bony ankylosis with complete loss of joint motion.

REFERENCES

1. Arend WP, Dayer J-M: Cytokines and cytokine inhibitor or antagonists in rheumatoid arthritis. Arthritis Rheum 33:305, 1990

2. Barth W, Drucky A, Kleesick K: L_2 macroglobulin proteinase complexes with L_1 proteinase inhibitor-elastase complexes in synovial fluids of rheumatoid patients. Arthritis Rheum 29:319, 1986

3. Beasley RP, Willkens RF, Bennett PH: High prevalence of rheumatoid arthritis in Yakima Indians. Arthritis Rheum 16:743, 1973

4. Cutolo M, Balleari E, Giusti M et al: Androgen replacement therapy in male patients with rheumatoid arthritis. Arthritis Rheum 34:1, 1991

5. Dayer J-M, Demczuk S: Cytokines and other mediators in rheumatoid arthritis. Springer Semin Immunopathol 7:387, 1984

6. Gran JT, Husby G, Thorsby E: The association between rheumatoid arthritis and HLA antigen DR4. Ann Rheum Dis 42:292, 1983

7. Guber B, Pozansky M, Boss E et al: Characterization and functional studies of rheumatoid mast cells. Arthritis Rheum 29:944, 1986

8. Harris ED Jr: Pathogenesis of rheumatoid arthritis. p. 905. In Kelley WN, Harris ED Jr, Ruddy S, Sledge CB (eds): Textbook of Rheumatology. 3rd Ed. WB Saunders, Philadelphia, 1989

9. Harris ED Jr: Pathogenesis of rheumatoid arthritis. Clin Orthop 182:14, 1984

10. Harvey J, Lotze M, Stevens MB et al: Rheumatoid arthritis in a Chippewa band. I. Field study with clinical servologic and HLA-D correlations. Rheumatology 10:28, 1983

11. Hench PS: The ameliorating effects of pregnancy on chronic atrophic (infectious) rheumatoid arthritis, fibrositis and intermittent hydrarthrosis. Proc Mayo Clin 13:161, 1938

12. Hoffman WL, Goldberg MS, Smiley JD: Immunoglobulin G_3 subclass production by rheumatoid synovial tissue cultures. J Clin Invest 69:136, 1982

13. Hollander JL, McCarty DL, Astorga G et al: Studies on the pathogenesis of rheumatoid joint inflammation. I. The rheumatoid arthritis "cell" and a working hypothesis. Ann Intern Med 62:271, 1965

14. Hopkins SL, Meager A: Cytokines in synovial fluid. II. The presence of tumor necrosis factor and interferon. Clin Exp Immunol 73:88, 1988

15. Houssian FA, Devogelaer J-P, Van Damme J et al: Interleukin-6 in synovial fluid and serum of patients with rheumatoid arthritis and other arthritides. Arthritis Rheum 31:784, 1988

16. Janossy G, Duke O, Poulter LW et al: Rheumatoid arthritis; a disease of T-lymphocyte of inducer and suppressor type occupy different microenvironments. Nature 287:81, 1980

17. Jasin HE, Dingle JJ: Human mononuclear cell factors mediate cartilage matrix degradation through chondrocyte activation J Clin Invest 68:571, 1981

18. Jasin HE: Autoantibody specificities of immune complexes sequestered in articular cartilage of patients with rheumatoid arthritis and osteoarthritis. Arthritis Rheum 28:241, 1985

19. Joffe I, Epstein S: Osteoporosis associated with rheumatoid arthritis; pathogenesis and management. Semin Arthritis Rheumatol 20:256, 1991

20. Lawrence JS: Rheumatoid arthritis: nature or nurture? Heberden oration, 1969. Ann Rheum Dis 29:357, 1970

21. Linos A, Worthington JW, O'Fallon WM, Kurland LT: The epidemiology of rheumatoid arthritis in Rochester, Minnesota; a study of incidence, prevalence and mortality. Am J Epidemiol 111:87, 1980

22. Mitchell D: Epidemiology of rheumatoid arthritis. p. 133. In Utsinger PD, Zvaifler NJ, Ehrlich GE (eds): Rheumatoid Arthritis: Etiology, Diagnosis, Management. WB Saunders, Philadelphia, 1985

23. Mundy GR, Altman AJ, Gondok MD, Bandelin JG: Direct bone resorption by human monocytes. Science 196:1109, 1977

24. National Center for Health Statistics. PHS Publication No. 1000, Series 11, No. 17. Government Printing Office, Washington, DC, 1966

25. Persellin RH: The effect of pregnancy on rheumatoid arthritis. Bull Rheum Dis 27:922, 1977

26. Reid DM, Kennedy NSJ, Smith MA et al: Total body calcium in rheumatoid arthritis; effects of disease activity and corticosteroid treatment. Br Med J 285:330, 1982

27. Robinson DR, Tashjian AH Jr, Levine L: Prostaglandin-stimulated bone resorption by rheumatoid synovia. J Clin Invest 56:1181, 1975

28. Rose HM, Ragon C, Pearce E et al: Differential agglutination of normal and sensitized sheep erythrocytes by sera of patients with rheumatoid arthritis. Proc Exp Biol Med 68:1, 1948

29. Ruddy S: Complement in the inflammatory response. p. 241. In Kelley WN, Harris ED Jr, Ruddy S, Sledge CB (eds): Textbook of Rheumatology. 3rd Ed. WB Saunders, Philadelphia, 1989

30. Solomon L, Robin G, Valkenberg HA: Rheumatoid arthritis in an urban South African Negro population. Ann Rheum Dis 34:128, 1975

31. Statsny P: Association of the B-cell alloantigen DRw4 with rheumatoid arthritis. N Engl J Med 298:869, 1978

32. Stuart JM, Townes AS, Kang AH: The role of collagen autoimmunity in animal models and human diseases. J Invest Dermatol, suppl 1, 79:121s, 1982

33. Tallon DF, Corcoran DJD, O'Dwyer EM, Greally JF: Circulating lymphocyte subpopulations in pregnancy. J Immunol 132:1784, 1984

34. Terato K, Hasty KA, Cremer MA et al: Collagen-induced arthritis in mice; localization of an arthri-

togenic determinant to a fragment of the type II collagen molecule. J Exp Med 162:637, 1985

35. Weismann G: Activation of neutrophile and the lesions of rheumatoid arthritis. J Lab Clin Med 100:322, 1982

36. Wingrave SF: Reduction of incidence of rheumatoid arthritis associated with oral contraceptives. Lancet 1:569, 1978

37. Wolfe F, Kleinheksel SM, Kahn MA: Prevalence of familial occurrence in patients with rheumatoid arthritis. Br J Rheumatol, suppl 2, 27:150, 1988

38. Wordsworth MB: The immunogenetics of rheumatoid arthritis. Curr Opinion Rheumatol 2:423, 1990

3

Clinical and Laboratory Features of Rheumatoid Arthritis

Charley J. Smyth

A definitive diagnosis of rheumatoid arthritis may be difficult in the early stages. All stages, however, require a reliable clinical history, joint examination, laboratory tests, roentgenograms, and the exclusion of other inflammatory joint diseases.

DIAGNOSIS

Perhaps the most important aspect of establishing a correct diagnosis is the interview; the physical examination and laboratory studies serve in large part to confirm a reliable history. Helpful guidelines, prepared by a committee of the American Rheumatism Association, list seven criteria. Four or more of them must be present to diagnose rheumatoid arthritis.

1. Morning stiffness for at least 1 hour and present for at least 6 weeks
2. Swelling of three or more joints for at least 6 weeks
3. Swelling of wrist; metacarpophalangeal (MCP) or proximal interphalangeal (PIP) joint swelling
4. Symmetric joint swelling
5. Hand roentgenographic changes typical of rheumatoid arthritis that include erosions or unequivocal bony decalcification
6. Rheumatoid nodules
7. Serum rheumatoid factor assayed by a method positive in fewer than 5 percent of normals[1]

The characteristic patient presents with complaints of pain and stiffness in multiple joints. As a rule, the onset is slow, insidious, and intermittent over several weeks or months. The onset and exacerbations are more frequent during the winter months. Symmetric small joints of the hands and feet with pain, swelling, tenderness, and warmth are the rule, although single joints occasionally are the first involved. When extension to other joints occurs, the joint(s) originally involved remains inflamed. Distal interphalangeal joints are seldom involved. From the beginning, range of motion is restricted, and function and muscle strength are diminished. The general physical examination is normal except for possible low grade fever, pallor, and general weakness. Most patients exhibit some degree of anxiety and concern.

Laboratory tests are helpful, but none is diagnostic. There is often a slight monocytic normochromic anemia and an elevated erythrocyte sedimentation rate; C-reactive protein is almost always present. A positive serologic test for rheumatoid factor is a reliable index but is often negative during the first several months of the illness. Elevated levels of α_1, α_2, and γ-globulins are often noted, and serum complement levels are normal or slightly elevated. Peripheral white blood cell (WBC) counts, urinalysis, and tests for kidney, hepatic, and metabolic functions are normal, as are antinuclear antibody and serum urate levels. Diagnostic arthrocentesis reveals synovial fluid that on gross inspection is straw-colored, slightly cloudy, and may contain flecks of fibrin. The WBC count varies from 5,000 to 35,000/cu mm, with 85 percent of these cells polymorphonuclear neutrophils (PMNs). These phagocytotic cells may contain immune complexes consisting of IgG, IgM, and C3. There are usually trace levels of C4 and C2, and C3 levels are normal. The synovial fluid glucose is often greatly depressed compared with serum glucose levels. No crystals are present, and cultures are negative.

Roentgenograms of affected joints of the hands, wrists, and feet are, in many instances, useful for establishing a diagnosis of rheumatoid arthritis. Soft-tissue swelling in the periarticular areas and subchondral osteoporosis are nonspecific early findings. These changes take on added significance if there is also diffuse osteoporosis involved in the PIP joints and over the wrist and dorsal tendon sheaths. Roentgenograms obtained during the first few months of the illness may be negative, but they are valuable as baseline films later as the disease progresses. Laboratory studies and roentgenograms in themselves do not prove the diagnosis but may support the clinical suspicion.

SITES AND PATTERNS OF JOINT INVOLVEMENT

The pattern of joint involvement is a helpful aid for establishing the diagnosis of rheumatoid arthritis. This disease is classically polyarticular with symmetric involvement. However, initially only approximately two-thirds of patients have paired joint involvement. The number usually rises to more than three-fourths of patients over the course of the first few years. In the typical patient, it is often the small joints of the hands and feet that first become symmetrically swollen, tender, and limited to motion. Frequently, in some hands this paired involvement is in the second and third MCP and PIP joints. In the feet, the middle three metatarsophalangeal (MTP) joints are apt to be the first involved.

Subsequently or concomitantly, the large joints (elbows, wrist, ankles, knees) also become symmetrically involved. However, any size

diarthroidal joint may be the first affected, with a tendency of the involvement to spread to additional joints, including the temporomandibular, sternoclavicular, and cricoarytenoid joints. The larger and more proximal extremity joints (wrists, elbows, ankles, knees) tend to become active somewhat later, with girdle joints (shoulders and hip), the spine, and sacroiliac joints much later.

Occasionally, just a single joint is involved, which may be falsely attributed to injury or infection. In such a case, the diagnosis is usually made only with the benefit of time when the patient develops a more characteristic pattern of joint involvement. In addition to involvement of a single joint, patients may present with a few involved joints (oligoarticular disease) and present the same problem in diagnosis as that of monarticular onset.

Another pattern of rheumatoid arthritis onset is recurrent attacks of severe painful arthritis and periarthritis that last a few hours or days with a return to normal between episodes. This pattern is the so-called palindromic type of presentation, and it occurs most commonly in the fingers, wrists, shoulders, and knees; in these cases laboratory results and roentgenograms remain normal for months to years before showing the characteristic changes of rheumatoid arthritis.[30] The ultimate outcome for patients with this palindromic rheumatism type onset who eventually develop rheumatoid arthritis does not differ from other patients with the disease.

Rarely, tenosynovitis, the carpal tunnel syndrome, or rheumatoid nodules develop prior to the onset of any arthritis and may persist for months or years before the patient develops polyarthritis and the diagnosis of rheumatoid arthritis can be made.

CLINICAL COURSE

The opinion of many physicians is that rheumatoid arthritis is always a chronic, progressive disease. On the contrary, the clinical course is highly variable and largely unpredictable.[7,17,33,34] The disease usually follows one of three common clinical courses (see Fig. 1-1). The first phase is a single period of activity that usually subsides after 12 to 18 months without permanent damage. An estimated 25 to 30 percent of patients have the monocyclic course and undergo permanent remission. If the initial attack of rheumatoid arthritis lasts longer than 2 years, the prospect of a spontaneous complete remission becomes less likely. A second group of patients, representing most of the patients with rheumatoid arthritis, experience chronic activity with periods of exacerbations interspersed with spontaneous remissions. In patients who have this polycyclic course, these periods of complete or incomplete remissions and relapses vary from a few to as many as 20 or more during a lifetime with the illness. This type of disease is usually mild, initially involving only a few joints followed by gradual spread to additional joints after periods of partial remission. The eventual clinical outcome involves bony erosive cartilage damage and other changes of the late stages of the illness. A third, progressive clinical course without remissions occurs in 12 to 18 percent of patients with relentless destructive changes leading to permanent disability. This group of patients with rapidly progressive, destructive disease involving multiple systems with several extra-articular changes are said to have "malignant" rheumatoid arthritis.

Using criteria for remission developed by an American Rheumatism Association Committee,[21] an outcome assessment of 458 rheumatoid arthritis patients was reported in 1985.[40] These investigators reported that the average remission lasted 10 months, rarely lasted more than 2 years, and was associated with the use of "remittive" drugs such as gold or penicillamine in 86 percent of the patients. In another long-term study[22] of 75 patients over 9 years, it was found that almost all had significantly lower functional capacity and increased mortality. This outcome occurred despite aggressive therapy begun shortly after the interval diagnosis. There is an urgent need for additional long-term outcome studies with the early use of drugs such as the immunosuppressive agents methobamate and azathioprine (Imuran) alone or in combination with one of the established disease-modifying drugs such as gold, penicillamine, or sulfasuxidine.

During the first several months of this illness, there are no reliable clinical features or laboratory tests to indicate which of several clinical patterns an individual patient will follow or to predict the rate of progression or the level of activity of the inflammatory or destructive changes. However, after the disease has been established for several months, a number of factors are helpful indicators of prognosis. A favorable outcome can be expected if (1) the onset is limited to one or a few proximal joints; (2) the patient is male and less than 30 years old; or (3) there is no rheumatoid factor (RF), nodules, or vasculitis. A protracted course and a more severe, aggressive, debilitating disease with an unfavorable outcome usually follows if RF is detected early and in high titer, if severe erosive changes occur in early disease, if nodules in the skin and other areas are present, or if extra-articular involvement develops, including vasculitis, peripheral neuropathy, and cutaneous ulcerations.

Joint Synovitis

Throughout this illness arthritis is the most prominent clinical feature, and it is manifested by pain, stiffness, swelling, and limited joint motion. Morning stiffness lasting 30 minutes or more is a characteristic symptom but is not specific. Pain limits joint motion at all stages of the disease, but in the later stages capsular fibrosis, muscle contractures, tendon laxity or rupture, and fibrous or bony fusion appear.

Rheumatoid arthritis can affect any diarthrodial joint; initially those most commonly affected are the small joints of the hands, the wrists, and the feet. As the disease becomes established, the more proximal joints are involved including the elbows, shoulders, sternoclavicular and subtalar joints, ankles, knees, and hips. Clinically significant involvement of the spine is usually limited to the upper cervical area. The characteristic joint deformities and subluxations of the hands include ulnar deviation at the MCP joint and felxor deformities at the PIP joint (boutonnière finger) or volar dislocation of this joint (swanneck finger) (Fig. 3-1).

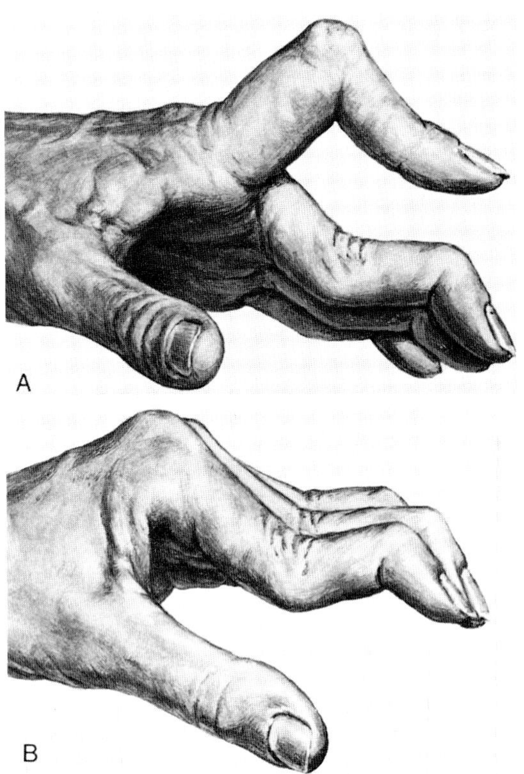

Fig. 3-1. (A) Typical finger joint deformities of the rheumatoid hand showing a boutonnière change in the index finger; three other fingers are dislocated in the volar direction (swan-neck deformity). (B) All of the fingers at the proximal interphalangeal joint are dislocated in the volar position, and the distal interphalangeal joint is flexed in the swan-neck deformity.

EXTRA-ARTICULAR MANIFESTATIONS

Certain systemic features of rheumatoid arthritis involving a number of nonarticular tissues are common and may predominate over those of the joints. These extra-articular manifestations have led some to prefer the term *rheumatoid disease* to rheumatoid arthritis in order to emphasize the multisystem nature of this illness. Gordon et al.[12] studied the extra-articular features of 127 hospitalized patients with rheumatoid arthritis and found that 37 percent had one and 42 percent had two or more systems involved. Rheumatoid lesions in tissues over and near joints include rheumatoid nodules, tenosynovitis, bursitis, synovial cysts, and nerve entrapment syndrome.

Rheumatoid Nodules

Subcutaneous nodules are the most frequent extra-articular features of rheumatoid arthritis, appearing at some time during the course of the illness in approximately 25 to 35 percent of patients with definite or classic rheumatoid arthritis. Their presence helps confirm the clinical diagnosis and is one of the criteria for this disease as established by the American Rheumatism Association.[1] Early lesions develop around small blood vessels; and mature nodules have a characteristic histologic picture, with a central area of necrosis rimmed by a corona of palisading and proliferating fibroblasts, macrophages making up most of the cells in this area. The collagenous capsule contains collections of chronic inflammatory cells.[20] They are almost always associated with seropositive RF in the serum and, in patients with the more severe and destructive changes, in the joints. These pathognomonic lesions are firm, round masses in the skin or deeper connective tissues, and they most commonly arise in areas subject to pressure or trauma, particularly over bony prominences, e.g., the olecranon process and the proximal portion of the ulna (Fig. 3-2). Rheumatoid arthritis nodules can also occur in the eyes, lungs, heart, vocal cords, tendons, muscles, and nervous system. Although freely movable, they may become firmly fixed to the underlying capsule or periosteum. They are frequently found in areas subjected to mechanical pressure and are especially common near the elbow in the region of the forearm or over the olecranon process. Other frequent sites include the Achilles tendon, occiput, and over the MCP and PIP joints of the hands and the MTP joints of the feet. These nodules may be mistaken for gouty tophi, basal cell carcinoma, xanthoma, or sebaceous cysts; a biopsy may be required to establish the diagnosis.

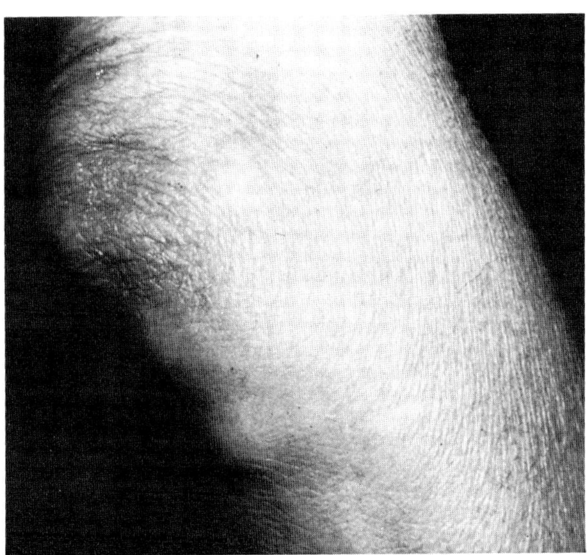

Fig. 3-2. Two subcutaneous rheumatoid nodules in the classic location on the extensor surface of the forearm just distal to the olecranon process of the elbow.

Nonarticular Synovitis

Rheumatoid inflammatory reactions of the extensor and flexor tendon sheaths about the wrists and ankles are frequent. On the volar surface of the wrist, swelling with the carpal tunnel underneath the transverse carpal ligament may cause pressure on the median nerve (carpal tunnel syndrome). Similar lesions with the ulnar tunnel at the wrist or at the medial side of the elbow may entrap the ulnar nerve and produce pain or tingling in that portion of the hand supplied by the ulnar nerve. Rheumatoid granulomas on the flexor tendons of the fingers and thumbs may produce painful triggering. On the dorsal surface of the wrist, the extensor tendons may be involved, and tendons may be invaded and eroded resulting in the sudden loss of extensor function of the involved digit(s) (Fig. 3-3).

Synovitis also occurs within the bursae that communicate with joints and in those that are adjacent to joints but do not communicate with them. In the knee, popliteal cysts (Baker's cysts) are common and are often asymptomatic. They usually communicate with the knee cavity in the popliteal space and may extend into the calf where they produce swelling but no pain. They cause pain most frequently when they rupture as a result of increased pressure such as squatting. Acute leaks result in sudden severe pain in the calf, with swelling, erythema, marked tenderness, fever, and the appearance of cellulitis or deep vein thrombosis. Arthrography may be used to confirm the presence of a cyst, its size, and if it has ruptured. A venogram confirms the patency of the calf veins.

Other commonly involved bursae include the subacromial of the shoulder, those adjacent to the first and fifth toes, and the Achilles area of the heels. In the feet, calluses commonly occur underneath the heads of the metatarsals (Fig. 3-4).

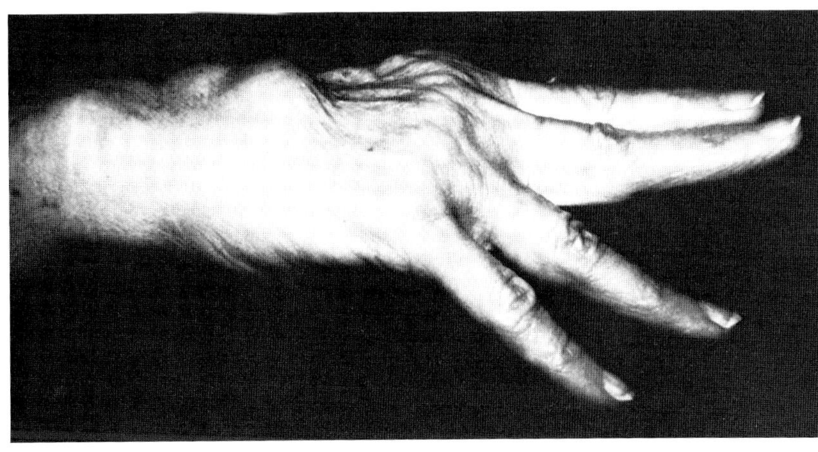

Fig. 3-3. Rheumatoid tenosynovitis of the extensor on the dorsum of the hand and rupture of the tendons to the ring and little fingers.

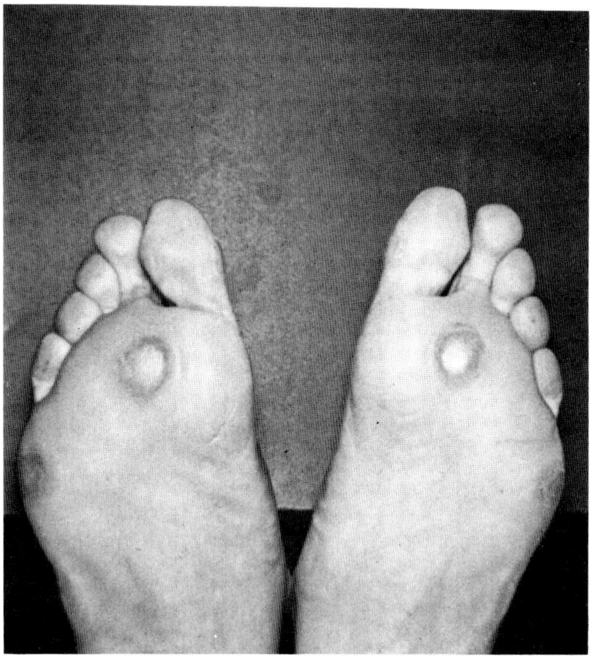

Fig. 3-4. Callous formation underneath the heads of each second metatarsal. Such lesions are common on the rheumatoid arthritic foot owing to loss of the transverse arch.

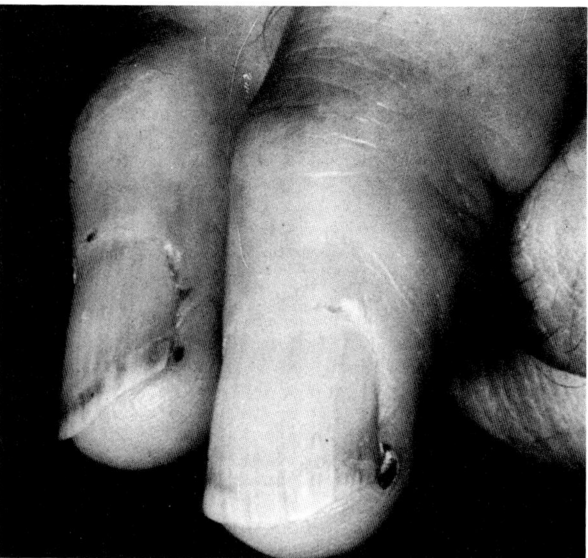

Fig. 3-5. Rheumatoid vasculitis with skin infarction involving small vessels around the fingernail folds.

Cardiovascular Manifestations

Cardiovascular involvement occurs in a wide spectrum of rheumatoid arthritis lesions including the small peripheral vessels, the medium and large arteries, and the heart. Vasculitic lesions of the small vessels of the nail folds and nail beds with infarction of the nutrient vessels to nerves, the pericardium, and arteries of viscera may occur (Fig. 3-5). Large indolent skin ulcers over the medial and lateral malleoli occur during the late stages of the disease. Acute generalized vasculitis may progress in a fulminating manner, with high fever, rapid disability, malnutrition, infections, and massive infarcts of the mesentery and cardiac chambers that may be fatal.[29] There is evidence that this widespread and progressive vasculitis is related to the precipitation of immune complexes.[8] Patients with this malignant form of vasculitis usually have low serum complement levels, antigen-antibody complexes in the circulation, and deposits of IgG, IgM, and C3 in the walls of the acutely inflamed vessels.[6] Although a variety of cardiac lesions are found in approximately one-half of rheumatoid arthritis patients at autopsy, clinically detectable heart changes attributable to rheumatoid disease is unusual. Pericarditis leading to thickening of the pericardium is the most common cardiac lesion. Less common is involvement of the myocardium, with fibrosis and thickening of the valves. Rarely, conduction defects occur, and nodules near the bundle of His have been observed. The presence of digital gangrene and widespread visceral lesions, including intestinal, cardiac, or renal involvement and mononeuritis multiplex, indicate extensive vasculitis and are associated with a poor prognosis.[9]

Pleuropulmonary Involvement

Rheumatoid arthritis may affect the pleura or the lung parenchyma. The pleural disease is usually asymptomatic. The characteristics of rheumatoid arthritis effusions are as follows: low glucose concentration (10 to 50 percent); protein 4 g/ml;

cells (mononucular) 1,000 to 3,000/cu mm; positive RF assay; markedly elevated lactic dehydrogenase level; and a depressed CH_{50} with C3 and C4 greatly decreased.

Rheumatoid nodules (0.5 to 5.0 cm) may be found on or near the pleura or distributed throughout the lung. These granulomatous lesions, which were originally described in Welsh coalminers as Caplan syndrome, are rarely found in patients in the United States. This serum RF assay of these patients is generally strongly positive. On rare occasions the nodules cavitate and may become infected or rupture into the pleural space, producing a bronchopleural fistula. Other patients develop diffuse interstitial fibrosis most frequently distributed at the lung bases. Roentgenographic findings include diffuse or patchy infiltrates, but later they may have a honeycomb appearance with bronchiolar ectasia. With these changes there is often a chronic production cough, crackling, rales, clubbed fingers, and decreased pulmonary function tests.

Eye Findings

Rheumatoid arthritis often produces a variety of ocular lesions including keratoconjunctivitis sicca, episcleritis, keratitis, iridocyclitis, scleromalacia, and scleromalacia perforans. The most common lesions are corneal and conjunctival, associated with Sjögren syndrome, which is a chronic inflammatory and anti-immune disorder characterized by dry eyes and dry mouth (the sicca complex), resulting in keratoconjunctiva sicca or xerostomia in approximately 10 percent of patients with rheumatoid arthritis. This syndrome may be associated with other connective tissue diseases, including systemic lupus, systemic sclerosis, and polymyositis, or it may occur in the absence of another connective tissue disease (primary Sjögren syndrome).[35] Eye problems tend to be bilateral and are generally accompanied by subcutaneous nodules, vasculitis, and other systemic manifestations. Rheumatoid arthritis nodules occasionally develop on the sclera. Ocular changes can result from the drugs used in this disease. Gold deposit in the cornea is a rare complication of this therapy. Posterior sub-

capsular cataracts may be caused by long-term corticosteroid therapy and corneal or retinal abnormalities following therapy with the antimalarial drugs chloroquine and hydroxychloroquine.

Lymphadenopathy, Splenomegaly, Felty Syndrome

Enlargement of lymph nodes is common with rheumatoid arthritis, and an enlarged spleen is found in 10 percent of patients. The combination of splenomegaly, leukopenia, and rheumatoid arthritis is called Felty syndrome. In addition, these patients have hyperpigmentation of the skin, leg ulcers, generalized lymphadenopathy, anemia, and thrombocytopenia. Most rheumatoid arthritis patients with this syndrome have active arthritis with fever, fatigue, anorexia, and weight loss, and they are almost entirely seropositive. HLA-DR4 has been reported in 95 percent of patients with this complication.[31] In this symptom complex, recurrent gram-positive infections are frequent with poor response to antibiotic therapy. Recurrent infections in patients with Felty syndrome are the major indication for splenectomy.

Neurologic Manifestations

A variety of neurologic complications involving the peripheral nerves are frequently encountered; the central nervous system is rarely affected. Subluxations at the level of the cervical spine occur in many patients during the late stages of the disease and are especially frequent at the C1-C2 level. This lesion may result in compression of the cervical cord with long-tract signs. The presence of this neurologic complication is of utmost importance in patients who require general anesthesia for reconstructive surgery. Any rheumatoid arthritis patient with long-standing illness who has headaches or severe neck pain and is being considered for general anesthesia should have roentgenograms of the cervical spine and neurologic evaluation for any evidence of cord compression or the likelihood of this serious complication developing.

Nerve entrapment syndromes due to the swelling of rheumatoid tenosynovitis occur frequently. A common site is underneath the volar compartment at the wrist, manifesting as the carpal tunnel syndrome. This neurologic complications is detected by the presence of burning pain with paresthesias commonly at night over the distribution of the median nerve. The symptoms may be reproduced by pressure over the median nerve at the wrist (Tinel sign). The diagnosis can be confirmed by electromyographic studies. Similar peripheral nerve entrapments occur behind the medial malleolus in the tarsal tunnel, and the ulnar nerve may be compressed within the ulnar tunnel at the wrist or at the medial side of the elbow. Less frequent neurologic lesions are a chronic sensory polyneuropathy and rarely an acute, severe sensorimotor peripheral neuropathy called "mononeuritis multiplex," which results from necrotizing angiitis of the vasa nervorum.

LABORATORY FINDINGS

There are relatively few crucial laboratory tests for the diagnosis of rheumatoid arthritis, and none is specific. Nevertheless, many nonessential laboratory tests are useful as confirmatory or supportive aids and serve as useful indices of disease activity and as gauges to the patient's response to therapeutic efforts.

Hematologic Tests

Mild anemia is the most common hematologic abnormality in rheumatoid arthritis, occurring in approximately 40 percent of cases. Typically, the anemia of chronic disease (hemoglobin 11 to 12 g%) is found with a low serum iron-binding capacity. Iron absorption is often slightly decreased, and bone marrow reserves are usually normal. The hemoglobin level is a fairly useful indicator of therapeutic response or increased disease activity. Anemia caused by chronic folic acid deficiency has been reported. The peripheral total and differential WBC count is usually normal, although the eosinophil count is occasionally increased. Patients with the acute systemic form of juvenile arthritis (Still's disease or its adult equivalent) characteristically have a strikingly elevated WBC count. With Felty syndrome (rheumatoid arthritis with hepatosplenomegaly and neutropenia) the patient may be profoundly leukopenic, with total WBC counts of less than 2,000/cu mm. An elevated platelet count may accompany highly active disease.

Acute Phase Reactants

The erythrocyte sedimentation rate (ESR) and C-reactive protein (CRP) are widely used to evaluate the degree of inflammation activity, as they closely parallel disease activity. The two commonly employed methods for measuring the ESR are those of Wintrobe and Westergren. The Westergren technique is generally accepted as the standard, with normal adult values of 15 mm/hr for men and 20 mm/hr for women. Values tend to be higher for aged patients. The serum level of CRP is the other reliable index of inflammation, and practically all rheumatoid arthritis patients have increased values (i.e., 5 mg/ml and usually in the 30 to 40 mg/ml range). In one report of 37 patients with rheumatoid arthritis, levels above 5 mg/dl (normal 0.6 mg/dl) predicted erosions, and the investigators regarded this test as an indicator of when to begin remittive therapy early in the course of the disease.[19]

Serologic Factors

The existence of antiglobulins called rheumatoid factors (RFs) in the sera of patients with rheumatoid arthritis was initially recognized during the 1940s by Waaler[39] and then Rose and coworkers.[27] Subsequent studies have resulted in a mass of information that establishes the existence of RF autoantibodies, which react with several classes of the hosts' own immunoglobulins, including IgG, IgM, and IgA. Because IgM molecules have multiple binding sites, this class is the one that is measured in the standard RF tests, which are based on the aggregation and precipitation of the RF that binds to standard IgG preparations. RFs are produced by lymphocytes and plasma cells in the synovial lining, accumulate in the synovial fluid, and spill over into the blood. The presence of RF has turned out to be a useful clinical test for rheumatoid arthritis, as RFs occur in the circulating blood of approximately 80 percent of patients with this disease. Although they appear most frequently and in the highest titer in rheumatoid arthritis patients, they are also found with various other connective tissue diseases, liver disease, sarcoidosis, tuberculosis, subacute bacterial endocarditis, syphilis, and some other chronic diseases. They are found as well in 1 to 5 percent of normal subjects, with the incidence increasing with advancing age. Thus a positive test is not diagnostic of rheumatoid arthritis, but its detection is a reassuring laboratory sign for the physician seeking a diagnosis. High titers of RF are generally associated with severe, active joint disease, the presence of nodules, vasculitis, and other systemic complications; their presence indicates a poor ultimate prognosis.

Studies have shown an association between seropositive rheumatoid arthritis and the major histocompatibility antigens in the D locus (HLA-D4/DR4). This association is generally absent with seronegative rheumatoid arthritis. The mechanism underlying these immunogenetic differences remains uncertain.

What role, if any, does RF play in the pathogenesis of RA? Investigations indicate that the immunoglobulins that are produced in the synovial lining combine with IgG to form immune complexes (ICs). These complexes then activate the complement system. PMNs and macrophages are chemotactically attracted to the joint, where they phagocytose the ICs and release lysosomal enzymes. These enzymes cause inflammation and joint destruction (see Ch. 2). Using reliable tests now available, it has been shown that ICs are ubiquitous in many diseases. Knowledge of ICs and rheumatoid arthritis has added greatly to the understanding of joint and extra-articular lesions but not to diagnosis or management. Another serologic finding in rheumatoid arthritis patients is the presence of antinuclear antibodies (ANAs) and lupus erythematosus (LE) cells in 10 to 50 percent of patients. Usually the ANA titer is low compared to that in systemic lupus erythematosus (SLE), and the number of LE cells are also less. High titers may occur in patients with severe, long-standing destructive disease, Felty syndrome, or juvenile rheumatoid arthritis. Hypocomplementemia is an infrequent finding and has been associated with severe systemic disease and vasculitis.

There is a correlation of IC concentration in the serum of rheumatoid arthritis patients with the presence of extra-articular manifestations of the disease as shown using C/q binding.[18] There is evidence based on the measurement of ICs by difference assays that the sensitivity, specificity, and predictive value are not sufficient to warrant their use in the management of the disease.[2]

Synovial Fluid

Analysis of the synovial fluid in patients with active rheumatoid arthritis synovitis may reveal several features to support the diagnosis, but no one finding is specific. The fluid is characteristically turbid and often green-tinged. The number of WBCs range from 5,000 to 60,000/cu mm, although counts higher than 100,000/cu mm may be seen. The predominant cells are PMNs, almost all of which harbor cytoplasmic inclusions (ragocytes) that contain immune complexes and complement. These cells are nonspecific and are found in inflammatory synovial fluids for almost any other disease.

The mucin clot (Ropes) test estimates the density and friability of the precipitate that forms when dilute acetic acid is added to joint fluid. A firm clot implies high-molecular-weight hyaluronic acid content. A friable or poor clot implies joint inflammation, but it is nonspecific. This test was formerly used as a criteria for rheumatoid arthritis but is no longer often used.

Analysis of rheumatoid arthritis synovial fluid has identified many other substances that reflect the inflammation of the proliferating synovium and pannus. They include a greatly diminished glucose level compared with the serum content; elevated total protein content; products of PMN phagocytosis and death (oxygen radicals, prostaglandins, thromboxanes, leukotrienes); diverse biologic mediators (interleukin-1, interleukin-2, neutral proteinases, γ-interferon, tumor necrosis factor, collagenoses, elastase); and components of the coagulation and kinin system and their product fibrin. These synovial fluid substances in rheumatoid arthritis patients have played an important role in investigations into the mechanism of the inflammation seen with the disease, but at this time there is no convincing reason to perform tests to identify any of the substances in a clinical setting.

RADIOLOGY AND RHEUMATOID ARTHRITIS

Radiography in Diagnosis

Radiographic changes are a key factor in the diagnosis of rheumatoid arthritis. With the most commonly used guides for the diagnosis of rheumatoid arthritis, the criteria of the American Rheumatism Association adopted in 1958,[26] the presence of typical radiographic changes of this disease is one of 11 findings considered when establishing this diagnosis. In the 1987 revision of these criteria, rheumatoid arthritis findings in conventional radiographs are given greater emphasis.[1] Hand roentgenograms with changes typical of rheumatoid arthritis, including erosions or unequivocal bony decalcification, represent one of seven diagnostic features.

Classification of Progression

Hand roentgenograms are useful for the determining the degree of damage in a patient. Based on conventional radiographs, four stages (or grades) can be defined. In the early (stage I) disease, there are no destructive changes on roentgenographic examination, but osteoporosis may be present (Fig. 3-6A). With moderate (stage II) disease there is roentgenographic evidence of osteoporosis with or without slight subchondral bone destruction and slight joint space narrowing. No deformities are present, and there may be adjacent muscle atrophy and extra-articular soft-

tissue lesions, e.g., nodules and tenosynovitis (Fig. 3-6). With severe (stage III) disease there is roentgenographic evidence of cartilage and bone destruction in addition to osteoporosis. Also, there are joint deformities (e.g., subluxations, ulnar deviation, or hyperextension) without fibrosis or bony ankylosis. Extra-articular soft tissue lesions such as nodules and tenosynovitis may be present as well (Fig. 3-6). In the terminal (stage IV) phase there is fibrous or bony ankylosis plus the abnormalities of stage III (Fig. 3-6).

CONVENTIONAL RADIOGRAPH IN RHEUMATOID ARTHRITIS

The pathologic changes in rheumatoid arthritis that are detected by routine roentgenograms are the keystone to establishing the diagnosis, staging the process, and managing the disease on a long-term basis. The characteristic findings of soft-tissue swelling, osteoporosis, joint space narrowing, and bony erosions are frequently sufficiently destructive to allow a tentative diagnosis to be made. However, none of the changes found by conventional radiograms is specific, but when combined with information from the clinical examination and laboratory tests they help to confirm the diagnosis. When more information is required for a definitive diagnosis, additional imaging examinations may be appropriate. However, these methods have only a limited role in selected patients with specific diagnostic problems in a routine clinical setting.

Soft Tissues

Examination of the periarticular structures, including joint fluid, synovial thickening, and joint space narrowing, is often helpful for establishing the diagnosis. Joint fluid often increases in the knees, fingers, feet, and wrists but is more difficult to detect in larger joints such as the hips and shoulders. In the small joints of the hands (PIP and MCP) and feet (MTP), swelling is symmetric and includes both synovial thickening and effusion. The enlargement in the fingers is characteristically fusiform or spindle-shaped. Films obtained in the lateral projection of the knees and ankles may demonstrate fluid in the suprapatellar pouch or the pre-Achilles regions. Subcutaneous nodules may be found in the extensor surfaces of the elbows, prepatellar areas, and points of pressure on the hands and feet. The lesions do not erode bone or calcify.

Osteopenia

Juxta-articular bone loss is a consequence of joint inflammation, and in rheumatoid arthritis it occurs bilaterally in symmetric joints and is an early sign of synovitis. The change is not specific for this disease, as it occurs also with pyogenic arthritis, Raynaud's phenomenon, and any localized acute inflammatory process. Generalized osteoporosis within a joint is a frequent finding of long-standing disease. Women with long-standing rheumatoid arthritis are likely to develop loss of bone substance in long bones distant from joints, as well as demineralization of the axial skeleton.[38] There are multiple factors that contribute, including age, sex, reduced physical activity, reduced dietary calcium intake, menopause, and in many patients the chronic use of

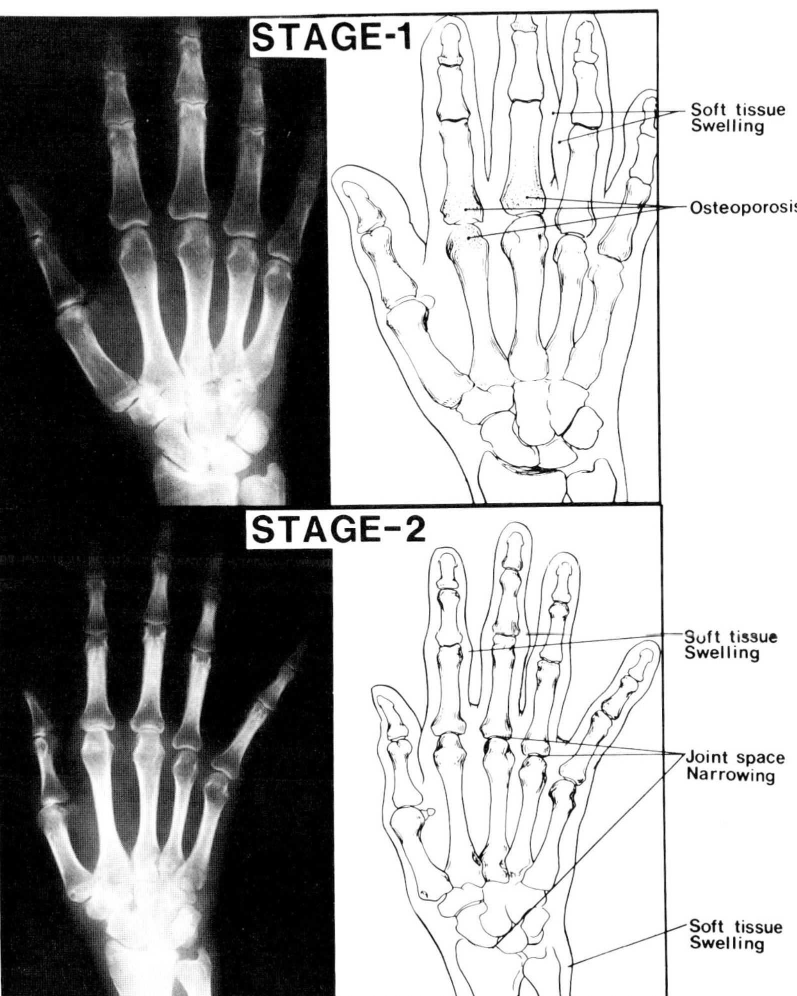

Fig. 3-6. Stages I, II, III, and IV of rheumatoid arthritis with characteristic roentgenographic changes of the hands and wrists. (*Figure continues.*)

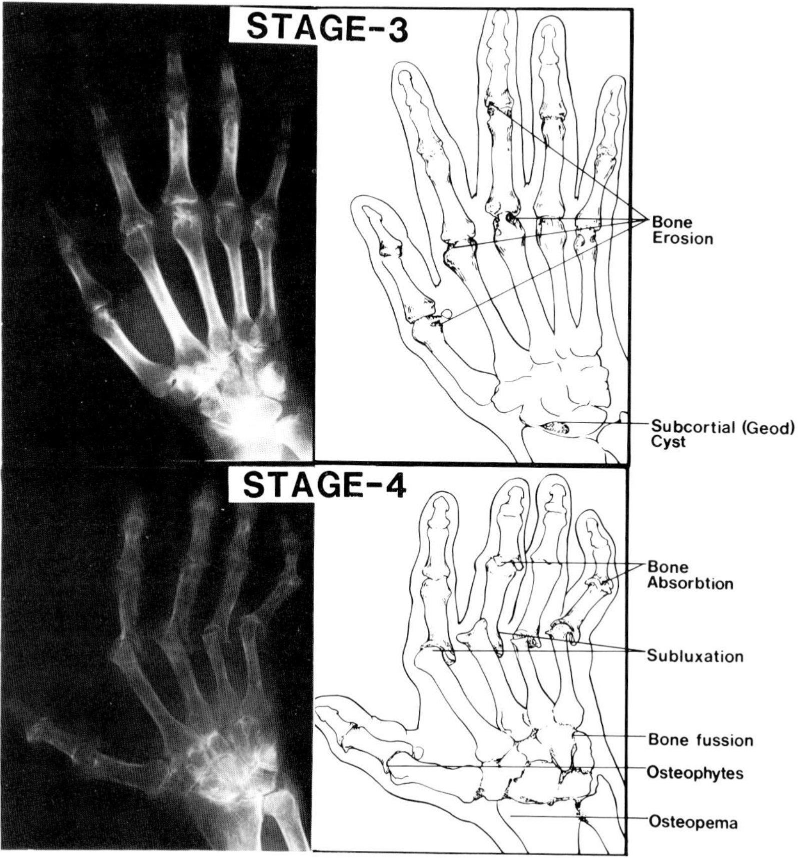

Fig. 3-6 *(Continued).*

corticosteroids.[28] All of these factors combine to produce a much higher frequency of stress fractures in this disease.

Osteolytic Lesions (Erosions)

Early in rheumatoid arthritis there are focal areas of cortical resorption of bone involving the metacarpal and metatarsal heads at the margin of the joints where cartilage ends and synovium begins. Later, the proliferating synovium and pannus erode the articular cartilage and eventually the subchondral bone. Early, the markings of these erosions are poorly outlined, irregular, and without sclerotic margins; however, with time and movement of the involved joint, the margins sclerose.

In advanced rheumatoid arthritis, showing malalignment and cartilage loss, pressure erosions may develop in the shaft of the bone adjacent to the diseased joint. Another type of bony erosion occurs when the articulating surface of the opposite bone destroys the cortex and invaginates one into the other, forming the pencil-in-cup deformity. Erosions may develop at either end of the clavicle or on the undersurface of the clavicle at the shoulder.

With more advanced cases, another common radiographic finding characteristic of rheumatoid arthritis is a subchondral radiolucent area in the ends of long bones and adjacent to large joints, variably described as cysts, pseudocysts, granulomas, or geodes. These lesions are usually small and without sclerotic margins; they are caused by the extension of pannus into bone, leading to bony destruction.[24] Erosions in the feet are most frequently found in the heads and underneath the calcaneal bone at the attachment of the plantar fascia. In the cervical spine, erosions are often found in the odontoid.

Periosteal Reactions

Along the cortex of bone near joints with active synovitis, thickening of the periosteum over the juxta-articular area is a frequent feature of roentgenograms of rheumatoid arthritis in children (juvenile rheumatoid arthritis). However, it is an infrequent finding in the adult form of the disease.

Joint Space

Diminution of joint space is an early, permanent radiographic feature of rheumatoid arthritis and implies destruction of articular hyaline cartilage. This narrowing is uniform, extending over the entire surface of the joint, and usually diminishes at the same rate and degree across the entire articular surface. It usually takes 3 to 6 months of active synovitis for this joint space loss to occur. Erosions at the margins usually appear within a short time after the reduction of cartilage space.

Malalignment of Bone

With late rheumatoid arthritis, flexion deformities of the small joints of the hands and hyperextension or flexion of the toes are commonly observed. These subluxations result from periarticular ligament and capsular laxity along with muscle imbalance. In the hands these changes occur at the MCP and PIP joints, producing the characteristic swan-neck and boutonnière deformities. The lack of associated erosions in such dislocated joints suggests the diagnosis of systemic lupus erythematosus. Another typical subluxation of the joints of the hands occurs with the fingers deviated toward the ulnar side, producing

the typical ulnar drift seen in rheumatoid arthritis patients.

In the feet, hallux valgus with plantar subluxation of the MTP joints is a characteristic deformity. Erosions of the involved joints in both the hands and feet usually are associated with deformities; such changes do not occur with other forms of arthritis.

In the cervical spine there may be relaxation of the transverse ligament at the C1-C2 level. Routine roentgenograms obtained at the lateral, oblique, flexion, and extension projections may determine the extent of this lesion. A clinically significant degree of atlantoaxial subluxation occurs when there is 3 mm or more space between the anterior surface of the odontoid process and the anterior surface of the anterior arch of the atlas. Computed tomography studies have provided additional information regarding attenuation of the transverse ligament and the presence or absence of spinal cord compression.[4] These authors and others, however, have stressed that plain roentgenograms, including full flexion views, and tomography should remain the primary radiographic means of evaluating the cervical spine in patients with rheumatoid arthritis.

Cartilaginous Joints

In addition to synovium-lined joints, rheumatoid arthritis may involve cartilaginous joints, including the symphysis pubis and discovertebral and sacroiliac areas. Sites of tendon and ligament attachments (enthesis) may also be involved, including the inferior surface of the calcanei, iliac wings, ischial tuberosities, and femoral trochanters. Radiographic findings in these areas include bony sclerosis, soft tissue swelling, cartilage space narrowing, bony erosions and proliferation, and bony ankylosis.[3]

Distribution of Roentgenographic Findings

When establishing the diagnosis, it is helpful to know which joints are involved. The PIP and

MCP joints are involved in the hands, and in the wrists the process usually involves the carpal bones and the ulnar styloid. In the feet, rheumatoid arthritis most often involves the middle three MTP joints; with advanced disease these toe joints are dislocated upward. Erosions frequently develop on the plantar surfaces of the calcaneus. In the spine, the most common radiographic changes are dislocation and fragmentation of the occipitoaxial joints, allowing forward dislocation of the odontoid. This complication is serious. It is rare to have the sacroiliac joints involved in adult rheumatoid arthritis, and if they do become involved it is usually late in the disease.

Chest roentgenograms of rheumatoid arthritis patients may show unilateral pleural effusions, and this extra-articular complication is usually associated with subcutaneous nodules. Another pulmonary finding that may be identified by roentgenography is fibrotic infiltration at the lung base. Rheumatoid nodules varying in size from 0.5 to 5.0 cm are seen in the pulmonary parenchyma (Caplan syndrome). Typical rheumatoid nodules may also be detected in the pleura.

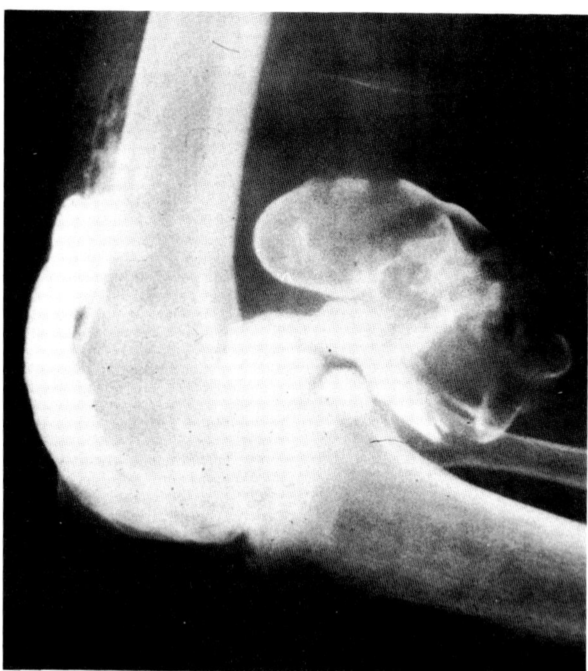

Fig. 3-7. Arthrogram of the knee with dye filling the suprapatellar pouch and extending posteriorly to fill a Baker cyst.

NUCLEAR IMAGING

Despite the application of radionuclide scintigraphs in rheumatology, the use of joint scanning with technetium 99m has not found a prominent place in clinical practice.[31] The injection of radiographic contrast material or air into the joint (arthrography) is of proved value in rheumatoid arthritis patients with a large effusion in the knee that has produced a popliteal or Baker's cyst. Sachs' lesions occasionally rupture and may descend into the calf and produce symptoms that mimic acute thrombophlebitis. With the use of radiopaque medium, it is possible to determine the size of the cyst and if it has ruptured into the calf (Fig. 3-7). In the shoulder, contrast arthrography has been useful for identifying surgically repairable soft-tissue damage due to rheumatoid arthritis involving that joint, e.g., rotator cuff tears.[23] This same technique may also provide a firm diagnosis of pigmented villonodular synovitis. Avascular necrosis of bone is a serious complication of long-term steroid therapy; radionuclide imaging is a far more sensitive method for detecting early disease than conventional roentgenograms.[5]

COMPUTED TOMOGRAPHY AND MAGNETIC RESONANCE IMAGING

The major role of computed tomography (CT) for assessing patients with rheumatoid arthritis is to establish the involvement and the extent of damage in the spine, especially in the cervical area. Abnormalities involving the occipital and C1-C2 joints are poorly visualized with conventional roentgenograms, and CT can better define this region.[15] Moreover, CT has been shown to supplement conventional roentgenograms to establish the presence or determine the degree of injury resulting from a variety of other conditions, among which are aseptic necrosis in rheumatoid arthritis patients receiving corticosteroids; temporomandibular and sternoclavicular involvement[36]; attenuation or tears of tendons or displacement in the shoulder joint; and the existence of synovial cysts arising from the knee joint.[32] High resolution CT has demonstrated abnormalities of the larynx in 72 percent of patients with rheumatoid arthritis, including erosions of the cricoarytenoid joint and adjacent soft-tissue swelling.[25]

In any patient with rheumatoid arthritis or another allied rheumatic disease, the occurrence of avascular necrosis (AVN), whether due to the disease itself or to long-term corticosteroid therapy, is a major complication. The early diagnosis of AVN is difficult because the radiographic findings due to late rheumatoid disease are similar to those of mottled sclerosis, subchondral osteoporosis, and collapse of adjacent bone that occurs with AVN. CT has been reported to be more sensitive than roentgenographs for detecting AVN but may be less reliable than radionuclide bone scans.[10]

Magnetic resonance imaging (MRI) is the newest diagnostic tool to have an established role in the assessment of rheumatoid arthritis. The advantages offered by this modality include the lack of ionizing radiation, its noninvasiveness, and its ability to detect early soft-tissue abnormalities and bony erosions before other imaging techniques, including conventional roentgenograms and CT scans. At present, the cost factor prohibits its use except in select situations. Its use is rarely the preferred procedure in patients with rheumatoid arthritis.

One of the unique advantages of using MRI in rheumatoid arthritis patients is that its image of joints and adjacent structures, by their different signal intensities, provide excellent identification of articular cartilage, ligaments, tendons, and fibrous capsule. By this superior resolution, it can separate synovial membrane from synovial exudate and distinguish cortical from medullary bone.[16] Another promising advantage is that data obtained by MRI can quantify inflammatory changes in these soft tissues at a much earlier stage in the disease than can be provided by any currently available method,[11] making it an invaluable tool for therapeutic decision-making

and for assessing response to interventional trials of new drugs or other promising therapeutic agents.

The results of two comparative studies of MRI, technetium 99m scintigraphy, and plain films indicate that MRI is the most sensitive and a relatively specific method for detecting early AVN.[14,37] MRI has also a place in locating ruptured Baker cysts and evaluating the response to local steroids in cysts associated with rheumatoid arthritis in large joints.[13]

REFERENCES

1. Arnett FC, Edworthy S, Block DA et al: The 1987 revised ARA criteria for rheumatoid arthritis. Arthritis Rheum 30:517, 1987
2. Bacon PA: Laboratory findings in rheumatoid arthritis. p. 750. In McCarty DJ (ed): Arthritis and Allied Conditions. 11th Ed. Philadelphia, Lea & Febiger, 1989
3. Ball J: Enthesopathy of rheumatoid arthritis and ankylosing spondylitis. Ann Rheum Dis 30:213, 1971
4. Braunstein EM, Weissman BN, Seltzer SE et al: Computed tomography and conventional radiographs of the craniocervical region in rheumatoid arthritis. Arthritis Rheum 27:26, 1984
5. Conklin JJ, Alderson PU, Zizic TM: Comparison of bone scan and radiograph sensitivity in detection of steroid induced ischemic necrosis of bone. Radiology 147:221, 1983.
6. Conn DL, McDuffie FC, Dyck PG: Immunopathologic study of sural nerves in rheumatoid arthritis. Arthritis Rheum 15:135, 1972
7. Duthie JJ, Brown PE, Truelove LH et al: Course and prognosis in rheumatoid arthritis. Ann Rheum Dis 23:193, 1964
8. Fisher M, Mielke H, Glaefke S, Deicher H: Generalized vasculopathology and finger blood flow abnormalities in rheumatoid arthritis. J Rheumatol 11:33, 1984
9. Geirsson AJ, Strufelt G, Truedsson L: Clinical and serological features of severe vasculitis in rheumatoid arthritis; prognostic implications. Ann Rheum Dis 46:727, 1987
10. Gillespy T III, Genant HK, Helsm CA, Richardson ML: Computed tomography and magnetic resonance imaging of articular disease. p. 318. In Katz WA (ed): Diagnosis and Management of Rheu-

matic Diseases. 2nd Ed. JB Lippincott, Philadelphia, 1988

11. Glikeson G, Polisson R, Sinclair H et al: Early detection of carpal erosions in patients with rheumatoid arthritis; a pilot study of magnetic resonance imaging. J Rheumatol 15:1361, 1988

12. Gordon DA, Stern JL, Broder I: The extra-articular features of rheumatoid arthritis and a systematic analysis of 127 cases. Am J Med 54:445, 1973

13. Hull RC, Harris EN, Gharavi AE et al: Nuclear magnetic resonance (NMR) tomographic imaging for popliteal cysts in rheumatoid arthritis. Ann Rheum Dis 43:56, 1984

14. Kalunian KC, Hahn BH, Bassett L: Magnetic resonance imaging identifies early femoral head ischemic necrosis in patients receiving systemic glucocorticoid. J Rheumatol 16:959, 1989

15. Kricun R, Kricun ME: Computed Tomography of the Spine: Diagnostic Exercises. Aspen, Rockville, MD, 1987

16. Kursunoghi-Brahme S, Ricco T, Weisman MH et al: Rheumatoid knee: role of gadopentetate-enhanced MR imaging. Radiology 176:831, 1990

17. Masi AT, Maldonado-Cocco JA, Kaplan SB et al: Prospective study of the early course of rheumatoid arthritis in young adults; comparison of patients with and without rheumatoid factor positively at entry and identification of variables correlating with outcome. Semin Arthritis Rheum 5:299, 1976

18. McDougal JG, Hubbard M, McDuffie FC et al: Comparison of fine assays for immune complexes in rheumatic diseases. Arthritis Rheum 25:1156, 1982

19. Nissinow S, Arnold WJ: Prognostic value of C-reactive protein (CRP) levels in rheumatoid arthritis. Arthritis Rheum 25:524, 1982

20. Palmer DG, Hogg N, Highton J et al: Macrophage migration and maturation within rheumatoid nodules. Arthritis Rheum 30:729, 1987

21. Pinals RS, Baum J, Foschick WM et al: Preliminary criteria for clinical remission in rheumatoid arthritis. Bull Rheum Dis 32:7, 1982

22. Pincus T, Callahan LF, Sale WG et al: Severe functional declines, work disability and increased mortality in 75 rheumatoid arthritis patients studies over nine years. Arthritis Rheum 27:864, 1984

23. Resnick D: Arthrography, tenography and bursography. p. 150. In Resnick D, Niwayama G (eds): Diagnosis of Bone and Joint Disorders. WB Saunders, Philadelphia, 1981

24. Resnick D, Niwayama G, Coutts RD: Subchondral cysts (geodes) in arthritic disorders; pathologic and radiographic appearance of the hip joint. AJR 128:799, 1977

25. Resnick D, Sartoris D, Cone RO III: Imaging. p. 656. In Kelley WN, Harris ED Jr, Ruddy S, Sledge CB (eds): Textbook of Rheumatology. 3rd Ed. WB Saunders, Philadelphia, 1989

26. Ropes MW, Bennett GA, Cobb S et al: 1958 Revision of diagnostic criteria for rheumatoid arthritis. Bull Rheum Dis 9:175, 1958

27. Rose HM, Ragan C, Pearce E, Olmstead L: Differential agglutination of normal and sensitized sheep erythrocytes by sera of patients with rheumatoid arthritis. Proc Soc Exp Biol Med 68:1, 1948

28. Saville PD, Kharmosh O: Osteoporosis of rheumatoid arthritis; influence of age, sex and corticosteroids. Arthritis Rheum 10:423, 1967

29. Schmid FR, Cooper NS, Ziff M, McEwen C: Arteritis in rheumatoid arthritis. Am J Med 30:56, 1961

30. Schumacher HR Jr: Palindromic onset of rheumatoid arthritis; clinical, synovial fluids and biopsy studies. Arthritis Rheum 85:361, 1982

31. Schumacher HR Jr (ed): Primer of Rheumatic Diseases. 9th Ed. Arthritis Foundation, Atlanta, 1988

32. Schwimmer M, Edelstein G, Heiken JP, Gilula LA: Synovial cysts of the knee: CT evaluation. Radiology 154:175, 1985

33. Sharp JT, Calkins E, Cohen AS et al: Observations on the clinical, chemical and serological manifestations of rheumatoid arthritis based on the course of 154 cases. Medicine (Baltimore) 43:41, 1964

34. Short CL, Bauer W, Reynolds WS (eds): Rheumatoid Arthritis. Harvard University Press, Cambridge, 1957

35. Talal N, Moutsopoulos H, Kassan S (eds): Sjögren's Syndrome: Clinical and Immunological Aspects. Springer-Verlag, Berlin, 1987

36. Thompson JR, Christiansen E, Hasso AN, Hinshaw DB Jr: Temporomandibular joints: high-resolution computed tomographic evaluation. Radiology 150:105, 1984

37. Totty WG, Murphy WA, Ganz WI et al: Magnetic resonance imaging of the normal and ischemic femoral head. AJR 143:1273, 1984

38. Vainio K: The rheumatoid foot; a clinical study with pathological and roentgenological comments. Ann Chir Gynaecol Fenn, suppl. 1, 107, 1956.

39. Waaler E: On the occurrence of a factor in human serum activating the specific agglutination of sheep blood corpuscles. Acta Pathol Microbiol Scand 17:172, 1940

40. Wolfe F, Hawley DJ: Remission in rheumatoid arthritis. J Rheumatol 12:245, 1985

4

Medical Aspects of Management of Rheumatoid Arthritis

Charley J. Smyth

The treatment of rheumatoid arthritis is steadily undergoing change as knowledge of the clinical course is revealed, medications become available, new regimens are attempted, and improvements are made in reconstructive surgery and rehabilitation. The most significant change in drug management since the mid-1980s has resulted from reports of the limited impact of the nonsteroidal anti-inflammatory drugs (NSAIDs) in altering the progressive and destructive changes of this disease during 2 to 3 years of continuous therapy, and the realization that the disease-modifying antirheumatic drugs should be given early rather than late when the short-acting agents have failed. In the area of orthopaedic surgical management of rheumatoid arthritis, the remarkable improvements in total joint replacement represent one of the greatest overall advances in the treatment of the patient with advanced disease.

This progress in the care of patients with rheumatoid arthritis has been accomplished by the team approach. By bringing the abilities and skills of all members of the health team—physicians, nurses, physical and occupational therapists, dietitians, social workers—to focus on the needs of the rheumatoid patient, it has been possible to improve the patient's comfort, functional ability, and overall well-being.

DEVELOPING A TREATMENT PROGRAM AND AIMS

As soon as the diagnosis is established, it is essential that the physician assess the patient's needs by obtaining a comprehensive medical history, determining the degree of joint damage and the extent of any extra-articular involvement. Performing selected laboratory and radiographic tests is the next order of business. These steps are essential for evaluating the extent of pathologic damage and functional capacity in order to use the criteria for "stage" and "class" established by the American Rheumatism Association.

During the development of a plan to treat the patient, it is important to recognize that rheumatoid arthritis is a systemic disease with variable onset, course, and outcome. Hence no single treatment plan is adequate. Rather, successful management requires a balanced program of many treatment modalities designed specifically for each patient and altered periodically as the disease progresses. The aim should be relief of discomfort, maintenance of good muscle strength and maximum joint motion, prevention of deformities, suppression of inflammation, and maintenance of proper nutrition and good general health by eliminating or controlling unrelated concurrent diseases.

KNOW THE PATIENT BEING TREATED

Physicians must evaluate the total needs of the patient, taking time to determine the patient's level of knowledge about the disease and his or her fears, foibles, concerns, and anxieties; physicians should also familiarize themselves with the patient's motivation, education, and willingness and ability to comply with instructions. The patient's socioeconomic status also needs consideration. It is essential that the primary physician appraise the patient's general health, including any concurrent or past diseases (e.g., diabetes, hypertension, gastrointestinal problems, anemia, renal and hepatic diseases). It is necessary when planning therapy to know what current or prior medications have been administered and the patient's response, including toxicities; in addition, knowledge of prior illnesses, accidents, and operations help to formulate a plan of management. Armed with this information, the responsible physician can avoid conflicts, anticipate complications, and eliminate any duplication of previously unsuccessful drugs or procedures. During this thorough evaluation, the physician will gain the confidence of the patient, an element essential to successful management.

NONDRUG THERAPY

Rheumatoid arthritis is a frustrating disease, not only for the patient and family but also for the physician. Although it is generally recognized that a cure for this illness has yet to be discovered, recent major advances in medical and surgical management are changing the former fatalistic attitudes, apprehensions, and anxieties among patients and families. It is incumbent on the primary physician and all members of the health team, from the moment of initial contact with the patient, to convey a *realistic optimism* and attempt to reverse the attitude that nothing can be done.

Education of Patient and Family

When informed early in the course of the disease about the nature of the illness, the symptoms to be expected, and the available therapeutic measures and their potential complications, a patient with rheumatoid arthritis is much more likely to be cooperative and compliant. Care of the rheumatoid arthritis patient is individualistic, and a patient may react differently to the same modality at different times during the course of the disease. Considerable time is required with the patient to explain the variable nature of this disease and the aims of therapy. Most patients can accept these facts, adjust to the disease, and lead as productive lives as possible. Given the knowledge, the patient is better able to deal with conflicting opinions about recommended remedies and nonscientific opinions.

Time spent with an occupational and physical therapist can also promote better understanding and awareness of how this disease affects daily activities and how adjustments can be made to make life easier. Examples of some useful modifications available to the disabled include built-up utensils and keys, grip cloths to open jars, modified door handles, rails to facilitate entering and exiting bathtubs, and elevated toilet seats.

Motivation and Compliance

The success of therapy often depends on whether the patient is motivated to deal with his or her disease. Even the strongly motivated patient may experience disappointing moments when encouragement by the physician is required. It is frequently a challenge to turn a discouraged patient around and instill the will, energy, and determination to conquer this disease. Here is where the team approach has distinct advantages in that the patient appreciates that not one but several professionals have a concerned interest and suggestions for making him or her feel better. Motivation therefore results from the patient's satisfaction of even minor degrees of pain relief and improved mobility, and must be nurtured by the physician and others who care about the patient.

In addition, success of any therapeutic plan for rheumatoid arthritis depends on patient compliance. If the patient has prior knowledge of the goals of therapy, as well as the limitations and potential adverse reactions, he or she is far more likely to follow the physician's recommendations. In studies of rheumatoid arthritis, the proportion of patients judged to be compliant with medications has ranged from 51 percent[6] to 78 percent.[11]

Rest and Activity

It is important that rheumatoid arthritis patients learn to limit or modify their activities to protect their joints, but not through total inactivity. Confinement to bed is neither necessary nor recommended. Reliable reports state that there are no substantial differences between the progress of hospitalized bedridden patients and those allowed activities.[23]

With acute generalized synovitis, fatigue is common, and periods of rest are particularly helpful. Also, rest of individual inflamed joints is important to relieve pain, prevent deformity, and allow the inflammation to subside. These goals may be achieved by avoiding weight-bearing and using removable splints, braces, and protective techniques. Wrist splints are especially helpful and may be worn at night to immobilize inflamed joints; they can be removed during the day when dexterity is necessary. A good general exercise program is recommended, and whirlpool or hot showers can help decrease muscle spasm, reduce pain, and permit exercise to improve tolerance.

Diet

The relation between diet and rheumatoid arthritis has received considerable attention in the lay press; despite intense interest, few well-designed scientific studies have been published to justify the use of any specific diet. There continues to be general agreement among rheumatologists that a nutritious diet to correct protein deficiency and a low-calorie weight reduction diet to assist the unloading of involved joints of the lower extremities do benefit these patients.

There is a popular notion among rheumatoid arthritis patients that foods are in some way related to their arthritic symptoms. The limited number of investigations that have been designed to establish a relation between immune-mediated rheumatic activity response and any restrictive or elimination diets have been short-term, involved few patients, and lacked control or blinded assessment. Thus results of these reports are considered uninterpretable.[33]

The other major interest in diet therapy for rheumatoid arthritis has been in the relation between this disease and the metabolism of arachidonic acid, the long-chain polyunsaturated fatty acids in fish oils. It has been shown in several studies that the dietary manipulation of polyunsaturated fatty acids (fish oils) alters production of the biologically active leukotriene B_4 in the synovial fluid of rheumatoid patients. Other clinical studies have reported that the reduction of this leukotriene is correlated with various indices of improvement in patients receiving large doses of fish oil[17] or primrose oil.[2]

Treatment of Concomitant Diseases

When treating rheumatoid arthritis in any patient, care must be taken to treat the associated illnesses as well. General symptoms of malaise, fatigue, weight loss, anemia, low-grade fever, chest pain, and headache may be due to some accompanying disease. Therefore it behooves the primary physician and orthopaedic surgeon to evaluate any complaint, particularly if it is new or if it occurs in an elderly patient who is being considered as a candidate for reconstructive surgery.

Other Considerations

Few people receive more free advice from well-meaning nonmedical sources—friends, neighbors, associates, family members, total strangers—than do patients with rheumatoid arthritis. Most authorities agree that almost all home remedies, spa type therapy, and manipulations are acceptable so long as they do no harm, are not expensive, and do not interfere with or delay the usual prescribed therapy. There is little evidence to justify advising a patient to move to a different climate. Separation from a stressful home or work environment may be more important.

DRUG THERAPY

Drug therapy plays a key role in the management of rheumatoid arthritis; and although a great variety of medications are available to aid these patients, their use should be kept to a minimum. All of the drugs and biologic agents are empiric and have potential harmful side effects. Three classes of medication are available for the management of this disease.

Analgesics and NSAIDs are considered the "first line" agents and are the most widely used by the 6.5 million Americans who suffer from rheumatoid arthritis. The slower-acting disease-modifying antirheumatic drugs (DMARDs) are the "second line" agents and are used when first line drugs do not control the activity of the disease. The immunosuppressive drugs alone or in combination are used more frequently but are still considered "third line" because they are prescribed when all others fail. As the benefit/risk ratio and long-time efficacy are established, this status may change. The benefits of systemic and intraarticular corticosteroids are adjuncts to any of the other drugs or modalities. The initial enthusiasm for the use of glucocorticoids has been tempered because the toxicity is high, but when used judiciously they still have a place in treating severe unremitting disease or life-threatening vasculitis and for intermittent intra-articular use.

Historical Background

Most of the pharmaceutical and other agents used for the treatment of rheumatoid arthritis during the first half of the twentieth century have been discarded because of inefficiency or toxicity. Only three drugs that were commonly administered during the years preceding the discovery of corticosteroids by Hench and his associates[13] in 1949 are still considered beneficial and are recommended for managing this disease. The first are the salicylates. Aspirin was shown to have remarkable benefits in rheumatoid arthritis patients a century ago by Hoffman, a German chemist who synthesized the compound when he gave it to his father, who had the disease.[12] The second group of drugs introduced early in the twentieth century, and that continue to be recommended, are gold salts. They were first used by Forestier[7] in France and were reported to be effective in 1929. He successfully treated rheumatoid arthritis patients using a gold compound (sodium aurothiopropanol, Allochrysine) based on the assumption that tuberculosis and rheumatoid arthritis might have a common infectious cause. The third drug that continues to be recommended for the treatment of rheumatoid arthritis and that was introduced during the precorticosteroid years is sulfasalazine. It was originally given to rheumatoid arthritis patients by Svarz[35] in Sweden in 1942 because she believed that this disease resulted from an intestinal bacterial infection. Only recently has there been a resurgence of interest in its use for patients with rheumatoid arthritis.

All of the numerous other drugs and biologic preparations that were used during the early decades of this century have been proved to be ineffective and are no longer recommended. A partial list of these agents includes various vaccines prepared from autogenous or stock vaccines; artificial fever (cabinet, hot tub, blanket packs, intravenous foreign protein, or typhoid vaccine); iontophoresis (using galvanic current to introduce transcutaneous vasodilating drugs (methacholine or histamine); parenteral sulfur; venom (bee or snake); vitamins (B complex, D, C); cinchophen; concentrated ozone; and multiple small whole-blood transfusions.

Discovery of Cortisone and ACTH

In May 1949 Hench and his associates from the Mayo Clinic presented a scientific paper[13] at the

International Congress on Rheumatic Diseases that described the dramatic effect of corticosteroids in 16 patients with moderately severe rheumatoid arthritis. The report captured the attention of the scientific world and especially of victims of this dreaded disease; it launched a new era in basic and clinical research regarding this long neglected, common rheumatic illness. Cortisone and its derivatives were immediately and enthusiastically accepted. For the next decade they became the treatment of choice and almost the only therapeutic drug used for the treatment of rheumatoid arthritis. Many were of the opinion that these agents might represent a cure. As is now well known, this optimistic view faded within a few years as the long list of toxicities associated with high doses and prolonged use of these agents became apparent. However, this revolutionary demonstration that the course of rheumatoid arthritis could be abruptly altered sparked an intensive worldwide search by pharmaceutical and clinical investigators into the cause(s) of rheumatoid arthritis and for better agents for its control.

During the four decades since this historical discovery, there has been a remarkable increase in knowledge of the mechanism of joint inflammation. An understanding of the relation involving immunologic reactions, biochemical mediators, and cellular responses in rheumatoid arthritis patients has created therapeutic approaches for controlling joint tissue destruction. As a result, there has been an increasing flow of nonsteroidal agents made available for clinical trials in patients with rheumatoid arthritis. Consequently, there were innumerable short-term trials beginning during the 1960s of the mechanism of these clinically unproved agents, conducted in the hope of finding products that are both effective and free of the side effects of the corticosteroids and to speed their release from the experimental laboratory to the stage of clinical use.

First Line Drugs: Salicylates and NSAIDs

It was 2 years after the striking effects of corticosteroids were announced before a new antirheumatic disease agent became available for the treatment of rheumatoid arthritis. In 1951 phenylbutazone (Butazolidin) was introduced, followed by indomethacin (Indocin) 10 years later. Since then, there has been a steady flow of short-acting NSAIDs approved by the Food and Drug Administration. To the salicylates has been added a list of more than 15 NSAIDs that are now accepted as first line agents for the management of this disease (Table 4-1).

Evaluation of Therapeutic Effectiveness

With the rapid increase in the number of promising agents came the need for a reliable means to evaluate their clinical efficacy. There was a wide difference of opinion regarding the best method for measuring benefit and safety in clinical trials, one that would provide reproducible data that could be statistically managed. The "activity index" of Lansbury,[20] proposed in 1958, was the plan most widely used. This plan and later modifications have been helpful but provided information mainly for short-term (2 to 3 year) studies. Evaluations of the long-term outcome of therapy for rheumatoid arthritis have revealed the limitations of the first line medications. Sharp,[28] using mean radiographic scores, reviewed long-term data indicating that when rheumatoid arthritis is firmly established progression of joint destruction is inexorable and inevitable, regardless of treatment. Further evidence that rheumatoid arthritis progresses despite long-term use of NSAIDs has been shown in the decline of work ability, severe functional ability, and increases in mobility and mortality. This evidence of poor outcome published during the 1980s has been reviewed by Pincus and Callahan.[24,25]

Clinical Use

It is generally agreed that one of the NSAIDs should be selected as the agent of first choice in every newly diagnosed patient with rheumatoid arthritis. Within a few days of administration, all of these agents effectively reduce symptoms and are the most effective quick-acting first line treatment for the illness. Their mechanism of action is to block the synthesis of prostaglandins and thromboxanes. There is lack of evidence that they have any influence on the basic chronic dis-

Table 4-1. Nonsteroidal Anti-inflammatory Drugs for Rheumatoid Arthritis

Drug (Trade Name)	Available Units (mg)	Recommended Dosage (mg/day)	No. of Doses/Day
Salicylates			
Acetylsalicylic acid (aspirin)	325	1,000—6,000	3–4
Sodium salicylate		1,000—6,000	2–4
Salsalate (Disalcid)	250	2,000—3,000	2
Diflusinal (Dolobid)	250/500	500—1,500	2
Choline magnesium trisalicylate (Trilisate)	750	3,000	1–2
Meclofenamate (Meclomen)	50/100	200—400	2–4
Sulfasalazine (Azulfidine)	500	1,000—3,000	2–6
Propionic acids			
Ibuprofen (Motrin, Advil, others)	300/400/600/800	1,200—3,200	3–4
Naproxen (Naprosyn)	250/375/500	250—1,000	2
Fenoprofen (Nalfon)	300/600	900—2,400	4
Ketoprofen (Orudis)	50/75	150—300	3–4
Phenylacetic acid			
Diclofenac (Voltaren)	50/75	150—200	2–3
Indoleacetic acid			
Indomethacin (Indocin)	25/50/75(SR)	75—150	2–3
Sulindac (Clinoril)	150/200	300—400	2–3
Tolmetin (Tolectin)	200/400	600—1,600	3–4
Oxicam			
Peroxicam (Feldene)	10/20	30—80	1–2
Phenylakanoic acid			
Flurbiprofen (Ansaid)	5/100	200—300	2–3

ease process. Also, it is not clear if any of these agents is consistently superior to another.

Patients with rheumatoid arthritis respond individually and unpredictably to a given NSAID, making it necessary to try one or a number of drugs in each patient. With the increasingly large number of preparations available—each with different size tablets, recommended daily dosages, and potential side effects—the physician is often confused about which NSAID to prescribe. Also, questions may arise about when to modify the amount, the interval between doses, and how to monitor their effects. There are some general guidelines about how to approach this treatment dilemma.

It is useful to begin with aspirin in doses of 2.4 to 3.6 g/day (8 to 12 five-grain tablets) in four divided doses. If this dosage is tolerated but symptoms persist after 5 to 7 days, an increase to 4.2 to 5.0 g/day (14 to 16 five-grain tablets) is appropriate. The dose required to obtain maximum anti-inflammatory results must be approached slowly. Blood salicylate levels between 20 and 30 mg% are desired.

In patients who develop gastrointestinal toxicity, enteric-coated or buffered aspirin may be tolerated. Sustained-release aspirin is useful in patients who are not compliant with the frequent dose schedule. Nonacetylated salicylates, including sodium salicylate, salalate, or choline magnesium salicylate may be less toxic. If intolerable pain, stiffness, or unacceptable side effects persist for 4 to 8 weeks after optimal doses of salicylates, one of the more recently approved NSAIDs may be selected.

Patient-related factors may influence this choice, as it appears that all available antirheumatic compounds of this class have proved to be at least as effective as aspirin for the treatment of rheumatoid arthritis and induce fewer untoward reactions. Indomethacin is usually avoided in the elderly, in whom shorter elimination half-life drugs may be preferable in order to reduce the levels of toxicity related to drug accumulation with underlying renal disease, congestive heart failure, or hepatic disease; sulindac is thought to be less deleterious. In patients receiving oral anticoagulants, the nonacetylated salicylates or an NSAID with a short elimination half-life is preferable. Patients may comply better with a drug requiring only one or two daily doses (compared with three or four). The cost factor of therapy should also be considered.

Second Line Drugs: DMARDs

There is another group of compounds described as second line agents, or DMARDs, for the treatment of rheumatoid arthritis. These agents have been clearly shown to produce improvement for short periods (several months to a few years), but highly critical appraisals of their use have failed to establish their long-term impact (5 to 20 years) on the course of the disease.[18,36] These so-called slow-acting drugs are parenteral and oral gold, the antimalarial hydroxychloroquine, penicillamine, sulfasalazine, and the immunosuppressive drugs azathioprine and methotrexate.

Gold

Among the drugs considered disease-modifying today, gold is the only one that was commonly used prior to the discovery of corticosteroids. During the 1930s Forestier[7] described his experience with more than 500 rheumatoid arthritis patients who benefited from using a 75 percent preparation of aurothiopropanol sodium sulfonate (Allochrysine). During the intervening years, the value of chrysotherapy has been confirmed by numerous carefully controlled clinical trials and years of experience by many rheumatologists. More than 50 years after the initial reports the use of gold salts has finally achieved acceptance as an important therapeutic intervention in the management of rheumatoid arthritis. Gold salts have become the standard for parenteral malate or gold sodium thioglucose given as a test dose followed by either of these compounds 50 mg weekly until the cumulative dose of 1 g or until toxicity or major clinical improvement develops. The recommended maintenance dose is 50 mg at monthly intervals. The orally absorbed gold complex auranofin is generally considered less effective than the intramuscular salts. There is no specific time limit to the course of gold therapy.

The toxic reactions to gold, which occur in about 30 percent of patients, include rashes, renal damage, and bone marrow depression. Permanent damage is rare, and these complications clear without residual if the drug is discontinued. It is of the utmost importance to recognize these reactions and to monitor each injection by at least a laboratory test of the hemoglobin level, white blood cell count, and urinalysis.

Antimalarial Drugs

The use of chloroquine for rheumatoid arthritis was first reported during the early 1950s and for a time enjoyed some popularity. With the continued use of this drug, there came an increasing number of reports indicating that it was deposited in the macular area of the retina, causing impaired vision. The drug was soon abandoned and replaced by hydroxychloroquine, which proved to be less toxic. When used, an eye examination every 3 months is required to detect any eye damage. It requires 4 to 6 weeks to obtain any antirheumatic results. Many investigators have been enthusiastic about the combined use of hydroxychloroquine and other remittive agents, but these combination regimens require additional controlled studies to establish their value.

Penicillamine

The DMARD penicillamine has been used successfully for the treatment of rheumatoid arthritis since it was first reported by Jaffe in 1963 and 1964.[14,15] Although a component of the penicillin molecule, it has no antimicrobial properties. It has been shown to be effective as injectable gold[14] and azathioprine[3] and is of particular value in rheumatoid arthritis-associated extra-articular manifestations such as vasculitis, lung infiltrations, Felty syndrome, and amyloidosis. It is not recommended for use during pregnancy and should be used with extreme caution in patients with concurrent renal disease. Traditionally, penicillamine has been used after chrysotherapy has failed.

The basic principle of therapy is to introduce the drug gradually, with the increments increased at intervals of 8 weeks or more. The recommended starting dose is 250 mg/day, with increases of 125 or 250 mg/day at intervals of 8 to 10 weeks. Doses of 500 mg/day or less are sufficient in most patients as a maintenance dose.

Untoward effects are numerous and diverse and have limited its clinical acceptance. These effects include hematologic changes (anemia, thrombocytopenia, leukopenia), proteinuria, nephrotic syndrome and myasthenia gravis, pemphigus, and Goodpasture syndrome. It is essential that a monthly complete blood count (CBC), platelet count, and urinalysis be done, as well as periodic renal function tests.

Sulfasalazine

During the 1980s sulfasalazine was rediscovered as an effective disease-modifying agent for rheumatoid arthritis. It was originally referred to as salazoprin and was used by Svarz in Sweden as an antimicrobial agent because of her belief that group B streptococci might cause this disease. She published her experiences of treating more than 400 rheumatoid arthritis patients between 1940 and 1946, with favorable responses in 63 percent.[35] The first account of its use in the United States, by Kuzell and Gardner[19] in 1950, supported Svarz' findings and reported suppression of arthritis in an animal model as well. However, during the years that followed highly variable results were reported in Europe, and great credence was given to a negative report by Sinclair and Duthie[30] of the prestigious Edinburgh Hospital arthritis unit. Probably the greatest cause for the temporary demise of sulfasalazine use in rheumatology was due to the explosive arrival of cortisone in 1949.

There has been renewed interest in this agent. A series of carefully conducted clinical investigations using open studies and randomized trials have found sulfasalazine to have the properties associated with other second line agents. The dose used in most of these studies starts with 0.5 g/day and increases by 0.5 mg weekly to reach a maintenance level of 2 g/day. Higher doses (2.5 to 3.0 g) have been used in some clinical trials. Its mode of action remains obscure. One study[31] involved 317 rheumatoid arthritis patients who received sulfasalazine with 5 years of follow-up evaluations of clinical parameters in conjunction with serial serum C-reactive protein (CRP) and erythrocyte sedimentation rate (ESR). A total of 163 patients received penicillamine, and 203 were given injections of gold sodium thiomalate. In each group there were significant improvements in clinical scores, CPR, and ESR at time points up to 30 months. The data showed that there was little difference among sulfasalazine, gold, and penicillamine in terms of clinical efficiency; serious adverse effects (rash and hematologic and renal parameters) were most common in the gold group (17.4 percent) and slightly less in patients given penicillamine (12.3 percent) or sulfasalazine (1.6 percent). The authors concluded that sulfasalazine appeared to be as well tolerated over long periods and was as effective as gold and penicillamine. It was also associated with fewer serious side effects and so was considered the agent of first choice.

Other reports have presented similar convincing evidence to document the efficiency of sulfasalazine in suppressing rheumatoid inflammation to a degree comparable with standard DMARDs.[40] The incidence of adverse reactions may occur in up to one-fourth of patients, but with few exceptions these reactions are readily reversible and not life-threatening.

Methotrexate

The latest second line drug to be made available for treatment of rheumatoid arthritis is methotrexate, which was approved in the United States in 1988. This antifolate agent was first introduced for use in treating malignancies; but during the 1980s it became one of the most widely used second line drug for the management of rheumatoid arthritis, and its use continues to rise markedly.

There have been numerous reports of short-term, carefully controlled clinical trials ranging from 3 to 4 years that clearly establish methotrexate as effective and with safety comparable to standard second line antirheumatic drugs. Scully et al.[27] treated 124 rheumatoid arthritis patients with this drug, followed them for 5 years, and compared their experience to the current studies in the literature with treatment durations longer than 12 months. In their study, methotrexate was found to be an effective and well-tolerated medication in 31 percent of the patients followed for 5 years. In their analysis of seven published reports on 486 patients, 283 (58 percent) continued with the drug at 2 years. At 3 years, five studies reported that 129 of 241 patients (54 percent) continued on the drug. At 4 years, three studies reported that 65 of 163 patients (40 percent) were continuing this medication. These authors and most experienced investigators who have reported their results of studies with methotrexate in rheumatoid arthritis patients agree that the potency and duration of action of the drug is equal or superior to that of other DMARDs. The significant literature concerning methotrexate for rheumatoid arthritis over a 5-year period was extensively reviewed in 1988.[10]

A major objective of rheumatoid arthritis therapy is suppression of joint inflammation, and one of the most reliable outcome measures of this change is radiographic evidence of change. Slowing of the progression of disease during methotrexate therapy has been shown radiographically in a limited number of studies, and others have shown no change. On the basis of the results of five open prospective studies of low-dose methotrexate, it was found that no definite conclusions could be drawn about the slowing effect of methotrexate on radiographic progression.[16]

The usual starting dose of methotrexate is 5.0 to 7.5 mg/week; at 3- to 6-week invervals the dosage can be increase in 2.5 mg increments up to 15 to 20 mg/week if a beneficial response has not occurred. After the therapeutic response has been achieved, the maintenance dose may be slowly reduced. The antirheumatic effect of this low-dose weekly methotrexate is often apparent within 4 to 6 weeks. Intramuscular doses of 5 to 15 mg/week are used by some and may prevent untoward gastrointestinal side effects associated with the drug using the oral route.[1] High-dose intravenous investigations are in progress.

Toxic effects have been a major factor in the acceptance of this agent and are the main reason for its discontinuation. The spectrum of side effects includes nausea, vomiting, anorexia, stomatitis, anemia, leukopenia, thrombocytopenia, alopecia, rash, abnormal liver function, hepatic fibrosis, and pulmonary infiltrates. In most reports the number of undesirable reactions is high. An analysis of the toxic reactions contained in five reports with follow-up periods of 2 to 3 years showed a prevalence of adverse reactions ranging from 57 to 93 percent.[27] Most patients on low doses for up to 2 years have had few serious reactions, and minor adjustments in the dose schedule have permitted continuation of therapy. The development of drug toxicity has limited long-term use of this agent in many studies.

Because of the frequent occurrence of adverse reactions, it is recommended that patients receiving methotrexate have screening tests (CBC, platelet counts, and hepatic function profiles) before and at intervals throughout therapy. During the first 24 weeks the CBC, platelet counts, and hepatic enzyme tests for liver toxicity should be repeated every 4 weeks and every 8 weeks thereafter. Concerns over hepatotoxicity have resulted from previous reports of the risk of cirrhosis in patients with psoriasis who were receiving this drug. These concerns have been allayed by the absence of reports of cirrhosis associated with the low-dose programs commonly used for rheumatoid arthritis patients. However, some observers recommend percutaneous liver biopsies after an accumulated dose of 1.0 to 1.5 g of the drug. Others recommend this procedure after 2 years of therapy and every 2 years thereafter. Daily folic acid supplements (1 mg/day) have been shown to reduce significantly the occurrence and severity of mucosal ulcerations and hematologic reactions without diminishing efficiency. The use of methotrexate is contraindicated in pregnant patients and in those with a history of renal disease or heavy alcohol intake.

Despite considerable knowledge of the influence of methotrexate on individual enzymes within the folate, immunologic, and inflammatory pathways, the exact mechanisms and site of action in patients with rheumatoid arthritis remain unclear. There is good evidence that it has both immunosuppressive and anti-inflammatory action.

Cytotoxic and Immunoregulatory Therapy

Refractory rheumatoid arthritis is being treated effectively by drugs, biologic preparations, and other procedures that modify the immune system. The drugs most commonly used are the glucocorticosteroids, azathioprine, cyclophosphamide, and cyclosporine. Other methods recently developed and applied to suppress some phase of the immunoregulatory cycle include plasma lymphoresis and total lymphoid irradiation. Although these agents and methods are especially potent suppressors of rheumatoid disease activity, this benefit is obtained at the expense of potentially serious side effects, and for this reason their place in the management of the rheumatoid patient is limited.[4]

Glucocorticoids

For the past four decades the corticosteroids have been used extensively and effectively in the management of patients with rheumatoid arthritis. The mechanism(s) by which these drugs exert beneficial effects on rheumatic diseases appears to be both anti-inflammatory and immunoregulatory. Among their actions are influences on the movement and immune function of leukocytes. They also are potent inhibitors of prostaglandin synthesis and of the production of many mediators of the immune response, e.g., interleukin-1.

Early in the cortisone years it became apparent that the clinical use of these powerful new therapeutic tools yielded undesirable, often severe, even fatal consequences. As a result, there was an immediate intensive search for, and the development and approval of, steroidal and nonsteroidal antirheumatic agents with fewer unfavorable reactions. This search and contentious production of new and beneficial anti-inflammatory and immunosuppressive therapeutic agents has continued to this day. Extensive experience over the years has defined an important role for the corticosteroids in rheumatoid arthritis. With low doses, the benefit/toxicity ratio has become acceptable, and it has been clearly shown that these agents are not curative nor do they prevent progressive joint damage. The initial and often dramatic beneficial effects are usually not maintained. There are, however, specific indications for their use.

Intra-articular injections are indicated and effective in controlling acute and subacute synovitis. These injections should not be repeated more than three or four times a year. It is important to rule out infection before using local steroid injections. A number of effective short- and long-acting synthetic steroids are available for intra-articular use. Corticosteroids may also be useful for the treatment of unremitting disease with acute exacerbations; they can be administered at high doses for short periods, with prompt tapering as the clinical flare-up subsides. Also, if the disease remains active despite adequate trials of NSAIDs, low-dose corticosteroids may be justified. At times steroids are required for socioeconomic reasons and while waiting for second line agents to become effective. The dose range should be 5 to 10 mg of prednisone or the equivalent. Severe, life-threatening vasculitis may require high doses of parenteral corticosteroid therapy.

Azathioprine

Azathioprine (Imuran), a cytotoxic agent, is an analogue of 6-mercaptopurine and acts by suppressing both primary and secondary immune resposes. It has an anti-inflammatory effect by inhibiting monocyte precursor proliferation and decreasing the entry of monocytes to the inflammatory site.

It is administered orally in doses of 1.0 to 2.5 mg/kg/day; it is usually started at a low dose (50 mg), which is gradually increased to the maintenance level of 100 to 150 mg/day over a 4- to 6-week period. There are numerous reports to show that azathioprine is an effective drug for the treatment of rheumatoid arthritis, as it has a steroid-sparing effect and the ability to retard the progression of radiographically demonstrable bony erosions. Based on comparative studies, it is as effective as gold, chloroquine, or penicillamine; like these second line agents, it has a gradual onset of response, requiring 6 to 8 weeks to produce a significant response. Maximal response may require 4 to 6 months.

In order of decreasing frequency, the major side effects are gastrointestinal problems, reversible mild leukopenia, and abnormal liver function tests. Despite these potential untoward reactions, azathioprine is generally well-tolerated short-term therapy. The major concern is with long-term therapy because of the potential for the induction of malignancies, especially lymphoma and leukemia. Acceptance of the use of this cytotoxic agent has been limited because of this fear of causing fatal neoplasms.

Cyclophosphamide

Cyclophosphamide (Cytoxan), an alkylating agent, has been shown by well-controlled studies to be effective in suppressing rheumatoid synovitis and to have a beneficial effect on the radiographically demonstrated progression of the erosions of this disease. In doses of 1.5 to 2.5 mg/kg/day, cyclophosphamide is often associated with leukopenia.

Despite its undisputed clinical value in rheumatoid arthritis patients and the fact that it may be the most potent of the available immunoregulatory agents for the treatment of this disease, its use is restricted by the high rate of occurrence of serious side effects associated with its use.[2] They include gastrointestinal intolerance, bone marrow suppression, alopecia, hemorrhagic cystitis, irreversible sterility, leukemia, and leukopenia. These toxic reactions have severely curtailed its use in the treatment of rheumatoid arthritis.

Cyclosporine

Cyclosporine, the newest immunoregulatory agent, was introduced into clinical practice in 1978 and since then has won an established plane in organ transplant clinics. Its action is to selectively modulate the immune system, particularly the subpopulation of immunocompetent T and B cells.[20] It is the latest of a growing number of agents being investigated for treatment of rheumatoid arthritis. Experiences with its use in autoimmune rheumatic diseases, including 53 patients with rheumatoid arthritis, was reported in 1985.[26] Two subsequent European reports, one controlled study involving 12 patients[8] and one double-blind trial of 52 patients with refractory rheumatoid arthritis,[5] confirmed the efficacy of this agent in this connective tissue disease. In a report of ten rheumatoid arthritis patients, all had adverse reactions that necessitated permanent withdrawal from the study of two patients, temporary discontinuation of treatment of seven, and dosage reduction for eight.[39] A comprehensive review of additional observations on the use of cyclosporine in rheumatoid arthritis patients by a large investigation has been published.[22] From this analysis of the available data it appears that the drug is effective in rheumatoid arthritis patients at doses of 5 mg/kg body weight, but that nephrotoxicity is clearly a major issue along with other frequent side effects.

These early clinical trials indicate that cyclosporine therapy, as with all other immunoregulatory agents, requires close monitoring. It remains to be seen whether it will be possible to administer these drugs safely for a sufficiently long time to determine if they can retard radiographic progression of rheumatoid arthritis.

Other Immunoregulatory Therapy

Other methods have been investigated as modifiers of the immune system for the management of rheumatoid arthritis, including total lymph node irradiation, plasmapheresis, lymphoresis and leukaphoresis, levamisole or γ-interferon administration, and clonal deletion. The preliminary clinical results with each of these methods involving short-term follow-up hve been described as moderately or highly successful. However, these procedures are expensive and require special facilities or hospitalization; and the long-term benefits and side effects are yet to be defined. At present they are considered experimental procedures. A brief account of several of these methods follows.

Untried and Promising Therapy

During the second half of the twentieth century, during the postcortisone years, there has been a steady and increasing flow of agents approved for treatment of rheumatoid arthritis. At present, a number of newly developed drugs and biologic preparations are in the early stage of evaluation and are undergoing extensive clinical trials. The final place of any of the following drugs or combinations will be measured by the benefit/toxicity ratio, i.e., the balance of their disease-suppressant effect against the frequency and severity of side effects.

Some of the most promising advances in therapy are being observed with agents that suppress precise immune reactions. An example of the immune-modulating drugs is cyclosporine, which acts by blocking the production of interleukin-2, a substance necessary for T- and B-lymphocyte differentiation and proliferation. It is being extensively investigated in patients with rheumatoid arthritis, and even at this early stage of drug evaluation the studies that have been completed clearly indicate that cyclosporin A is effective. Despite troublesome renal and other side effects, there are strong indications that, with small doses, it will ultimately prove beneficial. However, restriction posed by toxicities, particularly nephrotoxicities, remain to be defined.

Under investigation is another approach to modulating the immune system and producing therapeutic benefit in rheumatoid arthritis. It has involved the experimental use of monoclonal antibodies directed against lymphocyte surface markers. Preliminary clinical trials have been reported that involve the use of anti-CD4 (anti-helper-T-cell) monoclonal antibody. There was a dramatic reduction of CD4$^+$ cells; a significant reduction of the ESR, CRP, and rheumatoid factor (RF) concentration; improvement in grip strength; and decreased morning stiffness. Similar preliminary results have been reported when a marine CD5$^+$ monoclonal antibody was given to patients with rheumatoid arthritis. Both of these accounts are unconfirmed and require additional extensive clinical evaluation. It seems to be a promising alternative treatment for rheumatoid arthritis.

Radiotherapy

Total lymphoid irradiation (TLI) induces potent, prolonged suppression of the immune system in rheumatoid arthritis patients. It was first used effectively in patients with ankylosing spondylitis during the 1950s and acquired a high degree of popularity. Follow-up studies, however, showed that bone marrow aplasia or leukemia occurred in virtually all patients, and regeneration was incomplete for as long as 14 years. As a result, radiotherapy for this rheumatic disease has fallen into disrepute and has been abandoned by most authorities. Despite this experience, with the interest in immunosuppression as an approach in the therapy of rheumatoid arthritis, radiotherapy is being reevaluated. Two studies, one at Stanford[34] and the other at Harvard,[37] have made preliminary reports of the immunologic and clinical effects of TLI in patients with intractable rheumatoid arthritis. The Boston group used 3,000 rad over a period of 13 to 15 months, including 2-week rest periods; the Palo Alto group used 2,000 rad given continuously 4 to 5 days each week for 5 to 6 weeks.

The clinical results using conventional measurements were similar in the two groups, with improvement in 80 percent of patients after 6 months, a favorable change that lasted about 1 year in most patients. Other published clinical trials have contained similar beneficial results. The immunologic and other laboratory data, including such parameters as ESR and RF level, were similar in all studies. A profound and sustained lymphopenia was present and involved predominantly a depletion of T-helper cells and a decrease in the T-helper/T-suppressor ratio; also there was a decrease observed in the proliferative response of mononuclear cells. Other adverse reactions to TLI are common and serious, with marked and profound lymphopenia. The frequency and severity of these side effects are generally unacceptable. Moreover, the mortality rates have been disturbingly high, with 13 deaths among 108 patients reported in published studies from five centers from 1979 through 1987. These investigations using radiotherapy have greatly increased our understanding of the pathogenesis of RA and further established the prominent role of cell-mediated immunity in this disease, but this knowledge has been obtained at the expense of frequent or serious toxicities.

Many experienced clinicians are enthusiastic about the possibility of a relatively new concept of combining different antirheumatic medications to achieve greater efficacy in rheumatoid arthritis patients with lower toxicity. Various combinations have been reported, including sulfasalazine with penicillamine, azathioprine with hydroxychloroquine, and the triple combination of hydroxychloroquine, cyclophosphamide, and azathioprine. Perhaps it is not surprising that drug combinations in which an alkylating agent has been included are particularly effective.

One of the suggested plans of therapy is a "step-down bridge" concept, aimed at controlling inflammation as soon as possible and maintaining this control within the first year.[41] The plan is initiated with rapid-acting anti-inflammatory medications such as low dose (10 mg/day) prednisone to provide early control. If disease activity is not controlled within 1 month, these drugs are combined with slower-acting second line drugs such as methotrexate. When methotrexate has taken effect at about 3 months, the corticosteroid is stopped; and the methotrexate is discontinued at about 6 months.

Fries[9] recommended that one disease-modifying drug be administered continually throughout the illness and one of the nonsteroidal anti-inflammatory drugs (NSAIDs) be added frequently at the first sign of disease flare-up or increasing disability. This "saw-tooth" strategy has yet to be employed. Only after such studies can it be known if this approach and that of other combinations of medications will advance our ability to better manage patients with this potential crippling disease.

Constructing a Management Plan

In the foregoing section there is a review of a limited number of the wide variety of agents and modalities that are available or are being evaluated for treating rheumatoid arthritis. Each of these methods is empiric, and each has unique qualities, including dose schedules, duration of action, indications, contraindications, and requirements for monitoring to avoid side effects. The treatment of this complex, highly variable chronic disease with both articular and systemic components must be tailored to the individual. Different strategies must be used at different stages of the disease. It is important that the patient be informed that if treatment is not causing improvement within a certain period of time, changes will be made using other agents or methods or adding another drug.

Historical Perspective

During the years immediately following the introduction of cortisone and its analogues into clinical practice, these agents rapidly received worldwide acceptance and for a number of years became the most commonly used drugs for the treatment of rheumatoid arthritis. It became clear for the first time in history that it was possible to drastically alter the course of this disease that has crippled millions of people. Unfortunately, after only a few years it became evident that with the wonderful benefits there came undesirable and even fatal complications. It was soon realized that there was a real need for equally effective agents devoid of the high risk of toxicity. In response to this need, an intensive period of search began in many centers interested in rheumatic disease and in the pharmaceutical industry to produce an agent(s) to replace the corticosteroids.

During the early 1970s, two decades following the rapid rise and progressive decline in the popularity of the corticosteroids, there was an increase in the number of approved products for the treatment of rheumatoid arthritis, but without the undesirable toxicity that was associated with the steroids. Each of these new agents was introduced with claims of equal or superior qualities to existing measures. The practicing physician was faced with the question of which agent or method of treatment to use and when to prescribe it. There was added confusion because of the availability of many therapeutic options when only a few years before there had been almost nothing. In an effort to answer this therapeutic dilemma, based on the prevailing options of the most effective and safest approach to therapy a plan was proposed; the first therapeutic pyramid was reported in 1972 (Fig. 4-1).[32] The primary purpose of this plan was to bring some order out of the confusion that prevailed at the time.

Need to Remodel the Pyramid

During the years since the development of this plan, NSAIDs have been introduced for clinical

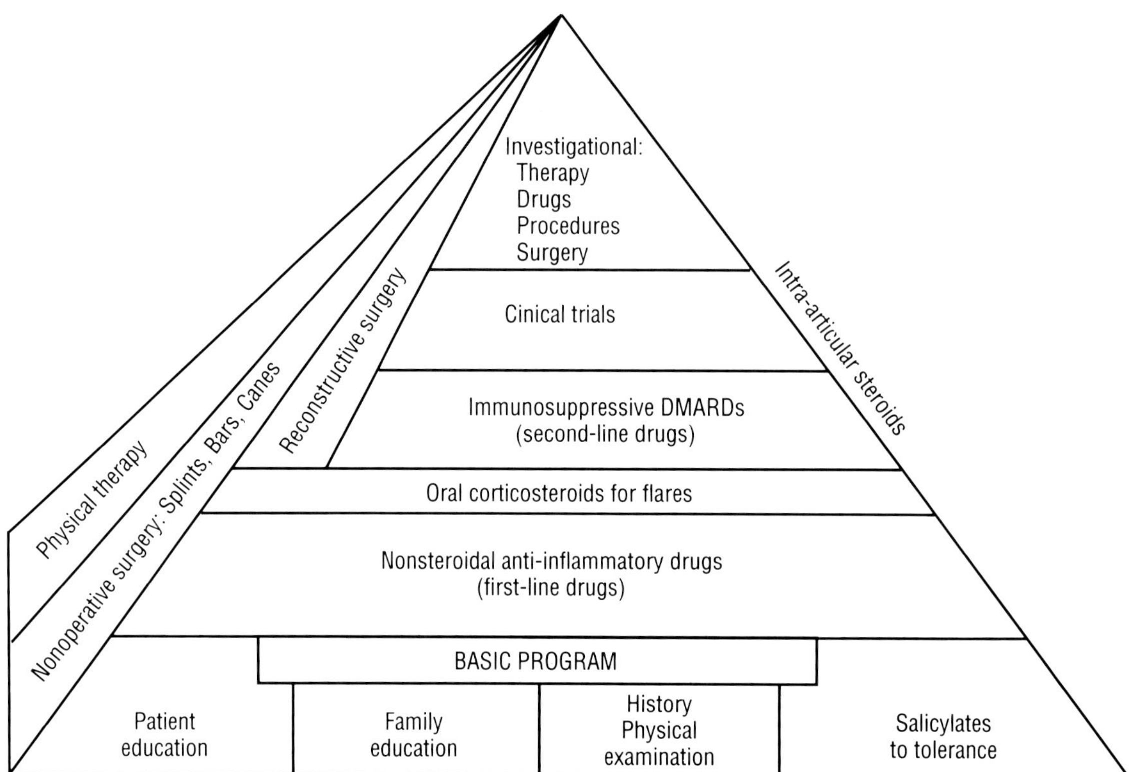

Fig. 4-1. Revised therapeutic approach combining physical therapy, nonoperative surgical methods, and systemic and intra-articular steroids throughout the disease with more aggressive drug therapy early in the illness.

use. During these same years there have been a number of carefully controlled long-term clinical trials of these drugs used in rheumatoid arthritis patients. These studies have produced reliable data about the highly variable clinical course of this disease, data showing a low prevalence of remissions (only 10 percent in a 2.5 year study of 458 patients[28]), reports of improved methods for evaluating drug responses, and recognition of the number, variety, and severity of adverse reactions associated with the use of new and established drug regimens. Other studies have shown by serial radiographs that there is an unexpectedly poor outcome of this disease with progressive joint destruction regardless of therapy.[28]

Articles published during the last few years have challenged the prevalent assumption that second line DMARDs are effective disease-modifying agents. In 1989 Kushner[18] summarized the results of several outcome studies in the litera-

ture and concluded that we are currently unable to influence the long-term outcome of rheumatoid arthritis. Others have also pointed out the short-term benefits of NSAIDs and DMARDs but agree that as currently used in long-term therapy there is inadequate evidence to show that joint destruction is being retarded.[38]

Suggested Therapeutic Approach

As a result of these long-term outcome observations that emphasize the weaknesses of traditional rheumatoid arthritis therapy, there have been a number of recommendations for earlier, more aggressive drug therapy for this disease. Among these suggested plans is the recommendation to begin with the slow-acting anti-rheumatic drugs (DMARDs), one of the immunosuppressive agents, or a combination of these

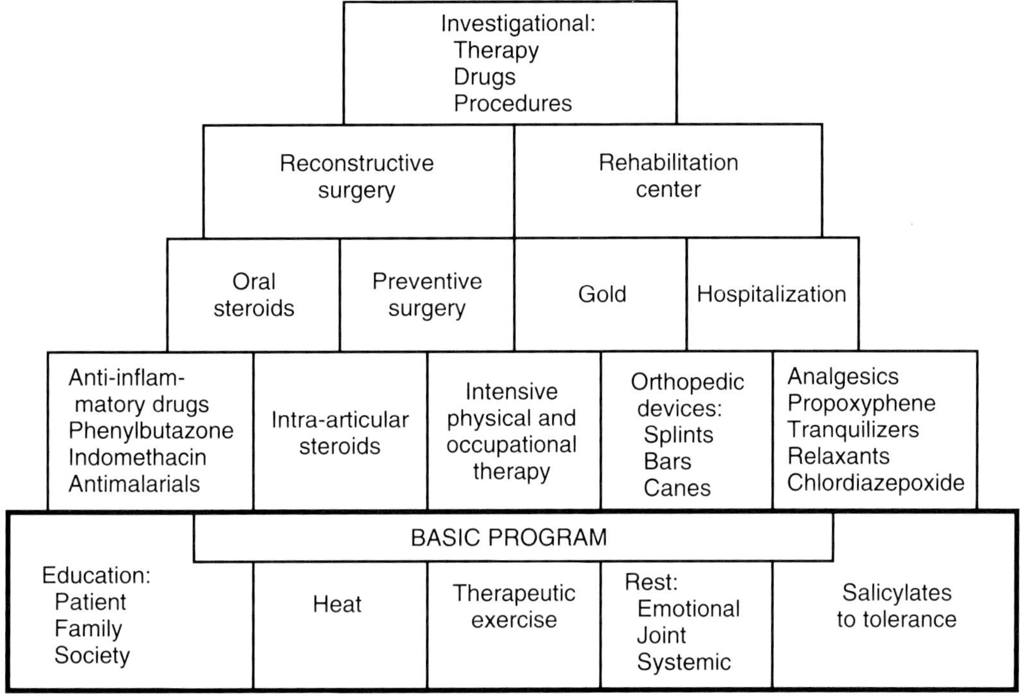

Fig. 4-2. First pyramid in print placed known therapies in perspective, suggesting a stepwise program beginning with more benign therapies ("Basic Program") and progressing to the dangerous and untried therapies at the top of the pyramid.

methods early in the course of the disease before structural joint damage has occurred.[21,24,41]

Presented here is a plan that retains much of the proved value of the traditional pyramidal approach to therapy and the established benefits of short-acting NSAIDs, while providing for the early use of slower-acting agents (DMARDs) and the current immunoregulatory agents or experimental combinations of these various agents (Fig. 4-2).

The initial step in this sequential treatment plan (Basic Program) is to emphasize to the patient and family the chronic nature of this disease, the slow improvement, and the important of compliance. There is general agreement that rest coupled with physical therapy and occupational counseling can maintain muscle strength and range of motion and assist the patient in job training, home modifications, overcoming disability, and preventing deformation. The plan provides for the initial use of the quick-acting NSAIDs as first line drugs. Oral corticosteroids are useful for short periods to control flare-ups in joint or systemic complications. The DMARDs have benefits above and beyond those of NSAIDs, but they are generally associated with greater therapy/rest period ratios; and their use raises the question of what justifies the risk. There is a growing consensus that more aggressive therapy with DMARDs be initiated early rather than later, and that if one of these agents fails another or some combination of these agents should be tried soon thereafter. Most authorities recommend that one of these agents be started when there is more than a mild degree of pain and synovitis in several joints, when function is compromised, and when erosive changes are first detected by roentgenograms.

Reconstructive surgery represents the greatest advance in the treatment of rheumatoid arthritis in recent years. Medicinal therapy is continued after surgery. Intra-articular steroids and physical and occupational therapy are helpful throughout the course of the disease.

REFERENCES

1. Andersen PA, West SG, O'Dell JR et al: Weekly pulse methotrexate for rheumatoid arthritis: clinical and immunological effects in a randomized double blind study. Ann Intern Med 103:489, 1985

2. Belch JJF, Ansell D, Madhok R et al: Effects of altering essential fatty acids on requirements for nonsteroidal anti-inflammatory drugs in patients with rheumatoid arthritis: a double blind placebo controlled study. Ann Rheum Dis 47:96, 1988

3. Berry H, Liyanage S, Durance R et al: Trial comparing azathioprine and penicillamine in the treatment of rheumatoid arthritis. Ann Rheum Dis 35:542, 1976

4. Decker JL: Toxicity of immunosuppressive drugs in man. Arthritis Rheum 16:89, 1973

5. Dougados M, Awada H, and Amor B: Cyclosporin in rheumatoid arthritis: a double-blind, placebo-controlled study of 52 patients. Ann Rheum Dis 47:127, 1988

6. Ferguson K, Bole GG: Family support, health beliefs and therapeutic compliance in patients with rheumatoid arthritis. Patient Counselling Health Educ 13:101, 1979

7. Forestier J: The treatment of rheumatoid arthritis with gold salts injections. Lancet 1:441, 1932

8. Forre O, Bjerkhoel F, Salvesen CF et al: An open, controlled, randomized comparison of cyclosporine and azathioprine in the treatment of rheumatoid arthritis: a preliminary report. Arthritis Rheum 30:88, 1987

9. Fries JF: Reevaluating the therapeutic approach to rheumatoid arthritis: the "sawtooth" strategy. J Rheumatol, suppl 22, 17:12, 1990

10. Furst DE, Kremer JM: Methotrexate in rheumatoid arthritis. Arthritis Rheum 31:305, 1988

11. Geersten HR, Gray R, Ward JR: Patient non-compliance within the context of seeking medical care for arthritis. J Chronic Dis 26:689, 1973

12. Goodwin JS, Goodwin JM: Failure to recognize efficacious treatments: a history of salicylate therapy in rheumatoid arthritis. Prospect Biol Med 25:78, 1981

13. Hench PS, Kendall EC, Slocumb CH, Polley HF: The effect of a hormone of the adrenal cortex (17-hydroxy-11-dehydrocorticosterone—compound E) and pituitary adrenocorticotrophic hormone on rheumatoid arthritis: preliminary report. Mayo Clin Proc 24:181, 1949

14. Jaffe IA: Comparison of the effect of plasmaphoresis and penicillamine on the level of circulating rheumatoid factor. Ann Rheum Dis 22:71, 1963

15. Jaffe IA: Rheumatoid arthritis with arteritis: report of a case treated with penicillamine. Ann Intern Med 61:556, 1964

16. Jeurissen MEC, Boerbooms AM, Levinus AB et al: Influence of methotrexate and azathioprine on radiologic progression in rheumatoid arthritis: a randomized, double-blind study. Ann Intern Med 114:999, 1991

17. Kremer J, Lawrence D, Jubiz W et al: Different doses of fish oil fatty acid supplementation in rheumatoid arthritis: a prospective, double-blinded, randomized study. Arthritis Rheum, suppl., 31:305, 1988

18. Kushner I: Does aggressive therapy of rheumatoid arthritis affect outcome? J Rheumatol 16:1, 1989 (editorial)

19. Kuzell WC, Gardner CM: Salicylazosulfapyridine (salazopyrin or azopyrin) in rheumatoid arthritis and experimental polyarthritis. Calif Med 73:476, 1950

20. Lansbury J: Report of a three-year study on systemic and articular indexes in rheumatoid arthritis: theoretic and clinical considerations. Arthritis Rheum 1:505, 1958

21. McCarty DJ: Suppress rheumatoid inflammation early and leave the pyramid to the Egyptians. J Rheumatol 17:1115, 1990 (editorial)

22. McCune WJ, Bayless GE: Immunosuppressive drug therapy. Curr Opinion Rheumatol 1:80, 1989

23. Mills JA, Pinals RS, Ropes MW et al: Value of bed rest in patients with rheumatoid arthritis. N Engl J Med 284:453, 1971

24. Pincus T, Callahan LF: Remodeling the pyramid or remodeling the paradigms concerning rheumatoid arthritis: lessons from Hodgkin's disease and coronary artery disease. J Rheumatol, suppl 12, 17:1582, 1990

25. Pincus T, Callahan LF: Reassessment of 12 traditional paradigms concerning the diagnosis, prevalence morbidity and mortality of rheumatoid arthritis. Scand J Rheumatol, suppl, 79:67 1989

26. Schindler R: Cyclosporin in Autoimmune Diseases. Springer, Berlin, 1985

27. Scully CJ, Anderson CJ, Cannon GW: Long term methotrexate threapy for rheumatoid arthritis. Semin Arthritis Rheum 20:317, 1991

28. Sharp JT: Radiologic assessment as an outcome measure in rheumatoid arthritis. Arthritis Rheum 32:221, 1989

29. Shevack EM: The effect of cyclosporin A on the immune system. Annu Rev Immunol 3:397, 1985

30. Sinclair RJG, Duthie JJR: Salazopyrin in the treatment of rheumatoid arthritis. Ann Rheum Dis 8:226, 1949

31. Situnayake RD, Grindulis KA, McConkey B: Long term treatment of rheumatoid arthritis with sulfasalazine, gold or penicillamine: a comparison using life-table methods. Ann Rheum Dis 46:177, 1987

32. Smyth CJ: Therapy of rheumatoid arthritis: a pyramidal plan. Postgrad Med 51:31, 1972

33. Sperling RE: Diet therapy in rheumatoid arthritis. Curr Opinion Rheumatol 1:33, 1989

34. Stober S, Tanay A, Field E et al: Efficacy of total lymphoid irradiation in intractable rheumatoid arthritis: a double-blind randomized trial. Ann Intern Med 102:441, 1985

35. Svarz N: Salazopyrin; a new sulfonamide preparation. Acta Med Scand 60:577, 1942

36. Symmons DMP, Darves PT: Outcome in rheumatoid arthritis. Br J Rheumatol, suppl 1, 27:1, 1988

37. Trentham DE, Belli JA, Bloomer WD et al: 2,000-CentiGray total lymphoid irradiation for refractory rheumatoid arthritis. Arthritis Rheum 30:980, 1987

38. Ward JR: Earlier intervention with second line therapies. J Rheumatol, suppl 25, 17:18, 1990

39. Weinblatt ME, Cablyn JS, Fraser PA et al: Cyclosporin-A treatment of refractory rheumatoid arthritis. Arthritis Rheum 30:11, 1987

40. Weisman MH (Chairman): Proceedings of conference on sulfasalazine in rheumatic diseases. J Rheumatol, suppl 16, 15:1, 1988

41. Wilske KR, Healey LA: Challenging the therapeutic pyramid: a new look at treatment strategies for rheumatoid arthritis. J Rheumatol, suppl 17, 17:4, 1990

II

SURGICAL PRINCIPLES IN RHEUMATOID ARTHRITIS

5

History of Surgery for Rheumatoid Arthritis

Mack L. Clayton

This short history of the development of surgery of rheumatoid arthritis is a personal opinion. Some readers may think there have been important omissions; if so, please note that it is not intended as a comprehensive literature review of the subject.

Synovectomy is the operation that is so unique to rheumatoid arthritis that the history of the disease really begins with this procedure.[8] In 1887 the German surgeon Schuller[23] reported four knee cases. He stated that cases of hypertrophic villous synovitis should be treated by early surgical removal rather than by spa therapy. He routinely divided the cruciate ligaments and either one or both collateral ligaments at their femoral insertions.

Goldthwait[10] in 1900 was the first in the United States to perform partial synovectomy for what he called hypertrophic villous synovitis. The procedure was limited to removal of protruding synovial fringes, which he believed mechanically blocked flexion to the joint.

In 1923 Swett[33] of Hartford, Connecticut, performed the first complete synovectomy for rheumatoid arthritis in the United States; he also popularized the procedure. In 1938 he published the results of surgery on 32 knees, stressing the selection of cases to ensure satisfactory results.[32] The popularity of this procedure, which has been in and out of favor since that time, was at a rather low ebb during the 1980s.

Hoffmann[13] of St. Louis reported an operation in 1911 for the relief of contracted and clawed toes by resection of all metatarsal heads through a curved plantar incision; 2 of his 11 cases were in rheumatoid arthritis patients (referred to as infectious arthritis at that time). The operation, with some modification, is still in widespread use today and has one of the longest histories of any continuously used reconstructive procedure.

In Chicago 1902, Murphy[19] used fascia for arthroplasty of the hip, knee, elbow, shoulder, and wrist. Arthroplasty of the elbow with fascia lata was described by MacAusland of Boston in 1921 and Campbell of Memphis in 1922. Many of the rheumatologic cases were complete ankylosis. The most successful of the large joint interpositional arthroplasties before the use of prostheses were done in the elbow; Vainio[34] of Finland has reported a large series of rheumatoid arthritis patients in whom skin was utilized as the interpositional material.

In 1929 Wilson[39] described posterior capsulotomy of the knee to correct common chronic flexion deformity. During the 1930s and 1940s, Smith-Petersen[24,25] had an assignment at the Massachusetts General Hospital to develop new operations for the relief of rheumatoid arthritis. In 1939 he described mold (cup) arthroplasty of the hip using a vitallium cup after reshaping the acetabulum and femoral head. It was the first successful use of a metallic interposition (Venable and Stuck[36] had introduced it for fracture fixation), and it is still in use today. Smith-Petersen had previously used glass and Bakelite without success.[25] The original idea was to have the cup as a mold to guide the shaping of the new joint and later remove the cup; however, he removed few of the cups. The procedure was further perfected by Law[15] and Aufranc[1,28] and was the operation of choice until total hip arthroplasty was introduced.

Smith-Petersen[24] described the ulnar approach for wrist fusion in rheumatoid arthritis patients, incorporating distal ulnar resection and utilizing the resected bone as a graft. In 1943, along with Aufranc and Larson, he described operative procedures for the upper extremity for relief of rheumatoid arthritis.[26] They included (1) partial acromionectomy and bursectomy in the shoulder, (2) excision of the radial head and synovectomy of the elbow, and (3) excision of the distal ulna with or without wrist fusion. This report was the pioneer article on upper extremity rheumatoid arthritis surgery, as well as the first documentation during the twentieth century for recommending reconstructive surgery while the disease is active and before extensive destruction had occurred. Smith-Petersen et al. were also the first to perform osteotomy of the spine for flexion deformity in ankylosing spondylitis[27] (then called rheumatoid spondylitis).

In 1948 Vaughn-Jackson[35] of London described rupture of extensor tendons at the wrist, which he treated by excising the distal ulna and performing tendon reconstruction. Straub and Wilson[30] of New York further refined the procedure, and early surgery was recommended before tendon rupture. Straub has remained one of the key figures in the development of rheumatoid surgery and founded the Committee on Arthritis of the American Academy of Orthopaedic Surgeons in 1961.

In 1958 Fowler of Nashville and Riordan of New Orleans reported jointly on resection arthroplasty of metatarsophalangeal (MTP) joints with realignment of the ulnar drift, thus initiating modern reconstruction of the rheumatoid digits.[6]

In 1959 in Iowa, Flatt[5] introduced press-fitted metallic hinge prostheses for finger joints, a modification of the Brannon prosthesis. These devices developed too many complications and were out of use within 10 years, but the early success gave impetus to further prosthetic development.[9]

Silicone hinge implants for finger joints were developed during the mid-1960s by Swanson[31] of Grand Rapids and by Niebauer of San Francisco. Swanson did not want fixation to the bone, whereas Niebauer did. The implants have improved the results of resection arthroplasty. The results of the Swanson and Niebauer prostheses are approximately the same; the technique of insertion is more important. Breakage had been a problem but is less now with a stronger silicone.

Silicone and metal to plastic (total wrist) replacements[18,37] were developed during the late 1960s and early 1970s. With modifications, they are still in use today. Wrist arthrodesis with intramedullary fixation remains a good procedure, particularly for late cases or for failed wrist arthroplasty.

Forefoot reconstruction by excision of MTP joints,[3] a modification of Hoffmann's procedure,[13] was developed during the 1950s into a widely accepted operation still in use today. Triple arthrodesis and ankle arthrodesis were also utilized.

In 1961 the Committee on Arthritis of the American Academy of Orthopaedic Surgery was organized under the chairmanship of Straub of New York. This was a key factor in educating physicians about rheumatoid surgery and the team approach.

During the late 1950s, Walldius[38] of Sweden and Young[40] of the Mayo Clinic developed the use of hinged knees to replace severely damaged rheumatoid knees. Other hinges were subsequently developed. These were not successful owing to high rates of infection and loosening. Cemented knee hinges were used for a time, but they also had problems with loosening and were perhaps worse than the uncemented hinges.

During the late 1950s, Charnley designed a low friction arthroplasty for the hip. A stemmed stainless steel femoral head replacement of 22 mm diameter was utilized against a Teflon acetabulum, and both components were anchored with methylmethacrylate. Early results were excellent; unfortunately, the Teflon rapidly showed wear, the minute particles soon caused a severe, painful reaction, and most cases failed. Charnley persisted, however, and during the early 1960s began using ultra-high-molecular-weight polyethylene (UHMWPE) for the acetabulum with success.[2] Practically all widely used modern total hip arthroplasties are a modification of the Charnley technique, and total hip arthroplasty is among the most successful of all rheumatoid surgical procedures for the patient, the rheumatologist, and the surgeon.

Others during the 1950s and early 1960s, e.g., McKeever[17] of Houston and MacIntosh[16] of Toronto, developed tibial plateau prostheses. Aufranc's group developed a distal femoral prosthesis with an intramedullary stem on an anatomic surface replacement.[14] This device had a remarkable resemblance to the femoral component of modern total knee replacements, and the results were better than with previous fascial arthroplasties. Then, in 1969, Gunston[12] developed a metal-plastic-cement total knee with ideas from Charnley's total hip arthroplasty (polycentric knee).

A number of bioengineered knees were developed and then disappeared. Gradually a resurfacing condylar, near-anatomic knee with patella emerged and is currently the common denominator for all others. A number of models have been designed with porous metal surfaces to enhance cement fixation or for bony ingrowth without cement. At this time there is no clear advantage to cementless fixation in rheumatoid arthritis patients.

Neer's group[20-22] developed a prosthesis for replacement of the humeral head and used it in rheumatoid arthritis patients during the 1960s. In 1974 Neer added a plastic glenoid, which has been the prototype for total shoulder replacement in rheumatoid arthritis patients.

Total elbow replacements with rigid (constrained) hinges were developed during the 1960s but have disappeared. Semiconstrained hinges or nonconstrained surface replacements, developed during the 1970s, have been successful and are gaining in use.[4]

In Europe a team approach with surgical emphasis was pioneered in Heinola, Finland. In 1950 Laine and Vainio,[34] as medical director and orthopaedic surgeon, respectively, cared for many patients and published excellent reports with follow-up studies. Vainio was one of the first orthopaedic surgeons to be made an honorary member of the American Rheumatism Association. At the Japanese Orthopedic Association meeting in 1983, he reported his 30 years of surgical experience.[34] Raunio succeeded Vainio, and now Hamilinenen is continuing the team approach to treating patients and training surgeons from around the world.

Other major contributors have been at Princess Margaret Rose Hospital in Edinburgh, starting with Savill and continuing with Lamb and Souter.[29] The Taplow unit, with surgeons Arden and Harrison and rheumatologist Ansell, also contributed importantly, especially in the area of juvenile rheumatoid arthritis. Gschwend[11] organized a team in 1962 in Zurich and published the first book on rheumatoid arthritis surgery in German in 1968 (later revised and translated in English). Pahle in Oslo was the leader in developing a unit similar to that in Heinola, and he played a key role in organizing the Norwegian Society of Rheumatoid Arthritis Surgery. Later he was the first president of the European Rheumatoid Arthritis Surgical Society (ERASS), an important educational force in Europe. Mori in Osaka, Heywood in Capetown, Mills in Melbourne, Zancolli in Argentina, Jakubowski in Warsaw, Tillman in West Germany, Brattstrom in Sweden, and many others from around the world have emphasized the need for utilizing a comprehensive team approach.

Brigham Hospital in Boston, under the leadership of Sledge, has seen an increasing volume of rheumatoid arthritis surgery and contributions to care of these patients. The Robert Breck Brigham Hospital was founded during the early 1900s and was the first hospital in the United States devoted soley to the care of arthritis patients. It recently joined with Peter Bent Brigham and the Boston Lying-In Hospital to form a megahospital, The Brigham and Women's Hospital.

Wilson, at the Hospital for Special Surgery in New York, recruited Freyberg to develop a Rheumatology Service there during the early 1940s. Straub and Freyberg continued to implement a strong team approach, which has made many contributions, including the first center to institute a fellowship in Orthopedics-Arthritis.

There are many examples of the team approach in the United States today, a number of which have developed into "arthritis centers" for the total care of arthritic patients. Most of the developments and refinements in surgical treatment of rheumatoid arthritis have come about through the team approach, which is emphasized in this book. We have cooperated in such an approach for more than 35 years.

The Arthritis Foundation has also become an important member of "The Team Approach" regarding education and research.

SUMMARY

During the early years of the twentieth century surgical and medical care of the rheumatoid arthritic patient was within the realm of orthopaedics. During the 1920s and 1930s, orthopaedic surgeons were instrumental in helping to create the rheumatologist as specialist, as so much more knowledge was developing and needed for treating this capricious, often devastating disease. (The American Rheumatism Association was founded during the mid-1930s and became the American College of Rheumatology in 1990. It is the largest such organization in the world and includes orthopaedic members.)

Since the 1950s, a team approach has yielded the major advances in treatment of severe cases of rheumatoid arthritis. The surgical procedures for this disease are not particularly different from those for other diagnoses; it is the rheumatoid patient who is different.

We believe that reconstructive surgery has been the most important advance in the treatment of the crippled rheumatoid arthritic patient over the last 35 years. Moreover, in answer to a questionnaire, rheumatologists ranked total joint replacement as the most important advance in 20 years, according to its importance for patients suffering from either rheumatoid arthritis or osteoarthritis.[7]

REFERENCES

1. Aufranc OE: Constructive hip surgery with the vitallium mold: a report of 1000 cases of arthroplasty of the hip over a 15-year period. J Bone Joint Surg [Am] 39:237, 1957
2. Charnley J: Low Friction Arthroplasty of the Hip. Theory and Practice. Springer, Berlin, 1979
3. Clayton ML: Surgery of the forefoot in rheumatoid arthritis. Clin Orthop 16:136, 1960
4. Ewald FC, Scheinberg RD, Poss R et al: Capitello-condylar total elbow arthroplasty. J Bone Joint Surg [Am] 62:1259, 1980
5. Flatt AE: The Care of the Rheumatoid Hand. CV Mosby, St. Louis, 1974
6. Fowler BF, Riordan D: Arthroplasty of metatarsophalangeal joints in rheumatoid arthritis. Presented at the American Orthopedic Association, Washington, DC, 1958
7. Fries JF: Advancement in the management of rheumatic diseases, 1965–1985. Arch Intern Med 149:1002, 1989
8. Geens S, Clayton ML, Leidholt JD et al: Synovectomy and débridement of the knee in rheumatoid arthritis. I. Historical review. J Bone Joint Surg [Am] 51:617, 1969
9. Girzadas DV, Clayton ML: Limitations of the use of metallic prosthesis in the rheumatoid hand. Clin Orthop 67:1186, 1969
10. Goldthwait JE: Knee joint surgery for non-tubercular conditions: a report of 38 operations for synovial fringes, injured semilunar cartilage, loose cartilage, coagula, exploratory incision, etc. Boston Med Surg J 143:186, 1900
11. Gschwend N: Surgical Treatment of Rheumatoid Arthritis. 2nd Ed. Verlag, Stuttgart, 1980.
12. Gunston FH: Polycentric knee arthroplasty; prosthetic stimulation of normal knee movement. J Bone Joint Surg [Br] 53:272, 1971
13. Hoffmann P: An operation for severe grades of contracted or clawed toes. Am J Orthop Surg 9:441, 1911
14. Jones WN, Aufranc OE, Kermond WL: Mold arthroplasty of the knee. J Bone Joint Surg [Am] 49:1022, 1967
15. Law WA: Late results in vitallium-mold arthroplasty of the hip. J Bone Joint Surg [Am] 44:1497, 1962

16. MacIntosh DL: Hemiarthroplasty of knee using space occupying prosthesis for painful varus and valgus deformities. J Bone Joint Surg [Am] 40:1431, 1958

17. McKeever DC: Tibial plateau prosthesis. Clin Orthop 18:86, 1960

18. Meuli HCh: Arthroplastie du paignet. Ann Chir 27:527, 1974

19. Murphy JB: Arthroplasty. Ann Surg 57:593, 1913

20. Neer CS: Articular replacement for the humeral head. J Bone Joint Surg [Am] 46:1607, 1964

21. Neer CS: Replacement arthroplasty for glenohumeral osteoarthritis. J Bone Joint Surg 56:1, 1974

22. Neer CS, Cruess RL, Sledge CB, Wilde AH: Total shoulder replacement: a preliminary report. Orthop Transact 1:244, 1977 (abstract)

23. Schuller M: Die Pathologie und Therapie der Gelenkentzundungen. Urban U. Schwarzenberg, Vienna, 1887

24. Smith-Petersen MN: A new approach to the wrist joint. J Bone Joint Surg 22:122, 1940

25. Smith-Petersen MN: Evaluation of mold arthroplasty of the hip joint. J Bone Joint Surg [Br] 30:59, 1948

26. Smith-Petersen MN, Aufranc OE, Larson CB: Useful surgical procedures for rheumatoid arthritis involving joints of the upper extremity. Arch Surg 36:764, 1943

27. Smith-Petersen MN, Larson CB, Aufranc OE: Osteotomy of the spine for correction of flexion deformity in rheumatoid arthritis. J Bone Joint Surg 27:11, 1945

28. Solomon L, Aufranc OE: Vitallium mold arthroplasty of the hip in rheumatoid arthritis. Arthritis Rheum 5:37, 1962

29. Souter WA: Planning treatment of the rheumatoid hand. Hand 11:3, 1979

30. Straub LR, Wilson EN: Spontaneous rupture of extensor tendons in the hand associated with rheumatoid arthritis. J Bone Joint Surg [Am] 38:1208, 1956

31. Swanson AB: Flexible Implant Resection Arthroplasty in the Hand and Extremities. CV Mosby, St. Louis, 1973

32. Swett PP: A review of synovectomy. J Bone Joint Surg 20:68, 1938

33. Swett PP: Synovectomy in chronic infectious arthritis. J Bone Joint Surg 5:110, 1923

34. Vainio K: History of surgery of rheumatoid arthritis in Europe. Scand J Rheumatol 12:65, 1983

35. Vaughn-Jackson OJ: Rupture of the extensor tendons by attrition at the inferior radio-ulnar joint: report of two cases. J Bone Joint Surg [Br] 30:528, 1948

36. Venable CS, Stuck WG: Electrolysis controlling factor in the use of metals in treating fractures. JAMA 111:1349, 1938

37. Volz RG: The development of total wrist arthroplasty. Clin Orthop 116:209, 1976

38. Walldius B: Arthroplasty of the knee using an endoprosthesis. Acta Orthop Scand [Suppl 1] 24, 1957.

39. Wilson PD: Posterior capsuloplasty in certain flexion contractures of the knee. J Bone Joint Surg 11:40, 1929

40. Young HH: Use of a vitallium prosthesis for arthroplasty of the knee. J Bone Joint Surg [Am] 53:1658, 1971

6

Status of Surgery for Rheumatoid Arthritis

Mack L. Clayton

Surgery for rheumatoid arthritis has the aims of relieving pain, improving function, and preventing further deterioration. Surgery must be a part of an overall combined medical care program that is carried on before, during, and after the operation. A team approach has been developed and is important to the care of the severely crippled rheumatoid arthritic. The team includes the patient, the treating physician (either family physician, internist, or rheumatologist plus the surgeon), anesthesiologist, and various allied health personnel, e.g., nurses, physical therapist, occupational therapist, and social worker, all of whom must be educated about the natural history of rheumatoid arthritis. There are now various arthritis centers in the United States.

Surgery for rheumatoid arthritis has a long history. Synovectomy and interpositional arthroplasty were described during the early years of this century.[31] As more and more became known about the generalized disease process of rheumatoid arthritis the medical speciality of rheumatology evolved during the 1930s.

Smith-Petersen et al.[1,31] (Fig. 6-1) had an assignment at the Massachusetts General Hospital during the 1930s and 1940s to find new operative procedures for the relief from rheumatoid arthritis and was the first modern physician to recommend surgery when the disease was still active and before joints were completely destroyed.

Surgery today is staged according to the individual patient and the involvement of the disease according to the roentgenographic staging (I, II, III, IV) of the American Rheumatism Association.

Stage I (early): normal roentgenogram, osteoporosis or soft tissue swelling
Stage II (early to moderate): slight joint narrowing only
Stage IIIa (moderate)
Stage IIIb (late): joint narrowing, erosions, and deformity
Stage IV (terminal): ankylosis or gross joint destruction

Surgery is rarely indicated for stage I because too many patients obtain remission. Relatively early surgery is indicated for stages II and IIIa, and arthroplasty is indicated for IIIb and IV. The operations in use today are as follows.

1. Synovectomy (tendon, bursa, or joint)
2. Osteotomy
3. Soft tissue release
4. Arthroplasty
5. Arthrodesis

Tenosynovectomy is an excellent procedure especially for early cases at the level of the wrist. Recurrences are few, and later rupture is rare (because of alteration of the environment with relative release of the tendon from a tight, closed space). Tenosynovectomy of the flexor tendons of the wrist and fingers[8] is also an excellent procedure that allows decompression of the median nerve when carpal tunnel symptoms are present (Figs. 6-2 and 6-3). Synovectomy of weight-bear-

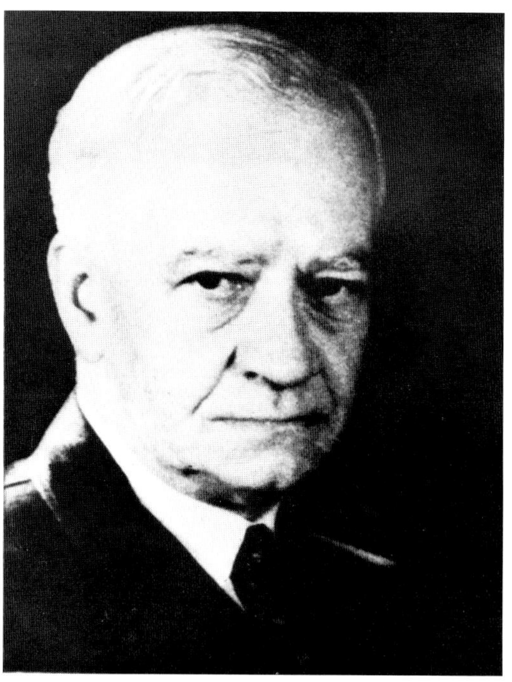

Fig. 6-1. M. N. Smith-Petersen, M.D., Chief of Orthopaedic Surgery at the Massachusetts General Hospital, 1929–1946. His assignment was to find new operative procedures for the relief of rheumatoid arthritis.

ing joints has had a decrease in popularity in the United States, especially for the knee (Fig. 6-4). Although two-thirds of the patients were improved at 3 years after synovectomy,[23,29] the morbidity, long recovery period, and unpredictability have made the procedure less popular. Arthroscopic synovectomy of the knee is increasing in popularity, and the early results of arthroscopic synovectomy are encouraging in terms of early relief of pain. Open elbow synovectomies have had the best results of all joint synovectomies.[22] Synovectomy is still occasionally indicated in the small joints of the hand. It is the only procedure we have to keep the patient's own joint functioning for an indeterminate length of time. We believe that, when evaluating a rheumatoid arthritis operation after 2 to 3 years, the result depends on the course of the disease. Total joint replacement is an exception because no articular cartilage remains.

Soft tissue release of contractures is rarely indicated as an individual procedure today but is often part of another procedure, e.g., release of the posterior capsule of the knee or subligamentous release during total knee replacement.

Osteotomy is not used for active rheumatoid arthritis of the weight-bearing joints at the time. For an occasional late, inactive, rheumatoid arthritic, osteotomy at the knee for angular deformity is indicated, as this disorder is really osteoarthritis.[12]

Excisional arthroplasty is widely used in the forefoot area.[6] Excisional arthroplasty plus implant (silicone) is also widely used in the hand and, in some cases, the great toe.[34]

Total joint replacement of the large joints with a metal-to-plastic articulation and anchorage with methylmethacrylate is the most common procedure in rheumatoid arthritis surgery.

Arthrodesis today is used mainly in the hindfoot and small joints of the hand and as a salvage procedure in the wrist and knee.

REGIONAL CONSIDERATIONS

Shoulder

The use of surgery of the shoulder has increased rapidly, and today total shoulder replacement of a nonconstrained type is the most common procedure (Fig. 6-5A).[20] It is performed through an anterior approach without release of the deltoid. The status of the rotator cuff is important, and reconstruction may be necessary. Resection of the acromioclavicular joint and anterior acromionectomy are frequently part of the procedure. A subacromial spacer is utilized occasionally, when the rotator cuff is irreparable.

Pain relief is excellent, and function is improved. The usual patient can elevate to a right angle and externally rotate 40 degrees, giving excellent positioning of the hand in space (Fig. 6-5B). The operative results are good, essentially equal to those of a total knee replacement.[11]

Elbow

The elbow is frequently involved in rheumatoid arthritis, but progress is slow. Involvement of

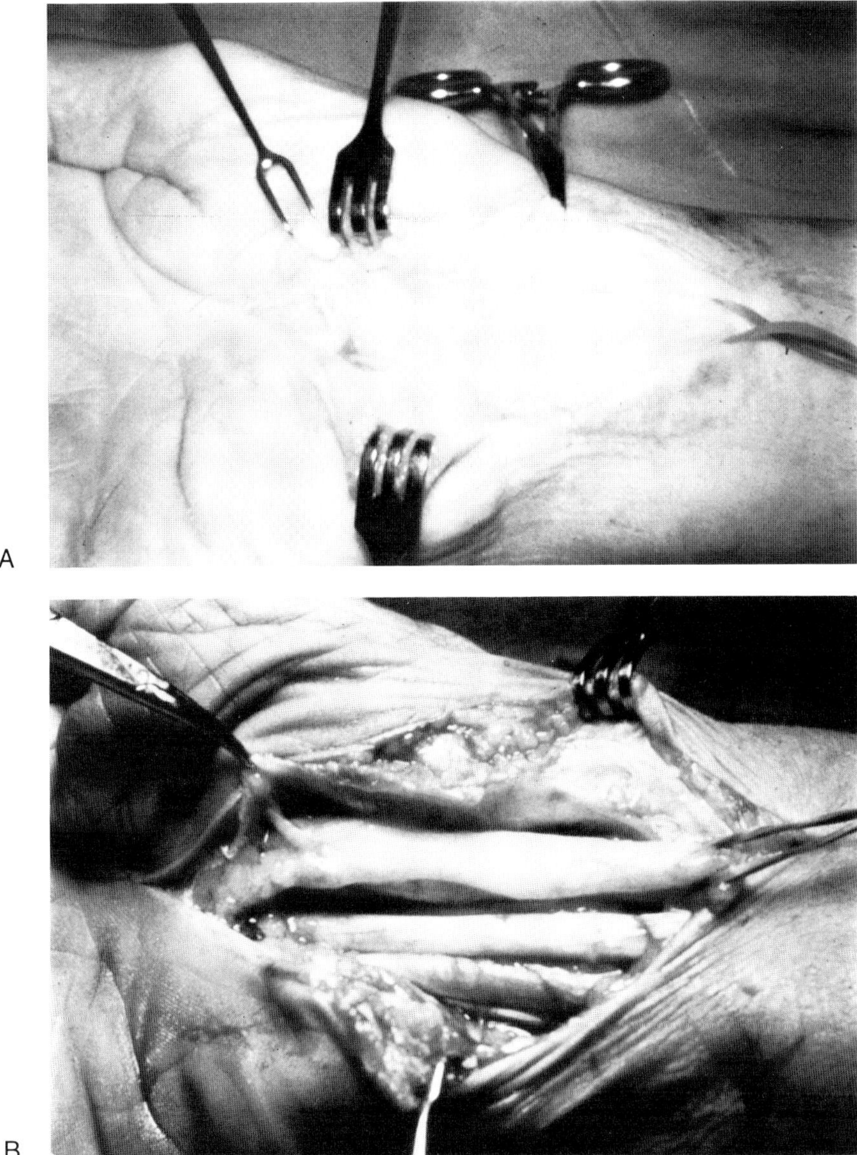

Fig. 6-2. (**A**) Flexor tenosynovitis at the wrist with compression of the median nerve underneath the transverse carpal ligament. This incision is longer than the incision utilized today, but it illustrates the pathology. Note the marked synovitis bulging proximal to the transverse carpal ligament, which is situated directly between the two tree-prong rake retractors. There is also some bulging of the synovium distally. (**B**) After removal of the marked bulging synovium the tendons are now grossly cleaned of the rheumatoid synovial tissues, and the median nerve is freed. Note the marked compression of the median nerve underneath the severed transverse carpal ligament. The motor branch of the median nerve is emerging directly from the midvolar aspect of the median nerve just opposite the hemostat in the upper corner of the figure.

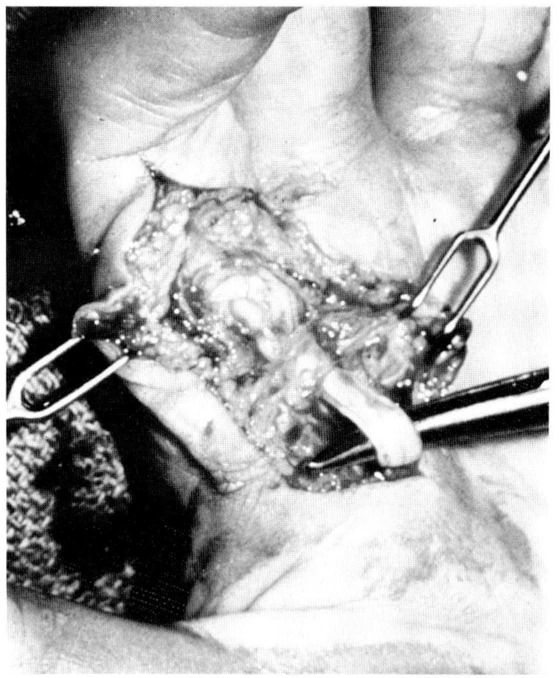

Fig. 6-3. Flexor tenosynovitis of the index finger. Note the large synovial nodule on the flexor tendon just distal to the annular A-1 pulley, which limits flexion and causes catching and limited motion of the finger with pain.

the elbow and shoulder cause great disability when positioning the hand. Synovectomy combined with radial head excision is a useful procedure even in some stage IIIb cases. If the range of motion is functional and the radio-ulnar joint smooth, clinically the operation is indicated.

A lateral incision is utilized, the radial head excised, and the joint cleared of synovium and bony spurs with rongeurs. The medial approach is elective and added if ulnar neuropathy is present. If pronation and supination are not restored, excision of the distal ulna is necessary. The results are excellent, and 80 percent of patients are improved at 5 years.[22] We have utilized a silicone radial head implant in certain cases, but the long-term results are no better,[22,35] and there have been complications.

For late cases total elbow replacement with a nonconstrained prosthesis (Ewald) is our preferred procedure in young patients.[17] (Fig. 6-6). Subluxation has been a problem in the past. Preservation of the medial collateral ligament is the key for prevention; our results are good.

Constrained elbows (hinges) have had high loosening rates. The second generation "lax"

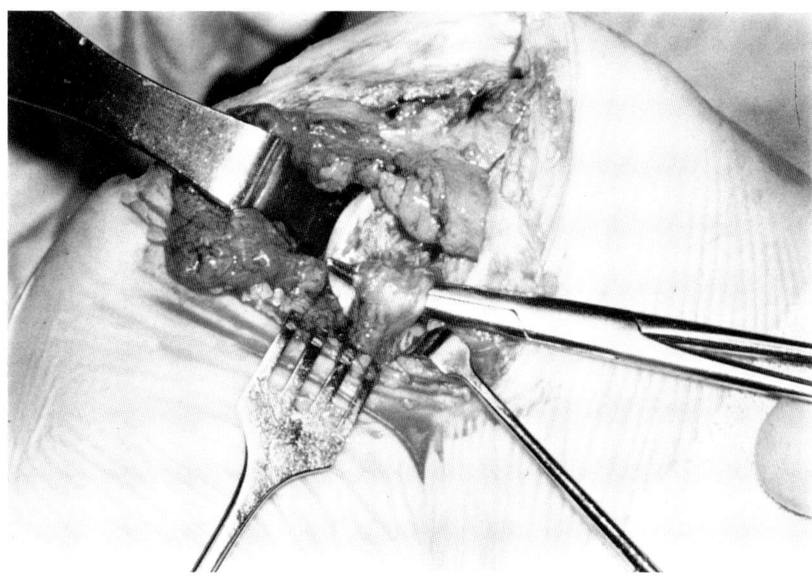

Fig. 6-4. Synovectomy of the knee. Note the good cartilage remaining, which improves the prognosis. This patient had an excellent result for more than 5 years.

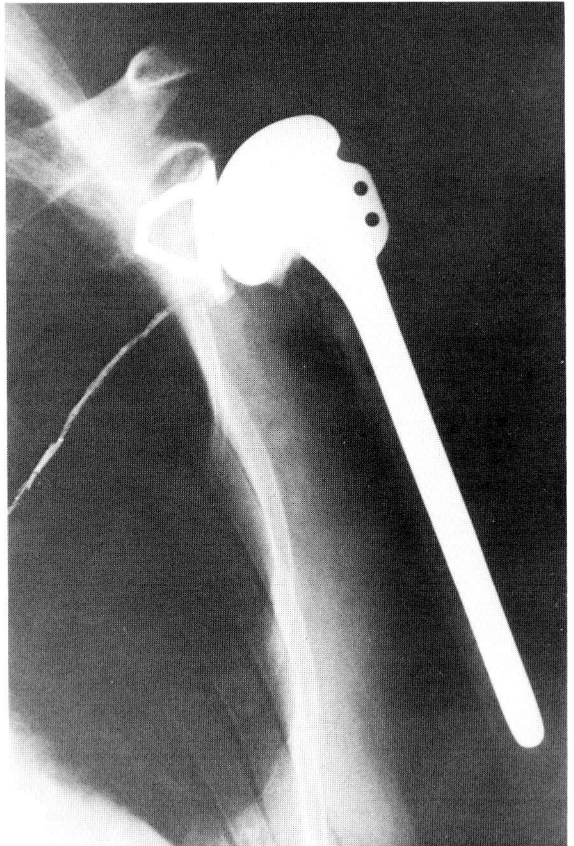
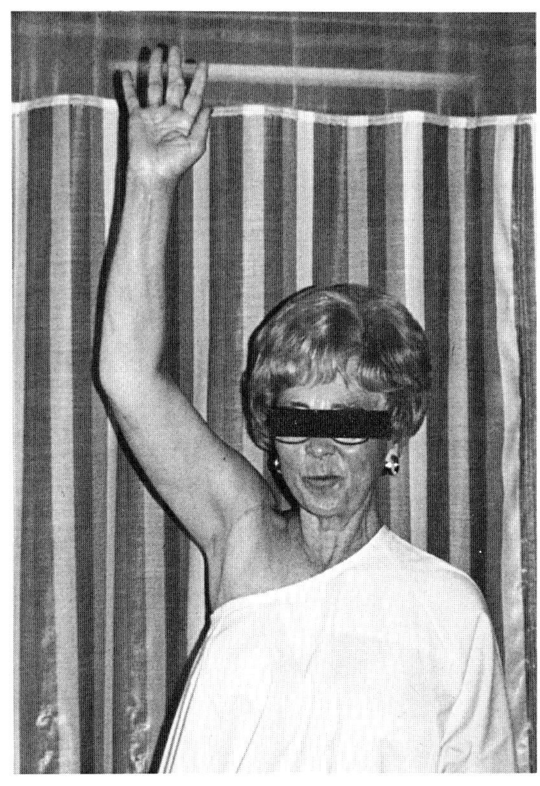

A

B

Fig. 6-5. **(A)** Roentgenogram of a Neer total shoulder with a metal-backed polyethylene glenoid and the stemmed humeral component. Both are anchored with methylmethacrylate. The white line shows the outline of the inferior scapular border. **(B)** Excellent result of the Neer total shoulder at 5 years.

hinges are promising and produce results equivalent to those with the nonconstrained elbows for several years.

Wrist

The wrist is the key joint to the hand. In early cases synovectomy, dorsal tenosynovectomy, and excision of distal ulna is an excellent procedure.[9,35] The key to correcting the supination deformity of the wrist is to reconstruct the radioulnar-carpal complex by suturing the ulnar lateral capsule and the dorsal retinaculum underneath the extensor carpi ulnaris to the dorsal ulnar border of the radius and realigning the extensor carpi ulnaris tendon[35] (Fig. 6-7). Tendon transfer is used only if necessary. Tendon reconstruction for rupture gives good results, but early surgery before rupture is better. At stage IIIb with intact wrist extensor tendons, wrist arthroplasty with total joint replacement has given patient satisfaction in more than 85 percent of cases[18,26] (Fig. 6-8). Silicone implants can also be used and are preferred when there is a lack of bone stock, but they are at more risk of breakage and a high failure rate.[25]

Arthrodesis is reserved for stage IV cases or salvage for other failures. Neutral position (0 degrees) is preferred, and pronation and supination

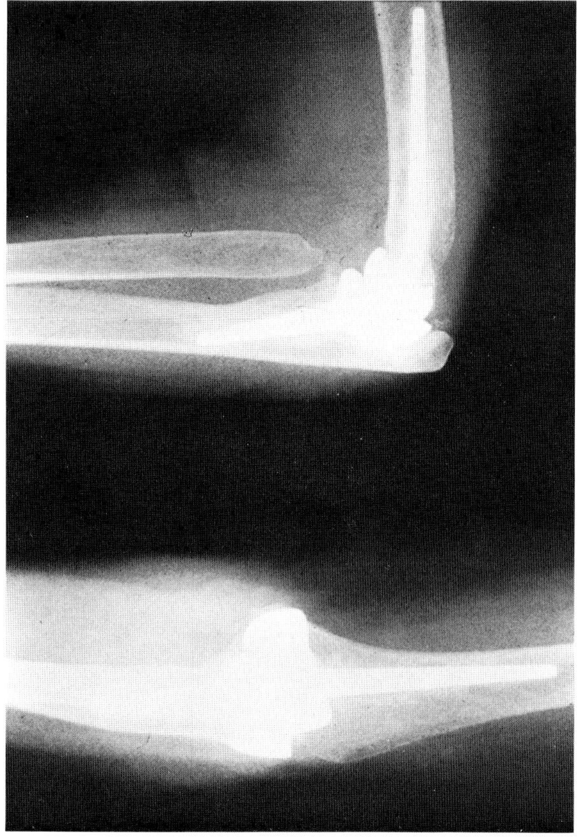

Fig. 6-6. Roentgenogram of an Ewald total elbow—a nonconstrained replacement of the elbow. The olecranon has a metal backing with polyethylene insert. The components are anchored with methylmethacrylate.

substitute well for palmar flexion or dorsiflexion.[3,8,10]

Metacarpophalangeal (MCP) fusion of the thumb (Fig. 6-9) is an excellent time-tested procedure. It generally is superior to reconstruction and is the most successful procedure used on the digits.[7,32] Synovectomy and MCP arthroplasty of the fingers with a silicone implant is the standard procedure.[34] Soft-tissue reconstruction and balancing are the keys to success along with proper aftercare and dynamic splinting to guide the encapsulation process (Fig. 6-10). Some deterioration may occur over the years. The newer high performance silicone has a lower, slower breakage rate.

Proximal interphalangeal silicone arthroplasty or arthrodesis is necessary for severe cases and aids in pinch and large grasp. Procedures other than at the wrist or thumb provide less increase in patients' overall function.[32]

Hip

The hip can cause more pain and disability than any other joint involved by rheumatoid arthritis. Today total hip replacement is the procedure of choice even in young individuals.[4,13,16] The loosening rate has been lower in rheumatoid arthritis than in osteoarthritis patients owing to the built-in restraint of the generalized disease.

The usual approach is by a lateral posterior route without removing the trochanter. A straight long-stem prosthesis is useful for filling osteoporotic bone space, and it ensures proper slight valgus alignment (Fig. 6-11); pressurization of cement in a low-viscosity state lessens radiolucent lines. This operation gives excellent pain relief and function and is the single best operation in terms of pleasing a patient.

Knee

Popliteal cysts (Fig. 6-12) also develops by extension from the knee joint and may become large and mimic thrombophlebitis.[27] Excision is often necessary with or without intra-articular surgery. Regarding the knee, synovectomy has been mentioned. Total knee replacement is now the most common procedure in rheumatoid arthritis surgery. There are many prostheses, but the common denominators are a metal femoral condylar component, a metal-backed plastic tibia, and a plastic or metal-backed plastic patella (nonconstrained) (Fig. 6-13). It is preferable to save the posterior cruciate ligament or provide a support for it. The most important factor is proper alignment of the leg at the mechanical axis, with the ankle, knee, and hip in a straight line. Late cases may require constrained prostheses.

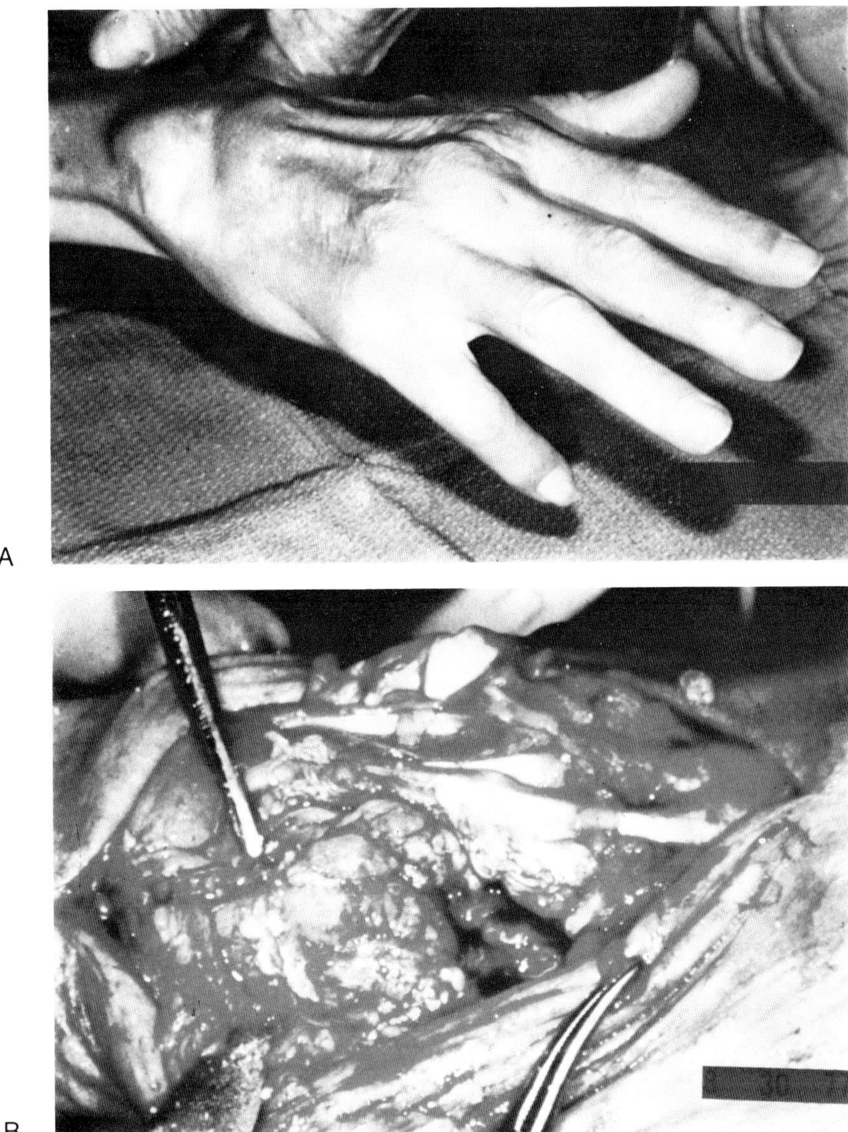

Fig. 6-7. (A) Dorsal tenosynovitis with rupture of the extensor tendons to the small finger. Note the bulging dorsal tenosynovitis just distal to the dorsocarpal ligament and the disappearance of the extensor tendons to the fifth finger. There is dorsal dislocation of the distal ulna and a supination deformity with descent of the ulnar side of the wrist; the extensor carpi ulnaris tendon is subluxed below the distal ulna. **(B)** After exposure the dorsocarpal ligament has been reflected radially like the page of a book. Note the irregular destroyed end of the ulna, which is underneath the two Hayes retractors, and that the irregular the end of the ulna is adjacent to the extensor tendon, which is the extensor to the ring finger. The ring finger and long finger extensors have been partially eroded over the irregular end of the distal ulna, and the small finger extensors have been completely ruptured. The distal ulna is about to be resected at this time.

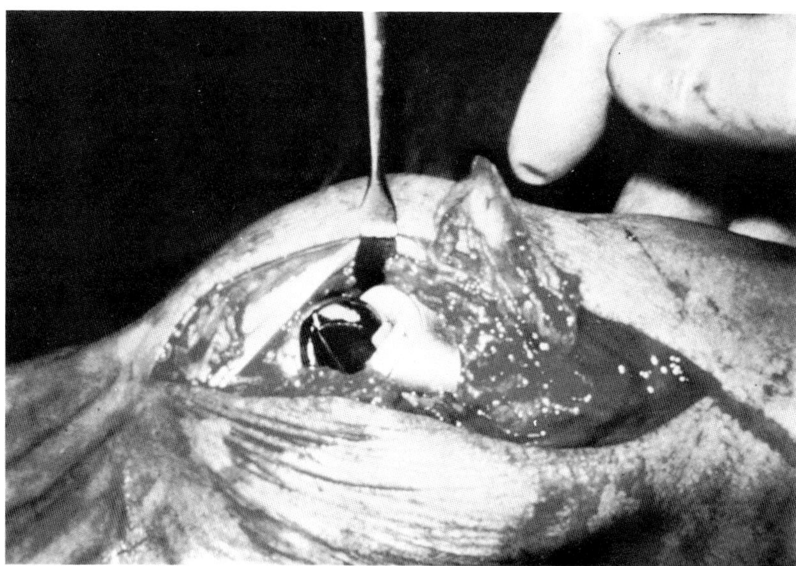

Fig. 6-8. Note the Volz wrist that has been inserted. The radial component has a metal backing to a polyethylene insert; and the distal component has a prong going into the third metacarpal. Both components are anchored with methylmethacrylate.

Replacement of the patella is advisable because recurrent rheumatoid synovitis has been noted in cases where articular cartilage has remained in the knee; this problem has not been noted with total replacement. Improved design and better instrumentation have helped obtain consistent alignment and increased range of motion up to as much as 135 degrees (our average is 113 degrees). Staged soft-tissue releases allow correction of angular deformity while maintaining taut collateral ligaments in full extension.[15]

Pressure injection of cement in a low-viscosity state has provided firm fixation and no radiolucent lines.[28] Total knee replacement is now as successful as total hip replacement.

A development has been the use of "continuous passive motion" after knee replacement. It is particularly helpful after a secondary operation. The pain is less, and motion is gained more rapidly (to about 90 degrees within 1 week); it also allows shorter hospitalization. It is not known if the final end result is better.

Ankle

Total ankle replacement (Fig. 6-14) has not been predictable and is not popular. A few patients are symptom-free with essentially normal walking, but others continue to have pain often due to hindfoot involvement. There should be improvement in the future, and a good total ankle is preferable to fusion in rheumatoid arthritis patients. Salvage of a failure is difficult. We cannot recommend total ankle replacement as a standard procedure at the present time; thus fusion remains the standard.

Foot

Surgery of the rheumatoid foot has a long record of success with stabilization of the hindfoot and resection arthroplasty in the forefoot. The talonavicular joint is the keystone in the arch of the foot, and arthrodesis of this joint alone relieves

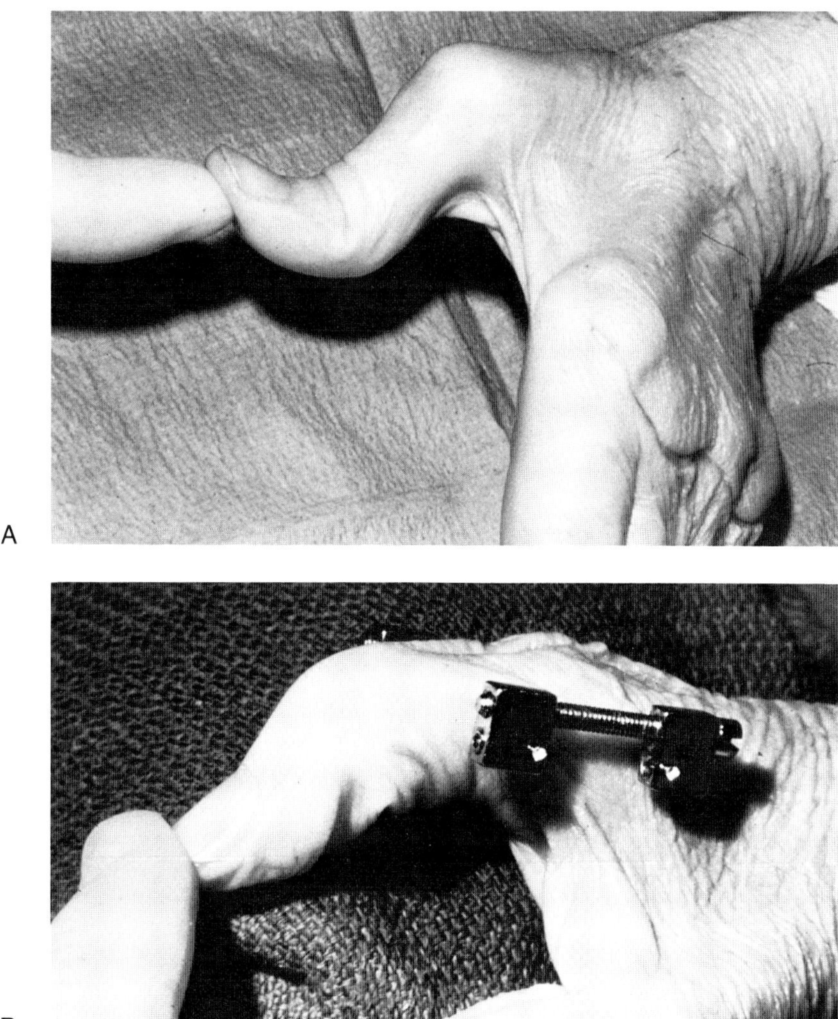

Fig. 6-9. (**A**) Metacarpophalangeal fusion of the thumb. Compression arthrodesis was used in this case. Note the free mobility of the IP joint and the collapse-type deformity of the thumb, which is accentuated by any pinching or pressure. (**B**) After fusion of the MCP joint, note the stable position for pinch at the time of surgery. (External fixation clamp remains 4 to 6 weeks.)

pain and prevents further collapse of the hindfoot.[19] If marked collapse has occurred, triple arthrodesis provides correction, pain relief, and stability, but with loss of motion[5] (Fig. 6-14).

Forefoot deformity of hallux valgus, bunions, splay foot, depressed metatarsal heads, and cock-up toes cause pain from intractable pressure problems. Resection of the metatarsophalangeal joints across the foot to realign weight-bearing is the basic procedure[2,5,6,33] (Fig. 6-15). Modifications to fit individual patients have been the use of intramedullary Kirschner wires for several weeks, a plantar plate arthroplasty with the plate interposed over the metatarsal head, and occa-

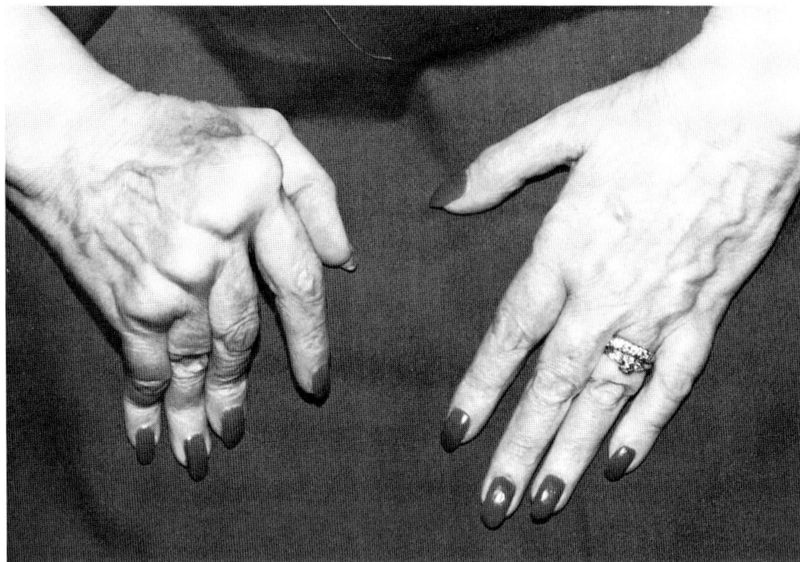

Fig 6-10. The hands were identical before undergoing MCP arthroplasties with silicone of the fingers and fusion of the MCP joint of the thumb on the left hand.

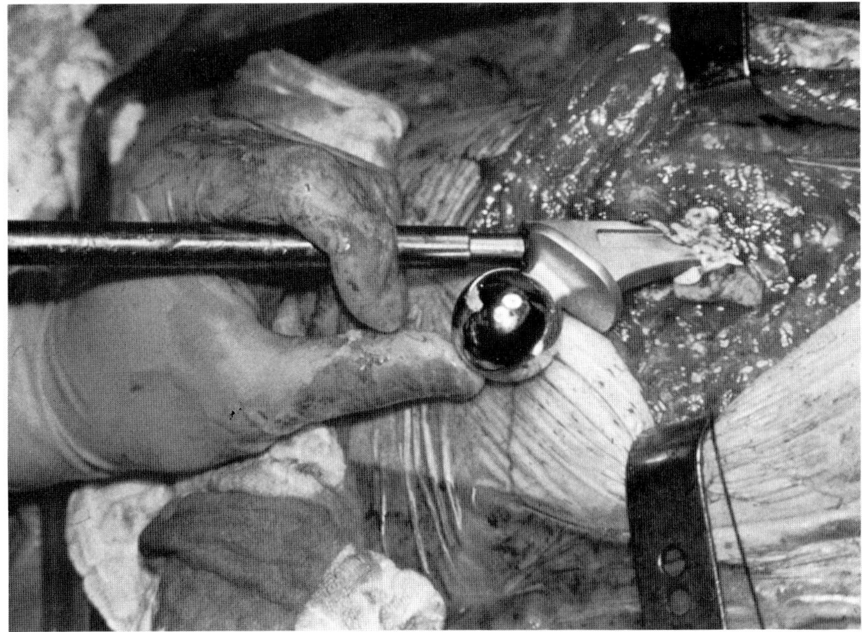

A

Fig. 6-11. (**A**) Insertion of a long, straight-stemmed femoral prosthesis. Bone cement has been injected into the femur, and the prosthesis is being positioned utilizing a driver and adjusting the neck for the proper amount of anteversion. The trochanter has not been removed, but excellent exposure has been obtained. (*Figure continues.*)

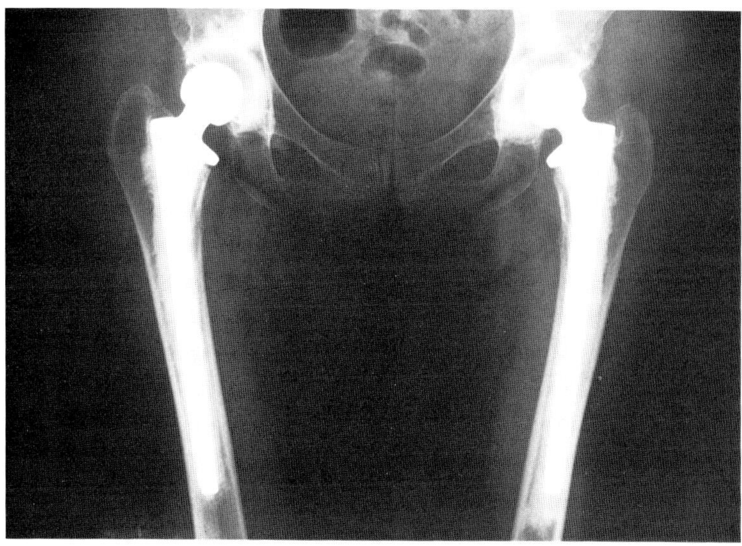

B

Fig. 6-11 (*Continued*). (**B**) Bilateral total hip replacements after 5 years on the right and 3 years on the left.

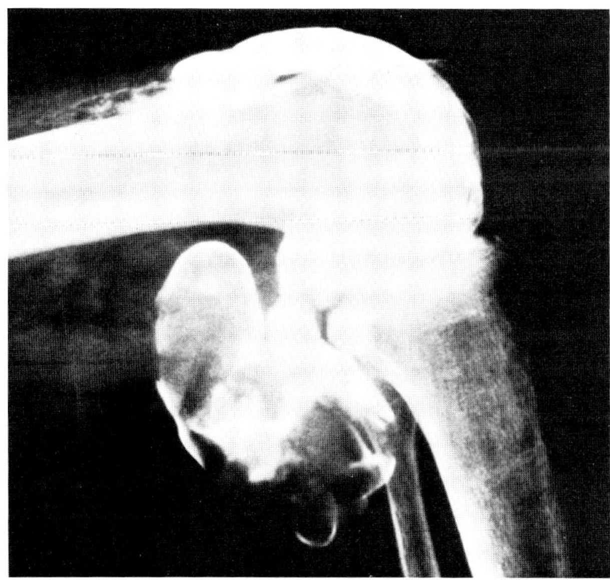

Fig. 6-12. Arthrogram with injection of dye into the knee joint. Note the extension of a large popliteal cyst from the posterior medial aspect of the knee joint.

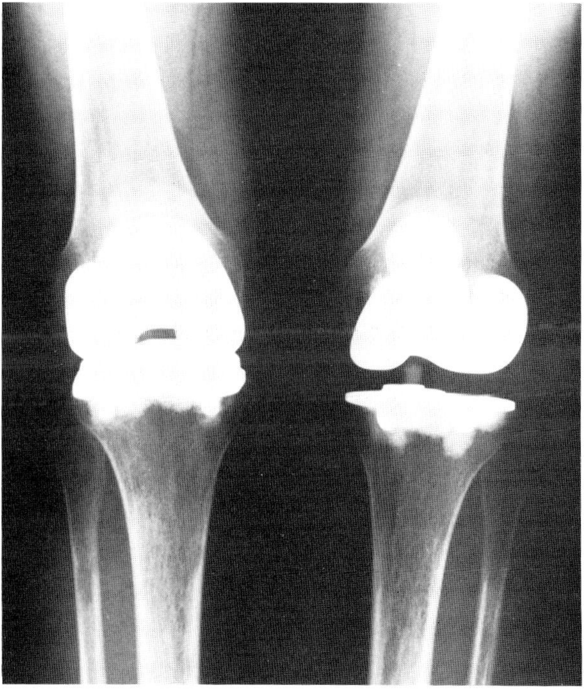

Fig. 6-13. Bilateral total knee arthroplasties of different types. Both are essentially nonconstrained, nonlinked prostheses anchored with bone cement. Note the excellent alignment in a neutral anatomic axis. Both knees are pain-free, function in a similar manner, and have motion of 115 degrees each.

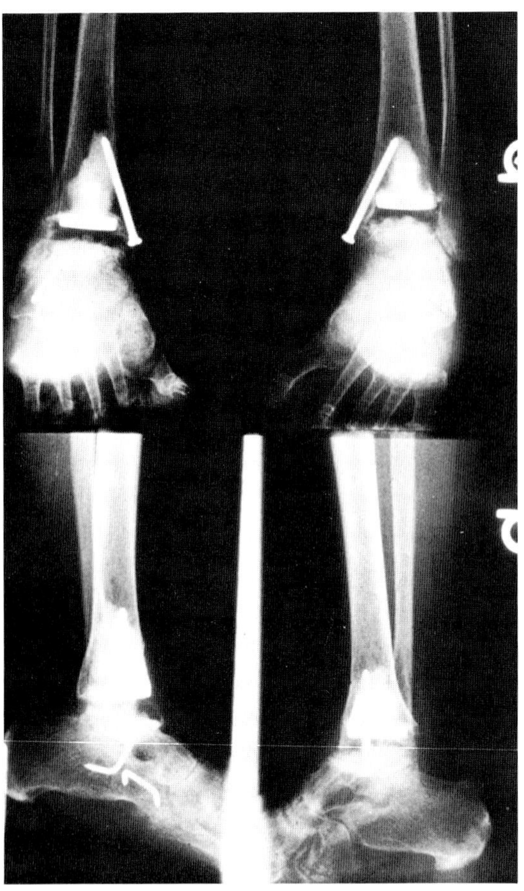

Fig. 6-14. Bilateral total ankle replacements that have been in place for 12 years plus a triple arthrodesis. Patient has no pain in either ankle and has about 30 degrees of motion on each side. It is an unusually good long-term result. (We do not recommend cemented total ankle replacements today.)

sional use of a silicone hinge arthroplasty for the great toe.[34]

Forefoot arthroplasty has retained its popularity, as is it a simple, dependable procedure that relieves pain and allows the patient to wear a reasonable shoe. It is the only lower extremity arthroplasty that has a success story of more than 30 years without a major change.

Spine

Spinal surgery for rheumatoid arthritis is mainly in the cervical area for subluxation and spinal cord compression. Treatment is usually by fusion,[21] a serious operation with high morbidity; it is usually indicated only if there are neurologic signs. Improved technique is now enlarging the indications, and it is becoming safer.

Multiple Procedures

Many patients require multiple procedures. The patient is usually most interested in the ability to walk and wants lower extremity surgery first. The ability to move about independently is important in modern society.

In a personal review of 21 patients with sevre rheumatoid arthritis who had had three or more

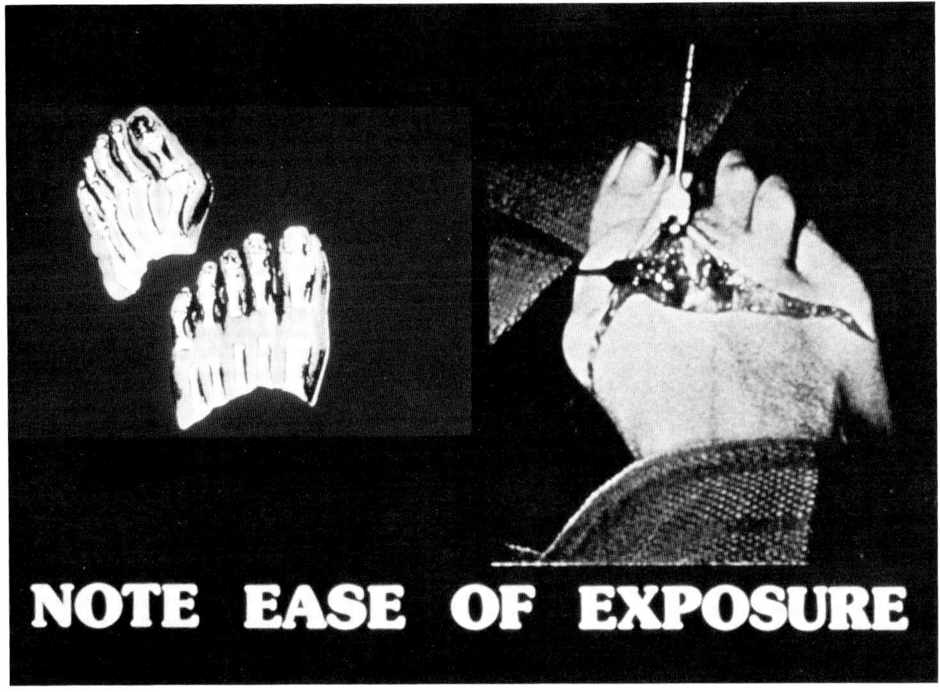

Fig. 6-15. Basic forefoot reconstruction utilizing a single dorsal transverse incision and excision of the metatarsophalangeal joints across the foot. It is a simple, dependable procedure.

lower extremity total joints, 19 became successful ambulators and all thought the procedures useful.[24]

Complications have been minimal, and rheumatoid patients have not had more complications than those with osteoarthritis. Wound healing has not been a problem, even with steroid medication. Skin and all tissues demand atraumatic technique. Perioperative antibiotics are used for 48 hours. Pulsatile air boots are used on hips and knees until the patient is ambulatory, along with aspirin; this method has been excellent for preventing thromboembolism without risk of anticoagulants.[14]

CONCLUSIONS

Although many procedures are utilized for surgery of rheumatoid arthritis in the United States today, most cases are total joint replacement. Although the long-term results are unknown at the present time, total joint arthroplasty has given the crippled rheumatoid arthritic patient a new horizon for relief of pain and increased function. Each of these procedures is discussed in detail in the following chapters of this book.

REFERENCES

1. Aufranc OE: Constructive hip surgery of the vitallium mold; a report of 1000 cases of arthroplasty of the hip over a 15 year period. J Bone Joint Surg [Am] 39:237, 1957
2. Aufranc OE, Larson CB: Surgery of the rheumatoid forefoot. Presented to the Boston Orthopaedic Club, 1949
3. Clayton ML: Arthrodesis of the wrist (position and technique). p. 352. In Strickland J (ed): Difficult Problems in Hand Surgery. CV Mosby, St. Louis, 1982

4. Clayton ML: Care of the rheumatoid hip. Clin Orthop 90:70, 1973

5. Clayton ML: Results of surgery in rheumatoid feet. Excerpta Med Int Congress Ser 165:107, 1967

6. Clayton ML: Surgery of the forefoot in rheumatoid arthritis. Clin Orthop 16:136, 1960

7. Clayton ML: Surgery of the thumb in rheumatoid arthritis. J Bone Joint Surg [Am] 44:1376, 1962

8. Clayton ML: Surgical treatment at the wrist in rheumatoid arthritis. J Bone Joint Surg [Am] 47:741, 1965

9. Clayton ML: The caput ulnae syndrome: update. p. 199. In Strickland J (ed): Difficult Problems in Hand Surgery. CV Mosby, St. Louis, 1982

10. Clayton ML, Ferlic DC: Arthrodesis of the wrist in the arthritic. Clin Orthop 187:89, 1984

11. Clayton ML, Ferlic DC, Jeffers PD: Prosthetic arthroplasties of the shoulder. Clin Orthop 164:184, 1982

12. Clayton ML, Leidholt JD, Gamble WE: Realignment osteotomy at the knee for chronic arthritis (degenerative and rheumatoid). J Bone Joint Surg [Am] 47:1284, 1965

13. Clayton ML, Stringer TL: Total hip arthroplasty with a new long-stem prosthesis. Clin Orthop 173:140, 1983

14. Clayton ML, Thompson TR: Activity, air boots and aspirin as thromboembolism prophylaxis in knee arthroplasty; a multiple regimen approach. Orthopedics 10:1525, 1987

15. Clayton ML, Thompson TR: Correction of alignment deformities during total knee arthroplasties; staged soft tissue release. Clin Orthop 202:117, 1986

16. Charnley J: Low friction arthroplasty. Clin Orthop 72:7, 1970

17. Dennis DA, Clayton ML, Ferlic DC et al: Long term follow up of capitella condylar total elbow arthroplasty. J Arthroplasty October Suppl 1990

18. Dennis DA, Ferlic DC, Clayton ML: Volz total wrist arthroplasties in rheumatoid arthritics; a long term review. J Hand Surg 11A:483, 1986

19. Elobar JE, Thomas WH, Weinfeld MS et al: Talonavicular arthrodesis for rheumatoid arthritis of the hindfoot. Orthop Clin 7:821, 1976

20. Ferlic DC, Clayton ML: Total joint arthroplasty of the large joints of the upper extremities. Colorado Med July: 262, 1981.

21. Ferlic DC, Clayton ML, Leidholt JD et al: Surgical treatment of the symptomatic unstable cervical spine in rheumatoid arthritis. J Bone Joint Surg [Am] 57:349, 1975

22. Ferlic DC, Patchett CE, Clayton ML et al: Elbow synovectomy in rheumatoid arthritis; long term results. Clin Orthop 220:119, 1987

23. Geens S, Clayton ML, Leidholt JD et al: Synovectomy and débridement of the knee in rheumatoid arthritis. J Bone Joint Surg [Am] 51:617, 1969

24. Harmon CE, Turner BD, Clayton ML et al: Multiple joint replacements (three or more) of the lower extremity in rheumatoid arthritis. Presented to the American Rheumatism Association, Boston, 1981

25. Jolly S, Ferlic DC, Clayton ML et al: Swanson silicone arthroplasty of the wrist in rheumatoid arthritis; a long term follow-up. J Hand Surg (in press)

26. Lamberta FJ, Ferlic DC, Clayton ML: Volz total wrist arthroplasty in rheumatoid arthritics; a preliminary report. J Hand Surg 5:245, 1980

27. Mack RP, Clayton ML: Synovial and bursal lesions around the knee. p. 3541. In Evarts CM (ed): Surgery of the Musculoskeletal System, 2nd ed. Churchill Livingstone, New York, 1990

28. Miller J, Clayton ML et al: Metal knee replacement. Presented to the Colorado Orthopaedic Association, Vail, CO, 1983

29. Mori M, Ogawa R: Anterior capsulectomy in the treatment of rheumatoid arthritis of the knee joint. Arthritis Rheum 6:130, 1963

30. Murphy JB: Hypertrophic villous synovitis of the knee joint; synovial capsulectomy. Surg Clin Chicago 5:153, 1916

31. Smith-Petersen MN, Aufranc OE, Larson CB: Useful surgical procedures for rheumatoid arthritis involving joints of the upper extremity. Arch Surg 46:764, 1943

32. Souter W: Planning treatment for the rheumatoid hand. Hand 11:3, 1979

33. Susman MH, Clayton ML: Surgery of the rheumatoid foot. Ann Acad Med Singapore 12:225, 1983

34. Swanson AB: Flexible Implant Resection Arthroplasty in the Hand and Extremities. p. 147. CV Mosby, St. Louis, 1963

35. Thirupathi RG, Ferlic DC, Clayton ML: Dorsal wrist synovectomy in rheumatoid arthritis; a long term study. J Hand Surg 8:848, 1983

7

Generalized Surgical Principles and Procedures

Mack L. Clayton

Surgical treatment for rheumatoid arthritis has become a recognized area of orthopaedic and hand surgery.[12] General physicians and rheumatologists using pharmaceutical and physical modalities realize that drugs accomplish little once the cartilage in a joint is destroyed. Joint replacement offers a great deal to the patient in a late stage of the disease (stages III and IV) who is facing life on crutches or in a wheelchair. These developments have occurred during the last 30 years with the greatest impetus during the 1970s and 1980s. Definite and gratifying progress has been made in reconstructive procedures that benefit selected patients with rheumatoid arthritis, and these significant advances in treatment by surgical means have occurred within only a few years.

Because this disease presents with the most awesome problems of the musculoskeletal system, no single operation is the solution. The analysis of the problem is comparable to that of a severely involved poliomyelitis patient of 40 years ago (before vaccine). The problem is compounded by the progressive and unpredictable nature of the disease and the fact that other joints will most likely be involved at some future time.

A number of general principles are important when treating chronic progressive rheumatoid arthritis. The generalized nature of the disease demands lifetime supervision and treatment by the rheumatologist or physicians specially trained in the care of the patients afflicted with this disease. It is the responsibility of the primary physician to supervise the general medical program, as described in earlier chapters. When progress is not being made, the orthopaedic surgeon should become involved and a team approach utilized. It is important that the rheumatologist be knowledgeable about what orthopaedic surgery has to offer and that the orthopaedist is aware of the natural history of rheumatoid arthritis and the medical rheumatologic treatments available. It is essential that the orthopaedic surgeon knows what can be accomplished by drugs and other measures and the limitations of each.

Surgery is just one incident, albeit often a dramatic one, in the comprehensive pyramidal approach to treatment of rheumatoid arthritis. At one time there was concern that a surgical procedure would exacerbate the disease activity, but it is now clear that surgery does not cause a flare-up of the disease and does not alter the general course of the disease. Many years ago temporary symptomatic improvement in rheumatoid activity was noted after general anesthesia, which at that time was commonly ether. It is now recognized that ether is the most stressful anesthetic on the adrenal glands, and that the temporary improvement was probably due to the increased corticosteroid output by the adrenal.

In view of the systemic nature of rheumatoid arthritis, certain principles and priorities are necessary when planning surgical intervention. Gschwend[11] has compared a body suffering from rheumatoid arthritis to a house on fire. Usually it is a long-lasting fire that can seldom be extinguished completely. The patient with destructive rheumatoid disease is like the burning house, and the pillars that support it—the bones and joints—must be saved to avoid its crashing. Furthermore, the owner's confidence must be gained if effective action is to be undertaken to save his house. As when fighting a house fire, the first steps taken must be successful.

PRIORITIES AND INDICATIONS FOR SURGICAL TREATMENT

The prognosis in an individual case is unpredictable even when all of the available laboratory tests are used. Repeated clinical evaluations done over a period of time plus serial roentgenograms and laboratory tests are the most important features to follow when deciding if surgery is indicated. Synovectomy during the early stages of the disease (stage II) has been recommended. Removal of the diseased synovium slows the disease temporarily, but with disease progression may come a return of pain within 2 to 3 years. Even though the patient is better than he or she would have been without surgery, that person is likely to be unhappy because of increased pain and may believe that "the pain is worse than before operation." There is now general agreement that synovectomy early in the disease has not proved to be the specific answer for rheumatoid arthritis. In selected cases where pain and recurrent effusion are prominent, relatively early synovectomy has been a well-accepted procedure,[10] but there is no perfect answer.

In the unusual monarticular case of rheumatoid arthritis of long duration, there is no problem with priorities for surgical consideration. In all cases of polyarticular involvement, the patient's major complaint is the most important factor. Patients generally are most concerned with pain, especially in weight-bearing joints. The ability to ambulate independently is important in modern society. One of the major concerns of physicians who treat the rheumatoid arthritic patient is to select those procedures that will keep the patient within the realm of social acceptance. To accomplish this aim, it is essential that the patient express his or her problems and the expectations about treatment. In complicated cases of multiple joint involvement, the team evaluation of family, social worker, and physical and occupational therapists can add much when planning surgical intervention.

When recommending one surgery or a series of surgical procedures, surgeons must consider their own past success with the operations. If that experience is limited, the surgeon must rely on the reports of others and weigh the risks and complications of surgery against the risk of not operating. The patient must understand the general procedure, the risks involved, the expected gains, the rehabilitation necessary, and the time factors. An effort should be made to keep expectations realistic. If results are better than those explained prior to surgery, the patient is happier. A number of patients seen by us had average postoperative results but were unhappy because of their unrealistically high expectations.

SURGICAL PROCEDURES AVAILABLE

Surgical procedures for rheumatoid arthritis are correlated to the stage of involvement; that is, the operation is tailored to the individual joint in the individual patient. A brief description of the available procedures may be found in Table 7-1.

Synovectomy

Synovectomy is indicated only for stage II and early stage III (good joint cartilage) when there is synovial proliferation in one or a few joints out of proportion to the generalized involvement despite several months of a basic general medical regimen. The indications are limited at this time, and patients must be selected with care. It is still the only procedure to keep the patient's own joint functioning for *x* years, and a major gain for patients is pain relief. The operation is essentially not indicated if there is no pain.

In many synovectomy cases *débridement* of secondary osteophytes is performed. These cases

Table 7-1. Surgical Procedures
Available for Rheumatoid Arthritis

Synovectomy
    Débridement
    Chemical synovectomy
    Tenosynovectomy
    Bursectomy
Release of contracture
Osteotomy
Arthroplasty
    Resection
    Fascial (interposition)
    Metallic hemiarthroplasty
    Plastic implant (silicone)
    Total joint arthroplasty
        Constrained or nonconstrained
        Bone cement anchorage (?)
        Metal to metal
        Metal to plastic
Arthrodesis

are at a later stage (IIIB), and the procedure often is not as effective in weight-bearing joints; but in the elbow and wrist it often gives good long-term improvement.[4,18]

The general activity of the disease is an important factor in terms of recurrence after synovectomy, and it is regrettable that markedly involved patients, who need help most, gain the least. A properly done synovectomy does not burn any bridges for later reconstructive procedures.

Chemical synovectomy has been tried for many years using various intra-articularly injected substances (steroids, nitrogen mustard, thiotepa, oxalic acid, and radioactive gold). Temporary improvement seems to be obtained, but no hard data are available. A radioactive isotope has been promising but is still investigational and not available for general use.[16]

Tenosynovectomy is a common procedure performed on the dorsum of the wrist, carpal tunnel, and flexor tendon sheaths in the fingers; additional regional bone and joint procedures are often done at the same time. The procedure has an excellent record for relieving pain, increasing function, and preventing tendon ruptures, particularly in the wrist and hand. The recurrence rate is low.

Bursectomy may also be useful. Nonarticular rheumatoid arthritis involves the tendon sheaths and bursae. Large bursal synovial cysts (or herniations from adjacent joints) often occur at the shoulder area, popliteal cysts at the knee[16] (see Fig. 6-12), iliopsoas cysts at the hip, and cubital cysts at the elbow. Large cysts should be excised and adjacent joint synovectomy performed if indicated. Synovectomy has been so closely identified with rheumatoid arthritis that a separate chapter has been devoted to the subject (see Ch. 8).

Release of Contracture

Release of contracture has been used mainly in the past for knee flexion contracture release. It is also useful for certain finger deformities. Today, however, it is generally part of an arthroplasty procedure.

Osteotomy

Osteotomy here refers to the correction of angular deformities of a joint by bony division and realignment. It has been most often used about the knee in the past; it is rarely utilized today because most rheumatoid patients require articular resurfacing as well as realignment. Osteotomy near the knee is still an excellent procedure for osteoarthritis with angulation and one-compartment arthritis. Osteotomy is useful in unusual "burned out" rheumatoid arthritis, as this type of rheumatoid arthritis is essentially an osteoarthritis.

There is no indication for osteotomy of the hip in those with rheumatoid arthritis today. However, there is a rare indication for osteotomy around the wrist or ankle to correct a deformity and change the arc of motion to a more functional one.

Arthroplasty

Arthroplasty has been utilized for many years in rheumatoid arthritis patients. The simplest type is an extension of synovectomy, where extensive débridement is performed, including smoothing of articular surface.

Resection arthroplasty is removal of the end of the bone of the involved joint. Its most successful use today continues in the forefoot, where metatarsophalangeal (MTP) joint resection is a well-accepted, time-tested procedure. It is often used in conjunction with other procedures, e.g., excision of the distal ulna, the radial head, and the outer clavicle. In certain areas resection arthroplasty has been improved by addition of a silicone implant.

Interposition arthroplasty utilizing neighboring structures or fasciae have been most successful in the elbow. These procedures are now generally falling by the wayside for rheumatoid arthritis and are being replaced by total joint replacement or implant arthroplasty. Sheets of cellophane, nylon, and silicone have also been used with no success in the past.

Metallic interposition arthroplasty is best exemplified by mold arthroplasty of the hip (cup arthroplasty), which was developed by Smith-Petersen in 1938 and perfected by Aufranc, Larson, and Law.[1,15]

Implant arthroplasty implies a resection arthroplasty with addition of an implant (silicone). This implant acts as a "spacer" to hold the resected ends apart and helps to maintain alignment while the arthroplasty is being formed and maturing. The soft tissue reconstruction around the implant is important, as is the prolonged aftercare with proper splinting to guide the capsule formation and obtain motion. The most successful areas are in the metacarpophalangeal (MCP) joints of the hand. Swanson[19] and Neibauer have been the leaders in developing this type of arthroplasty. Swanson used an implant that allows the stem to glide and form a "large synovial cavity"; Neibauer utilized rough Dacron on the stems to enhance adherence to the medullary canal.

There is now a stronger, more durable silicone elastomer, so breakage and wear should be less of a problem. Many "fractures" are essentially asymptomatic, as a firm joint capsule has formed and functions well.

At the present time, *total joint arthroplasty* is best exemplified by hip, arthroplasty, which has been the most successful. The most generally used prostheses are modifications of Charnley's device, with a plastic (high density polyethylene) acetabulum and a metallic femoral prosthesis that fit together in an unconstrained ball and socket manner. Charnley had developed his prosthesis by 1963, but biomechanical improvements have occurred.[2] The total replacements in general are classified as constrained (hinge knees), nonconstrained (most hips and total knees with separate tibial and femoral components), or semiconstrained.

Charnley[2] developed the use of polymethylmethacrylate, which is utilized in most total joint replacements today. It would be wonderful if a living, reproducible physiologic anchorage of metals and plastic to bone were available. Research is in progress, but nothing has proved to be any better than "bone cement" in adult rheumatoid arthritis today.

Metal-to-plastic causes less friction and less wear and is the most widely used combination. There is much room for improvement, however, and there is need for a substitute for articular cartilage with its cushioning effect for impact absorption.

Wear and loosening may occur over a long period owing to the amount of use and force. Total joints are generally not recommended in young patients. However, most rheumatoid arthritics who require joint replacement have a generalized disease that limits their overall activity, and they need to reduce the mechanical stress on the joint. Total joint replacement is often indicated in young patients with rheumatoid arthritis when no other procedure can produce as useful a result.

Arthrodesis

Arthrodesis is a useful procedure for the wrist and digits in late cases and is particularly useful for the thumb. It is widely utilized in the hindfoot as a talonavicular or triple (subtalar, talonavicular, and calcaneocuboid) correction, as well as in the ankle. It is considered a salvage procedure for severe failed knee arthroplasty and is used for instability in the spine.

Total joint arthroplasty has given crippled rheumatoid arthritic patients a new horizon for pain relief and function, allowing them the ability to remain an active and independent part of modern society.

EVALUATION OF SURGICAL PROCEDURES

The initial surgical procedure should be as successful as possible ("a winner"). Souter[18] has had a wide experience in rheumatoid arthritis surgery and has evaluated the most frequently performed surgical procedures of the hand according to pain relief, functional improvement, durability, cosmesis, and complications. Gschwend[12] has enlarged the evaluation to other rheumatoid surgical procedures commonly performed.

INDICATIONS FOR SURGERY

When planning surgical treatment of the patient, there are certain indications that take priority and are not elective (and thus are not rated).

1. C1–C2 subluxation with neurologic signs (requires fusion and possible decompression)
2. Rupture of a tendon or threatened rupture (wrist, volar, or dorsal)
3. Compression neuropathy due to rheumatoid synovitis, e.g., carpal tunnel syndrome
4. Infected or troublesome rheumatoid nodules or infection of a joint

The elective procedures are considered following "operations of necessity." The overall outcome evaluations by patients and surgeons are shown in Table 7-2 on a 100 point score based on our personal experience. The procedures rated below 75 need careful consideration and are sometimes unpredictable, particularly in terms of long-term results. However, there is sometimes no alternative, a fact the patient must realize.

Some percentage ratings are slightly higher for the lower extremity because these procedures of-

Table 7-2. Rating of Common Elective Rheumatoid Arthritis Procedures[a]

Procedure	Rating
Total hip arthroplasty	95
Forefoot reconstruction	90
Total knee arthroplasty	90
MCP thumb fusion	90
Dorsal wrist reconstruction (synovectomy, tenosynovectomy, excision of distal ulna)	85
Flexor tenosynovectomy of hand or wrist	85
Total shoulder arthroplasty	85
Elbow synovectomy	85
Triple arthrodesis (or talonavicular arthrodesis)	85
Total wrist arthroplasty	80
Total elbow arthroplasty	80
MCP arthroplasty	80
Wrist fusion	80
Knee synovectomy	75
Ankle fusion	75
MCP synovectomy	70
PIP synovectomy or arthroplasty or fusion	70
Hip (salvage) girdlestone	60
Knee (salvage) fusion	60
Total ankle	NR

Note: In general, procedures rated 80 and above are the best procedures for the patient and surgeon. Ratings are based on a 100-point scale according to the following categories/point scale.

Pain relief	40
Function	20
Prevention	10
Cosmetic	10
Complications	10
Longevity	10

NR = not rated.
[a]Cervical spine operations require different rating, as they concern life-threatening problems.

ten do more for the patient's overall function in daily life and social involvement. Upper extremity surgery, however, is just as important in individual cases.

Total hip arthroplasty is rated as the most successful arthroplasty, with the knee a close second. The hip is the joint that can be so painful day and night that the patient's life is ruined; and giving narcotics for pain relief places the patient at risk of addiction. In such a case, total hip arthroplasty is a dramatic operation for the patient and the treating team.

The total knee has just as good long-term results now as the total hip, but the patient must work harder to obtain the best results. Rheumatologists have rated total joint replacement as the number one advancement in the treatment of rheumatoid arthritis in 20 years.[9]

SELECTING THE SURGICAL PROCEDURE

The most important considerations are the patients' major complaints, even if there are multiple problems. Moreover, the initial operation should be a "winner" for the patient and the surgeon. For example, if feet and knees need surgery, the best initial procedure is usually a bilateral forefoot reconstruction, which is highly rated and requires minimal effort from the patient to obtain a good result. If the patient and surgeon are not satisfied by the initial procedure, other elective procedures may not be done or may be postponed. Total hip replacement is an excellent beginning procedure because of its superb pain relief and need for only moderate rehabilitation effort by the patient. Total knee replacement requires much more cooperation to obtain a good result—a reason the hip is rated higher than the knee. Total ankle replacement (cemented) is not rated because of the unpredictability and the difficulty of salvage by fusion if it fails and has to be removed; the operation is rare today.

When considering upper extremity procedures, the wrist should be corrected before the digits if the hand is the major problem and the shoulder and elbow allow reasonable function. The dorsal wrist reconstruction using tenosynovectomy, synovectomy, and excision of distal ulna is a prime initial procedure.[20] At a later stage wrist replacement[14] and wrist arthrodesis[4] are good beginnings. In this extremity, after the wrist, the next best operation is the thumb MCP fusion. This procedure has received a top rating

for more than 30 years.[3] MCP and interphalangeal (IP) finger procedures do not rate as high because the patient's overall function is not changed as much. Furthermore, they require a great deal of cooperation during rehabilitation to achieve maximum benefit.

If the surgery has an additional prophylactic element, e.g., dorsal wrist reconstruction for preventing tendon rupture, the patient should be urged to have surgery. If the shoulder is so painful and limited that the hand cannot be positioned, shoulder arthroplasty should be the first operation selected.[5] If the elbow is painful and stiff (e.g., the hand cannot reach the face), elbow arthroplasty takes precedence. Sometimes a good elbow arthroplasty can defer the need of shoulder surgery. When planning a series of procedures, it is highly desirable that each procedure provides a gain for the patient even if the next planned procedure must be deferred.

If upper and lower extremity procedures are indicated, it is better to finish lower extremity procedures that will require crutches before upper extremity procedures, which may be harmed by using crutches. One of the greatest gains in the results from upper extremity reconstructive surgery is due to such fine total hip and knee replacements that crutches are not necessary.

General complete examination of the patient is necessary before progressing to indications for a single procedure. It is for this reason that a surgeon who is limited to one region may be at a disadvantage when treating this disease. Many rheumatoid patients in the later stages of their illness have destructive changes in multiple joints of the upper extremities and frequently the lower extremities as well. Thus it is imperative that the status of all joints be evaluated to determine which joint will benefit from reconstructive surgery. Only then can a decision be reached regarding a single joint.

The decision about surgery is ultimately made by the patient. If the surgical indications are there and the problem interferes with his or her way of life, surgery should be a serious consideration. Discussion with a patient who has had the procedure may help in the decision. After a team evaluation, the surgeon must make the operative recommendations, but it is the patient who makes the final decision and accepts the responsibility for doing so.

Contraindications do exist. The patient's general preoperative condition must be evaluated. Other disease processes may exist, but the activity of rheumatoid arthritis is itself not a contraindication to surgery. Any infection must be cleared before surgery. For example, urinary infection in the female patient may be asymptomatic but must be treated, particularly for hip surgery, where there is an overlap in lymphatic drainage, and spread of infection could be local as well as hematogenous. Tooth infections or surface skin infections must also be cleared. The treating physician makes the responsible decision about the general risks and in all major cases should also treat and follow the patient as necessary through the surgical hospitalization (team approach).

If the procedure is purely elective, e.g., total hip or forefoot reconstruction, there is less hurry. It can be performed at any time so long as bone stock is preserved and there is no infection.

PLANNING FOR MULTIPLE JOINT PROCEDURES

Despite the best available medical care, physical therapy, and a cooperative patient, active inflammation and the resulting destruction in multiple joints may continue in certain patients. Surgery plays an important part in management once joint destruction has occurred and reconstruction must be considered. The aim of surgical therapy in these patients is the relief of symptoms and restoration of function so the patient may lead an active, self-sufficient, productive life. The indications, goals, and timing of surgery must be tailored to the patient. The status of all of the joints must be reviewed when selecting the initial operation and, equally important, when planning the order in which multiple joints are to be approached. For example, if total joint replacements are needed for the hips or knees, the patient will need adequate function of the upper extremities to be able to use a walker or crutches during the recovery period following the lower

extremity procedure. Frequently, surgery may be performed on two joints during one operative session, or several procedures may be safely done during the same hospitalization in order to lessen the need for repeated anesthetics and to provide adequate rehabilitative measures. These decisions should be shared by the primary physician, surgeon, and patient.

MULTIPLE PROBLEMS OF UPPER EXTREMITY

The shoulder positions the hand in space in rheumatoid arthritis. Most patients are not interested in or able to throw a ball or to effect other forceful motions that are important to some others. Shoulder motion, of course, is a combined action of scapulothoracic and glenohumeral motion, and it makes no difference which one moves. Pain at the acromioclavicular joint may limit motion in either joint. The shoulder and elbow joint function together, and either can supplement the other.

A painful shoulder can make distal function of the hand impossible; whereas if glenohumeral motion is limited but painless, scapulothoracic motion can provide useful function.

Ninety degrees of forward elevation with external rotation produces a functional global arc of motoin when positioning the hand; in fact, it gives more than 80 percent of the useful arc of motion, whereas 90 degrees elevation with fixed internal rotation gives an arc of only 50 percent. Obviously, external rotation in the shoulder should be maintained or obtained, but the most important activities of daily living are fulfilled if the hand can reach comfortably to the top of the head and both ends of the gastrointestinal tract.

The elbow is a hinge joint, and reasonable mobility is absolutely necessary for upper extremity function. Flexion to 100 degrees or more is necessary to reach the face, and extension to 40 degrees is necessary to reach the perineal area. Essentially full motion of the elbow can compensate for much loss of shoulder motion for activities of daily living.

Forearm rotation is another important function

in combination with the wrist. The wrist is the key joint to the hand. Pain or malposition can seriously compromise hand function. The "position of function" of 20 to 30 degrees dorsiflexion is erroneous for most activities of daily living for rheumatoid arthritis. Flexion is important for many functions that are awkward in dorsiflexion. Neutral position is the most universally functional position if the wrist is fused, provided free pronation and supination are preserved. Rotation then provides a substitute for palmar flexion, dorsiflexion, and a global arc of about two-thirds of normal, whereas 25 degrees dorsiflexion provides almost a zero arc as the axis of rotation passes through the pinching of the thumb and index finger.

In the rheumatoid arthritic hand, the thumb provides about 50 percent of the function necessary for pinch or grasp, depending on its length and the stability of the distal joints and free mobility at its base. The fingers need to open for large grasp, must oppose the thumb for pinch, and must flex a varying amount for small grasp or hook.

The outlined functions of the upper extremity provide the key to timing surgical procedures. If the shoulder and elbow can reasonably position the hand, hand surgery is indicated first. The wrist, being the key joint to the hand, should be corrected before the digits.

In early cases dorsal wrist surgery consisting of tenosynovectomy, synovectomy, and excision of distal ulna gives excellent results.[20] In later cases, joint replacement or even fusion provides good results compared to the preoperative status. The common denominator is excision of distal ulna. If free rotation is not obtained, elbow surgery with excision of the radial head is indicated.

If the wrist is functional, the next most important worthwhile area for surgery is the thumb, as it is responsible for half of the hand function. The surgery is usually simple for both the surgeon and the patient, and it is predictably successful. Thumb MCP fusion is the best operation available on the digits (Table 7-2).[3]

If the fingers require surgery, e.g., MCP arthroplasty for pain and ulnar drift, the fingers should be corrected before the thumb or at the same time to ensure best position for opposition. Sur-

gery of the fingers does not provide as much functional gain as surgery of the thumb; and often surgery on four MCP joints is necessary.

Proximal interphalangeal (PIP) joint surgery requires careful selection, as the gain is usually limited and requires careful individual selection. Arthroplasty is often indicated when one finger has pain and limited motion, as one stiff finger in an otherwise mobile hand limits function of the entire hand. Fusion of three or four badly damaged PIP joints in functional position can greatly improve function.

Tendon involvement must be considered and treated during or before joint reconstruction. Dorsal tenosynovitis is an indication for early surgery, as tendon rupture is common in untreated cases and is rare after dorsal wrist reconstruction (1 percent).[20] Also, flexor tenosynovitis of the carpal tunnel is important to relieve median nerve compression and prevent ruptured tendons.

Flexor tenosynovitis of the fingers leads to lack of active flexion with further passive flexion.[7] Early surgical correction yields good long-term results. With marked deformity it should be corrected before MCP joint reconstruction; in mild cases it can be corrected through the volar plate at the time of MCP arthroplasty.

A number of the wrist cases require elbow surgery at the same time as radial head excision in order to provide free pronation and supination, which is even more important in an involved rheumatoid arm, as compensatory motion is limited by a painful shoulder.[7] Wrist and elbow synovectomy with resection of the distal ulna and radial head can be performed at the same time (the postoperative rehabilitation can easily be combined), or they can be performed separately.

If elbow synovectomy is indicated,[13] it should be performed before shoulder arthroplasty, as it is a lesser procedure with an easier recovery and predictably good results. However, if shoulder and elbow replacement arthroplasty are indicated, the shoulder should usually be done first, particularly if external rotation is limited, as some elbow replacements have probably loosened owing to rotational strain on the humeral component.

Synovectomy of the shoulder by arthroscopy is

a procedure that shows promise. The entire joint is more accessible than the knee, and minimal hospitalization is necessary. Morbidity is no more than that associated with diagnostic arthroscopy.

The most common operation on the rheumatoid shoulder today is total joint arthroplasty.[5] It is a good procedure, with results equal to those of total knee arthroplasty; but it is a meticulous, time-consuming operation with a slow, lengthy rehabilitation period.

All of the major reconstruction operations performed to maintain or gain motion do much better with closely supervised rehabilitation by the surgeon and an educated therapist as well as continued proper medical treatment ("team approach").

MULTIPLE PROBLEMS IN THE LOWER EXTREMITY

In general, patients who have major lower extremity problems want help with them before upper extremity surgical treatment. It is because reasonable ambulation is necessary in order to function independently in society today.

Lower extremity procedures are of great importance, particularly with the success of hip and knee joint replacement. Actually, lower extremity surgery has a higher percentage of success with greater predictability than upper extremity surgery.

An evaluation of the major procedures for lower extremity surgery (Table 7-2) places total hip arthroplasty at the top with a 95 rating by all evaluations by patient and surgeon; forefoot reconstruction by MTP resections is 85 to 90 and has a successful record for over 30 years, longer than any other widely used procedurein the lower extremity today.

Total knee arthroplasty is the most common arthroplasty today, with a rating of 90, almost equal to that for the hip. Other procedures, such as synovectomy of the knee and ankle, are done less frequently today. Their success ratio is approximately 50 percent improvement at 5 years, but

the procedure is unpredictable in individual cases.

Hindfoot arthrodesis (talonavicular or triple) gives relief of pain and improved ambulation but with sacrifice of motion. Ankle fusion relieves pain at the expense of motion but may accelerate pain and destruction of the subtalar and talonavicular joints. Total ankle arthroplasty does not always relieve pain, as the pain is often due to hindfoot involvement. Also, loosening is high owing to concentration of high forces with normal walking (up to eight times body weight); it is not a standard procedure today.

If there is a choice of first operation, consideration should be given to the operation most likely to succeed and the patient's major complaint. If surgery is necessary in feet, knees, and hips, a good beginning is bilateral forefoot reconstruction at one sitting if the hindfoot is properly aligned or has motion to compensate later. This operation is easy on the patient and requires minimal effort for success. If the patient and the surgeon cannot succeed with this procedure, further surgery is rarely indicated. If there is fixed hindfoot deformity requiring triple arthrodesis, hips and knees should be treated first, hindfoot arthrodesis (for a plantigrade foot) second, and forefoot reconstruction last (see Ch. 17).

If hips and knees require arthroplasty, the hips should be corrected first unless the knee flexion deformity is so severe that nursing and postoperative mobilization would be difficult. The patient could be partially sitting in bed to correct hip flexion problems if necessary. Hip and knee procedures can be performed unilaterally or bilaterally at one sitting as necessary. This decision often depends on the judgment of the surgeon, as one must perform the procedure with which one is most comfortable and confident. At the present time we prefer to do one major joint at a time if other joints do not interfere with the rehabilitation. In some cases bilateral knee replacements are performed simultaneously using two teams, and the results are the same with considerable saving of hospital time.

The procedures are planned with a staged sequence. The second procedure is performed after the success of the preceding procedure is established; often more than one is necessary to achieve the ultimate aim. However, each procedure should provide a gain for the patient even if for some reason the chain is interrupted; no planned procedure should leave the patient worse if the next one is canceled. For example, total hip arthroplasty can relieve pain and allow easier sitting and sleeping even if the knees prevent ambulation and for some reason further surgery to correct the knees is contraindicated. The other extreme would be straightening of a flexed knee in a wheelchair patient, which would not help appreciably unless both knees were straightened and the hips corrected to allow walking.

In general, lower extremity reconstruction that requires crutches should be completed before upper extremity surgery. Procedures not requiring crutches can often be performed simultaneously by two operative teams: bilateral forefoot reconstruction by one team and a hand or wrist procedure by another. The surgeon must know the patient well before undertaking such extensive procedures.

Upper extremity procedures are important at each end of the spectrum. The patient who can ambulate will want further improvement, and the nonambulator will look for improved use of the hands because of chair confinement.

Patients who seek out the orthopaedic surgeon on their own usually do so because they want to walk better. Modern society requires that one must be an independent ambulator, and one of our most important tasks as surgeons is to keep the rheumatoid patient involved in the society.

Patients seen for upper extremity problems have usually seen another patient who has had surgery, or they are referred by their physician. Most upper extremity surgery is even more elective than lower extremity surgery and demands careful planning and timing.

A study was done to determine the outcome in terms of the benefits versus the risks of three or more joint replacements of the lower extremity in patients with rheumatoid arthritis.[21] Twenty-one patients (16 classic rheumatoid arthritis patients and 5 adults with the juvenile form of the disease) received a total of 81 joint replacements. The mean age was 50 years with a disease duration of 23 years (average follow-up 4.5 years).

The American College of Rheumatology classification of rheumatoid arthritis is as follows.

Class I   complete functional ability
Class II   adequate but restricted ability
Class III   limited ability
Class IV   confined to bed or wheelchair

Six of eight class III patients improved to class I, and one improved to class II. The one remaining patient deteriorated to class IV. All 13 class IV patients improved, with two to class I, ten to class II, and one to class III.

Of the 21 rheumatoid patients with multiple joint replacements, 19 had both subjective and objective improvement of pain and function. There were relatively few complications (15 percent) resulting from the total 81 procedures. Better results were obtained when one or two joints were operated when indicated and additional joints added as the disease progressed. Patients confined to wheelchairs who needed three or more total joint replacements to walk created a more serious problem. Comments from patient questionnaires were uniformly favorable, with 20 percent of 21 patients satisfied with the surgical results in terms of decreased pain, increased function, and continued improvement. Some revisions have been necessary. Multiple total joint replacements have added a new horizon for the severely crippled rheumatoid arthritic patient.[7]

ANESTHESIA

General anesthesia is most commonly used. Cervical spine or jaw problems frequently complicate endotracheal intubation. Maintaining an airway without a tube is also difficult. The cervical spine should always be handled with care and caution, as if there is a C1-C2 subluxation of fragile spine. If there is marked limitation of motion, neck pain, or spinal cord neurologic signs, a preoperatively cervical spine roentgenogram should be obtained including lateral views in flexion and extension. Routine cervical spine roentgenograms are not necessary on all patients. A soft collar worn to the operating room and postoperatively can prevent excessive flexion and, more importantly, warns personnel to handle the neck with care. All rheumatoid arthritic patients must be handled with extra care.

Stiffness of the temporomandibular joint makes visualization of the larynx difficult, especially in those with juvenile rheumatoid arthritis and a small mandible. In difficult cases, intubation under local anesthesia by one trained to use the fiberoptic laryngoscope has been the best solution.

Cricoarytenoid rheumatoid involvement leads to hoarseness and immobility of the vocal cords. Patients with chronic hoarseness should have their vocal cords checked before general anesthesia. It is important to recognize potential problems and to *plan ahead* by including the anesthesiologist on the team.

With general or spinal anesthesia, steroid-dependent patients should have steroid support. Recommended amounts vary. For general anesthesia, hydrocortisone (Solucortef) 100 mg IM is given with the preoperative medication, 100 mg IV during surgery, and another 100 mg IV slowly in a continuous infusion over the next 24 hours (100 ml/hr). This regimen has been utilized with repeated success. The infusion is continued until medication can be taken orally, at which point the preoperative dosage is resumed. The patient who has been off steroids for more than 1 year does not need extra support. For the patient who has been off steroids for only a few months, support is necessary and should be tapered off over a period of several days.

Regional anesthesia such as axillary block can be safely done by continuing the patient's maintenance dosage of steroid. In our opinion, it is better to err on the side of extra support than too little. Regional blocks are excellent for rheumatoid surgery. Some anesthesiologists (and patients) do not like the long periods the patient is "lying uncomfortably on the table." These individual problems must be dealt with by "the team." For example, a wrist block (or finger block) is excellent for some hand procedures, as active motion can be tested during the procedure with the patient awake but comfortably sedated.

Anesthesia is never "routine" for the rheumatoid patient. We have enjoyed superb cooperation with anesthesiologists and have had no major anesthesia complications over the last 30 years. Difficult cases demand preliminary discussion with the anesthesiologist ("team approach").

BLOOD TRANSFUSIONS

Autologous blood is obtained in advance for major procedures during which blood transfusions are usually necessary (e.g., total hip replacement) if the general condition of the patient and the distance involved permits. It can also often be obtained in another city through blood bank cooperation. *Note*: In some patients with severe, active rheumatoid arthritis, the general condition, often with chronic anemia, does not permit autologous blood banking, and the treating physician can make this decision. We have used this system for over 16 years and generally obtain three units of blood in less than 25 days.

PREOPERATIVE TRAINING

At the same time patients are preparing for surgery they are undergoing physical therapy training by the therapist for the important postoperative care. A knowledgeable physical or occupational therapist is essential for obtaining the best possible result from the surgery.

Perioperative antibiotics (usually intravenous cephalosporin) are utilized in practically all cases. For total joint replacement, it is usually continued for approximately 48 hours. In other cases, one postoperative dosage 8 hours later is used. This practice has resulted in an infection rate of less than 1 percent in rheumatoid arthritis patients. Thromboembolism prophylaxis is indicated in many cases, particularly for total hip and total knee arthroplasties. We prefer early activity, compression air boots, and aspirin.[6] Surgeons should use the prophylaxis with which they are most comfortable.

In long-standing cases, tissues often are atrophied and thinned, particularly skin and subcutaneous tissues. For surgery of large or small rheumatoid joints, all tissues must be handled with care ("atraumatic technique"). Wound healing is the common denominator of all surgical procedures. The basic surgical principles are the key to obtaining the best results through the team approach.

REFERENCES

1. Aufranc OE: Constructive hip surgery of the vitallium mold; a report of 1000 cases of arthroplasty of the hip over a 15-year period. J Bone Joint Surg [Am] 39:237, 1957
2. Charnley J: Low friction arthroplasty. Clin Orthop 72:7, 1970
3. Clayton ML: Surgery of the thumb in rheumatoid arthritis. J Bone Joint Surg [Am] 44:1976, 1962
4. Clayton ML: Surgical treatment at the wrist in rheumatoid arthritis. J Bone Joint Surg [Am] 47:741, 1965
5. Clayton ML, Ferlic DC, Jeffers PD: Prosthetic arthroplasties of the shoulder. Clin Orthop 164:184, 1982
6. Clayton ML, Thompson TR: Activity, air boots and aspirin as thromboembolism prophylaxis in knee arthroplasty; a multiple regimen approach. Orthopedics 10:1525, 1987
7. Fergesen HE, Poss R, Sledge CB: Bilateral total hip and knee replacements in adults with rheumatoid arthritis: an evaluation of function. Clin Orthop 137:120, 1978
8. Ferlic DC, Clayton ML: Flexor tenosynovectomy in the rheumatoid finger. J Hand Surg 3:364, 1978
9. Fries JF: Advancement in the management of rheumatic diseases, 1965 to 1985. Arch Intern Med 149:1002, 1989
10. Geens S, Clayton ML, Leidholt JD, et al: Synovectomy and débridement of the knee in rheumatoid arthritis. I. Historical review. II. Clinical and roentgenographic study of thirty-one cases. J Bone Joint Surg [Am] 51:617, 1969
11. Gschwend N: General surgical principles in rheumatoid arthritis; priorities. Can J Surg 26:410, 1983
12. Gschwend N: Surgical Treatment of Rheumatoid Arthritis. Georg Thieme Verlag, Stuttgart, 1980
13. Harmon CE, Turner BD, Clayton ML, Smyth CJ: Multiple joint replacements (three or more) of the lower extremity in rheumatoid arthritis. Presented to the American Rheumatism Association, Boston, 1981
14. Lamberta FJ, Ferlic DC, Clayton ML: The use of the Flatt hinge prosthesis in the rheumatoid thumb. Hand 10:94, 1978
15. Law WA: Late results in vitallium mold arthroplasty of the hip. J Bone Joint Surg [Am] 44:1497, 1962
16. Sledge CB, Archer RE, Shortkroff S et al: Intra-articular radiation synovectomy. Clin Orthop 182:37, 1984
17. Sledge CB, Walker PS: Total knee arthroplasty in rheumatoid arthritis. Clin Orthop 182:127, 1984
18. Souter WA: Planning treatment of the rheumatoid hand. Hand 11:3, 1979
19. Swanson AB: Flexible Implant Resection Arthroplasty in the Hand and Extremities. CV Mosby, St. Louis, 1973
20. Thirupathi RG, Ferlic DC, Clayton ML: Dorsal wrist synovectomy in rheumatoid arthritis; a long term study. J Hand Surg 8:848, 1983
21. Turner B, Harmon C, Smyth CJ, Clayton ML: Multiple joint replacements of the lower extremity. Presented to the American Rheumatism Association, Boston, 1981

8

Synovectomy

Mack L. Clayton

Rheumatoid arthritis is an inflammatory disease characterized by its involvement of the synovial tissues throughout the body and particularly in the joints. In a similar process it also involves the tendon sheaths and bursae. The surgical procedures of synovectomy and tenosynovectomy are discussed.

In joint surgery, synovectomy refers to removal of the inflamed involved synovial tissue within a joint. The objective is to relieve the patient's pain, remove the inflammatory tissues, preserve function in the joint, and prevent further changes of destruction to the articular cartilage of the joint.

REVIEW OF THE LITERATURE

Credit for the first report of complete synovectomy in the joints of rheumatoid arthritis patients belongs to the German surgeon Schuller,[19] who in 1887 reported four cases of knee synovectomy. The same cases were described again in more detail in 1893.[20] Schuller thought that the cases of hypertrophic villous synovitis should be treated by early synovectomy rather than by spa therapy. Muller,[16] another German author, described in 1894 a 4-year follow-up of a successful synovectomy on a rheumatoid knee. Both of these surgeons recommended extensive exposure to remove the largest amount of synovial tissue and divided the cruciate ligament and collateral ligaments as necessary.

In the United States, Goldthwait[12] was the first to report the use of this operation in 1900, performing a partial synovectomy for what he called hypertrophic villous arthritis. The procedure was limited to removal of protruding synovial fringes that would mechanically block function of the joint. Complete synovectomy in two cases of monarticular hypertrophic villous arthritis was reported by Murphy[17] in 1916.

However, Swett[23] provided the main impetus to standardize and popularize the procedure by performing complete synovectomies in rheumatoid arthritis patients. During the second and third decade of the twentieth century, he published a number of articles and reported the results of surgery in 32 knees, stressing the importance of proper selection of candidates to ensure satisfactory results. He stressed the fact that they should have reasonable range of motion and good articular cartilage remaining.

Many other reports followed that by Swett, but unfortunately only a few of the investigators analyzed their results. Moreover, some of these authors mixed the results of synovectomy for a variety of conditions. It was an era during which rheumatoid arthritis was called by a number of names—before there was general agreement on a specific name for this disease process.

In 1941 Ghormley and Cameron, at the Mayo Clinic, reported an incidence of almost 50 percent poor results with synovectomy of rheumatoid knees.[10] Use of the operation was gradually discontinued, and it was rarely performed from 1940 until the mid-1950s. In 1955 an excellent statistical study was reported by London[14] in which he demonstrated the reliability of preoperative roentgenograms as a prognostic criterion for final results.

About this time, increasing interest in surgical procedures for the relief of problems associated with rheumatoid arthritis spawned a number of reports, and a new wave of enthusiasm popularized the procedure worldwide. There was some enthusiasm for early synovectomy as a prophylactic means of preventing joint damage, distinct from palliative synovectomy at a later stage of the disease.

Throughout these early years the main interest had been in synovectomy of the knee, but the procedure was applied to almost every joint during the first half of the twentieth century. A thorough historical review of synovectomy was published by Geens[8] in 1969.

SYNOVECTOMY USING THE KNEE AS MODEL

It has been stated repeatedly that synovectomy should be performed early in the course of rheumatoid arthritis, i.e., during the period of synovial proliferation prior to bone invasion or cartilaginous destruction (synovial stage). However, most published studies do not allow one to draw conclusions as to the true value of the synovectomy performed.

Results of a consecutive series of patients in 1969[9] were described in sufficient detail to allow such conclusions to be drawn. Only patients with classic progressive rheumatoid arthritis with multiple joint involvement and an advanced degree of involvement of the knee were included. The results were quantitatively scored with respect to the degree of disability and disease activity of the knee; roentgenographic evaluation was included. Postoperatively selected patients underwent arthroscopy for visual evaluation of the regenerated synovium, biopsy for light and electron microscopic examination, and tissue and fluid retrieval for enzyme analyses.

Twenty-eight synovectomies in 20 adult patients were evaluated (14 women, 6 men). The average age was 45 years (range 25 to 70), and the average duration of follow-up of the 28 knees was 23 months (range 7 to 49 months). All adults had classic rheumatoid arthritis, and in all but two the disease had run a progressive course with a persistently elevated erythrocyte sedimentation rate (ESR).

The activity of the disease process, based on the number of joints showing severe inflammation and destruction, was high in five, moderate in nine, and low in six. Most patients were in the later stages of the disease, with 24 knees beyond stage II and with moderate or marked joint narrowing. Most patients had stage III disease; only one was at stage I. All patients were on basic medical regimens. Almost all had taken steroids at some time during the course of the disease, and eight were still taking steroids at the time of surgery. These patients had been treated with gold injections. The other patients received various anti-inflammatory agents; aspirin was used by all.

Methods

All patients were examined by one orthopaedic surgeon who had not performed the surgery.

1. Each patient was asked to estimate the present condition of the knee and to grade it as excellent, good, fair, or poor. Using our 100 point scale, quantitative ratings of knee disability were obtained before synovectomy and at the time of review[9] (Table 8-1).
2. The value of synovectomy as a prophylactic procedure was tested utilizing a local inflammatory activity index based on 10 criteria derived from the 30-point scale of the American Rheumatism Association (ARA) Committee in

Table 8-1. Average Functional Score with Estimates of the End Result by the Patient[8]

Patient's Estimate	No. of Knees	Preop. Score	Postop. Score	Gain/ Loss
Excellent	9	61	90	+29
Good	8	50	81	+31
Fair	5	46	72	+26
Poor	6	52	41	−11

Diagnostic and Therapeutic Criteria. Again, comparable scores were obtained before synovectomy and at the time of rating.

3. The examiners' estimated result was based on eight criteria, including activity and functional scores, range of motion, pain, swelling, instability, flexion contracture, and progression of the disease seen roentgenographically. Arbitrary leads were determined for each of these eight criteria, and the results were classified accordingly as excellent, good, fair, or poor. Roentgenographic progression was evaluated by comparing pre- and postoperative films and analyzing cartilage destruction (erosions, impacting of condyles or plateaus, and deformity—posterior or lateral subluxation or malalignment).

Joint narrowing as a roentgenographic criterion and joint instability as a clinical criterion were found to give the most accurate evaluation of the condition of the joint. (Weight-bearing anteroposterior films are necessary.) These criteria called for a subdivision of stage III into early and late, as two-thirds of the patients were in stage III at the time of synovectomy.

Surgical Technique

A transverse skin incision at the level of the inferior pole of the patella with L-shaped longitudinal division of the capsule of both sides of the patella and a small posterior incision just behind the medial collateral ligament were made. All synovium was excised, including the retropatellar fat pad, proliferations in the intercondylar notch, posterior compartments, and popliteus tendon. Care was taken to preserve the fatty tissue underneath the synovium in the suprapatellar pouch overlying the distal end of the femur. The menisci were generally removed as indicated by invasion and destruction or when an underlying erosive lesion had to be excised. Roughened areas in the femoral condyles were excised level with the surrounding surface. Marginal synovial overgrowths were "rubbed off" the cartilage and cauterized at the articular margins; mar-

ginal osteophytes were removed. (In a few cases the classic median parapatellar approach was chosen, but the posterior compartment was not reached). Medial and lateral skin incisions may be used if preferred to transverse incisions. (A horseshoe incision was chosen in a few cases, which lifted the tibial tubercle and provided excellent exposure: but in one case the block was reinserted and fixed with a screw, and the tendon was pulled out of the bone. Reoperation was unsatisfactory, and infection occurred. Lifting the tibial tubercle is not recommended in rheumatoid arthritis patients.)

At this time one should consider that a total knee arthroplasty may be necessary in the future and plan incisions accordingly. No skin problems have occurred with secondary procedures. An important factor is that synovectomy should include the posterior compartment if it is involved.

Postoperative Management

A suction drain was inserted. The knees were splinted in full extension, and quadriceps exercises were started immediately. Motion was started at 4 days, and most knees were gently manipulated to 90 degrees at 7 to 10 days under general anesthetia or intravenous diazepam (Valium); usually the weight of the leg was sufficient force. At the present time continuous passive motion (CPM) is recommended immediately after surgery: Voluntary motion is obtained in a few days, and hospitalization is shortened.

Night splinting in extension was utilized until full active extension was present. Crutch walking with partial weight-bearing was started with mobilization and full weight-bearing with crutches about 4 weeks after surgery. Crutches were recommended for at least 6 weeks, as some studies have reported alterations in cartilage metabolism for 6 to 8 weeks after synovectomy. A few patients with considerable instability were fitted with long leg braces for 3 to 6 months.

Complications were few. One patient had a deep venous thrombosis without untoward effects. The patellar tendon detachment that occurred has already been mentioned.

Analysis of Clinical Results

Of the 28 synovectomies (average follow-up 23 months), 20 knees (71 percent) were rated as improved by the patient compared with 18 knees (64 percent) rated improved by the examiner. Clinical arrest of local disease activity was obtained in 25 knees; in 13 knees there was a recurrence (either definite or probable). Definite recurrence of synovitis with a marked effusion and a boggy synovium was found in eight knees. Of these eight, three were bilateral and two unilateral; in the latter two patients, the opposite knee (not operated on) was involved also. One additional knee was considered to have a definite recurrence as evidenced by deterioration seen on the roentgenograms, but there was no definite hypertrophic synovial tissue to palpation. Synovial fluid was obtained from five knees showing recurrences, and the findings were compatible with rheumatoid arthritis. They differed in no way from the usual preoperative findings.

Four knees demonstrated persistent effusion, but synovial hypertrophy could not be palpated. Although the true significance of these findings is not known, these knees were considered potential failures and were classified as probable recurrences. It is interesting to note that when synovectomy was done bilaterally at an identical stage of destruction, the result in both knees was almost identical in seven of eight patients.

In the patient's estimate of satisfactory improvement, pain and functional improvement are the chief determining factors, with pain as the patient's first concern. Indeed, a patient might rate the result excellent in the presence of a recurrence provided there was no pain. It was surprising to find that pain was relieved in most of the patients experiencing a recurrence. Five knees had more pain at follow-up than before the operation. Results in all of these patients were poor. However, the other eight knees with recurrences obtained pain relief of various degrees. Because pain was successfully relieved in the patient with the ankylosed knee, she classified the result fair instead of poor. In general, there was a return of some pain over a period of time, but it was usually considerably less than before the op-

eration. None of the patients in this series mentioned a change in the character of the pain.

Functional improvement was the second beneficial effect of synovectomy, and five patients were moved from class III to class II. In general, the patient's own estimate correlated with the functional score reached. Functional gain remained high throughout the series, provided the joint damage preoperatively was not severe. In a number of patients with recurrences, functional improvement was considerable. In the group of patients grading their results as excellent, the average gain was not higher than in the group with good or fair results. The earlier that synovectomy is done, the less one should expect with regard to subjective improvement. Indeed, 15 knees had a functional score of 50 or more before surgery and the average gain was only 14 (scores of 63 and 77). Conversely, 13 knees did not reach 50 before synovectomy, but their postoperative gain averaged 31 (scores 40 and 71). This seemingly minor improvement is due to the fact that the disability and pain of early arthritis are less severe.

Range of motion was not significantly affected in this group of knees when early motion was encouraged after synovectomy. Significant loss of flexion is certainly not to be feared after synovectomy if a vigorous postoperative regimen is followed utilizing manipulation or CPM in many cases. The average change in the series was less than 2 degrees change in flexion and less than 2 degrees change in extension. Loss of extension of any appreciable degree over 15 degrees was associated with clinical and roentgenographic deterioration of the joint. However, the total range of motion was unrelated to the result; and indeed in many patients with poor results the total range of motion was still surprisingly good. Also, the range of motion after synovectomy was not related to the course of the disease and did not decrease with time. The average range of motion in the group of knees followed more than 2 years was significantly better than in knees followed for less than 2 years.

Roentgenographic progression (joint narrowing, bone destruction, and joint deformity) has taken place in nine knees, of which eight had a moderate of marked loss of joint space (at least half the normal width). In addition, these eight knees were moderately or markedly unstable. All six subjective failures are included in this group. Progression was found to correlate with recurrence in seven and preexisting angular deformity in two.

None of the patients experienced a beneficial effect on the general disease or on the condition of other involved joints. Instability had not improved when compared to the preoperative status, and it was significantly increased in three knees that had a preexisting varus deformity antedating the rheumatoid process. In some cases the patients thought that the stability in the knee was improved as a result of better muscle control because of the lack of pain.

Determining Factors

It is generally accepted that the quality of the final result is determined primarily by the extent of rheumatoid involvement. The patient's and examiner's estimate of the results were compared with the extent of joint destruction at the time of surgery. Five knees had slight narrowing and either no or mild instability. All but one was subjectively improved, and only two had persistent effusion without certain evidence of progressive rheumatoid activity. On the other hand, recurrences were seen most frequently in knees with moderate or marked instability and joint narrowing (11 of 17 knees). Five of the six poor results belong in this group. All results were subjectively satisfactory when the joint was no more than slightly narrowed. With moderate joint narrowing 77 percent of the patients expressed satisfaction with the results, whereas with marked narrowing only 28 percent were satisfied. Seven of the eight knees with marked anterior and posterior instability due to complete instability of the cruciate ligaments had a recurrence. Two were rated by the patients themselves as excellent, three fair, and three poor. Instability appeared to bear just as heavily on the final result as joint narrowing. There was only one knee in the series that was done in the early stage of the disease (stage I). In this patient, synovectomy was performed within 1 year after the knee had become involved. Early synovectomy was done with the intention of preventing it from becoming as badly destroyed as the opposite knee. There is convincing evidence that a synovectomy performed in a late stage with marked joint space reduction and instability accomplishes little.

A particular problem is presented by a knee with a preexisting angular deformity unrelated to the rheumatoid disease. The deformity often increases rapidly as soon as the knee becomes involved by arthritis, and this progression is not arrested by synovectomy. In this series, two patients had known bilateral genu varum before the onset of the disease. Synovectomy of three of the affected knee joints did not stop progression of the deformity, and recurrence was apparent in both knees of one of these patients.

The extent of joint damage, however, cannot be blamed for all recurrences. Of eight knees in five patients with a highly active disease, the results in five were poor, fair in two, and good in one. All knees had recurrences: seven definite and one probable. There was one probable recurrence in the group with low disease activity. There was only one poor result in the group of patients with moderate and low disease activity. The course of disease is an important determining factor for the result of synovectomy in rheumatoid arthritis patients.[7]

An attempt was made to correlate results of the findings of rheumatoid nodules—either distinctive palpable subcutaneous nodules or nodules found histologically in excised synovial membrane. Findings were inconclusive, and the widely accepted opinion that nodules bear a particularly unfavorable prognostic significance was not substantiated.

The duration of rheumatoid involvement prior to synovectomy had no effect on the results, as excellent results were obtained with synovectomies on knees with more than 10 years' involvement, and poor results were obtained in some involved for 1 to 5 years. The time lapsed after synovectomy appears to be significant. Indeed, in this series of 28 knees the results are better in the patients with shorter follow-up. If the knees operated on are divided into three groups according to the time of follow-up, good and excellent subjective results were found in 60 percent of the whole group; however, only 46 percent in the group were studied for more than 2 years, 73 percent in the group were followed for less than 2 years, and 100 percent in the group for less than 1 year. Percentages of recurrence in the same order are for the whole group 46.5 percent, more than 2 years 72 percent, less than 2 years 24 percent, less than 1 year 14 percent.

RHEUMATOID SYNOVIUM REGENERATION

Thirty-one synovectomized knees (25 patients) were included in the following study,[18a] and the average postsynovectomy evaluation was performed at 31 months. Average patient age was 43 years (range 20 to 62 years), and the average number of years the patient had rheumatoid disease prior to surgery was 10.7 years. All patients underwent both an anterior and a posterior compartment synovectomy of the knee, and the stages of the knee were recorded: 17 in stage II and 14 in stage III. In addition, 70 biopsy specimens for the knee synovial membrane were obtained from various control groups. All patients with rheumatoid arthritis in the synovectomized group were evaluated as follows.

1. Outpatient arthroscopy was performed under local anesthesia, and photographs of the gross appearance of this regenerating synovium were obtained.
2. Synovial biopsy specimens were obtained for light and electron microscopy study under direct vision so the most involved area could be biopsied.
3. Aspirated synovial fluid was obtained to assay for lysosomal glycosidase activity.
4. Clinical examination and functional evaluation were done to search for evidence of recurrence or radiographic progression at any time during the postsynovectomy period.

The microscopic specimens were examined for changes considered to be characteristic of rheumatoid arthritis, and electron microscopy was performed on the specimens as well. The synovial fluid enzymes were evaluated and clinical status results recorded.

The gross appearance of the regenerating synovial membrane revealed that there were four architectural patterns noted. Group 1 displayed a pale, smooth, nonvillous synovium often resembling fibrous tissue. Group 2 was mainly hyperemic smooth synovium with an occasional large villus. Group 3 showed a pale villous synovium, and group 4 had a hyperemic villous synovium. In most cases the gross appearance of the regenerating synovium was closely correlated with the histology. In one patient, the synovium at 5 years after synovectomy seemed grossly like dense scar tissue, although microscopically the lining was hyperplastic. Another patient's synovial membrane after a second synovectomy grossly showed areas of both smooth and villous hyperemic synovium.

Evaluations of the histologic appearance were based on two criteria for diagnosis of active rheumatoid arthritis: (1) hyperplasia and hypertrophy of the lining layer; and (2) the presence of collections of perivascular plasma cells and lymphocytes. Ninety percent of the biopsy specimens from rheumatoid patients not operated on were positive, whereas only 6 percent of the clinically nonrheumatoid controls contained the elements described previously. Using the same criteria for diagnosis of rheumatoid activity in the postsynovectomy group, only 60 percent had positive biopsy specimens.

Only two of the biopsy specimens obtained between 0 and 11 months after surgery met the criteria for active rheumatoid arthritis, but there were far fewer plasma cells in them in comparison with later biopsy specimens.

One month postsynovectomy, the membrane contained large lining cells somewhat oriented toward the joint space. At 2 months the lining cells were more numerous, large, and sometimes multinucleated. In addition, there were numerous capillaries with large endothelial cells. Areas of fibrin-like material were present among the lining cells. The findings at 3 months revealed more pronounced abnormalities of the vessels, and at 4 months large deposits of fibrin-like material were seen covering the hypertrophic lining cells. At 5 months a recurrence was seen in one biopsy specimen, and another showed only a fibrotic synovium. Thus histologic diversity was seen in different patients during the same time period and in the same patient in different areas of the joint. A more severe recurrence was seen in one patient 10 months postsynovectomy.

Fibrin-like deposits were noteworthy. Multinucleated cells were found in about half the cases of rheumatoid arthritis, and they were found as frequently in the unoperated patients. The small vessels in the subintimal space were abnormal in most patients. There was an increase in number, size, and erythrocyte content of the small vessels.

Results of the enzyme studies were recorded. The recurrence of active synovitis was marked by synovial fluid enzyme levels more than twice the levels of those seen in degenerative joint disease for at least three of the four enzymes studied (α-N-acetylglucosaminidase, β-galactosidase, β-glucuronidase, mannosidase.)

It is apparent that, as the interval after synovectomy increases, the activity of lysosomal glycosidases increases. For the most part, in the group between 36 and 120 months, the values obtained are nearly equivalent to those shown for rheumatoid arthritis in general. This fact suggests that 2 to 3 years postsynovectomy patients suffering from rheumatoid arthritis whose general joint disease is active have a high incidence of recurrent active synovitis in the operated knee.

Results

Of the 32 regenerated rheumatoid synovial membranes, 20 (88 percent) were classified microscopically, showing recurrence of the rheumatoid process in 18 of 21 specimens 12 months or more after synovectomy. Only 25 of the 31 synovectomized knees (46 percent) demonstrated clinical recurrence, but among the patients followed 12 months or longer 66 percent had clinical evidence of recurrence. Seventy-five percent had elevated lysosomal activity, and 81 percent of those seen 12 months or more after synovectomy demonstrated elevated lysosomal activity. Roentgenographic progression of the disease was

noted in 71 percent of patients 12 months or more after synovectomy. In the knees followed 24 months or more after synovectomy, roentgenographic evidence of progression of the disease, clinical recurrence, histologic recurrence, and elevated lysosomal enzymatic activity correlated exactly in 83 percent of the knees studied.

From this study it appears that, with time after synovectomy, the regenerating synovium in the knees of patients with rheumatoid arthritis tends to become histologically and enzymatically indistinguishable from that of rheumatoid patients who were not operated on. Cruickshank[1] has emphasized the variable histologic appearance of the synovial membrane in patients who have had the disease for less than 2 years. In the study by Patzakis et al.,[18a] the arthroscope permitted biopsy of grossly active areas in the joint, which accentuated the findings of early recurrence. The synovial fluid enzyme assays, on the other hand, are indicators of average disease activity in the entire knee. Despite this difference, there was a close correlation between the histology and the assay of synovial fluid enzyme activity in our study.

Goldie[11] reported that there were only minimal differences in histopathologic appearance of original and regenerated synovial tissue from 26 patients 1 to 3 years postsynovectomy. Ranawat et al.[18] reported that 7 of 12 patients, 6 months to 2 years postsynovectomy, had either definite recurrence of the rheumatoid inflammation or features characteristic of rheumatoid synovium.

Results of Patzakis et al.,[18a] demonstrated that the synovial membrane that re-forms after synovectomy of rheumatoid joints is abnormal as early as 1 month after surgery. At 1 to 4 months after synovectomy, large frequently multinucleated lining cells appear, as do many capillaries and venules with abnormal endothelial cells. These features probably constitute more than just a reaction to tissue injury because they are not seen in synovial membranes obtained from knees that have been injured. The biopsy specimens taken 5 to 18 months postsynovectomy showed wide variation. Some evidenced areas of fibrous replacement of the lining layer, and others had definite synovitis. In specimens removed 24 to 60 months after synovectomy, there was a progressive increase in perivascular plasma cells and lymphocytes and an increase in the size and number of lining cells.

Changes described in the postsynovectomy biopsy specimens are comparable to those reported for early synovitis, except for the added variable of the operative trauma of synovectomy. Although the biopsy specimen in rheumatoid arthritis is nonspecific, it was thought that the simple histologic criteria were available and present in only 6 percent of the control biopsy specimens. The use of the specific type of sections allowed lymphocytes and plasma cells to be more easily distinguished from fibroblast macrophages and pericytes. With respect to the lysosomal glycosidases, the levels in synovial fluid enzyme activity were representative of the general degree of disease activity in the joint cavity. This relation of lysosomal hydrolase in synovial fluid and activity of clinical disease has been well documented. This hydrolase probably has its origin from two sources: (1) the inflammatory leukocyte infiltrate, and (2) the metabolic turnover of the hyperplastic, hypertrophic inflammatory synovial lining. Therefore the more active the recurrent disease activity, the higher is the level of enzyme activity, even if the involvement is focal in distribution.

Finally, the analysis of our series showed that 85.7 percent (18 of 21) of the regenerated synovial tissue specimens obtained more than 12 months after synovectomy met the criteria for rheumatoid synovium, and in the synovial fluid from these joints the lysosomal enzyme activity was elevated in 81.2 percent (13 of 16) of the specimens. The only difference in gross and histologic appearance between the rheumatoid synovium not operated on and the regenerated rheumatoid synovium was the increased amount of scarring present in the latter.

Summary

The visual, histologic, and enzymatic characteristics of the regenerated rheumatoid synovium were evaluated in 31 synovectomized knees. Of the 21 synovial biopsy specimens obtained from regenerated rheumatoid synovium 12 months or longer after synovectomy, 18 (85.7 percent) were classified as rheumatoid synovium, and 18 of 24 (75 percent) of synovial fluids obtained from the patients were found to have elevated lysosomal enzyme activity. In the fluids of 13 of 16 patients (81.2 percent) followed 12 months or more after synovectomy, there was elevated lysosomal activity. Lysosomal glycosidase activity reflects the development of active inflammatory synovitis often before it becomes clinically significant. Also, 14 of 21 (66.6 percent) were found to have a clinical recurrence, and roentgenographic progression of the disease was noted in 15 of 21 knees (71.4 percent).

Conclusions

Synovectomy of the knee should be considered a palliative procedure, not a curative one. It is not surprising that such a high recurrence rate was found in the enzymatic and microscopic changes in the regenerated synovial membranes. If the study was carried further and a microanalysis was performed of the body's connective tissue, all tissues would be found to be rheumatoid, as this disease is generalized.

A joint synovectomy removes the active synovial membrane with its areas of inflammation, relieves pain, and allows a new membrane to form. It is well known that in practically all cases of rheumatoid arthritis certain joints are not clinically active. Yet it is a generalized disease, and the patient's joints must have some rheumatoid-type tissue in it. The goal of synovectomy is to make an active joint fall into the category of one of the inactive joints in the same patient. It is obvious that the patient with severe, progressive, active, continuous rheumatoid arthritis cannot benefit from synovectomy for long, which is unfortunate because it is this patient who needs most to have a satisfactory outcome.

Current Conclusions About Synovectomy

Based on the two previous studies, which included follow-up of all possible parameters and represented a thorough study on postoperative results following knee synovectomy, certain conclusions have been drawn.

Synovectomy in rheumatoid arthritis is followed by regeneration of synovium that in time generally becomes typical rheumatoid synovium. This outcome is not illogical, as rheumatoid arthritis is a generalized disease.

In a clinical knee series,[9] 79 percent were rated by the patient as improved (pain relief was the most important factor), compared with 65 percent rated improved by the examiner, despite a clinical recurrence rate of 46.5 percent overall (Table 8-2). Eighty-five percent of synovial biopsy specimens obtained from regenerated synovium after 1 year were classified as rheumatoid. Lysosomal glycosidase levels were elevated and rose with time to those consistent with rheumatoid arthritis.

The results and incidence of microscopic recurrence were not always reliable for predicting the chances of pain relief. Angular deformity antedating involvement tends to progress rapidly with onset of the arthritis. Moderate to marked instability or translatory subluxation (a form of instability) is also a poor prognosis. Weight-bearing roentgenograms are necessary for evaluating the knee.

Recurrence does not always become apparent during the first few months after synovectomy and may be a relative matter; for example, after 36 hours of rest the knee may be essentially normal to examination, but after 8 hours of standing there is a marked effusion and warmth but no pain. Many patients reported that the knee treats them as well as they treat it.

In advanced stages of destruction, synovectomy provides short-term relief of pain and minimal functional improvement; synovectomy alone is not indicated when there is severe instability and loss of articular cartilage. Synovectomy is strongly indicated for a knee that has shown persistent involvement of short duration and there is advanced joint destruction of the opposite knee (a poor host-disease relation has been demonstrated, and the second knee will probably follow the course of the other without intervention).

With CPM and a persistent, supervised physical therapy regimen, the range of motion is not significantly affected and does not correlate with the final subjective and objective result in most patients. Loss of significant extension (more than 15 degrees) has a poor prognosis.

The above conclusions are based on studies of the knee as a key weight-bearing joint (Table 8-2). Upper extremity joints often have a more favorable course regarding pain relief and function even if they have considerable joint narrowing and some instability, particularly in the elbow[5] (78 percent good or excellent results after 7 years). In a thoroughly documented series of synovectomy of the MCP and PIP joints of the hand, Flatt[6] reported a recurrence rate of 50 percent, similar to the knee series, but clinical improvement was higher.

Table 8-2. Frequency of Recurrence in Selected Studies Reported in the Literature

		Recurrence		
Year	Author(s)	%	No. of Knees	Follow-up
1926	Swett	22	7/32	
1929	Allison & Coonse	10	2/19	
1930	Boon-Itt	10	4/41	Av. 3 yr
1938	Inge	39	10/26	
1941	Ghormley & Cameron	44	21/47	
1951	Magnusson	54	9/15	Av. 6 yr
1964	Aidem & Baker	8	2/26	Av. 4 yr
1964	Mori	5	3/60	
1965	Torppi & Heikkinen	8	2/24	
1966	Gariepy et al.	6	3/56	Av. 6.5 yr
1966	Marmor	0	0/34	3 mo–3 yr
1966	Stevens & Whitefield	9	9/100	3 mo–2 yr
1966	Vainio	25	50/201	Av. 2.5 yr
1969	Geens, Clayton et al.	46.5	13/28	2 yr plus

With the present knowledge, there is no place for the term "prophylactic" synovectomy. Synovectomy must be considered a palliative procedure, not a curative one. Synovectomy is rarely indicated in the patient with highly active disease where most joints are involved and the disease has a rapid downhill course despite general medical treatment. Synovectomy here helps the least where it is needed the most.

Synovectomy is indicated for the patient with moderate or low activity in a slowly progressive disease where one or a few joints are painful and involved out of proportion to the whole; it is also indicated in patients who have not responded to a good basic medical regimen within about 6 months. One must delineate between time of involvement of a joint and time of total disease duration. Synovectomy should rarely be considered during the first year of the disease because of the high number of remissions. Pain should be present, and we are reluctant to advise synovectomy earlier than when pain is a major complaint. Synovectomy is an excellent pain reliever, and patients relate their results more to pain relief than to any other factor. Good range of motion must also be present. In the weight-bearing joints there should be articular cartilage remaining (the more the better) as well as reasonable alignment and stability (no actual bone loss). In the upper extremity, synovectomy is more successful in later stages. Synovectomy of individual areas is discussed further in regional chapters.

Despite its drawbacks, synovectomy should not be discarded.[7] It is the only procedure that retains the patient's own natural joint functioning with less pain for an indefinite period of time; the period depends more on the general activity of the disease than any other single factor. General medical treatment must be continued, and if some remission is obtained the result of synovectomy is much better. Synovectomy does not "burn any bridges"; and later reconstructive surgery can be performed if necessary.

Synovectomy of the knee has become an uncommon operation in the United States today because of its unpredictability and long recovery period, and total knee arthroplasty has become an excellent and reliable procedure. Arthroscopic synovectomy of the knee has been in use for several years, and its use is increasing. The advantages are short hospitalization, low morbidity, rapid regain of motion, and loss of pain. One study found better results with arthroscopic synovectomy than with open synovectomy of the knee at a 10-year follow-up.[15] However, if pain is alleviated and motion is regained for even 1 to 2 years, it is a worthwhile procedure that can be repeated if necessary.

Synovectomy is often combined with excision of synovial cysts that occur around the joints. Occasionally they represent individual bursal involvement. The most common is the popliteal cyst at the knee, but they are also noted anterior to the hip, in the shoulder area either in the subdeltoid bursa or distally along the long head of the biceps, or at the elbow along the neck of the radius.

Sledge et al.[21,22] have reported encouraging results with intra-articular radiation synovectomy. An investigation that is not generally available, it does give hope for the future. The subject of synovectomy has been reviewed by Gschwend, President of the European Rheumatoid Arthritis Surgical Society and a respected leader in arthritis surgery. His chapter is recommended as another review with an extensive bibliography.[13]

TENOSYNOVECTOMY

The synovium around the tendon sheath becomes involved in the same way as the synovium in a joint; pathologically, there is no difference. Clinically, tenosynovitis originates in a closed space, e.g., in the carpal tunnel or flexor tendon tunnel sheath of the fingers or underneath the dorsocarpal ligament on the dorsum of the wrist. It can originate also in the same area around the foot and ankle.

At any point were rheumatoid synovium can enlarge and is inflamed, it can invade the bone, cartilage, or tendon where it is in a closed space under pressure. The tendon involvement can progress to a constriction with aseptic necrosis, leading to tendon rupture. Tendon rupture can also result from direct invasion of the tendon or erosion on the edge of a ligament (retinaculum) or on irregular bony spicules such as the distal ulna at the wrist.

Tenosynovectomy with removal of the involved tendon sheath is a satisfactory procedure with a minimal recurrence rate. The latter is true because the environment is usually altered with the procedure; for example, at the dorsum of the wrist the dorsal carpal ligament is folded back like the page of a book, and at the finish it is passed underneath the wrist extensor tendon, leaving the tendons resting in a bed of healthy fat[4] (see Fig. 6-7). The rheumatoid process, as noted before, damages tendons in a closed space under pressure, and with this alteration of the environment it is rare to have recurrent disease of tendon rupture. Tenosynovectomy is a popular procedure and has had a successful record for 30 years.[2,3,24] Articular synovectomy can be performed at the same time, as indicated. Individual procedures of tenosynovectomy are discussed in other chapters.

REFERENCES

1. Cruickshank B: Interpretation of multiple biopsies of synovial tissue in rheumatic diseases. Ann Rheum Dis 11:137, 1952
2. Ferlic DC, Clayton ML: Flexor tenosynovectomy in the rheumatoid finger. J Hand Surg 3:364, 1978
3. Ferlic DC, Clayton ML: The shoulder in rheumatoid arthritis. p. 203. In Strickland J (ed): Difficult Problems in Hand Surgery. CV Mosby, St. Louis, 1982
4. Ferlic DC, Clayton ML: Synovectomy of the hand and wrist. Ann Chir Gynaecol, suppl, 198:26, 1985
5. Ferlic DC, Patchett CE, Clayton ML, Freeman AC: Elbow synovectomy in rheumatoid arthritis; long term results. Clin Orthop 220:119, 1987
6. Flatt AE: The Care of the Rheumatoid Hand. 3rd Ed. CV Mosby, St. Louis, 1974
7. Gariepy R, Demers R, Laurin DA: The prophylactic effect of synovectomy of the knee in rheumatoid arthritis. Can Med Assoc J 94:1349, 1966
8. Geens S: Synovectomy and débridement of the knee in rheumatoid arthritis. I. Historical review. J Bone Joint Surg [Am] 51:617, 1969
9. Geens S, Clayton ML, Leidholt JD et al: Synovectomy and débridement of the knee in rheumatoid arthritis. II. Clinical and roentgenographic study of thirty-one cases. J Bone Joint Surg [Am] 51:626, 1969
10. Ghormley RK, Cameron DM: End results of synovectomy of the knee joint. Am J Surg 53:455, 1941
11. Goldie I: Pathomorphologic features in original and regenerated synovial tissues after synovectomy in rheumatoid arthritis. Clin Orthop 77:295, 1971
12. Goldthwait JE: Knee joint surgery for non-tubercular conditions; a report of 38 operations for synovial fringes, injured semilunar cartilage, loose cartilage, coagula, exploratory incision, etc. Boston Med Surg J 143:286, 1900
13. Gschwend N: Synovectomy. In Kelly WN, Harris ED Jr, Ruddy S, Sledge CB (eds): Textbook of Rheumatology. 3rd Ed. WB Saunders, Philadelphia, 1989
14. London PS: Synovectomy of the knee in rheumatoid arthritis; an essay in surgical salvage. J Bone Joint Surg [Br] 37:392, 1955
15. Matsui N, Taneda Y, Ohta H et al: Arthroscopic versus open synovectomy in the rheumatoid knee. Int Orthop 13:17, 1989
16. Muller W: Zur Frage Der Operativen Behandlung Der Arthritis Deformans Und Des Chronischen Gelenkrheumatismus. Arch Klin Chir 47:1, 1894
17. Murphy JB: Hypertrophic villous synovitis of the knee joint; synovial capsulectomy. Surg Clin Chicago 5:155, 1916
18. Ranawat CS, Straub LR, Freyberg R et al: A study of regenerated synovium after synovectomy of the knee in rheumatoid arthritis. Arthritis Rheum 14:117, 1971
18a. Patzakis MJ, Mills DM, Clayton ML et al.: A visual histological and enzymatic study of regenerating rheumatoid synovium in the synovectomized knee. J Bone Joint Surg 55A:287, 1973.
19. Schuller M: Die Pathologie und Therapie der Gelenkentzundungen. Urban U. Schwarzenberg, Vienna, 1887
20. Schuller M: Chirurgische Mitteilungen Uber Die Chronisch Rheumatischen Gelenkentzundungen. Arch Klin Chir 45:153, 1893
21. Sledge CB, Archer RE, Shortkoff S: Intra-articular radiation synovectomy. Clin Orthop 182:37, 1984
22. Sledge CB, Zuckerman J, Shortkoff S: Synovectomy of the rheumatoid knee using intra-articular injection of dysprosium-165-ferric hydroxide macroaggregates. J Bone Joint Surg [Am] 69:970, 1987
23. Swett PP: A review of synovectomy. J Bone Joint Surg 20:68, 1938
24. Thirupathi RG, Ferlic DC, Clayton ML: Dorsal wrist synovectomy in rheumatoid arthritis: a long term study. J Hand Surg 8:848, 1983

III

REGIONAL SURGICAL CONSIDERATIONS

9

Management of the Rheumatoid Shoulder

Donald C. Ferlic

Considering the amount of material written on surgery for rheumatoid arthritis, there are few publications relating to the surgical and orthopaedic management of the rheumatoid shoulder, and few operative procedures are performed on the shoulder compared to other joints. Of our patients who have undergone surgery for rheumatoid arthritis, only 4 percent had shoulder surgery.[5] Surgery to the shoulder is frequently not necessary because decreased glenohumeral function can often be compensated for by normal scapulothoracic motion; shoulder involvement is usually insidious, and patients with multiple involved joints often draw attention to other joints. Nonoperative treatment includes physical therapy, an occasional steroid injection, and rest.

Lower extremity surgery may be considered first in the patient with many joints involved, as it puts less demand on the shoulder for crutch-walking and perhaps removes the need for performing surgery. The patient who most likely requires shoulder surgery is the one who has multiple upper extremity joint involvement with pain and needs the shoulder to position the hand. If multiple joints in the upper and lower extremities are involved with accompanying pain and limitation of motion, some priority in treatment must be established before considering surgery. Such judgment is based on the predictability of results as well as preventing further, more devastating complications, e.g., paralysis due to cervical spine dislocation and rupture of extensor tendons in the wrist. We have established our treatment priorities, in order of importance, to be the cervical spine with neurologic signs and symptoms, forefoot resection, hips, knees, wrist, hand, and finally elbow or shoulder. Although the shoulder is our last priority, there are a number of patients in whom surgery is definitely indicated.

ANATOMY

The shoulder is composed of four joints: sternoclavicular, acromioclavicular, glenohumeral, and scapulothoracic. Rheumatoid arthritis may affect any of the first three diarthrodial joints. The scapulothoracic bursa is not involved in rheumatoid arthritis, and thus some motion may be preserved even in patients with severe destruction in the glenohumeral joint (Fig. 9-1). There is motion in all four joints upon movement, with 60 degrees in the sternoclavicular and 60 to 70 degrees at the acromioclavicular joint when the scapula rotates.[25] There is a rhythm between the scapular and humeral movements upon shoulder motion, with 1 degree of upward scapular rotation for each 2 degrees of movement at the glenohumeral joint after 30 degrees of abduction and a similar rotation after 60 degrees of flexion.[10]

The tendons about the shoulder make up the rotator cuff, which inserts on the neck of the humerus. These muscles are the subscapularis, supraspinatus, infraspinatus, and teres minor (Fig.

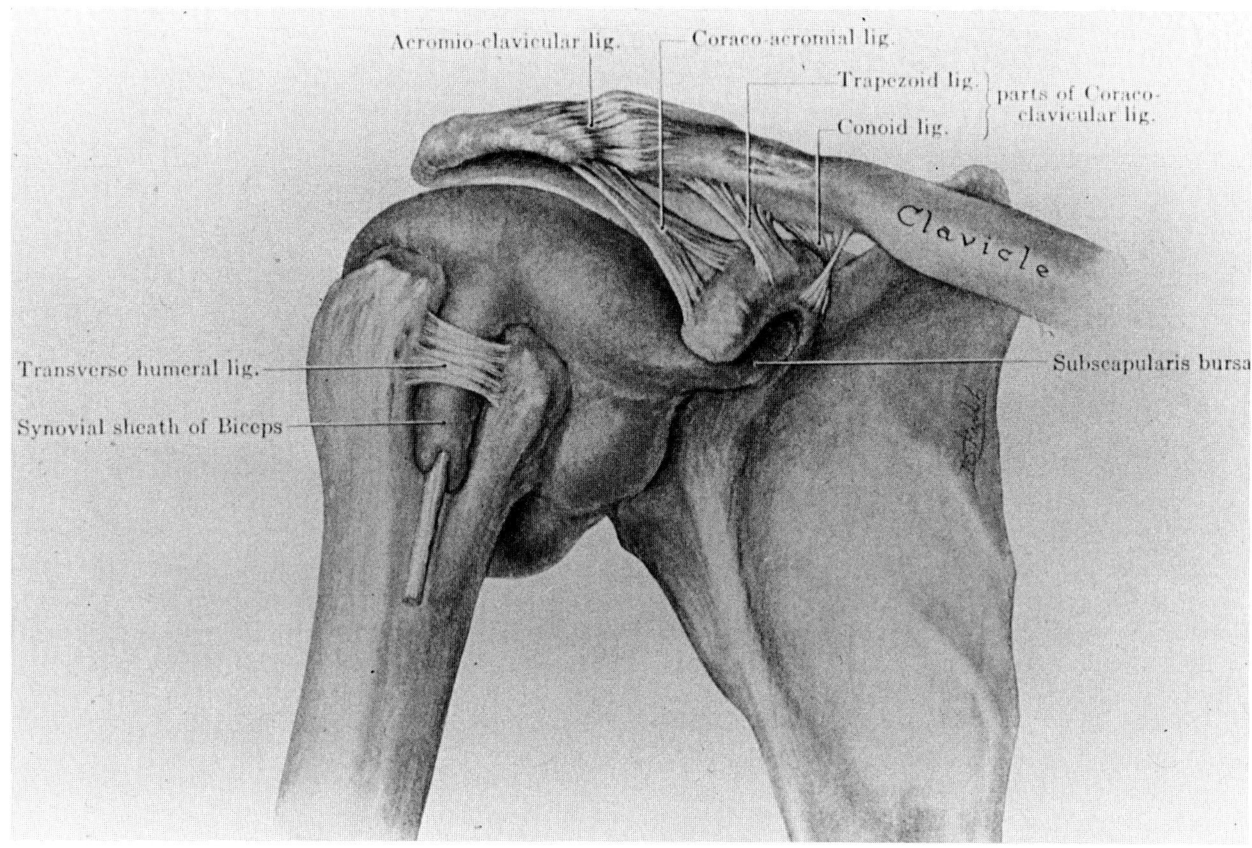

Fig. 9-1. Anatomy of the shoulder. (From Grant,[8b] with permission.)

9-2). Rheumatoid involvement of the shoulder may cause rupture of the rotator cuff, usually the supraspinatus, which results in pain and a decrease in active motion, although passive motion may be maintained. Considerable forces act on the glenohumeral joint, measured to be 10.2 times the weight of the extremity when the arm is abducted 90 degrees,[12] although Post et al.[22] stated that the compressive forces are greatly diminished when the muscle power is weak, which may be the case in rheumatoid arthritis.

INDICATIONS AND CONTRAINDICATIONS

Patient selection is important when considering major reconstructive shoulder surgery. A considerable amount of physical therapy is necessary to obtain optimal results, and surgery in an unmotivated patient is sure to bring disappointment. The patient must understand and be willing to participate in the exercise program. Surgery should be considered when pain is not controlled by good medical management and is unresponsive to conservative measures. Surgery has been successful in relieving pain, but caution should be exercised when considering shoulder surgery in the rheumatoid patient for decreased range of motion without pain, as prosthetic arthroplasty may produce little gain in motion.[5] A moderate gain in motion in some patients with multiple joint involvement, however, may be enough to increase their functional capacity by allowing the patient to fulfill the most important function of the shoulder, i.e., reaching the top of his or her head and both ends of the gastrointestinal tract.

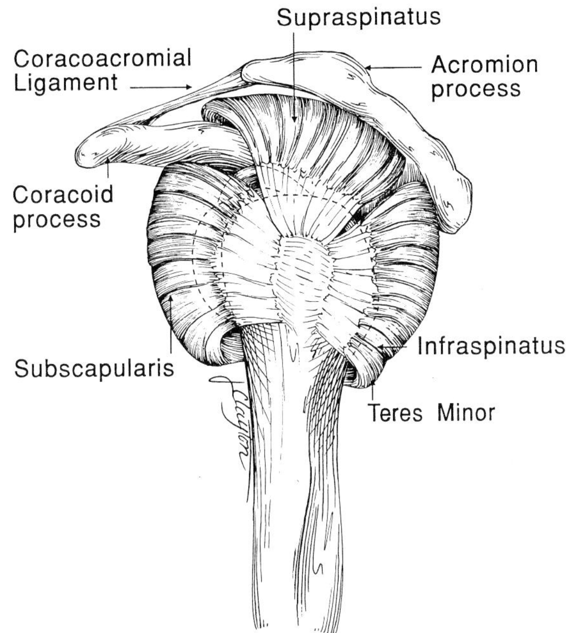

Fig. 9-2. Anatomy of the rotator cuff.

PREOPERATIVE EVALUATION

Our preoperative radiologic evaluation includes auteroposterior (AP) views in internal rotation, axillary views, and Grashey views in external ro-

tation of the shoulder. The Grashey view is obtained with the roentgenographic tube angled 35 degrees to the patient's shoulder (Fig. 9-3). This positioning opens the glenohumeral joint, making evaluation of the articular surface possible (Fig. 9-4). The standard AP view is necessary to evaluate the acromioclavicular joint, and the axillary lateral view demonstrates subluxation and loss of glenoid bone stock. If the shoulder is subluxed, an alternative procedure may be indicated. Arthrograms may be helpful when a larger rotator cuff tear is suspected so the operative procedure can be better planned. They are also useful to review the postoperative exercises before surgery so the patient has a good idea of what will follow. Range of motion, function, and pain are recorded preoperatively. Range of motion is measured in forward elevation and external and internal rotation. Active motion should be recorded in the standing position. Forward elevation instead of abduction is measured because elevation and external and internal rotation are much more useful motions for daily living. Abduction also places excessive force on the glenoid and impingement at the acromion, and it is therefore not recommended.

Preoperative function is recorded on a 100-point Denver Orthopedic Clinic evaluation sheet. Ten points are assigned to each modality

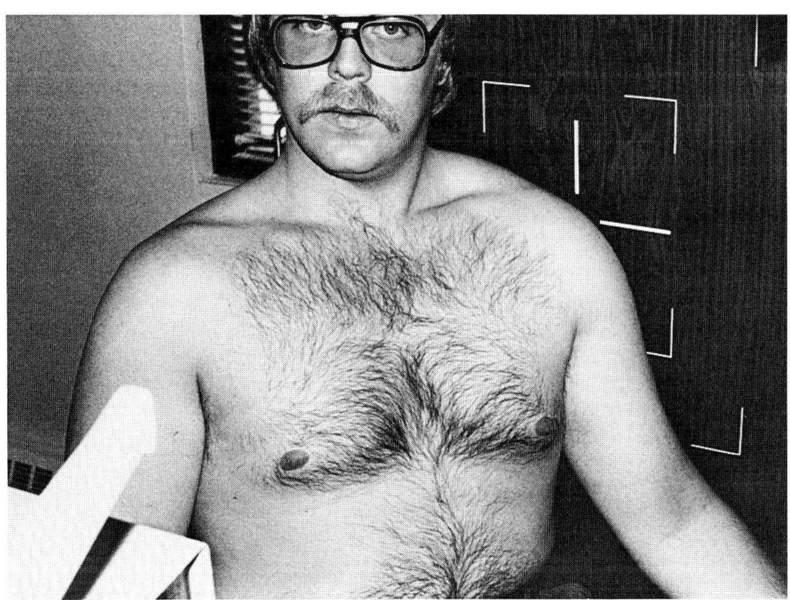

Fig. 9-3. Method of obtaining a Grashey view of the shoulder with the roentgenogram beam 35 degrees to the shoulder. (From Ferlic and Clayton,[8a] with permission.)

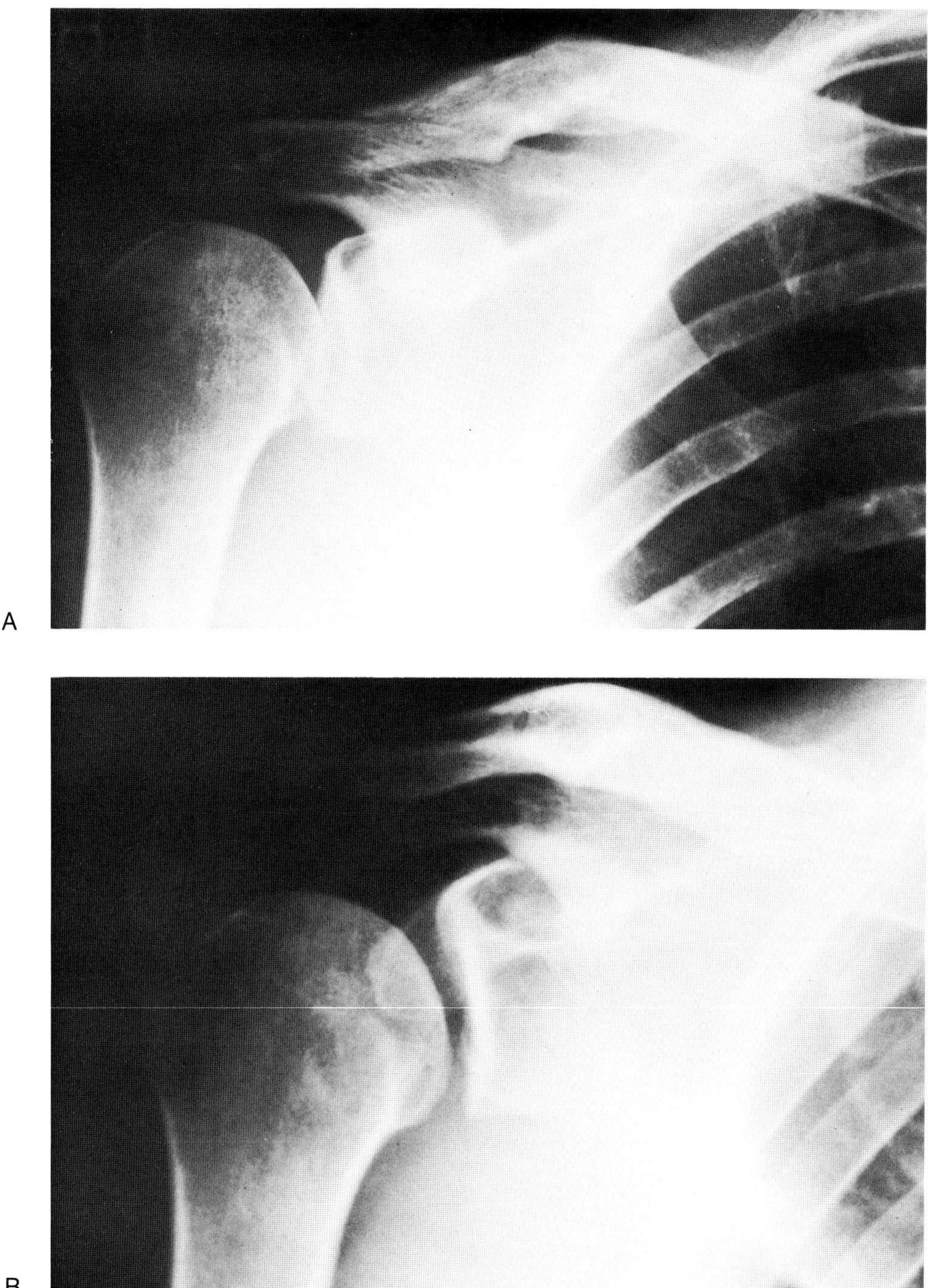

Fig. 9-4. **(A)** Standard anteroposterior view of the shoulder. **(B)** Grashey view showing the articular surface of the shoulder joint. (From Ferlic and Clayton,[8a] with permission.)

Table 9-1. Denver Orthopedic Clinic
Shoulder Function Evaluation

1. Comb hair
2. Dress
3. Use arm at shoulder level
4. Take care of hygiene
5. Reach to pocket, brassiere strap
6. Eat
7. Carry 20 pounds or more at side
8. Use arm above head
9. Sleep on the involved shoulder
10. Participate in nonviolent sports

of function if essentially normal, six points if difficult but done without assistance from the opposite extremity, three points if assistance is needed, and only one point if the task can be done only occasionally or not at all (Table 9-1). Amount of pain is measured, and patients are categorized as having no pain, mild pain (does not limit activities), moderate pain (intermittent pain at rest and with activity but still can carry out activities of daily living), and severe pain (continuous pain even at rest).

TREATMENT OPTIONS

The most recent emphasis of surgery of the rheumatoid shoulder has been on prosthetic arthroplasty, just as it has been for other joints.[1,5–7,13,15–17,19–23] It is important that other procedures are not forgotten, as they might be useful in earlier stages of the disease before prosthetic arthroplasty is indicated.

Any of the several bursae about the shoulder may become inflamed and swollen. Painful bursitis can be treated with a local steroid injection, but excision may be necessary. The subdeltoid bursa is the most commonly affected and may become large and painful (Fig. 9-5). At the time of excision, coracoacromial ligament and anterior acromionectomy is performed. Resection of the distal end of the clavicle[4,6,8,17] may be all that is necessary to relieve pain if it can be shown that the pain originates from the acromioclavicular joint (Fig. 9-6). This area is sometimes the site of symptoms, even though there are roentgenographic changes in the glenohumeral joint. An injection of local anesthetic into the acromio-

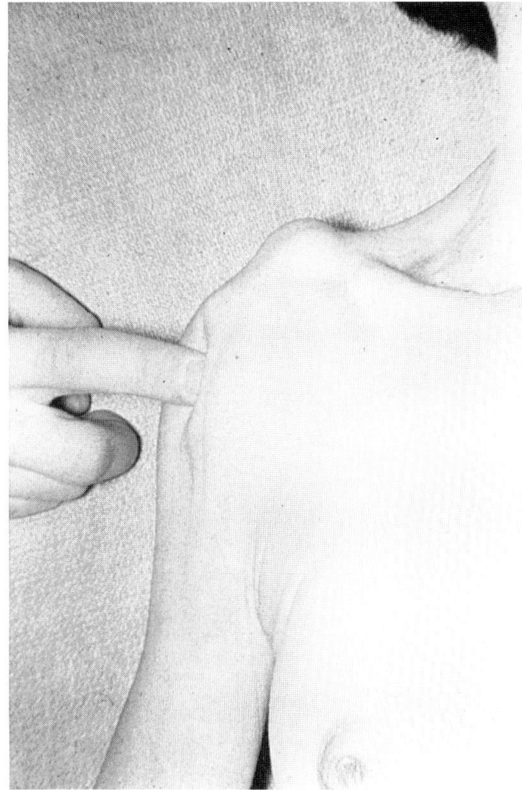

Fig. 9-5. A 36-year-old woman with continued active juvenile rheumatoid arthritis. Note the swelling of the deltoid area due to a large rheumatoid bursa.

clavicular joint may help diagnose the location of the pain.

Synovectomy and Acromionectomy

Synovectomy for stage II disease may relieve pain and retard the destructive process.[4,11,23,24] Synovectomy of the bursa and glenohumeral joint is occasionally successful and may be indicated in a patient to relieve pain when there is good motion and preservation of articular cartilage. We have performed a few shoulder synovectomies arthroscopically, a procedure that is less traumatic and has a shorter rehabilitation period. Time will tell whether this procedure can have a long-standing impact on the disease. Total acromionectomy has been shown to relieve pain in stage III patients, with excellent range of motion resulting[4,9] (Fig. 9-7), but this procedure

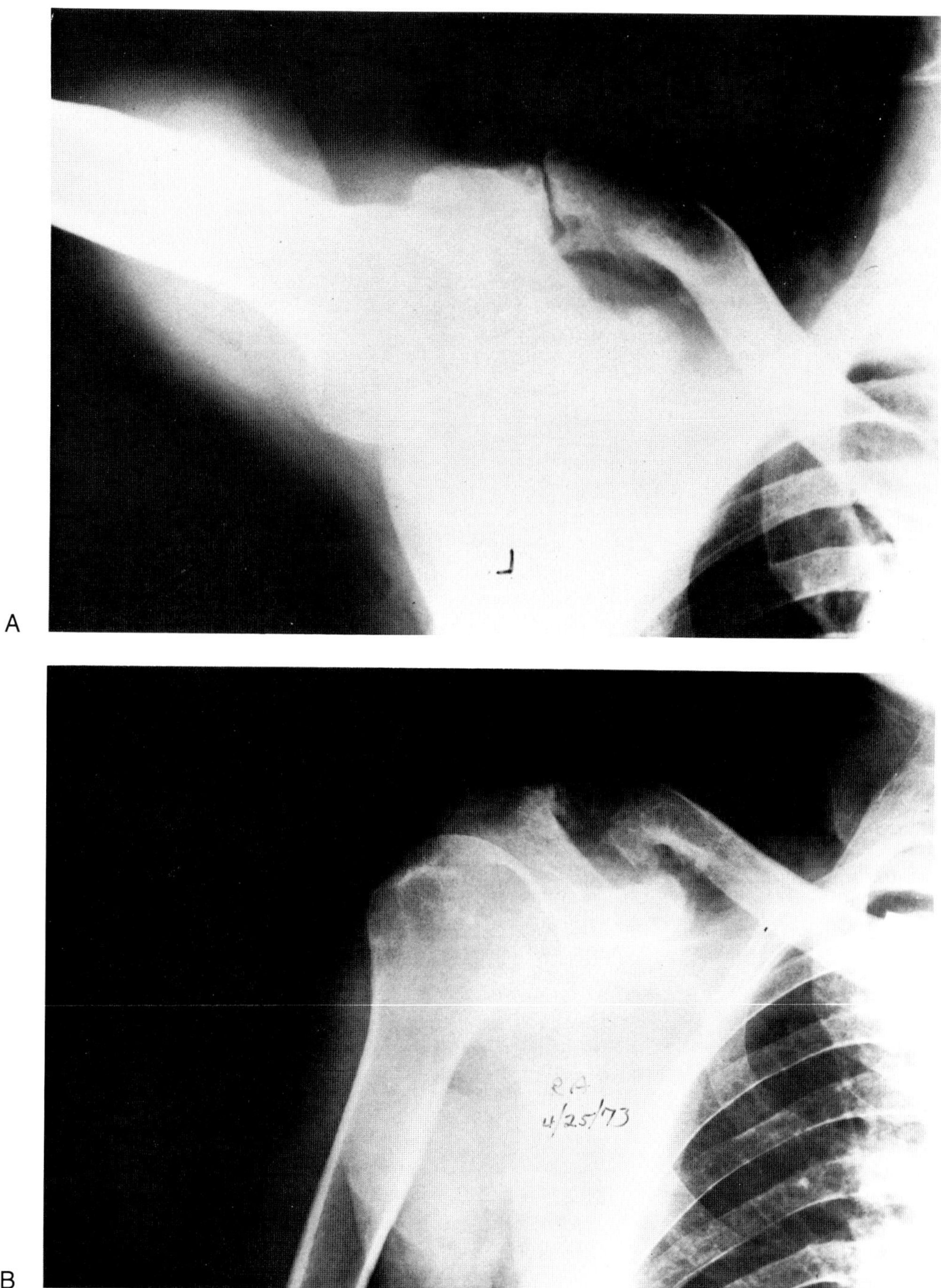

Fig. 9-6. (**A**) Preoperative roentgenogram of a rheumatoid patient's painful shoulder with narrowing in the acromioclavicular joint. (**B**) Postoperative roentgenogram showing bone resection from the distal clavicle. Pain has been relieved.

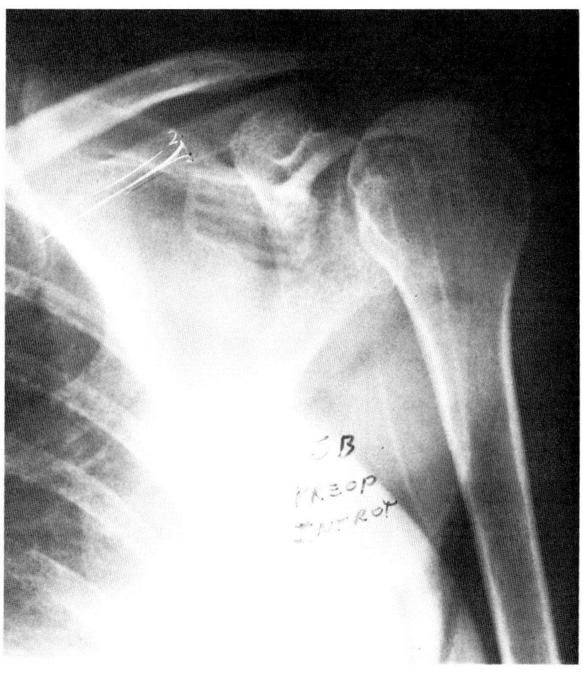

A

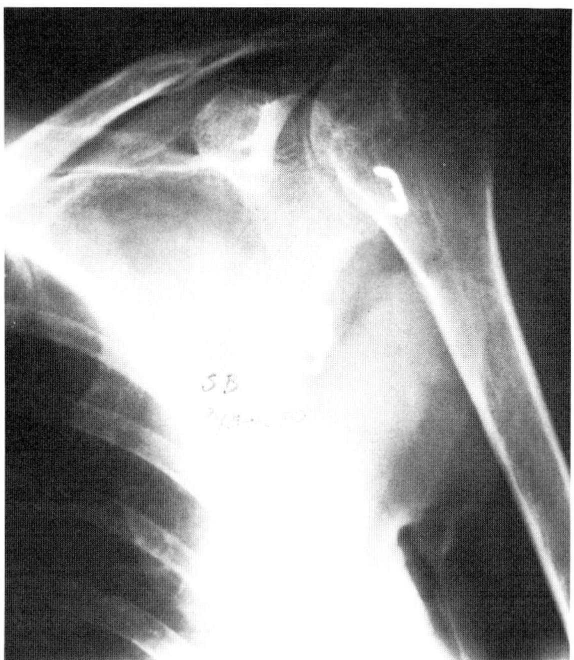

B

Fig. 9-7. (A) Preoperative roentgenogram of a patient treated with total acromionectomy and synovectomy. (B & C) Three-year postoperative roentgenograms showing full range of motion after acromionectomy. This patient did well for 10 years before joint replacement was needed. (B) Arm at side. (C) Arm in full abduction. (From Clayton,[4] with permission.)

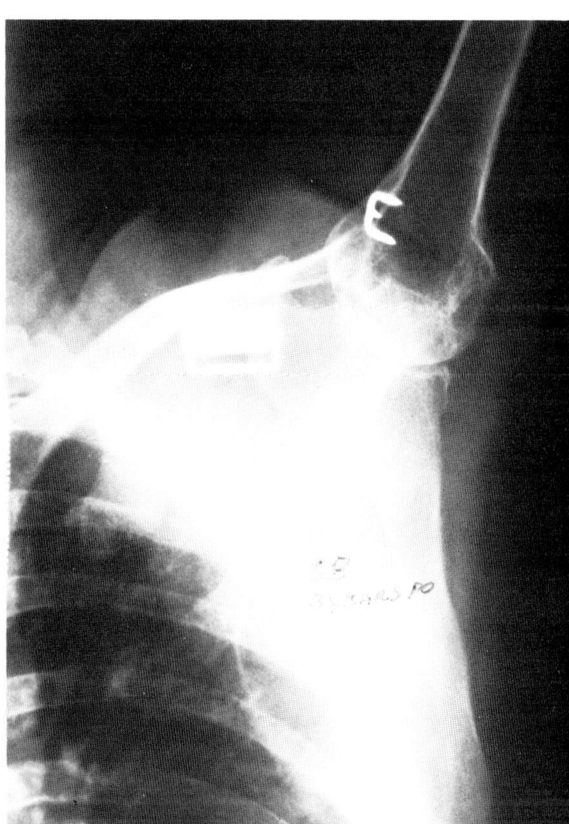

C

should rarely be done because the deltoid power is weakened, shoulder stability is diminished, and crutch-walking, which may be necessary in the rheumatoid patient, may be difficult.

Neer and Marberry[18] studied 30 patients who underwent previous radical acromionectomy. All had poor results. Twenty-seven percent experienced persistent pain, and all had marked weakness of the shoulder. None of these patients could raise the arm above the horizontal level. Although most in this series were not rheumatoid patients, Neer concluded that radical acromionectomy was not an effective procedure in any diagnostic category. Instead, the anterior acromioplasty, as advocated by Neer,[14] which eliminates the above objections, is used. The bicipital tendon may become inflamed, frayed, or ruptured. The intra-articular portion of this tendon may need to be resected and the remainder of the tendon decompressed from underneath the transverse humeral ligament.

Rotator Cuff Repair

The rotator cuff is a frequent source of symptoms in the rheumatoid shoulder. Simple tendinitis can often be treated with anti-inflammatory medications or an occasional steroid injection, but frequent injections are not used because of an increased incidence of tendon rupture and articular cartilage degeneration. Tendinitis and bursitis may give rise to impingement at the coracoacromial arch, and decompression is indicated by excising the coracoacromial ligament and beveling the undersurface of the acromion. Small holes in the rotator cuff may require repair, but large rotator cuff tears may be more difficult in the rheumatoid patient because of attenuation of tissue. There are some cases of rotator cuff rupture that are irreparable even with extensive mobilization of the supraspinatus, superior transposition of the scapularis, or use of a bicipital tendon patch. A subacromial spacer for these cases has been developed with the help of Peter Giammichele (Fig. 9-8). It was designed to depress the humeral head, thereby giving the deltoid a better mechanical advantage and, enabling it to initiate abduction and act as a rotator cuff. In addition, the spacer changes the relative position of the articular surfaces, a result similar to that achieved by performing an osteotomy. The first spacer was manufactured from chrome–cobalt alloy and was used without any humeral replacement.

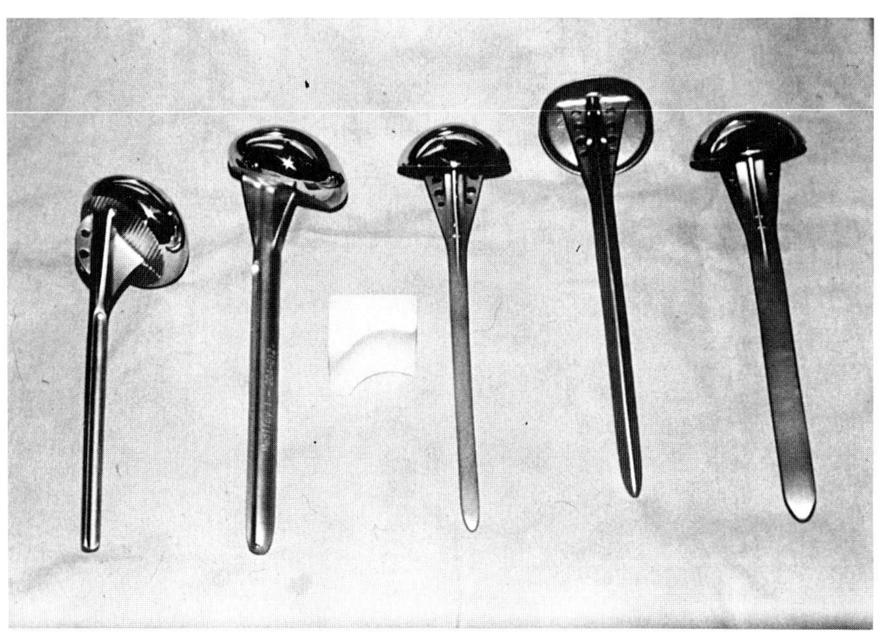

Fig. 9-8. Subacromial spacer with Neer prostheses. (From Clayton,[4] with permission.)

Case Report 1

A 56-year-old woman had a 16-year history of rheumatoid arthritis with multiple joint involvement. The patient had previously undergone multiple surgical procedures in both upper and lower extremities. Because of pain, decreased motion, and crepitation, a synovectomy was done, and a specially designed metallic prosthesis was inserted. Postoperatively, her pain was greatly reduced. She can use her arm much more easily and has a markedly increased range of motion (Fig. 9-9).

The spacer successfully relieved pain; but in order to use it the acromion and a functioning deltoid must be present. The coracoacromial ligament is also helpful (Fig. 9-10).

The metal spacer has been used alone successfully in nonrheumatoid patients with massive irreparable rotator cuff ruptures. Most of our experience is with the spacer composed of polyethylene and used with a humeral metallic implant. We are not using the spacer at this time, as other devices and techniques have become available.

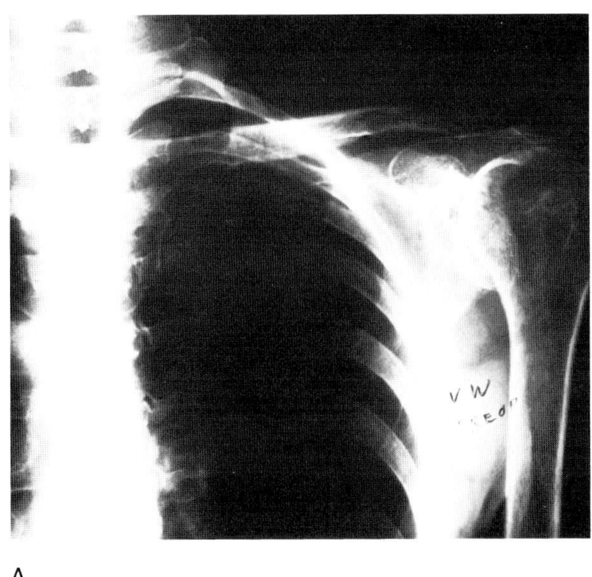

A

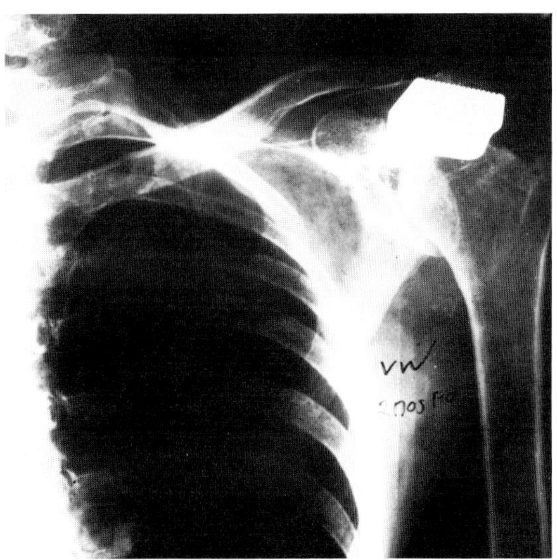

B

C

Fig. 9-9. (A) Preoperative roentgenogram of patient reated with a vitallium subacromial spacer. Note the severe destruction of the glenohumeral joint with a high-riding humerus, suggestive of a large rotator cuff rupture. (**B & C**) Postoperative roentgenograms with arm at side (**B**) and in abduction (**C**). (From Clayton,[4] with permission.)

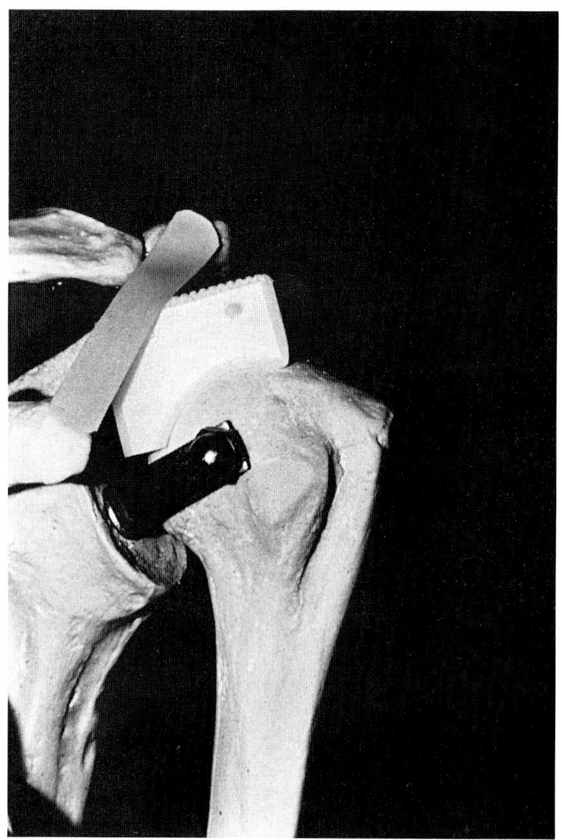

Fig. 9-10. Subacromial spacer in place showing the anterior buttress of the coracoacromial ligament. The spacer is fixed with sutures, and no cement is used.

Osteotomy and Glenoidectomy

Three other procedures in particular must be mentioned regarding surgery of the rheumatoid shoulder. Osteotomy of the glenoid and humeral neck (double osteotomy) has been shown by Benjamin et al.[2] to relieve pain and improve the roentgenographic picture. We have had no experience with this operation. The second is glenoidectomy, which is not as good as a total shoulder arthroplasty but has been effective for relieving pain.

Case Report 2
A 65-year-old woman presented in 1978 because of severe pain in her right shoulder. She had a 30-year history of rheumatoid arthritis and marked involvement of almost all her joints. She had been using a wheelchair for 9 years. The patient is right-handed and had become further incapacitated because of the shoulder involvement. Her preoperative roentgenogram (Fig. 9-11) showed severe destruction of the joint with considerable loss of bone stock of the glenoid. The humeral head was subluxed superiorly with impingement of the inferior rim of the glenoid against the shaft of the proximal humerus. Her motion was 45 degree active and 70 degrees passive forward flexion, external rotation 45 degrees, internal rotation 90 degrees, and abduction 0 degrees.

The shoulder was surgically explored in August 1978. Complete loss of the rotator cuff was found, and the glenoid was markedly degenerated. The posterior rim of the glenoid was abutting against the shaft of the humerus, which was dislocated superiorly, touching the acromioclavicular joint. Because of the severe destruction, it was not thought possible to insert a prosthesis. Therefore the glenoid was resected along with the distal clavicle (Fig. 9-12). Postoperatively she did well, with relief of pain and better function.

Arthrodesis

The third procedure is arthrodesis. There is no place for shoulder fusion in rheumatoid arthritis,[2,4] because of the multiple joint component of the disease, although Cooney and Bryan[8] stated that if other joints in the extremity are mobile and the disease is quiescent arthrodesis may be considered. We have seen one such patient in whom arthrodesis was performed. Other joints became debilitated later, and the stiff shoulder, though painless, proved to be a marked hindrance.

Arthroplasty

Prosthetic replacement is now the mainstay of shoulder surgery for rheumatoid arthritis (Fig. 9-13). All of the preceding procedures are occasionally useful by themselves as well as in conjunction with replacement surgery. Prosthetic replacement of the shoulder joint has been

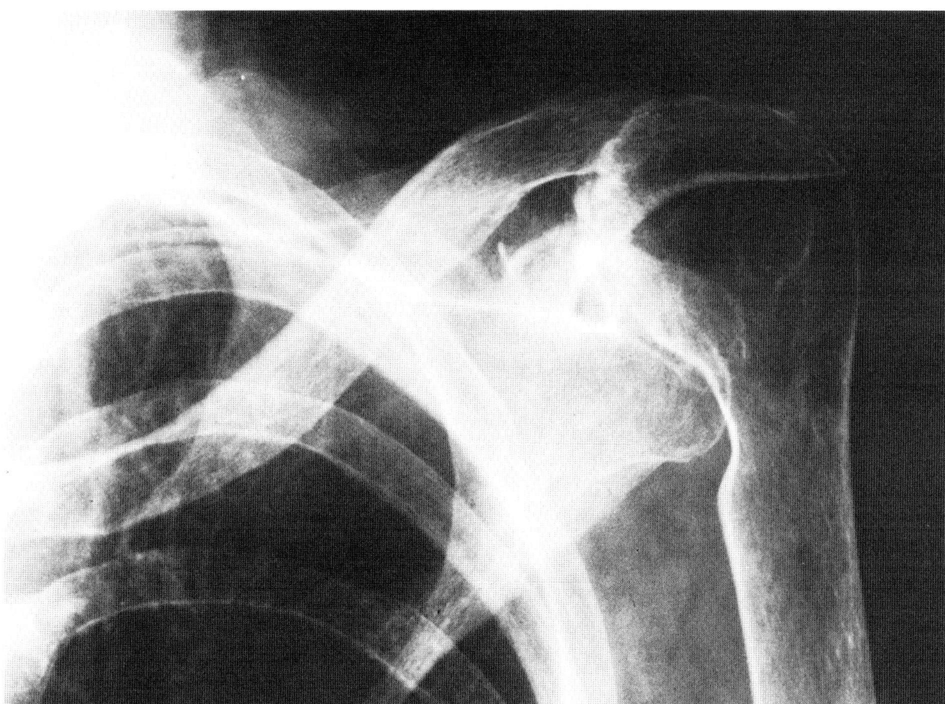

Fig. 9-11. Preoperative roentgenogram of a patient with severe destruction of the shoulder, bone loss of the glenoid, and impingement of the humeral shaft against the glenoid.

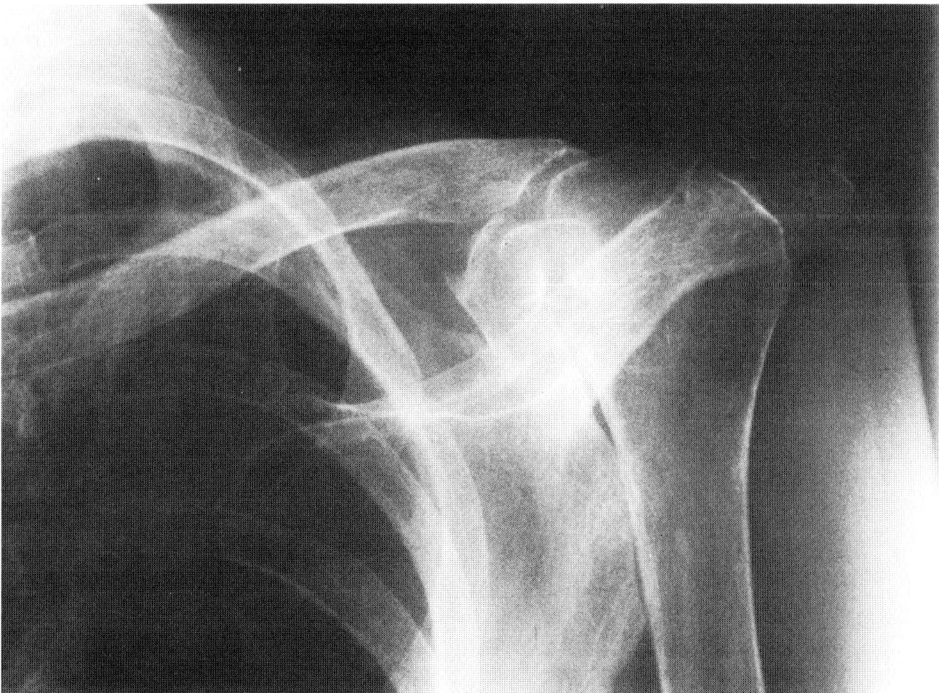

Fig. 9-12. Postoperative roentgenogram of the shoulder treated with glenoid resection arthroplasty, which helped relieve the pain.

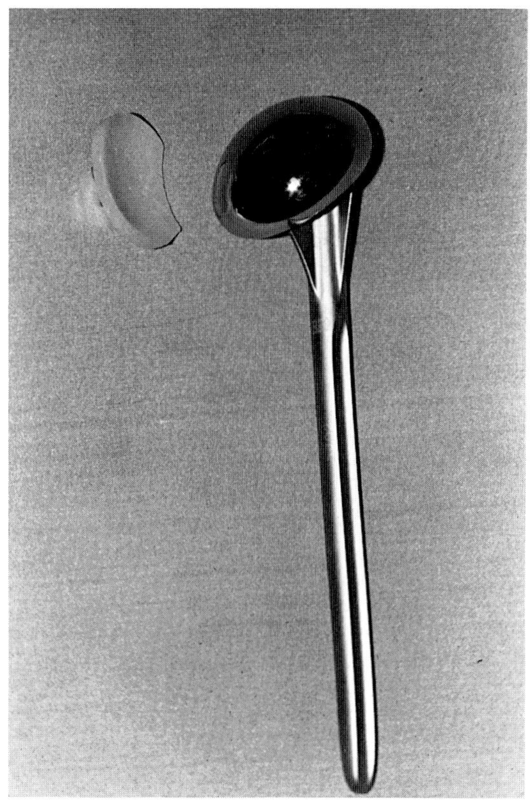

Fig. 9-13. Neer total shoulder.

developed because less radical procedures, e.g., resectional arthroplasties and arthrodeses, have consistently failed to produce satisfactory results.

Neer[15] developed a nonconstrained prosthesis for shoulders with reparable rotator cuffs and good muscle. Cofield[6,7] reported 25 procedures using this prosthesis, with all patients attaining satisfactory pain relief and stability. Marmor[13] described ten patients in whom hemiarthroplasty resulted in good pain relief and a "modest" gain in shoulder motion over an average follow-up period of 4.5 years. In 1974 Neer[16] reported good results with hemiarthroplasties in 41 of 47 shoulders where pain relief and postoperative range of motion was consistently good, although it was not specified whether it was active or passive motion. There were no infections, dislocations, loosening or settling of the prostheses, or evidence of intrusion or resorption of the glenoid. A later abstract from a multicenter study[19] emphasized

poor muscle reconstruction and inadequate postoperative rehabilitation as the cause of 21 of 83 unsatisfactory results.

In 1982 Neer et al.[20] reported 273 metal to plastic total shoulder replacements, of which 69 were done for rheumatoid arthritis. There were no instances of clinical loosening, but radiolucent lines were seen in 30 percent (Fig. 9-14). Twelve patients required further surgery. Neer developed two categories of patients: One included patients for whom a full exercise program was indicated, and the other, a "limited goals" category, included the 20 percent in his series who had a massive deficiency of bone or muscle. Of the patients in the full exercise program, 86 percent achieved an excellent or satisfactory rating, and those with good muscles often attained essentially normal motion and function. Fifty shoulders in Neer's rheumatoid group were followed for more than 24 months. Seven patients with massive rotator cuff tears were successfully treated on a limited goals basis. Among the remaining 43 patients, the clinical results were excellent in 28, satisfactory in 12, and unsatisfactory in 3. Rehabilitation time was generally much longer than in the osteoarthritic group.

Occasionally, there is a need for the constrained shoulder (e.g., with dislocation, irreparable rotator cuffs, or paralysis), but we think that the incidence of failure due to loosening and dislocation is high. Post et al.[21] reported on 43 shoulder joint replacements using a constrained joint, only four of which were done for rheumatoid arthritis. They reported 12 material failures in the first series of 22 shoulders, but only 2 in the second modified series of 21 shoulders. There was no loosening of the humeral component, although radiolucent lines were observed around some of the components.

Cofield[6] reviewed the Mayo Clinic results of constrained Bickel and Stanmore prostheses and compared them with the results of the nonconstrained Neer replacement arthroplasties. He found that the nonconstrained prostheses allowed greater postoperative motion, preserved bone stock, and eliminated mechanical failure if the rotator cuff was intact or could be repaired. We prefer to use a nonconstrained shoulder such as the Neer or Gristina, and lately we have been

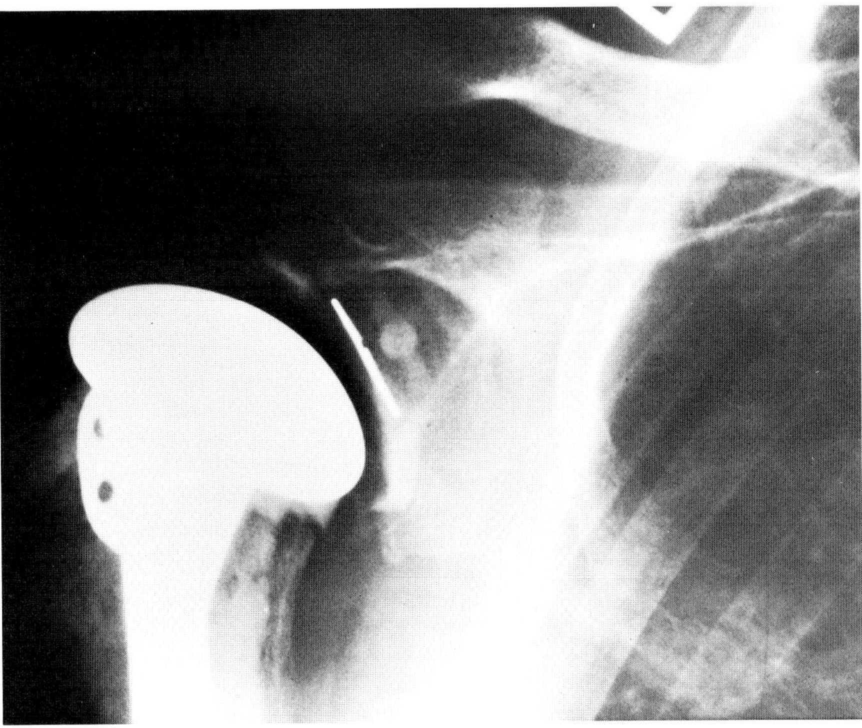

Fig. 9-14. Total shoulder with a radiolucent line at the cement–bone interface at the inferior aspect of the glenoid. This picture indicates possible loosening, although it is asymptomatic; this line has not progressed over 5 years.

using a modular device with various size heads and stems.

The Denver Orthopedic Clinic has divided shoulder prosthetic arthroplasties into three groups: Group I includes those in which the Neer humeral replacement was used alone; group II includes those with the humeral replacement used in conjunction with subacromial spacer; and group III includes those with the humeral component and the glenoid replacement. The glenoid component has been used in all of the recent humeral implants for rheumatoid arthritis owing to the erosion of the glenoid occasionally seen after several years when the vitallium humeral head has been left to articulate with the articular cartilage of the glenoid. The most recent cases have been done with modular components (Fig. 9-15).

Operative Technique

An incision extending from the acromioclavicular joint to the axilla is generally used, but additional exposure is obtained by making an incision beginning 0.5 inch inferior to the distal third of the clavicle and extending down the humerus to the deltoid insertion (Fig. 9-16). The deltopectoral groove is developed *from clavicle to deltoid insertion*, but the deltoid is not released from its bony origin, as it would significantly delay rehabilitation. The rotator cuff is examined, and small defects are later repaired directly. The superior portion of the subscapularis can be advanced superiorly to aid in repair of a defect (Fig. 9-17A & B). The tendinous portion of the subscapularis is divided, leaving enough tendon attached distally for later repair.

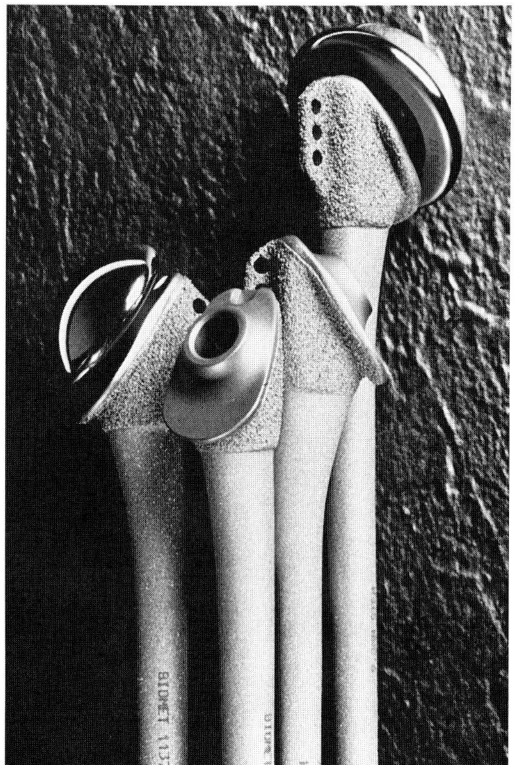

Fig. 9-15. Modular humeral components.

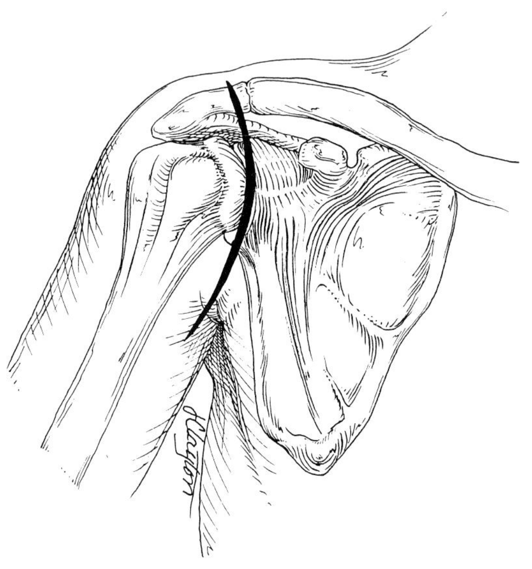

Fig. 9-16. Skin incision for shoulder replacement. (From Clayton,[3a] with permission.)

If the shoulder has an internal rotation contracture, the subscapularis is divided by beveling the tendon so it can be lengthened when closing. The capsule of the shoulder joint is opened and the joint inspected.

An anterior acromionectomy is carried out by removing a minimal wedge of bone if it is impinging on the rotator cuff. Extensive acromionectomy is unnecessary and is contraindicated because of its later effect on deltoid function. If there are arthritic changes in the acromioclavicular joint, the distal clavicle is excised. It may be necessary to remove osteophytes from the inferior surface of the joint. A synovectomy is carried out if boggy synovium is present. The bicipital tendon helps to stabilize the shoulder and is left in place if possible; but if it has already torn, the intra-articular portion is excised. This tendon can sometimes be used to aid in the repair of a rotator cuff tear. The humeral head is then dislocated and the articular surface excised, making the cut in 35 degrees of retroversion, which allows proper seating of the prosthesis (Fig. 9-17C).

Care should be taken to preserve as much of the humeral neck as possible. At this point, we have to make our final decision as to what type of arthroplasty is needed. If the glenoid articular surface is uninvolved, we prepare the intramedullary canal of the humerus with rasps and high-speed burrs. Trial reductions begin with a small stemmed humeral component. Once we have determined the proper size, a larger-stemmed component is used. This method may result in a tight press-fit, but we do not hesitate to use cement fixation if there is any question of component stability.

All of our recent rheumatoid arthritis patients with shoulder involvement have undergone total shoulder replacement. In this situation, the humeral implantation is the last step in our procedure. The coracoacromial ligament if left intact.

Osteophytes are trimmed as necessary, allowing visualization of the true glenoid. A high-speed burr prepares the glenoid surface. The surgeon defines the scapular neck with his or her fingers and carefully burrs a seating hole in a position to accept the stem of the glenoid component. Only the cartilage is removed from the re-

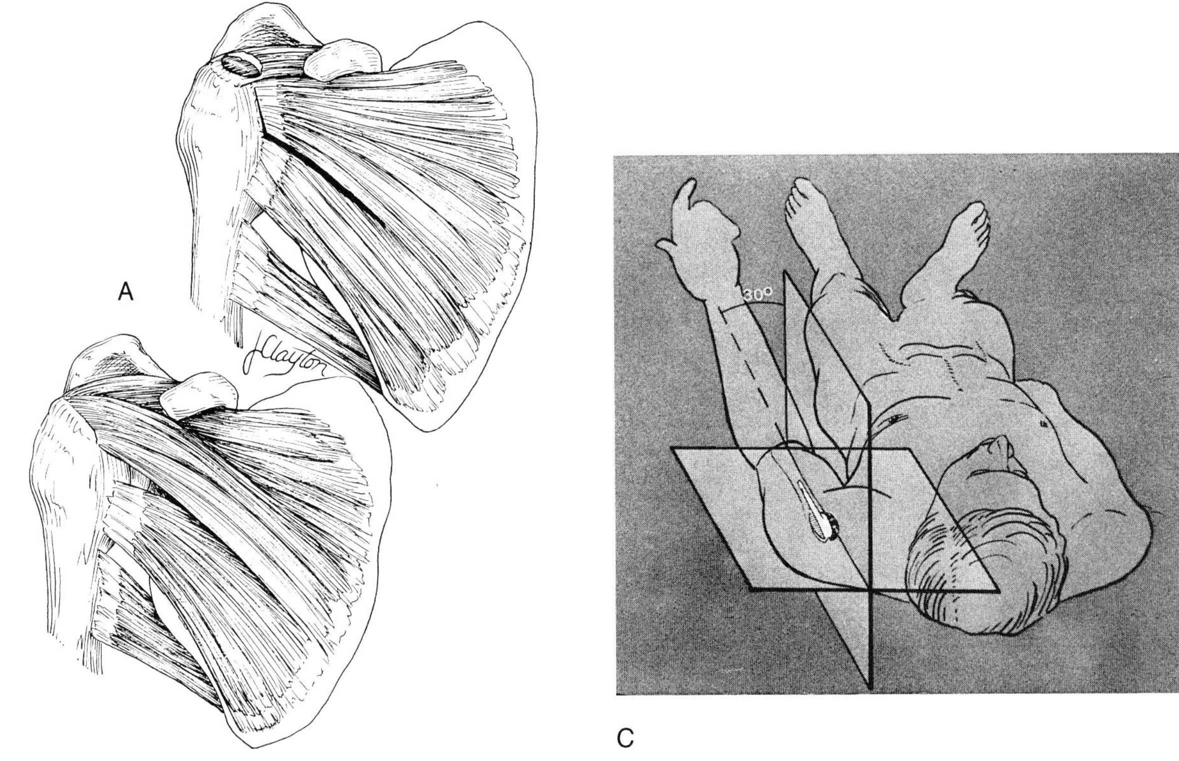

Fig. 9-17. (A) Repair of a rotator cuff defect by superior shifting of the subscapularis. (B) Humeral head is excised at 30 to 35 degrees of retroversion.

mainder of the glenoid; the subchondral bone is not removed. The component is cemented in place using low-viscosity, pressurized cement. The humerus is prepared, and trial reductions of both components are completed. If cement is to be used, the humerus is plugged just distal to the stem. The cement is injected and the humeral component cemented. If the rotator cuff must be repaired, the long head of the biceps tendon may be taken down from its glenoid insertion and used for repair. It can be widened by longitudinal splitting if the defect requires a larger graft. The biceps stump is reattached distally. The subscapularis can also be used for rotator cuff reinforcement by dividing a portion and advancing it superiorly and distally, or it can be lengthened if the internal rotation contracture limits external rotation to the neutral position. The wound is closed, and the patient is placed in a sling and swathe, unless it was necessary to perform an extensive rotator cuff repair. In these cases, a hu-

meral foam rubber splint or an airplane splint is used to keep the arm in 60 degrees of forward flexion.

Postoperative Rehabilitation

Patients are encouraged in hand, wrist, forearm, and elbow motion for the first 3 days after surgery. Therapy is divided into three stages. Stage I lasts 4 days to 3 weeks. In this stage, only passive and gentle assisted exercises are done. Pendulum exercises and passive range of motion are begun on the fourth day. Motion, especially external rotation exercise, is limited only by the integrity of the repair when tested at the time of surgery. The subscapularis repair is protected by internally rotating and adducting the arm for all forward flexion exercises. At the end of 1 week, the sling may be discarded during the daytime, and active assisted exercises are begun. A knowledgeable therapist checks the patient on a daily basis for a minimum of 3 weeks, at which time active assisted exercises with the aid of pulley and stick are instituted.

Stage II is from 4 to 6 weeks. In addition to active assisted exercises, gentle active exercises may be started, depending on the patient's musculature, needs, and strength of repair. Active motion is started at the beginning of the fourth postoperative week. If the deltoid muscle had not been detached at the time of surgery, active motion quickly progresses. Although the group of our patients in whom the deltoid was not taken down progressed more rapidly, the ultimate outcome was not different in the two groups.

Stage III starts 6 weeks after surgery. Active resistive exercises are added to the active exercise program.

Note: It is *important* to treat each patient as an individual and adjust the rehabilitation schedule according to the specific surgical repair.

Results

Good pain relief can be expected, but there may be limited increase in motion. Therefore if replacement arthroplasty is done for the painless, stiff shoulder, the end result may disappoint the patient. In our series with a minimum of 2 years' follow-up evaluation, the rheumatoid arthritic patients with a hemiarthroplasty gained an average of 11 degrees elevation (64 to 75 degrees), 12 degrees external rotation (30 to 42 degrees) and 7 degrees internal rotation (74 to 81 degrees). The total shoulder group gained 35 degrees elevation (59 to 94 degrees), 12 degrees external rotation (34 to 46 degrees), and 3 degrees internal rotation (87 to 90 degrees). The spacer group gained 40 degrees elevation (38 to 78 degrees), 28 degrees external rotation (5 to 33 degrees), and 15 degrees internal rotation (75 to 90 degrees). From these figures we cannot single out any one operative procedure as being better in terms of increasing range of motion. Although we anticipated less satisfactory results in patients in whom a spacer was used for an irreparable rotator cuff and the tissues were generally of poorer quality, it was not found to be the case. Pain relief was

satisfactory, and 86 percent achieved good or excellent relief at the end of 2 years. We have also seen two patients with hemiarthroplasties who started to erode the glenoid after 5 years. One of these patients developed shoulder pain after 5 years, and we believe that the erosion may be causing the pain. In a more recent study,[3] we reported 92 percent survivorship at 11 years of unconstrained total shoulder arthroplasties in patients with rheumatoid arthritis.

Case Report 3

A 32-year-old woman with rheumatoid arthritis from 8 years of age, multiple joint involvement, and numerous previous surgeries to her wrists, feet, knees, and hips presented with severe right shoulder pain and marked crepitation. She could actively elevate her right shoulder 70 degrees, although passively it could be brought up 128 degrees with considerable crepitation. External rotation reached 40 degrees, and she could internally rotate to where she could place her hand behind her back. The left shoulder showed limited abduction to 35 degrees. Roentgenograms showed marked destruction of the right shoulder joint (Fig. 9-18A).

On October 29, 1972, a Neer prosthesis was inserted into the right shoulder. The rotator cuff was torn, but repair was possible by rotating the superior half of the subscapularis to fill the deficit. In December 1972 she could elevate the shoulder 150 degrees, abduct 60 degrees, and externally rotate 45 degrees. In January 1974 the shoulder had active elevation to 90 degrees, and she could get her hand behind her head and low back (Fig. 9-18B). In May 1978 she could elevate her shoulder passively 135 degrees and actively 110 degrees; she could externally rotate 25 degrees; and she could reach behind her back and head. In 1979 the same motion was maintained, but roentgenograms showed some glenoid invagination (Fig. 9-18C). She has maintained good function up to now and has better motion than the unoperated left shoulder, which is painless.

Note: Another patient's shoulder was subluxed inferiorly preoperatively, and postoperatively she was kept in a Kenny-Howard type of acromioclavicular splint, which kept the shoulder reduced until the capsule tightened up and the

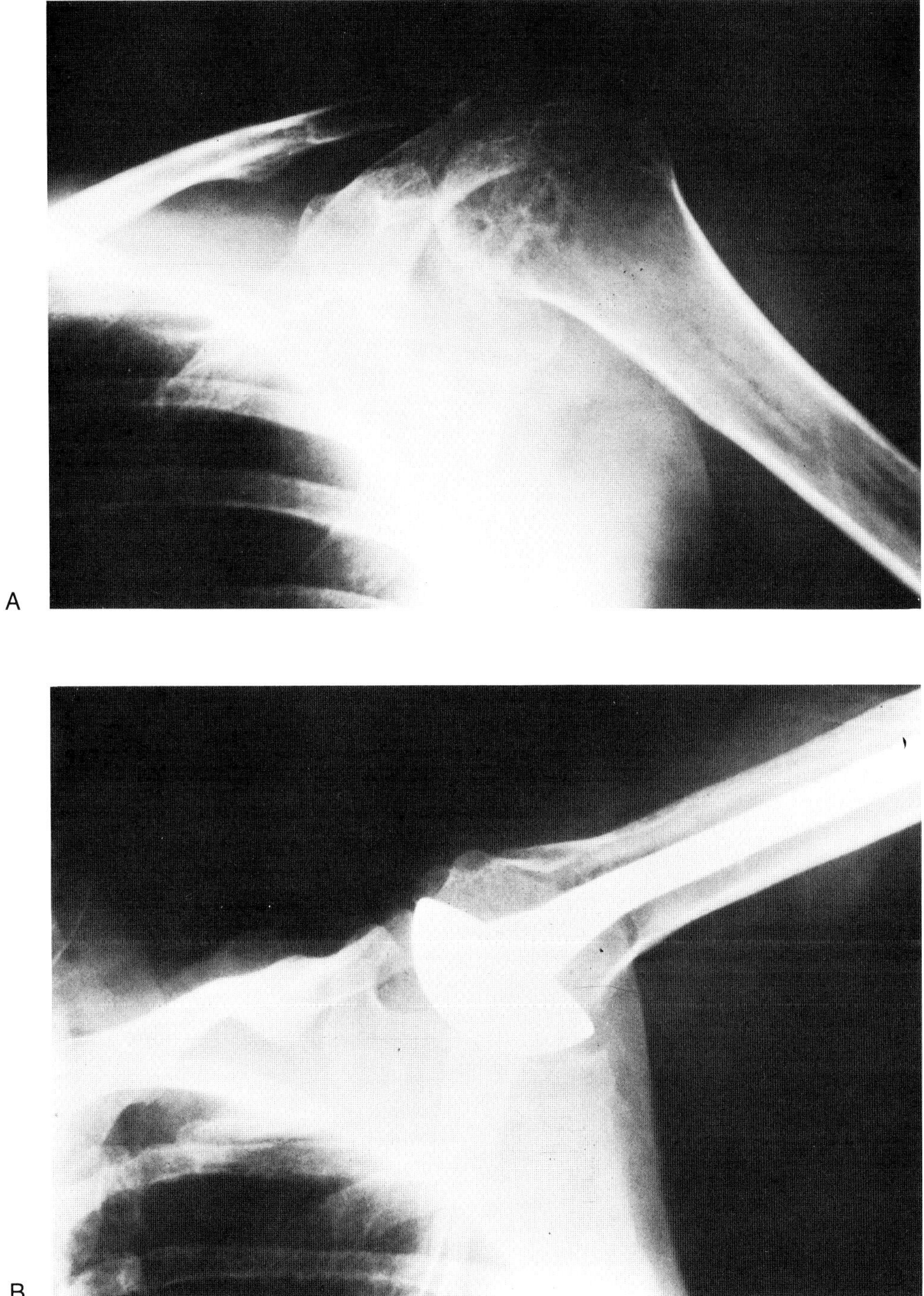

Fig. 9-18. (**A**) Preoperative roentgenogram of the right shoulder showing marked arthritic involvement. (**B**) Immediate postoperative roentgenogram with arm abducted, showing the position of the prosthesis in relation to the glenoid. (*Figure continues.*)

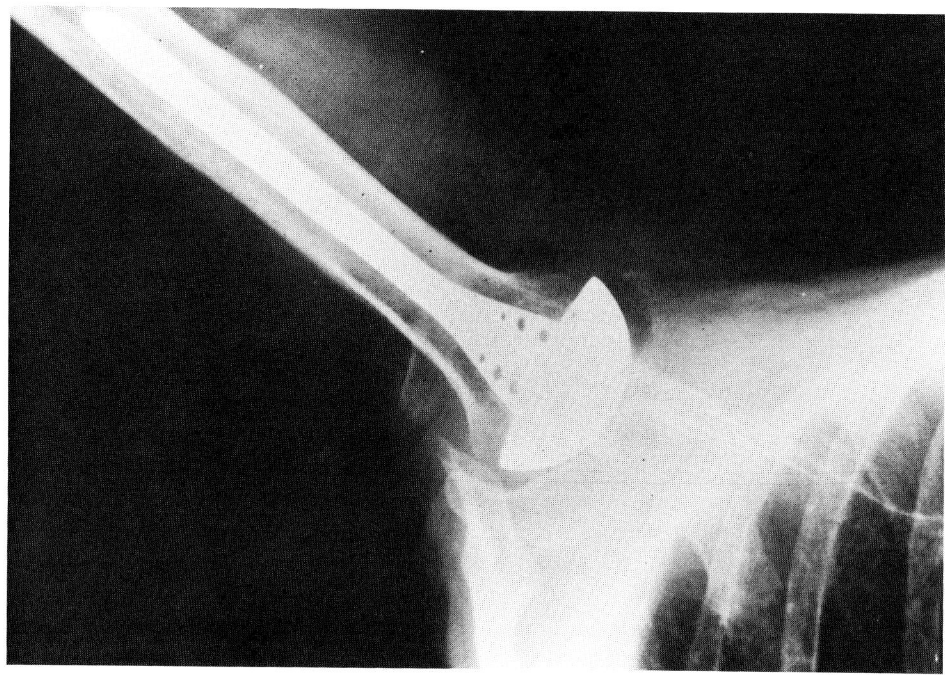

C

Fig. 9-18 (*Continued*). (**C**) Five-year postoperative roentgenogram showing erosion of the glenoid.

shoulder girdle musculature was rehabilitated. This operation thus produced a good result.

Case Report 4

A 54-year-old woman who had had rheumatoid arthritis for 30 years presented in May 1977 with pain and limited motion of her right shoulder of 1 year's duration. She had been on cortisone, gold, and many nonsteroidal anti-inflammatory medications in the past. The shoulder pain was unresponsive to an intra-articular steroid injection.

Examination of the shoulder revealed considerable muscular atrophy with marked crepitation and pain on motion. Active forward elevation was 65 degrees, external rotation 60 degrees, and internal rotation to where she could put her hand behind her buttocks. Roentgenograms showed irregularity of the glenohumeral joint, with narrowing and inferior subluxation of the humeral head (Fig. 9-19A).

On July 5, 1977 a Neer total shoulder replacement was performed. Postoperatively she had some persistent inferior subluxation of the prosthesis (Fig. 9-19B), which was treated in a Kenny Howard type of acromioclavicular dislocation splint until her shoulder girdle musculature could be strengthened.

Roentgenograms showed good position of the prosthesis 2 years later (Fig. 9-19C). Motion showed elevation to be 170 degrees, external rotation 55 degrees, and internal rotation to where she could ge her hand behind her back. She is still functioning but has mild pain due to a loose glenoid.

Note: Functionally, our patients averaged a more than 100 percent increase in score compared to the preoperative level.[5]

Case Report 5

A 26-year-old woman with juvenile rheumatoid arthritis from the age of 5 developed an increasing amount of pain and limitation of motion of both shoulders to the extent that they markedly inhibited her daily activities. Previous surgery consisted of bilateral total hip replacements. When first seen in March 1981, examination of

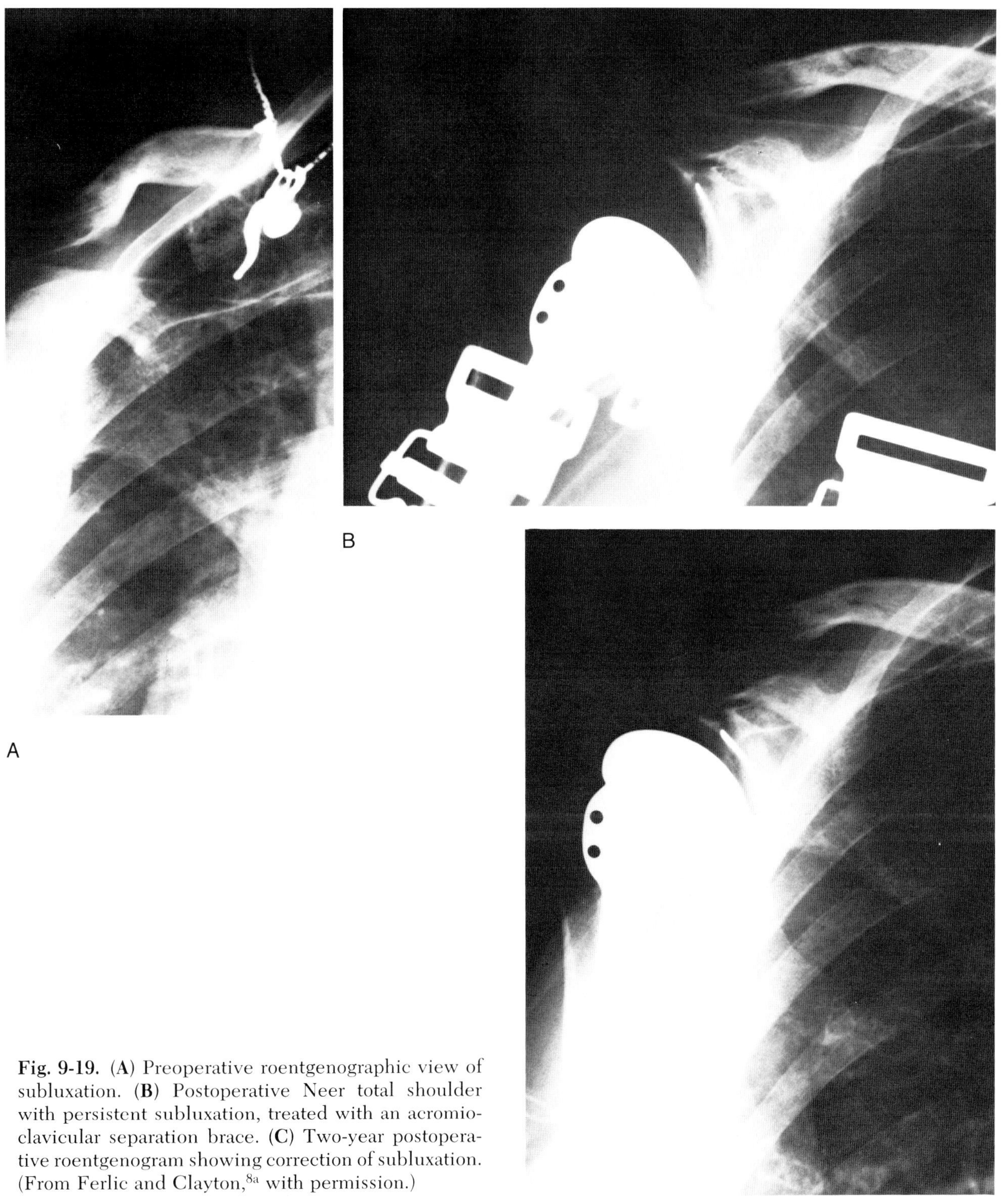

Fig. 9-19. (**A**) Preoperative roentgenographic view of subluxation. (**B**) Postoperative Neer total shoulder with persistent subluxation, treated with an acromioclavicular separation brace. (**C**) Two-year postoperative roentgenogram showing correction of subluxation. (From Ferlic and Clayton,[8a] with permission.)

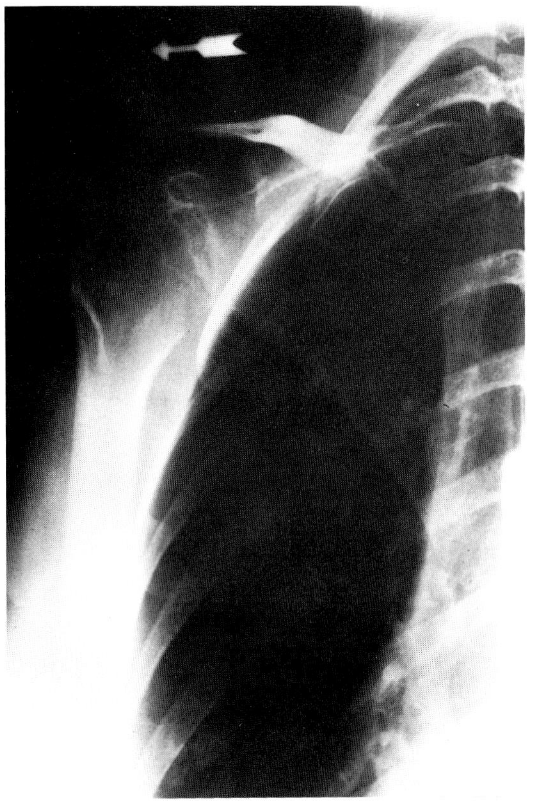

A

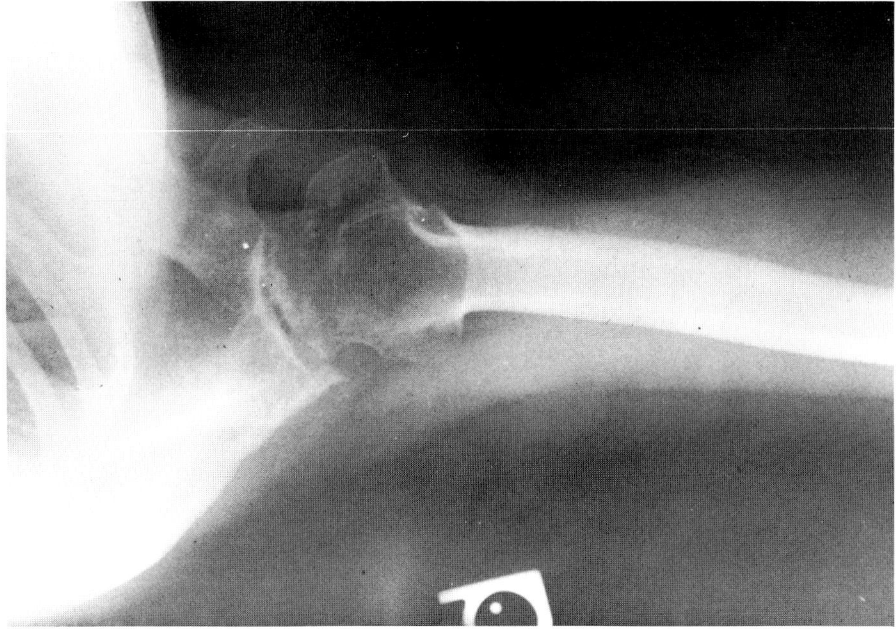

B

Fig. 9-20. Preoperative anteroposterior (**A**) and axillary lateral (**B**) roentgenograms of the right shoulder in a patient with juvenile rheumatoid arthritis showing severe destruction of the glenohumeral joint with the small size of the bones. (From Clayton et al.,[5] with permission.)

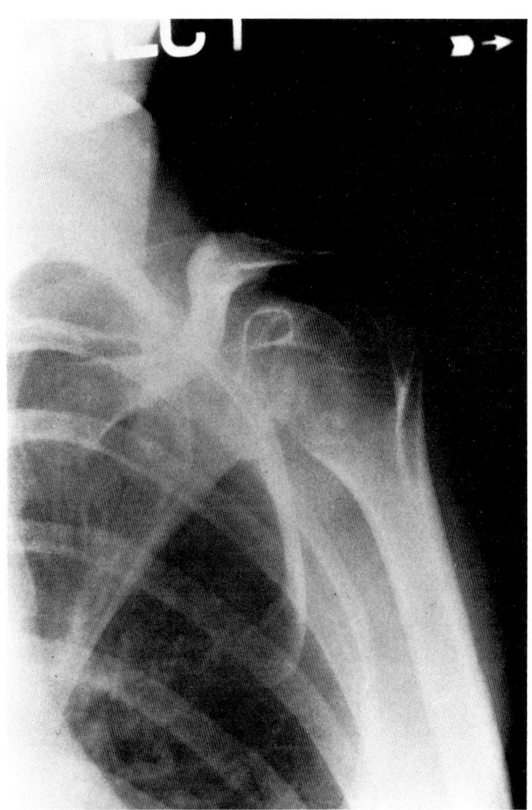

A

Fig. 9-21. Preoperative anteroposterior (**A**) and axillary lateral (**B**) roentgenograms of the left shoulder with severe destruction and small size of the medullary canal.

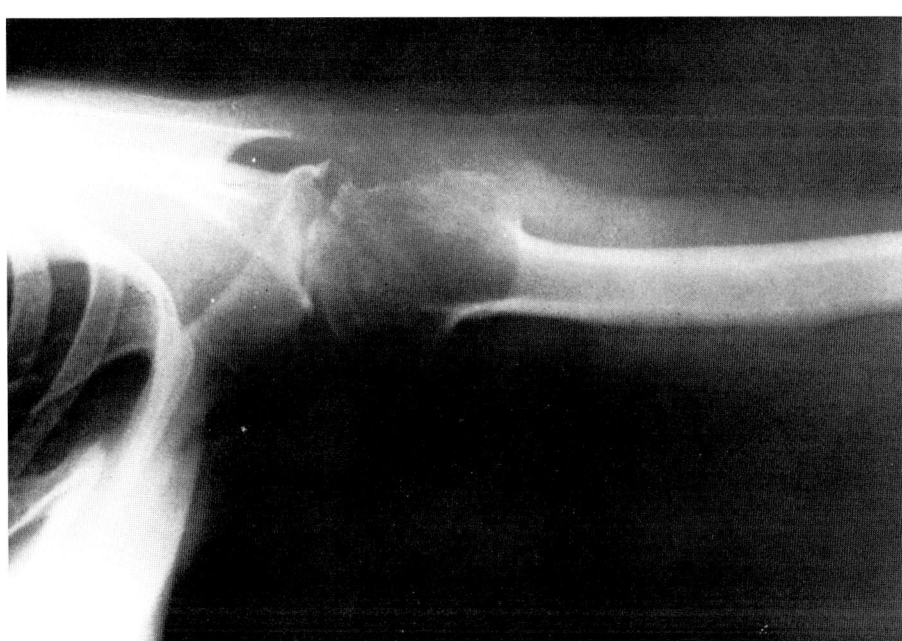

B

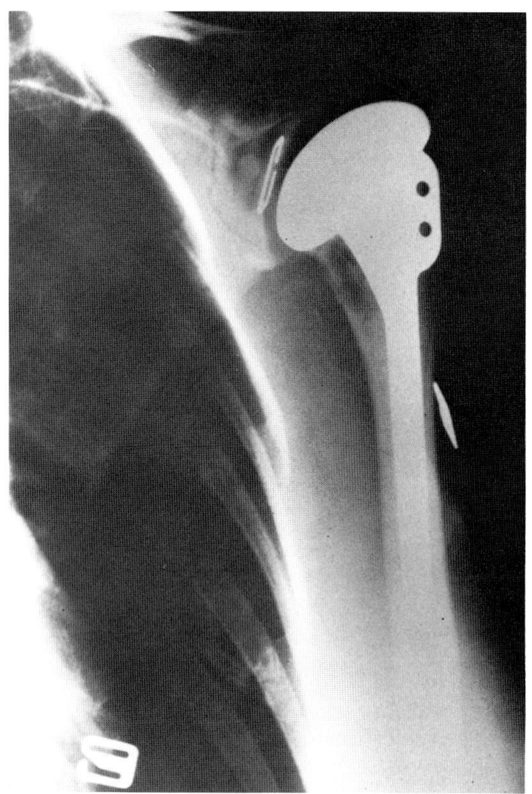

A

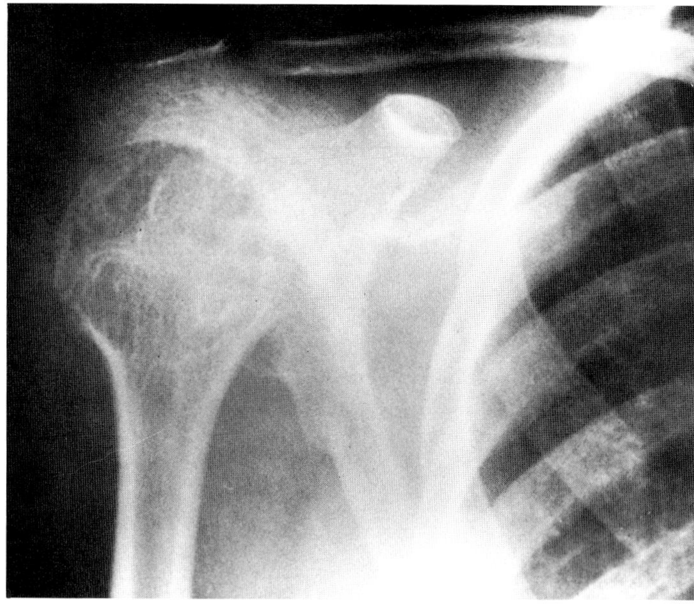

B

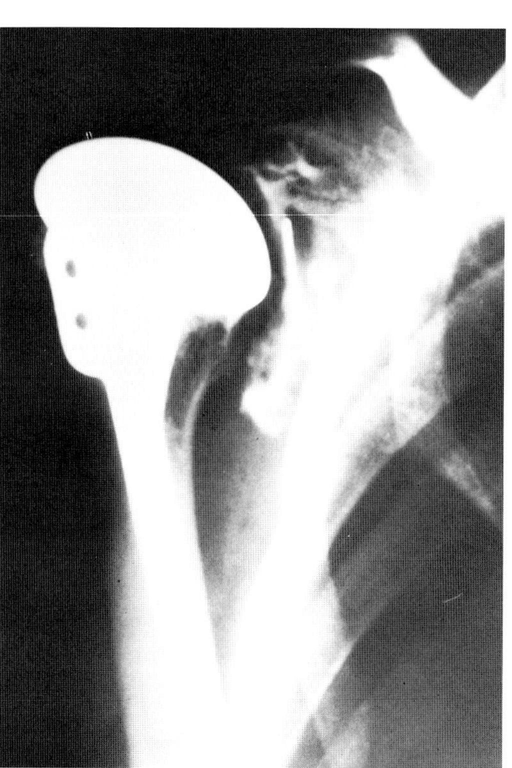

C

Fig. 9-22. (A) Postoperative anteroposterior roentgenogram of the left shoulder showing the total shoulder replacement. The proximal end of the stem needed to be cut off in order to fit it in the medullary canal. There is a radiolucent line around the glenoid. (B) Another patient with juvenile rheumatoid arthritis showing the small size of the humerus. (C) Postoperative total shoulder with small humeral components.

the right shoulder showed active elevation to 75 degrees and external rotation 30 degrees; she could internally rotate her arm so she could put her hand behind her back. Her left shoulder showed active elevation to 65 degrees, external rotation 40 degrees, and internal rotation to the point where she could place her hand behind her lumbar spine. Roentgenograms showed complete narrowing of both shoulder joints (Figs. 9-20 and 9-21). The medullary canals were noted to be small.

In April 1981 a total shoulder replacement of the left shoulder was carried out, and the right shoulder was replaced in August of that year (Fig. 9-22A). Because of the small size of the canal and the curve of the humerus, it was not possible to place even the smallest stem into the humerus, and the distal 1.5 inches of the humeral component stem was cut off using a sharp grinder. [A short stem prosthesis is now available (Fig. 9-22B & C).]

In May 1982 the patient was pleased with her shoulders. She could elevate the right one 90 degrees and the left one 95 degrees. External rotation reached 30 degrees bilaterally, and she could internally rotate to where she could get both hands to her lumbar spine.

Complications

Basically, shoulder replacements are divided into constrained and nonconstrained types; both have their complications. There have been many types of constrained shoulders that have subsequently been modified or abandoned because of loosening or failure of the components. The Michael Reese shoulder, however, has been an exception. Post et al.[21] reported 43 shoulder replacements (three for rheumatoid arthritis and one for juvenile rheumatoid arthritis). Of these three, one failed because of infection (this rheumatoid patient was the only infection in the series). Of the entire group, there were 14 major complications related to the design of the prosthesis. Subsequently, the design was changed part-way through the series. There were four dislocations and six broken and two bent prosthetic humeral necks. Post et al. emphasized that this technique is a salvage procedure, and they now

do more nonconstrained than constrained shoulders. Post has made a great contribution by his careful development and regular reporting of the Michael Reese shoulder. Most other constrained shoulders have already "come and gone."

The nonconstrained resurfacing Neer prosthesis has been associated with other complications. Neer et al.[19] reported that of 153 patients with rheumatoid arthritis who underwent a total of 153 procedures 61 had minimal complications. Of the 28 operations done for rheumatoid arthritis and followed for more than 1 year, 11 were excellent and 8 satisfactory.

In 1982 Neer et al.[20] reported on 273 shoulder arthroplasties, among which 69 patients had rheumatoid arthritis. Of the total, 30 percent showed a radiologic line around the implant but no clinical loosening. There were 24 complications, of which 12 required further surgery. One patient with old trauma had a wound infection that necessitated prosthesis removal. There were four instances of dislocation. All were reduced and immobilized 3 to 6 weeks, and only one of these patients has recurrent subluxation. Two shoulders subluxed postoperatively owing to loss of humeral bone. Five patients who sustained subsequent injuries experienced disruption of the rotator cuff, which allowed the implant to sublux, although it remained intact. One patient with a nonunited greater tuberosity and aseptic necrosis was not relieved of pain. The humeral component and wire fixing the tuberosity were eventually removed, but there was no improvement in pain status. Of three patients with spontaneous late breaking of wires used to fix the tuberosity, two required wire removal. Two patients had roentgenographic evidence of loosening of the humeral components, but neither presented symptoms that would require revision. One paraplegic patient required an anterior acromioplasty for symptoms of subacromial impingement. Three patients experienced unexplained pain, and two of these patients underwent further surgery without relief of pain.

In 1977 Cofield[6] reported on the status of total shoulder replacement, using various types of shoulder, at the Mayo Clinic. The Stanmore constrained total shoulder was used in nine patients, four of whom had rheumatoid arthritis. Of these patients, three had significant pain, and one of the three shoulders became infected and was subsequently converted to a resectional arthroplasty. The other two painful shoulders loosened their glenoid component, and one dislocated. Two patients (one rheumatoid arthritic and one osteoarthritic) underwent satisfactory results with the Michael Reese constrained shoulder. Twenty-five patients underwent replacement with the Neer resurfacing prosthesis. Nine of these operations were done for rheumatoid arthritis; and satisfactory pain relief and stability was achieved in all cases. There was one axillary nerve paralysis and one with no motion after heterotrophic bone formation; neither was done because of rheumatoid arthritis.

In our group of shoulder arthroplasties done for both rheumatoid arthritis and osteoarthritis, we used the Neer humeral endoprostheses alone in the earliest cases, but later added the glenoid replacement. In patients with an irreparable rotator cuff tear, we used the polyethylene subacromial spacer in the earlier cases.

There were no infections, nerve problems, or cases of clinical loosening in our series, even though some of the humeral components were not cemented in place. The patients in whom only the humeral head was replaced showed erosion of the glenoid 5 years later, and one of them developed arthritis-type pain.

One should expect the results from limited surgery to the shoulder for rheumatoid arthritis to be satisfactory if done for the proper indications, e.g., resection of the distal clavicle for limited acromioclavicular disease or anterior acromioplasty for impingement condition or synovectomy for early disease. Rheumatoid arthritis is a progressive disease, and one should expect that the eventual outcome in the shoulder will lead to replacement arthroplasty. Therefore limited surgery that will preclude replacement arthroplasty at a later time should not be done.

Replacement arthroplasty has been successful, with 90 percent patient satisfaction, a figure equal to the results of total knee replacement.

Case Report 6

A 68-year-old woman with long-standing rheumatoid arthritis presented in 1971 with severe right shoulder pain and the inability to use her

right arm due to pain and shoulder stiffness. Examination revealed swelling, tenderness, and crepitation in the shoulder with only 20 degrees flexion.

Roentgenograms showed severe destruction of the humeral head, which was riding high in the glenoid underneath the acromion (Fig. 9-23A). An arthrogram revealed a massive tear of the rotator cuff (Fig. 9-23B).

Surgery was performed in July 1972. The rotator cuff was torn and frayed, and repair was not possible. The articular surfaces of the glenohumeral joint were destroyed. A Neer humeral head prosthesis and a polyethylene subacromial spacer were inserted (Fig. 9-23C & D). Postoperatively, pain was relieved; she had attained 90 degrees of elevation and could reach the top of her head and behind her back.

Pain has generally been relieved by these procedures, but there have been complications. Of all the procedures of this type, all of which have been followed more than 2 years, there was one case of recurrent dislocation. This patient had the only poor result in the group.

Case Report 7

A 65-year-old woman with rheumatoid arthritis for 10 years presented because of disabling left shoulder pain. She had multiple joint involvement and had already undergone several operations, including synovectomies and tendon repairs on her hands.

Examination showed 90 degrees of motion in her left shoulder, but it was both glenohumeral and scapulothoracic motion. Preoperative roentgenograms showed marked destructive changes.

Exploration of the shoulder revealed the presence of a considerable amount of fibrinous material and thickened synovial fluid in and about the joint space. The rotator cuff proved to be markedly attenuated, and articular cartilage was absent from both the humeral head and the glenoid face. It was not thought possible to repair the badly deteriorated rotator cuff. A Neer humeral head prosthesis and a subacromial spacer were inserted to help prevent the humerus from riding up.

Although the surgical wound healed without problems, the patient did not do as well as

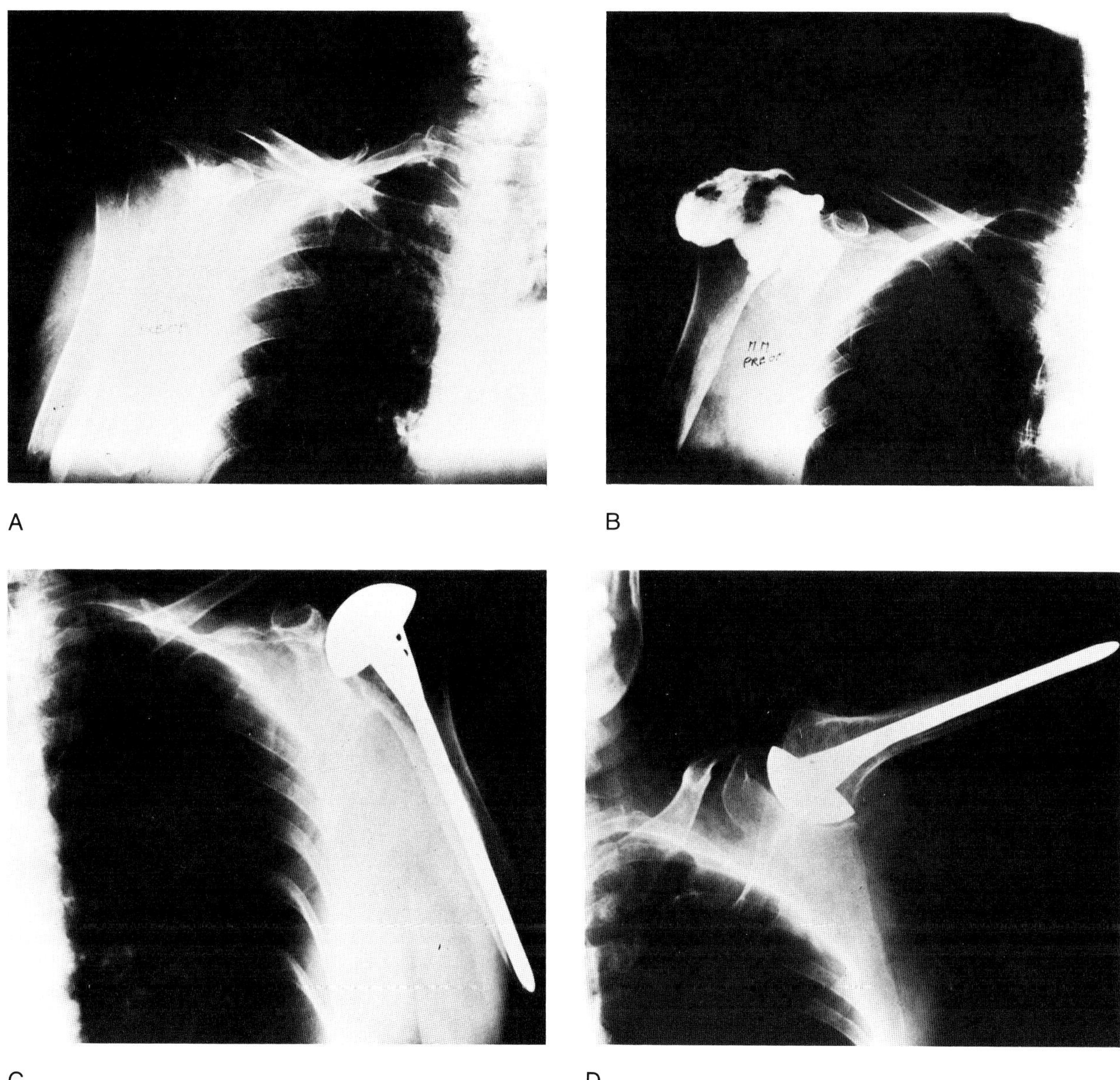

Fig. 9-23. (**A**) Preoperative roentgenogram showing severe destruction of the shoulder with the humerus riding high. (**B**) Preoperative arthrogram showing a rotator cuff tear. (**C & D**) Postoperative roentgenograms with arm at the side (**C**) and in abduction (**D**). A polyethylene subacromial spacer was used, but it is not visible because there was no radiographic marker in the early models.

hoped. During the course of her exercise program, it was found that when she contracted the deltoid with the arm forward flexed the humerus tended to sublux posteriorly. These subluxations were initially painless and comparatively infrequent, but with time they became both painful and frequent. Ultimately, the patient was comfortable only when her arm was immobilized. Surgical revision was advised, but the patient refused further surgery.

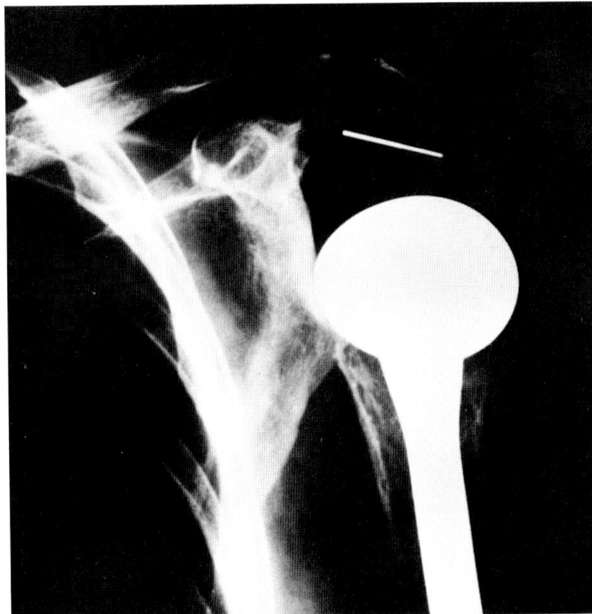

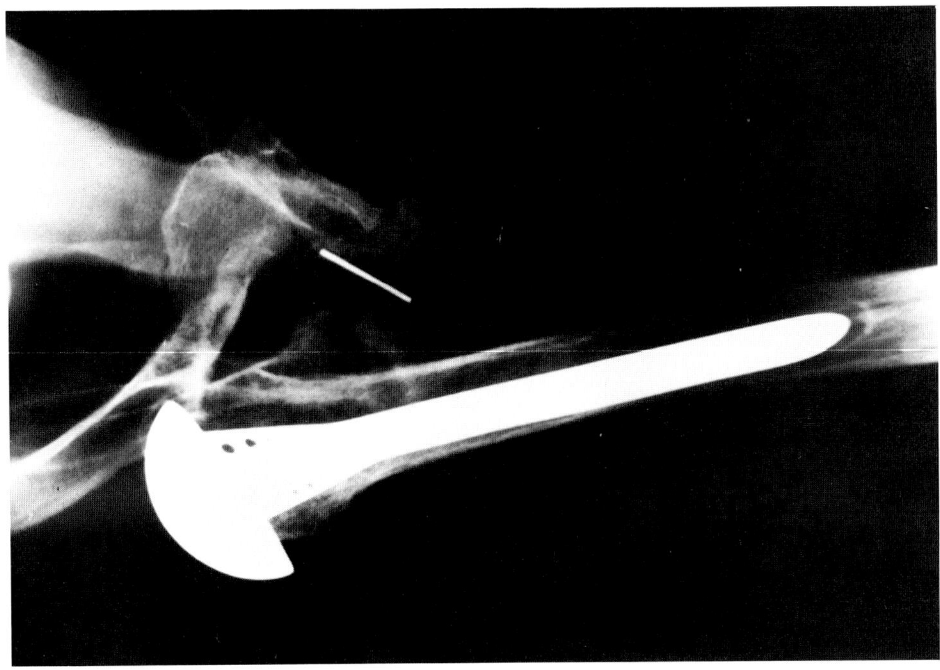

Fig. 9-24. Postoperative roentgenograms showing inferior (**A**) and posterior (**B**) dislocation of the prosthesis.

Postoperative shoulder roentgenograms showed posterior dislocation in the lateral view; the anteroposterior view indicated that the subacromial spacer was not properly seated but had subluxed anteriorly (Fig. 9-24). This case emphasizes the importance of obtaining an axillary view roentgenogram before surgery to determine posterior subluxation or a posterior sloping glenoid. In such a case, another method of reconstruction may be necessary, such as a constrained prosthesis or bone graft as described by Neer et al.[20]

SUMMARY

There are few operations done on the shoulder of patients with rheumatoid arthritis. It is not because surgery is not successful but because problems in other joints take precedence; moreover, conservative treatment is often successful. The emphasis on treatment has been on replacement arthroplasty, which has been effective for the control of pain in the shoulder with severe destruction due to rheumatoid arthritis. Lesser operative procedures, such as synovectomy, partial acromionectomy, or bursa resection, may also produce good results in patients with earlier stages of the disease.

REFERENCES

1. Averill R, Sledge C: Neer total shoulder arthroplasty. Presented to the annual meeting of the American Academy of Orthopaedic Surgeons, Atlanta, February 1980
2. Benjamin A, Herschowitz D, Arden GP: The treatment of arthritis of the shoulder joint by double osteotomy. Int Orthop 3:211, 1979
3. Brenner BC, Ferlic DC, Clayton ML, Dennis DA: Survivorship of unconstrained total shoulder arthroplasty. J Bone Joint Surg [Am] 71:1289, 1989
3a. Clayton ML: Surgery of the rheumatoid shoulder. p. 229. In Bostwick JA (ed): Current Concepts in Hand Surgery. Lea & Febiger, Philadelphia, 1983
4. Clayton ML, Ferlic DC: Surgery of the shoulder in rheumatoid arthritis. Clin Orthop 106:166, 1975
5. Clayton ML, Ferlic DC, Jeffers PD: Prosthetic shoulder arthroplasties. Clin Orthop 164:184, 1982
6. Cofield RH: Status of total shoulder arthroplasty. Arch Surg 112:1088, 1977
7. Cofield RH, Morrey BF, Bryan RS: Total shoulder and total elbow arthroplasties: the current state of development. JCE Orthop Patient 1:14, 1978
8. Cooney WD, Bryan RS: Rheumatoid arthritis in the upper extremity: treatment of the elbow and shoulder joints. AAOS Instr Course Lect 28:247, 1979
8a. Ferlic DC, Clayton ML: Rheumatoid arthritis of the shoulder. p. 3:97. In Evarts CM (ed): Surgery of the Musculoskeletal System. Churchill Livingstone, New York, 1983
8b. Grant, JC: An atlas of anatomy. Williams & Wilkins, Baltimore, 1943
9. Hammond G: Complete acromionectomy in the treatment of chronic tendinitis of the shoulder. J Bone Joint Surg [Am] 44:494, 1962
10. Harmon PH: Surgical reconstruction of the paralytic shoulder by multiple muscle transplantation. J Bone Joint Surg [Am] 32:583, 1950
11. Linscheid RL: Surgery for rheumatoid arthritis: timing and techniques: the upper extremity. J Bone Joint Surg [Am] 50:605, 1968
12. Lucas DB: Biomechanics of the shoulder joint. Arch Surg 107:425, 1973
13. Marmor L: Hemiarthroplasty for the rheumatoid shoulder joint. Clin Orthop 122:201, 1977
14. Neer CS II: Anterior acromioplasty for the chronic impingement syndrome in the shoulder. J Bone Joint Surg [Am] 54:41, 1972
15. Neer CS II: Articular replacement for the humeral head. J Bone Joint Surg [Am] 46:1607, 1964
16. Neer CS II: Replacement arthroplasty for glenohumeral osteoarthritis. J Bone Joint Surg 56:1, 1974
17. Neer CS II: The rheumatoid shoulder. In Gruess RE, Mitchell N (eds): Surgery of Rheumatoid Arthritis. JB Lippincott, Philadelphia, 1971
18. Neer CS II, Marberry TA: On the disadvantages of radical arcomionectomy. J Bone Joint Surg [Am] 63:416, 1981
19. Neer CS II, Gruess RL, Sledge C-B, Wilde AH: Total shoulder replacement: a preliminary report. Orthop Trans 1:244, 1977 (abstract)
20. Neer CS II, Watson KC, Stanton FJ: Recent experiences in total shoulder replacement. J Bone Joint Surg [Am] 64:319, 1982
21. Post M, Haskee S, Jablon M: Total shoulder replacement with a constrained prosthesis. J Bone Joint Surg [Am] 62:327, 1980

22. Post M, Jablon H, Singh M: Constrained total shoulder joint replacement: a critical review. Clin Orthop 144:135, 1979
23. Ranawat CS, Tulyasathien X, Straub LR, Inglis A: Synovectomy and Neer prosthetic replacement of the shoulder in rheumatoid arthritis. Presented to the Annual Meeting of the American Academy of Orthopaedic Surgeons, Dallas, 1974
24. Smith-Petersen MN, Aufranc OE, Larson CB: Useful surgical procedures for rheumatoid arthritis involving joints of the upper extremity. Arch Surg 46:764, 1943
25. Steindler A: The reconstruction for upper extremity in spinal and cerebral paralysis. AAOS Instr Course Lect 6:120, 1949

10

Management of the Rheumatoid Elbow

Donald C. Ferlic

The elbow joint is made up of the distal humerus articulating with the proximal ulnar and radius, which also articulate together. These articulations are enclosed in a common fibrous sheath. The synovial lining is continuous with all components of the joint, so a synovitis presenting in the radiohumeral portion of the joint is not limited to that area. The bones about the elbow are held together by a ligamentous network with a particularly strong anterior band of the medial collateral ligament.

The elbow is commonly thought of as strictly a hinge joint, with the radius rotating about the capitellum and the radial notch of the ulna. Detailed studies have attempted to define the kinematics of the elbow, some in an attempt to directly explain the high incidence of loosening of uniaxial total elbow replacements. These studies have produced conflicting results.

Fischer[13] found a locus of instant centers about 1 to 3 mm in diameter near the center of the trochlea. Ewald[9] described a pathway of instant centers for elbow flexion. Morrey and Chao[26] described a locus of instant centers near the center of the trochlea for flexion and extension, a linear decrease in the carrying angle that progressed from a valgus angle at full extension to a varus angle at full flexion and axial rotation of the forearm on the humerus during flexion. Dempster[7] described a change in the carrying angle during elbow flexion, but it followed an oscillatory rather than a linear pattern. Von Meyer[35] described an axial rotation of the forearm during flexion, but in the opposite direction than that reported by Morrey and Chao. London,[21] in an attempt to design a better total elbow, found a more basic pattern of motion and concluded that flexion and extension occurred about a single axis. It is a sliding type of motion, except at the extremes of flexion and extension when it changes to a rolling motion. London found that the carrying angle of the elbow remains constant as the elbow flexes.

Forearm rotation has likewise been said to involve only the radial-capitellum articulation, but Ray et al.[28] have shown that there is some motion of the ulna during rotation of the forearm with 8 to 9 degrees of lateral abduction of the distal end of the ulna with full supination and pronation.

EXTRA-ARTICULAR CONSIDERATIONS

Rheumatoid elbows are frequently plagued with superficial problems, e.g., olecranon bursae that become painful and inflamed (Fig. 10-1). The olecranon bursa does not normally communicate with the elbow joint, but in rheumatoid arthritis it occasionally does; infection of the joint sometimes presents as a draining olecranon bursa. The clinical factor to consider is a bursitis with copious drainage.

Bursae tend to recur or drain after excision. To prevent this problem we insert a drain, excise the

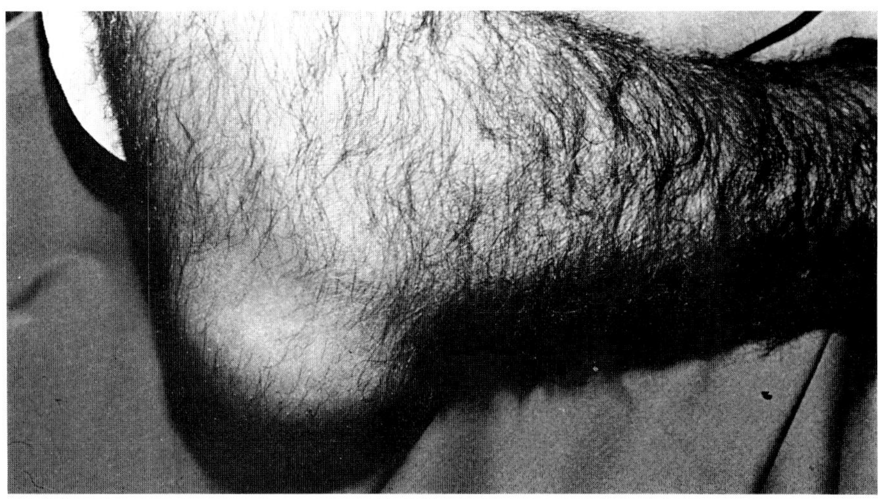

Fig. 10-1. Olecranon bursa in the rheumatoid elbow.

redundant skin, and splint the elbow 2 to 3 weeks after surgery. Prominent rheumatoid nodules about the bony surface of the olecranon (Fig. 10-2) may also be painful and ulcerate. Although they require removal, it is important to warn the patient that these nodules frequently recur; rheumatoid arthritic patients are hypersensitive to pressure, and most nodules are related to pressure. Antecubital cysts in the rheumatoid elbow are similar to Baker cysts in the knee and occasionally must be removed because of pain or nerve impingement.

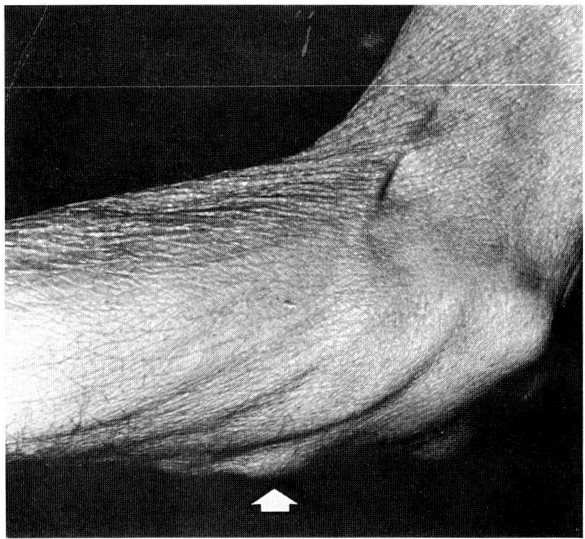

Fig. 10-2. Rheumatoid nodules.

A relation exists between elbow and hand/ wrist problems; therefore when a patient is examined for a hand problem, it is always necessary to consider the elbow as well. One should keep three things particularly in mind: forearm rotation, ulnar nerve problems, and posterior interosseous nerve palsy resulting from elbow synovitis. A patient with limited forearm rotation may indeed have problems with the distal radioulnar joint, but the rotation may also be limited at the proximal radioulnar joint and necessitate radial head resection in addition to removing the distal ulna to restore rotation. Seventy-five percent of our patients who have undergone elbow synovectomy/radial head resection have also had distal ulnar resection and synovectomy of the wrist. Elbow problems are closely linked to shoulder problems. Good elbow function often provides compensation for limited shoulder motion. The general function of the shoulder and elbow is to position and move the hand in space.

When a rheumatoid patient presents with the inability to extend the fingers, the pathology may be in the hand, wrist, or elbow; and there may well be a problem differentiating between posterior interosseous nerve palsy at the elbow (Fig. 10-3), subluxation of the extensor tendons off the metacarpophalangeal (MCP) joints in the hand, or even ruptured extensor tendons at the wrist. This problem can be correctly diagnosed only if one is aware of these possibilities. A hand with posterior interosseous nerve palsy can often be

Fig. 10-3. Hand with posterior interosseous nerve palsy due to rheumatoid invasion at the elbow. The position of the hand and fingers is strikingly similar to a hand with a triple rupture of the extensor tendons of the fingers and the hand where the patient is unable to extend the fingers due to synovitis of the MCP joints and subluxation of the extensor tendons off the metacarpal heads. (From Ferlic,[10a] with permission.)

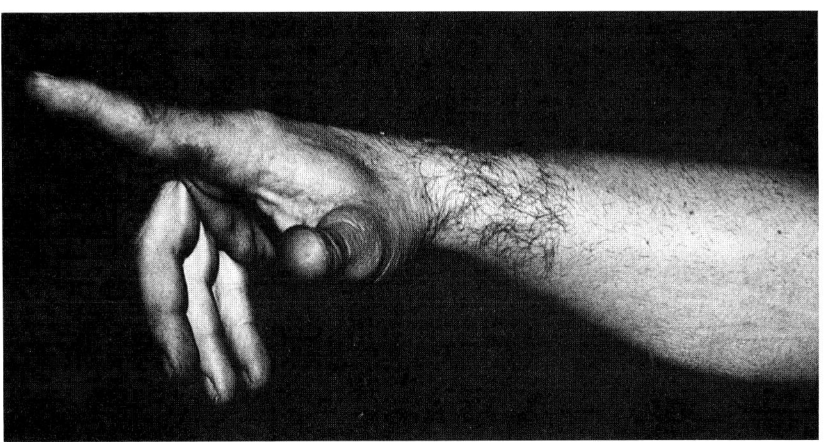

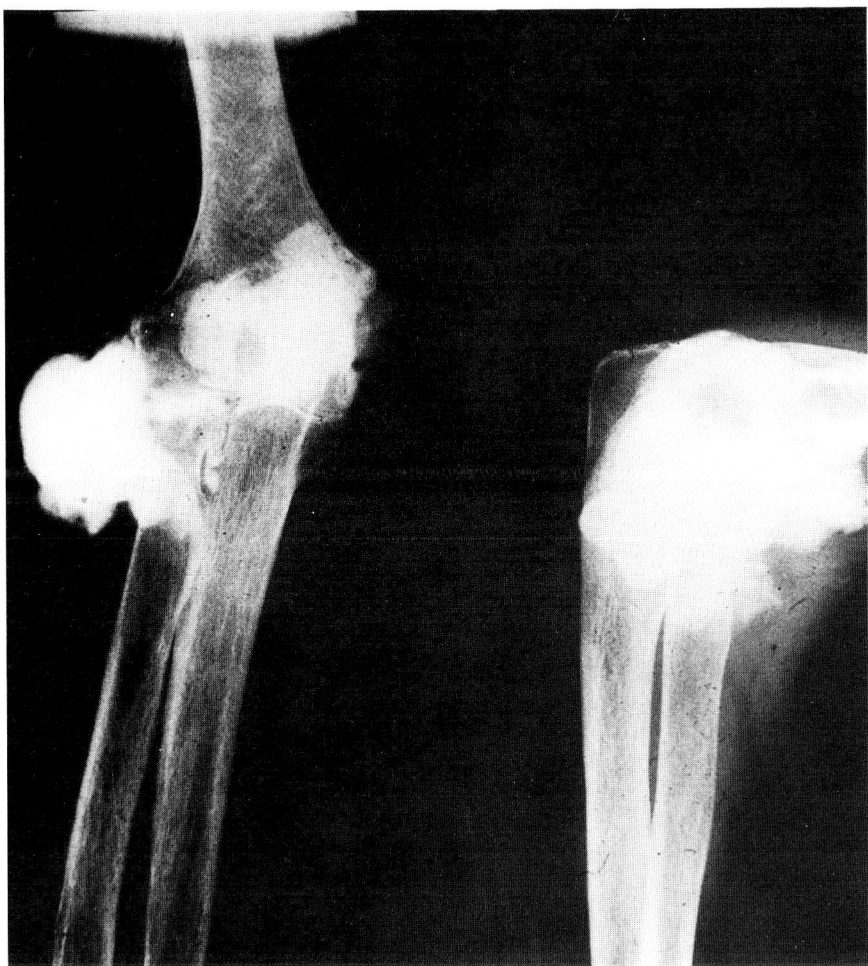

Fig. 10-4. Arthrogram of a rheumatoid elbow showing synovial cysts.

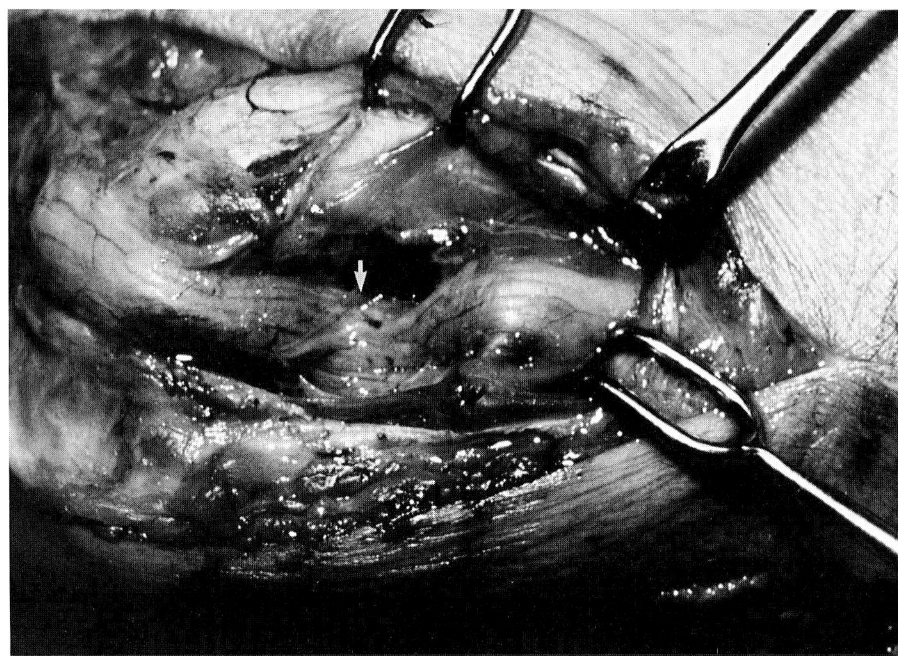

Fig. 10-5. Compression of the ulnar nerve at the elbow by a bony spicule due to bony erosion in rheumatoid arthritis. Arrow points to nerve.

differentiated by demonstrating a positive tenodesis effect. When the wrist is flexed, the intact extensor tendons should extend the fingers; but if the wrist or MCP joints are stiff, the tenodesis effect is not apparent and thus presents an additional problem in diagnosis.

An arthrogram of the elbow may reveal a large antecubital cyst pressing on the posterior interosseous nerve (Fig. 10-4). A steroid injection into the elbow may resolve the inflammation, but synovectomy and nerve decompression may also be necessary.

The rheumatoid patient may develop ulnar nerve palsy at the elbow. Bony deformities, erosions, or synovitis contribute to its cause (Fig. 10-5). Moore and Weiland[24] have even reported a case of bilateral attrition rupture of the ulnar nerves at the elbow in a 56-year-old woman with severely deforming rheumatoid arthritis. Such patients may present with numbness and paresthesias in the ulnar nerve distribution in the hand or just weakness and lack of hand dexterity (Fig. 10-6). This clinical picture often is interpreted as symptoms of arthritic involvement of the hand, but one must consider neuropathy of the ulnar nerve at the elbow. It is best treated by decompression and rerouting of the nerve anteriorly.

SURGICAL INDICATIONS

Most large series of patients undergoing surgery for rheumatoid arthritis include relatively few who have elbow operations, although the elbow is frequently involved in rheumatoid arthritis. Laine and Vainio[18] found two-thirds of their patients with rheumatoid arthritis to have elbow involvement. Severe elbow problems necessitating surgery arise later in the disease because (1) the onset of elbow symptoms is generally insidious; (2) patients may be unaware of disability until destruction is advanced because range of motion is aided by gravity, which helps to maintain extension, and the activities of daily living help to maintain flexion; (3) loss of pronation is compensated by shoulder motion, so the patient is not

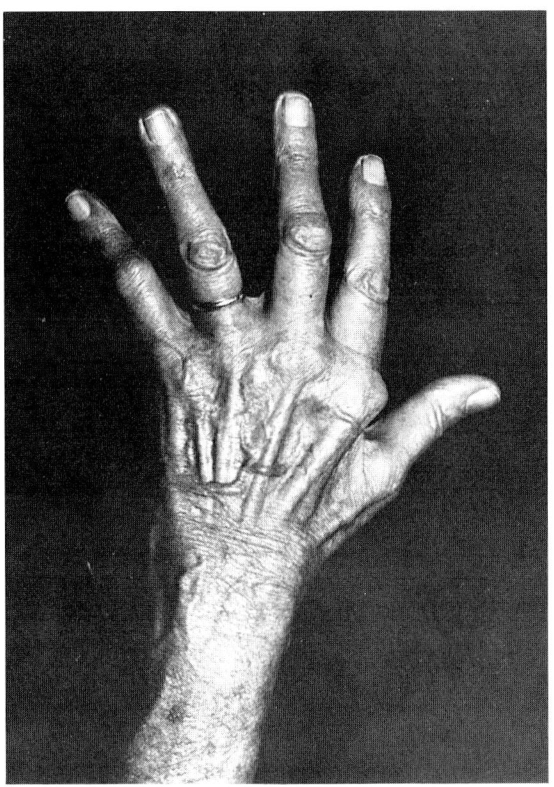

Fig. 10-6. Hand of a patient with ulnar neuropathy at the elbow. Note the profound wasting of the intrinsic musculature.

aware of the elbow problem until shoulder and wrist motion also become limited; (4) the elbow frequently responds well to conservative measures such as rest, splinting, and analgesics.

Elbow synovectomy and débridement was first reported in 1893.[29] Since then, there have been many reports citing good results.[1,11,15,16,18–20,23,31,32,34,37,39] Although it is generally agreed that this procedure is not necessary during the early stages of rheumatoid arthritis, physicians disagree as to the best surgical approach. Smith-Petersen et al.[30] described the basic procedure of radial head excision and synovectomy that is most widely used today. Inglis and associates[15] have advocated a transolecranon approach. Others[27,29] have recommended lateral and medial incisions, and many[1,20,23,34] recommended only a lateral incision.

The transolecranon approach is reported to produce good pain relief but significant complications associated with fixation of the bone. Reports on the lateral and medial approach[27,38,39] relate ulnar neuropathy postoperatively, with Wilson et al.[39] stating that three of eight patients who had had a routine medial approach developed ulnar nerve symptoms. We favor the lateral approach only, as adequate synovectomy can be carried out on both medial and lateral sides through one lateral incision. Indications for synovectomy and radial head resection are pain, swelling, and reasonable range of motion for the elbow with an American Rheumatology Association (ARA) classification of stage II or III. Painful crepitus over the radial head with rotation with less crepitus on ulnohumeral motion is a favorable sign.

Synovectomy

A posterior lateral incision extending from the posterior border of the ulnar 4 cm distal to the tip of the olecranon to a point 4 cm proximal to the lateral epicondyle of the humerus is made, keeping the forearm pronated to protect the radial nerve (Fig. 10-7). A fascial incision is made along the line between the anconeus and common extensor tendon origins to the triceps tendon posteriorly. The common extensor tendons are detached by sharp dissection from the lateral condyle and retracted upward. The radial head is excised, synovectomy carried out, and the ulna subluxed to remove the synovium from the posterior and medial sides. By flexing the elbow, the anterior recess can be cleared, and in extension the olecranon fossa is similarly exposed. A rongeur is a useful instrument for removing the synovium. The coronoid process is partially excised if it limits flexion, and bone from the tip of the olecranon may be excised if necessary.

A silicone radial head prosthesis can be inserted in an attempt to prevent proximal migration of the radius or valgus deformity and to modulate the forces across the elbow (Fig. 10-8). Use of a radial head implant, however, is not accepted by all surgeons, and we have stopped using this implant in this type of elbow unless the elbow is

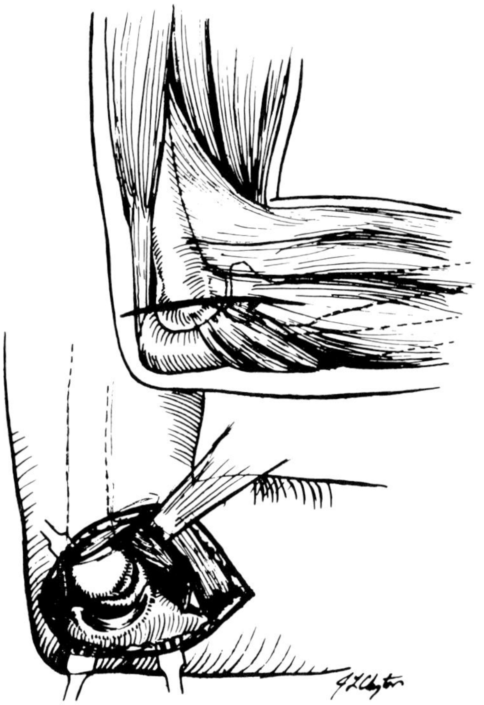

Fig. 10-7. Incision for synovectomy of the elbow and subluxation of the olecranon after the radial head has been removed. This method allows adequate room for a synovectomy to be performed in the posterior and medial compartments as well as in the lateral compartment.

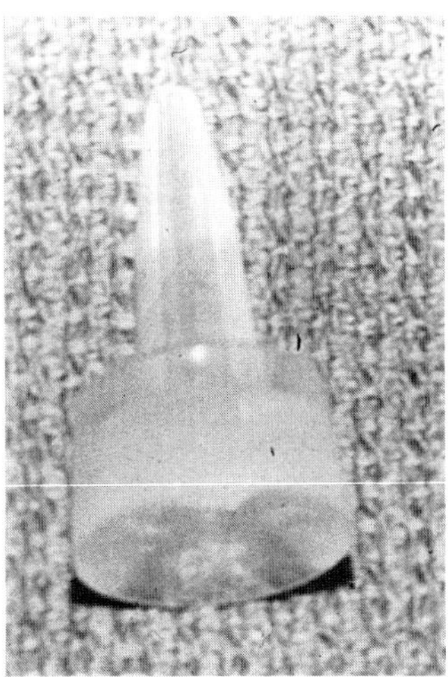

Fig. 10-8. Silicone radial head implant.

unstable after the radial head has been excised. Walker[36] demonstrated in biomechanical studies that the amount of force exerted must reach 9.8 kg before the force is absorbed by the radiohumeral joint. It does not seem that the rheumatoid patient with marked involvement and weakness can achieve such force, but if their lower extremities are involved they are apt to exceed this force when they are using crutches or a walker. In addition, there is a considerable lever effect in the forearm when the elbow is flexed 90 degrees, creating a joint reactive force often magnified at least 20 times. Many of these patients have lax joints, and the radial head is important for preventing extremes of valgus angulation about the elbow,[22] particularly if the medial collateral ligament is unstable. The radial head implant acts as a spacer and "shock absorber" to help unload the ulnohumeral joint.

If there is excessive medial pain or ulnar neuropathy, a medial incision is made over the tip of the medial epicondyle 5 cm distal and proximal to the joint. The ulnar nerve is isolated and transferred anteriorly. The muscles originating from the epicondyle are reflected, and the capsule is incised and the synovium removed; the important anterior medial collateral ligament is preserved. Care must be taken to avoid injuring the median nerve passing over the anterior aspect of the joint. A bulky dressing with a posterior splint is applied postoperatively, and active and passive motion is begun within 3 to 4 days.

In our series of 46 patients,[12] we performed 57 procedures. This group included 41 women with an average age of 48 (range 21 to 74). Six had juvenile rheumatoid arthritis, and 36 of the 40 patients had suffered from the disease for more than 10 years.

In our first published series[11] of 34 elbow synovectomies in 29 patients, we showed an average gain of 9 degrees in the flexion-extension arc and a gain of 22 degrees rotation. Four elbows decreased in flexion/extension, and three lost rotation. Twenty elbows were pain-free, and nine had less pain preoperatively; two patients' pain levels remained unchanged, and three experienced more pain than before the surgery. The follow-up period ranged from 4 to 85 months with an average follow-up of 35 months. The results of synovectomy in the elbow are the best for any joint, probably due to the non-weight-bearing status and the decompression effect obtained with radial head excision.

Case Report 1

A 56-year-old woman with long-standing chronic rheumatoid arthritis of 8 years' duration complained of pain on motion of her elbow. Examination revealed she had the "loose type" of rheu-

matoid arthritis with full rotation of the right elbow and motion from 0 to 150 degrees. There was painful crepitation around the radial head and nodules over the olecranon. Roentgenograms (Fig. 10-9A) showed slight narrowing of the articular space with some mild irregularity.

She underwent synovectomy of the elbow, débridement, radial head resection, and excision of the rheumatoid nodules in 1967. Postoperatively she was relieved of pain, could flex from 0 to 135

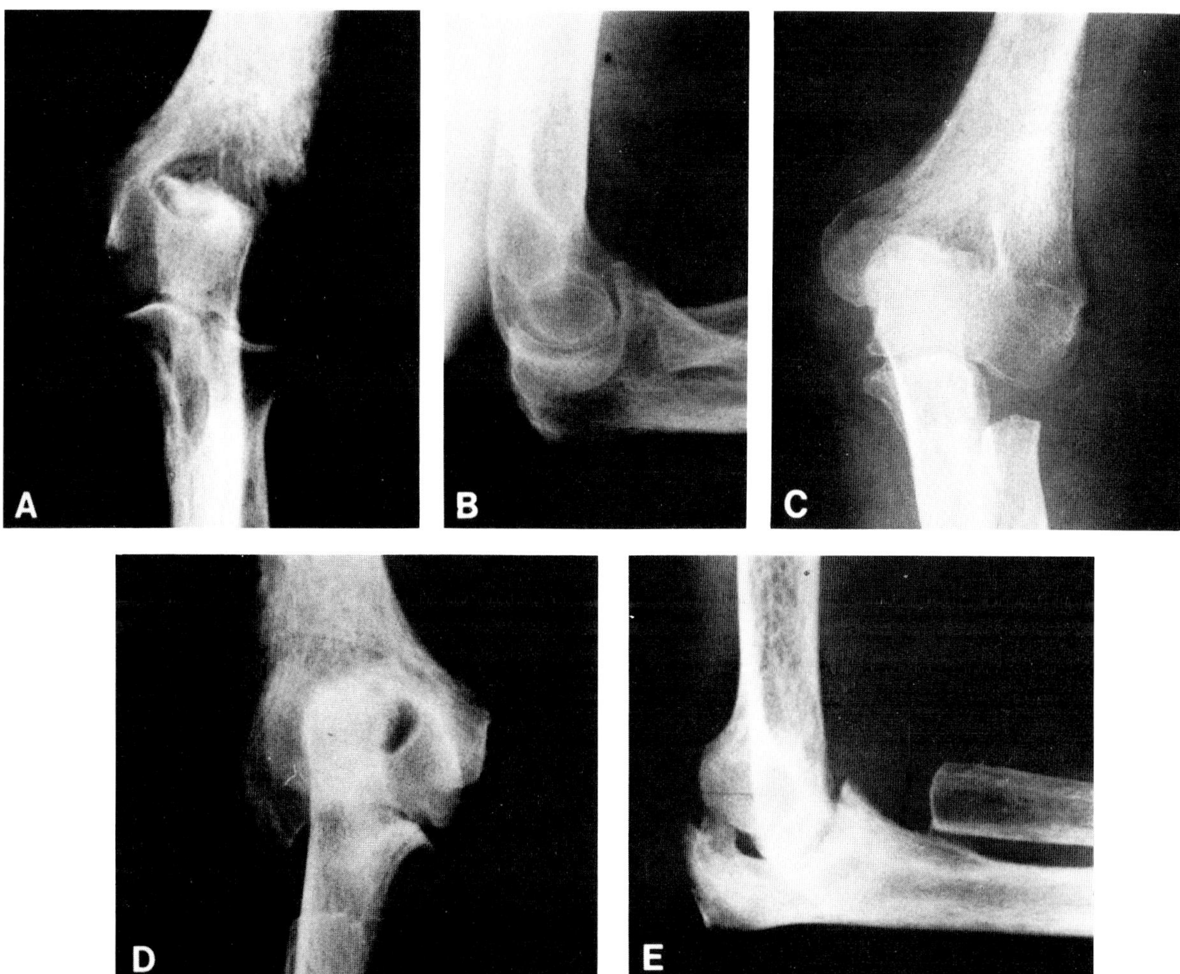

Fig. 10-9. (**A**) Preoperative anteroposterior roentgenogram of the elbow showing slight narrowing of the articular space with mild irregularity. (**B & C**) Recent postoperative roentgenograms showing amount of bone resection and minimal amount of destruction in the elbow. (**D & E**) Roentgenograms 11 years postoperatively show an increase in the destruction of the elbow, although the elbow functions well and is pain-free.

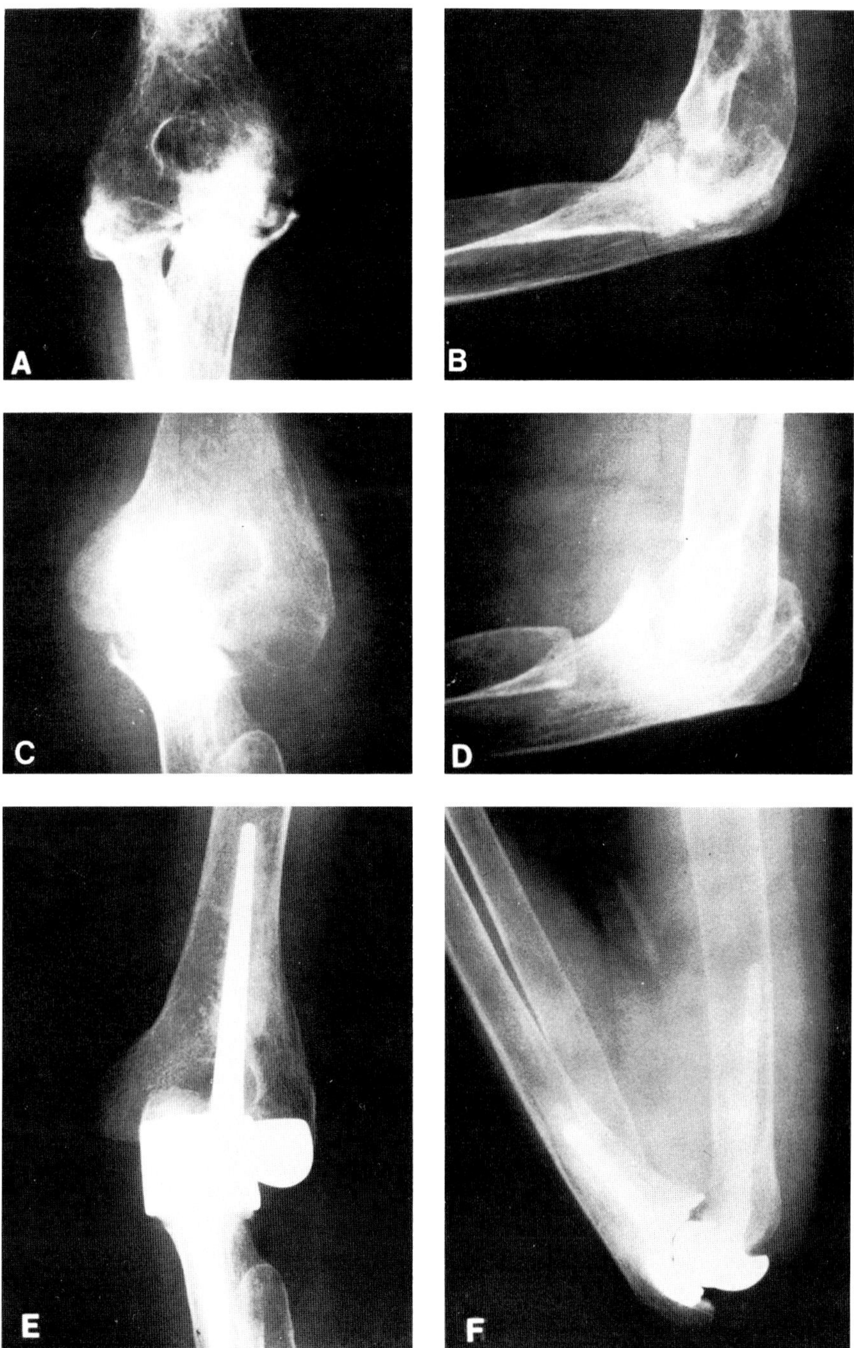

Fig. 10-10. (**A & B**) Preoperative roentgenograms showing late stage III changes. Synovectomy and radial head resection were carried out, but with an unsatisfactory result owing to the advanced destruction of the elbow. (**C & D**) Roentgenograms 2 years after surgery show an increase in destruction. (**E & F**) Ewald total elbow arthroplasty was carried out with good relief of pain.

degrees, and had full rotation. Roentgenograms shortly after the surgery (Fig. 10-9B & C) showed the amount of bone resected. Seven years later she had motion from 10 to 135 degrees with full rotation and minimal medial pain in the elbow. Roentgenograms obtained 11 years after the surgery (Fig. 10-9D & E) showed some destruction of the joint, but the result remained excellent. She was able to use a walker or crutches during much of the time (required because of multiple lower extremity operative procedures done for rheumatoid deformities).

Case Report 2

A 69-year-old woman with a 40-year history of rheumatoid arthritis presented because of upper extremity involvement with multiple joint complaints and severe pain in the left elbow. Motion was from 35 to 120 degrees with 70 degrees supination and 20 degrees pronation. Roentgenograms (Fig. 10-10A & B) showed advanced changes of rheumatoid arthritis.

She underwent synovectomy, débridement, and radial head excision in 1976. Three months after surgery, motion was from 20 to 130 degrees with 75 degrees pronation and supination. She was pleased with the relief of pain, even though there was slight discomfort.

Two years after surgery she developed marked pain and diminished motion. Examination showed the elbow to be painful and swollen, with motion from 15 to 115 degrees, supination 90 degrees, and pronation 20 degrees. Roentgenograms 2 years after surgery (Fig. 10-10C & D) showed a progression of the destructive changes. A total elbow arthroplasty was performed with excellent relief of pain and motion (Fig. 10-10E & F). It is 4 years after operation at this time. Although the good results in this patient were short-lived, synovectomy does not burn any bridges for future reconstruction should it be necessary.

Arthroplasty (Without Implant)

For the elbow with more advanced disease, interpositional arthroplasty has been performed using fascia, dermis, Gelfoam, or silicone. Fascial arthroplasty for rheumatoid arthritis was first performed by Murphy in 1902.[16] Souter[31] stated that there were 10 to 50 percent unsatisfactory results with this operation. Indications for fascial arthroplasty vary from bilateral ankylosis to partial ankylosis with disabling pain.[4,15,20]

Fascia is preferred in our clinic when performing an interposition arthroplasty in the elbow of a rheumatoid patient. Indications are a late stage III or IV elbow with adequate bone stock so stability is not compromised.

A posterior incision is made just lateral to the elbow midline, extending distally 10 cm and then curving to the medial side and extending proximally 10 cm (Fig. 10-11). The ulnar nerve is transposed anteriorly, the triceps reflected in a V fashion (Fig. 10-12), the joint dislocated, the radial head excised, the semilunar notch of the olecranon deepened, and the trochlea deepened in such a manner as to provide medial and lateral bony stability (Fig. 10-13). A strip of fascia lata is sutured over the semilunar notch. Postoperatively, bulky dressings and a posterior splint are applied, and active and passive motion is started in 3 to 4 days. We have obtained favorable results

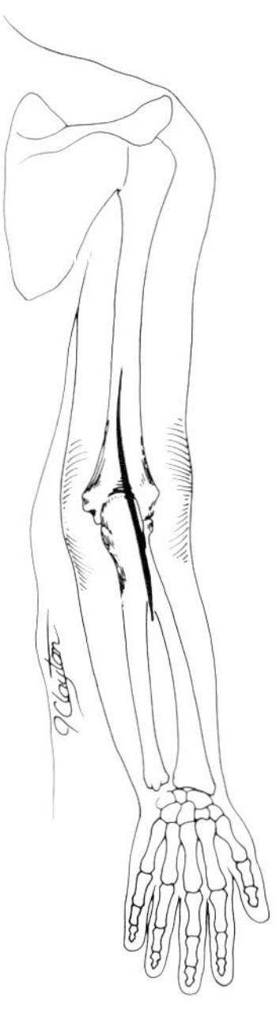

Fig. 10-11. Skin incision for fascial arthroplasty. (From Ferlic,[10a] with permission.)

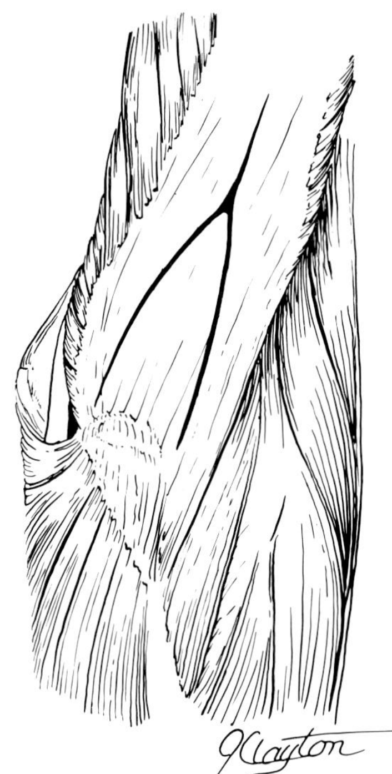

Fig. 10-12. Method of triceps incision. (From Ferlic,[10a] with permission.)

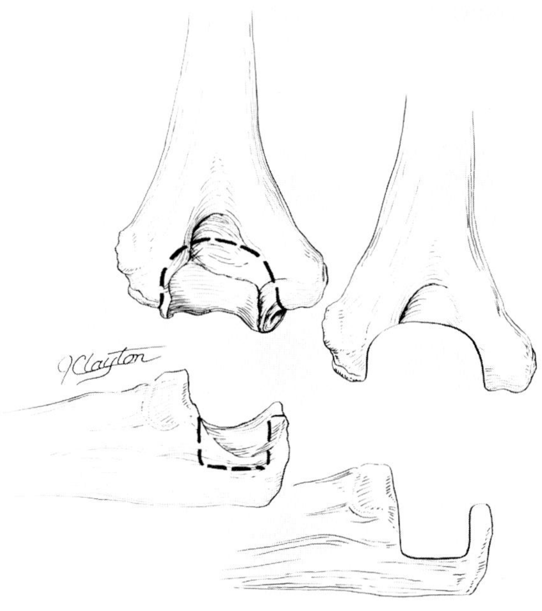

Fig. 10-13. Amount of bone resected from the semilunar notch of the olecranon and trochlea. (From Ferlic,[10a] with permission.)

in the small number of rheumatoid patients in whom we performed this operation, with a marked decrease in pain and an average range of motion of 100 degrees flexion-extension arc. Failure has been due to further absorption of bone exhibited by some rheumatoid patients.

Case Report 3

A 56-year-old woman with long-standing rheumatoid arthritis presented in 1966 with severe pain in the elbow. Examination showed crepitation and pain with motion. Motions was 45 to 150 degrees with supination 30 degrees and pronation 65 degrees. Preoperative roentgenograms (Fig. 10-14A & B) showed severe elbow destruction.

A fascial arthroplasty was carried out in 1966. The olecranon and humeral notch were deepened to obtain stability (Fig. 10-14C & D). Postoperatively she maintained motion from 25 to 130 degrees and was pain-free. This period included the time she was ambulating on crutches because of a fractured hip. She died of metastatic breast carcinoma 4 years after the elbow arthroplasty.

Arthrodesis

Arthrodesis of the elbow in the rheumatoid patient is rarely, if ever, indicated. This procedure relieves pain but markedly interferes with function of the upper extremity. The single exception may be in an infected or otherwise failed total elbow arthroplasty where there is not enough bone stock for another procedure or where resection arthroplasty is not acceptable. Surgeons in our clinic have never arthrodesed a rheumatoid elbow.

Total Elbow Arthroplasty (With Prosthesis)

There have been numerous reports of total elbow arthroplasty resulting in a high complication rate and frequent withdrawal of the components for redesign. In 1974 Street and Stevens[33] reported

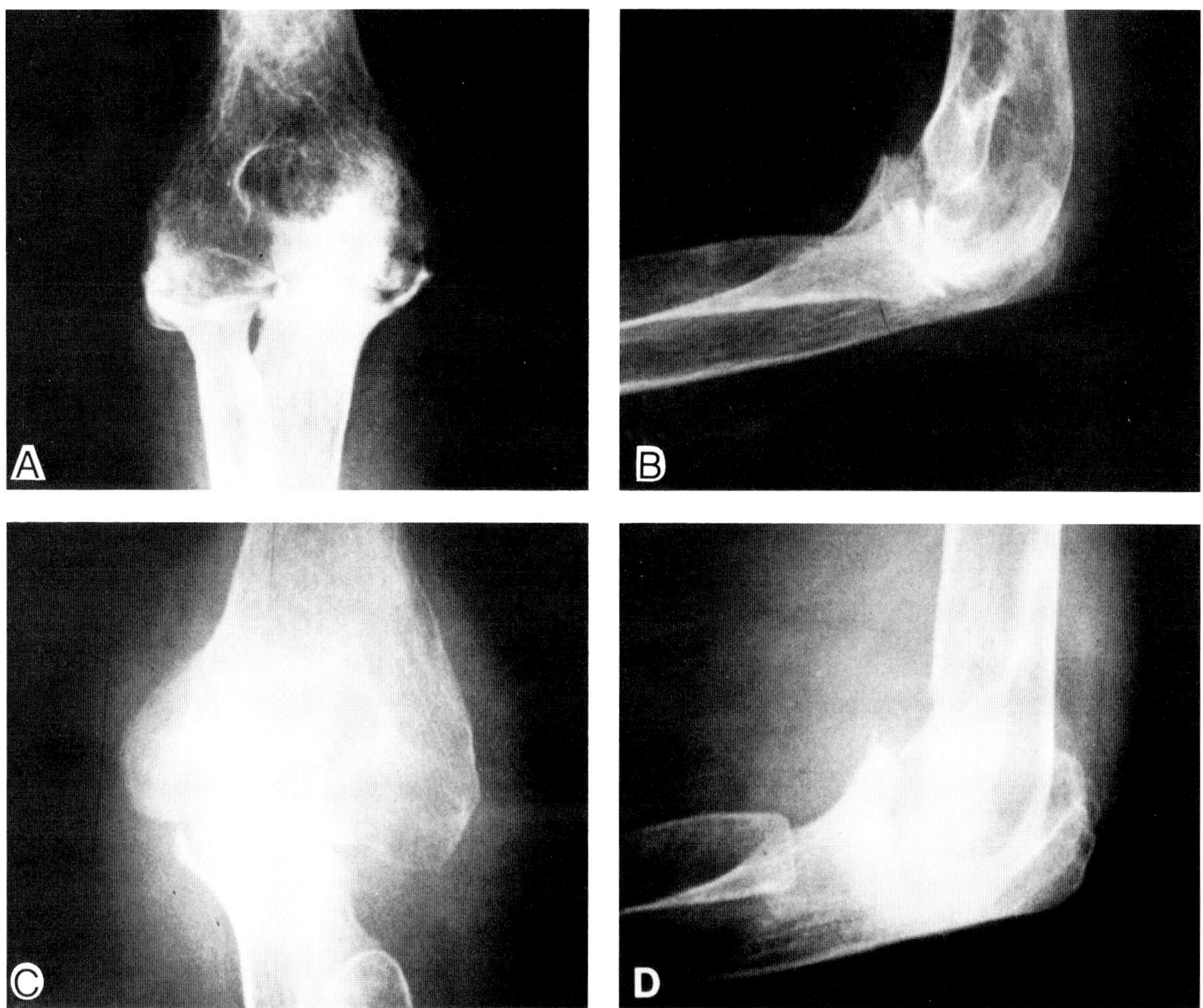

Fig. 10-14. (A & B) Preoperative roentgenograms of an elbow with late stage rheumatoid disease that was treated successfully with fascial arthroplasty. (C & D) Postoperative roentgenograms show the amount of bone resected from the humerus and olecranon in order to obtain stability with a mortise effect.

on their use of a metallic distal humeral resurfacing device in ten patients. Three were for rheumatoid arthritis, and results in two of these three were unsatisfactory. One of the two experienced complete ankylosis of the elbow and a transient ulnar neuropathy. The other unsatisfactory result was due to elbow dislocation with skin erosion on the medial side, necessitating removal of the prosthesis with ankylosis resulting (Fig. 10-15).

Silicone hinge arthroplasty at the elbow has also been tried but has been abandoned because

of breakage (Fig. 10-16). The results with the rigid hinges have likewise been disappointing. Cooney and Bryon[4] tabulated results with a combination of 111 Schiers, Dee, McKee-Dee, GSB, and Coonrad elbows, with 24 percent having poor results. Cofield et al.[3] tabulated the complications in 346 hinge total elbow replacements of both constrained and semiconstrained types and found loosening in 13 percent, fracture or wound problems in 9 percent (each), infection in 5 percent, ankylosis in 4 percent, neuropathy in 6 per-

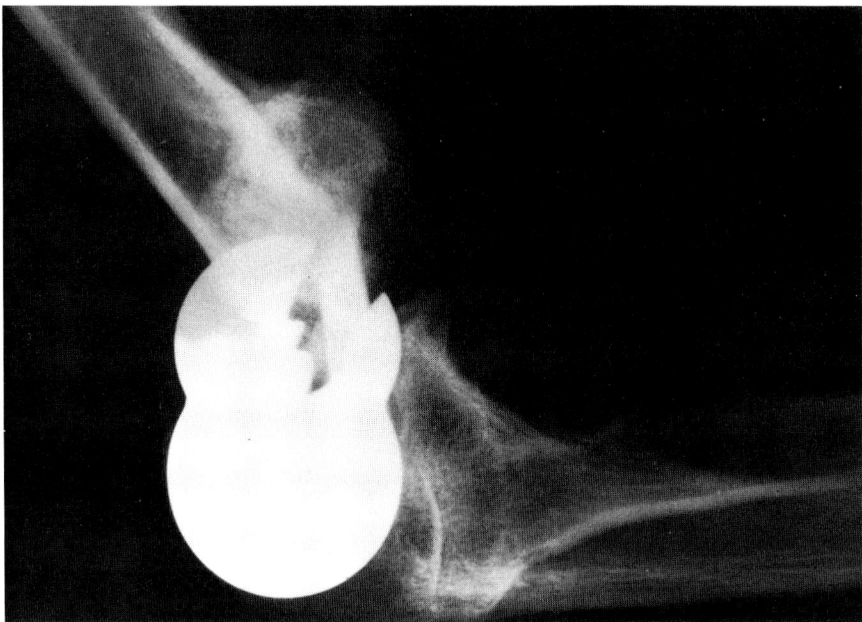

Fig. 10-15. Roentgenogram of an elbow with the Street-Stevens distal humeral resurfacing component, which failed owing to fracture of the distal humerus.

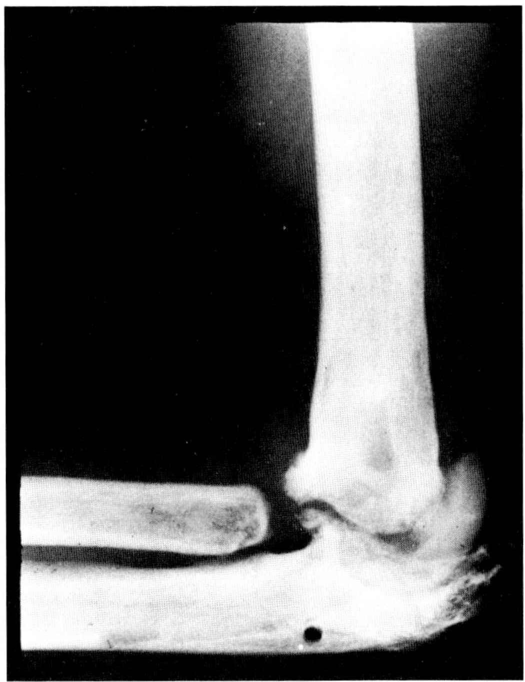

Fig. 10-16. Failed, broken silicone elbow arthroplasty.

cent, and triceps rupture in 2 percent. Twelve required revision.

Coonrad[5] reported on 150 elbows with rheumatoid arthritis done in a multicenter study with 95 percent good results (Fig. 10-17). There were only six failures: four due to loosening and two to infection, although 12 percent of patients had loosened humeral stems. Coonrad concluded that it was a good procedure for rheumatoid arthritis but not for trauma. His original elbow design was a rigid hinge and was modified to allow some lateral motion. The humeral stem was also lengthened. The results of this modified prosthesis were even more promising than the earlier model. Coonrad[6] however, reported two deep infections in 14 elbows he personally had to replace.

Ingles and Pellicci[14] reported on 36 semiconstrained elbow replacements followed for a minimum of 2 years and found a 53 percent complication rate, but only one-fourth of the complications affected the outcome. The first 17 in this series were done with a semiconstrained Pritchard-Walker elbow (Fig. 10-18) and the rest

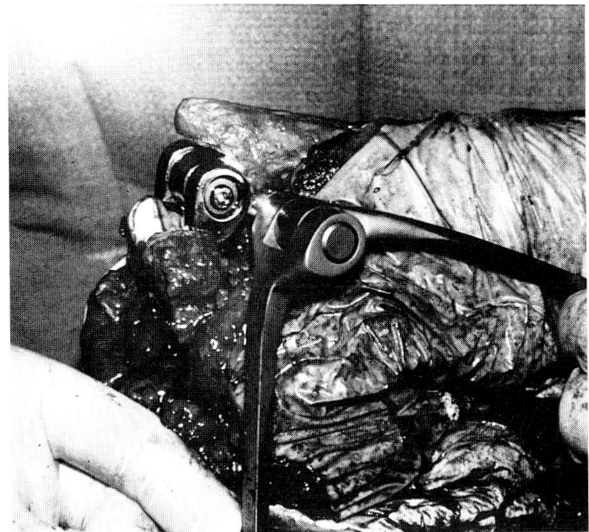

Fig. 10-17. Coonrad hinge elbow.

with the triaxial prosthesis. There were 22 rheumatoid patients who did generally better than the post-traumatic group. Of the 19 complications found in this group of 36 patients, there were wound hematomas in four, loosening in two, two fractured humeri, two ulnar neuropathies, two

triceps ruptures, two with skin slough, two with broken components, one fractured olecranon, one infection, and one cementophyte.

The Mayo Clinic[3,4] obtained satisfactory results in 75 percent of cases with total elbow replacement for rheumatoid arthritis. The rheumatoid patients again showed better results than the patients with post-traumatic arthritis.

The nonconstrained elbows were introduced in hopes of alleviating the loosening problem, but these prostheses have been associated with a high complication rate. Kudo et al.[17] reported 24 elbow replacements done for rheumatoid arthritis using a resurfacing prosthesis and found 14 excellent and 3 poor results. Two elbows failed to regain useful motion: One had proximal migration of the humeral component, and one had persistent subluxation with pain and instability.

Ewald et al.[10] reported 60 prosthetic replacements (Fig. 10-19) for rheumatoid arthritis and found 87 percent good or excellent results. He reported a 39 percent complication rate, with eight requiring revision of the arthroplasty: four

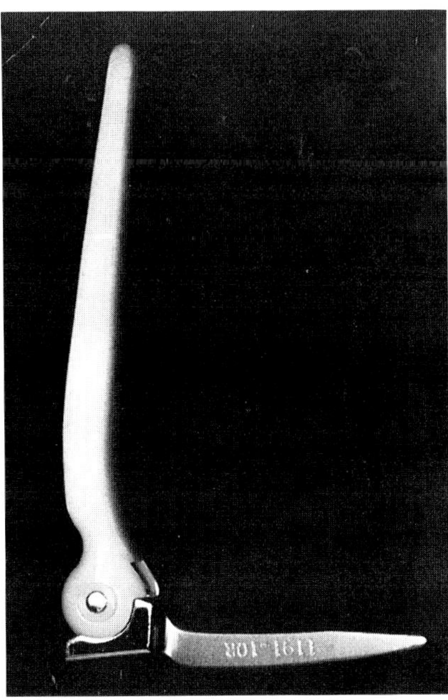

Fig. 10-18. Pritchard-Walker hinge elbow.

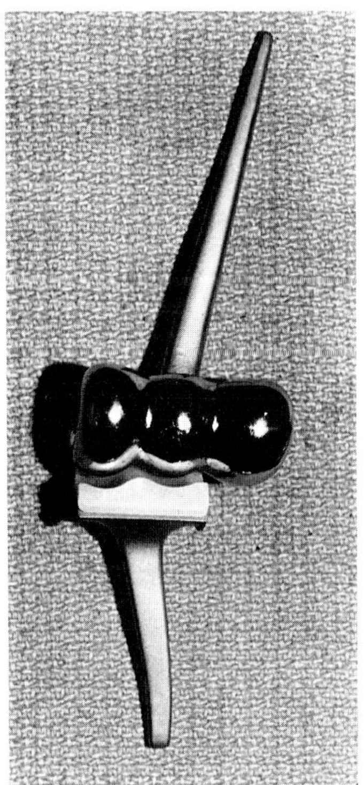

Fig. 10-19. Ewald total elbow.

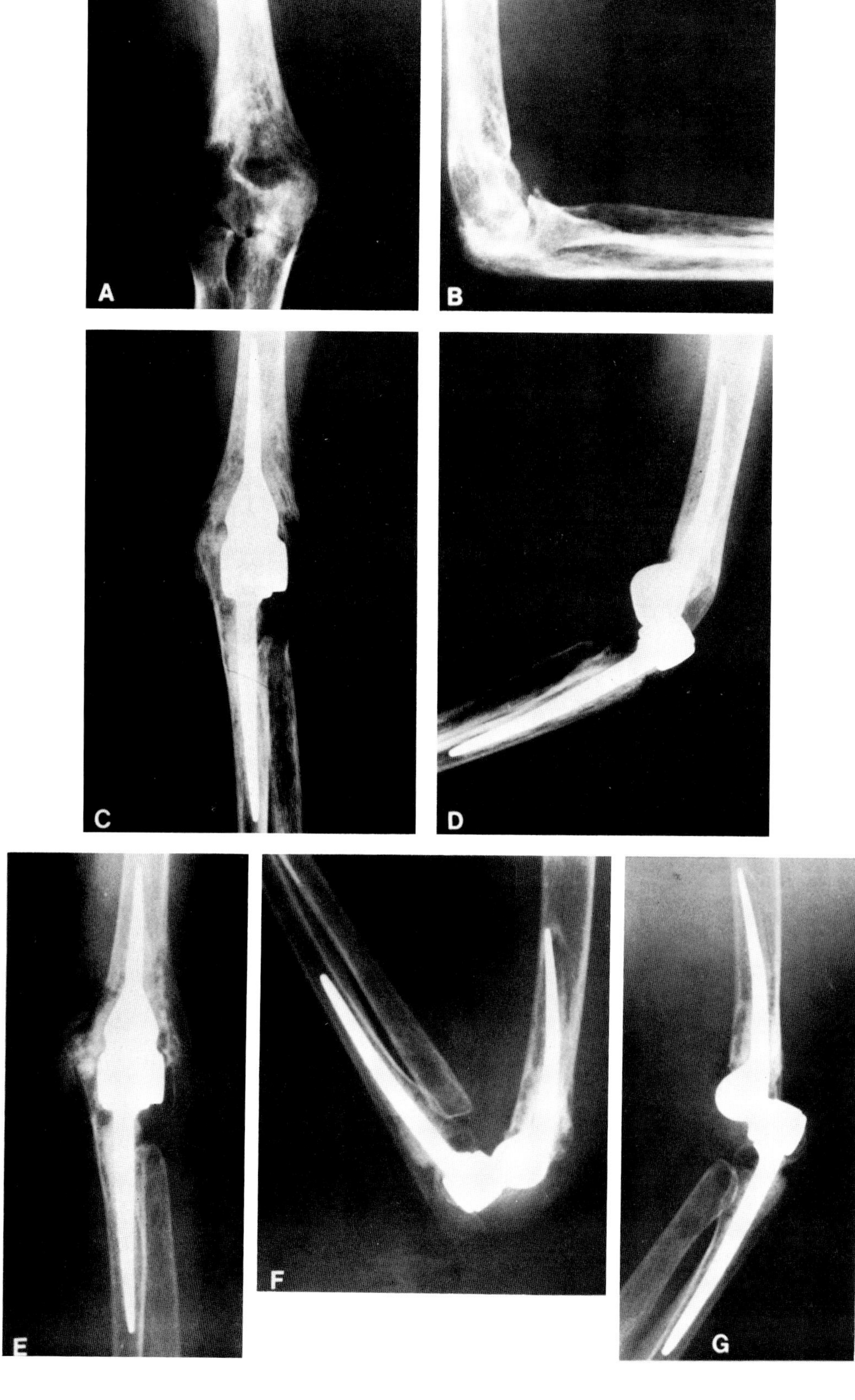

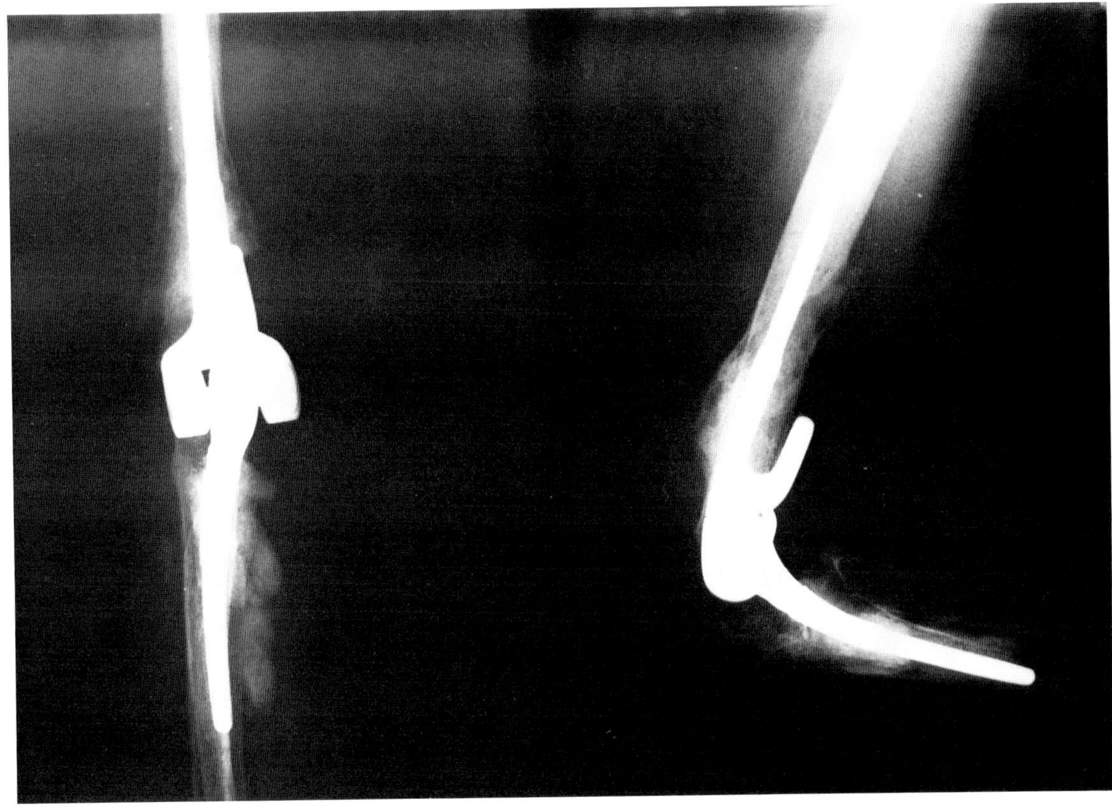

Fig. 10-20. (A) Preoperative anteroposterior roentgenogram of the elbow shows severe narrowing and destruction of the elbow joint. (B) Lateral roentgenogram. (C) Roentgenogram 8 months after insertion of the GSB elbow shows good position and function. (D) Lateral roentgenogram. (E) Anteroposterior roentgenogram 6 years after surgery shows fracture of the medial condyle with bone resorption and loosening. (F) Lateral rotengenogram shows amount of fixation. (G) Lateral roentgenogram shows extension. (H) Postoperative Coonrad-Morrey elbow, anteroposterior and lateral views.

for dislocation, two for sepsis, one for loosening, and one for fracture. Five experienced recurrent dislocation, and there were five permanent and six transient ulnar nerve palsies. Three fractures occurred: two of the olecranon and one of the humeral shaft. Three elbows demonstrated some degree of wound breakdown and skin loss.

Clark and Weiland[2] reported 16 Ewald elbows for rheumatoid arthritis, with pain relief in all cases. Complications included one patient who required additional surgery owing to subluxation and one patient with ulnar neuropathy. Judging from all of these reports, we conclude that elbow replacement should not be performed by the "occasional elbow" surgeon.

We have performed 16 total elbow replacements, all on rheumatoid patients. Four were done with rigid hinges: three GSB and one Coonrad. The first was performed in 1971, and two are still excellent results. Flexion and extension arc is between 104 and 140 degrees, and all have had full rotation. We chose the GSB initially because we thought that its small size would preserve bone stock so if the device had to be removed a fascial arthroplasty with stability was still possible. These four patients were followed between 22 and 84 months. One of the elbows loosened after 6 years and is painful now. One GSB elbow did well for 7 years before developing a deep wound infection that necessitated operative treatment; this elbow is still functioning well 6 months later.

Case Report 4

A 53-year-old woman with an 18-year history of rheumatoid arthritis presented in 1976, complaining that she had developed an increasing amount of pain in the left elbow. She had already had numerous operative procedures for rheumatoid deformities.

Motion was from 25 to 150 degrees with full rotation. There was marked pain and crepitation with motion. The elbow was unstable. Roentgenograms showed marked destruction of the elbow joint (Fig. 10-20A & B).

In April 1976 a GSB total elbow was inserted. Postoperative roentgenograms (Fig. 10-20C & D) 8 months after insertion of the GSB elbow showed good position and fixation. The patient did well with motion from 0 to 140 degrees and full rotation until October 1982, when she developed mild elbow pain. Her motion was 30 to 145 degrees with full rotation. There was no tenderness or swelling but mild crepitation medially along a small, movable fragment. Roentgenograms (Fig. 10-20G) showed fracture of the medial condyle and bone absorption with loosening. Flexion and extension motion remained excellent. It was revised to a Coonrad-Morrey semiconstrained hinge with a good result (Fig. 10-20H).

Case Report 5

A 48-year-old woman with a long-standing history of rheumatoid arthritis with severe involvement of the left elbow presented in 1977. The elbow was painful with decreased motion. She could flex from 65 to 110 degrees with 80 degrees supination and 40 degrees pronation. Preoperative roentgenograms (Fig. 10-21A & B) showed severe destruction of the elbow joint.

In September 1977 she underwent an Ewald total elbow arthroplasty (Fig. 10-21C & D). Her

postoperative course was complicated by acute cholecystitis, renal failure, gram-negative septicemia, respiratory failure, and skin breakdown over the olecranon (Fig. 10-21E). A flap was rotated over the defect, and she was doing well 2 months postoperatively with no pain on motion and no evidence of loosening or bony destruction. Motion was 45 to 115 degrees with 40 degrees supination and 60 degrees pronation.

Six months after the original surgery, the elbow started draining and was painful, necessitating removal of the prosthesis and conversion to a resection arthroplasty (Fig. 10-21F & G).

She had another episode of infection 3 years after removal of the elbow that was treated with antibiotics and suction irrigation. The elbow is pain-free, but it is unstable and lacks active extension. She is prone to developing blood-borne infections, as are certain severe rheumatoid arthritic patients. This patient died 1 year later owing to repeated infection elsewhere in her body.

Complications

Because of the high rate of hinge loosening reported with the original rigid GSB, we started using the Ewald capitellocondylar nonconstrained elbow if there are adequate ligaments and bone stock preoperatively. Our series[8] of the first consecutive 20 cases showed 95 percent satisfactory results, but the complications have been numerous and significant, making us proceed with great caution if we are to continue with this procedure. Eight of the 20 cases experienced twelve complications: subluxation (two patients) (Fig. 10-22), dislocation (one), posterior interosseous neuropathy (one), ulnar neuropathy (one), skin necrosis (two), failure due to infection, late (one), rupture of triceps repair (two).

One patient with ulnar neuropathy underwent nerve decompression and anterior transposition with return of normal function. The other two resolved spontaneously. Of the subluxators, one was splinted for an extended period; the elbow

Fig. 10-21. (**A & B**) Preoperative roentgenograms showing severe destruction of the elbow. (**C & D**) Postoperative roentgenograms showing placement of the Ewald elbow. (**E**) Skin breakdown over the olecranon. (**F & G**) Prosthesis was removed because of infection. It left the patient with an unstable elbow, but it was painless and she could flex to her face.

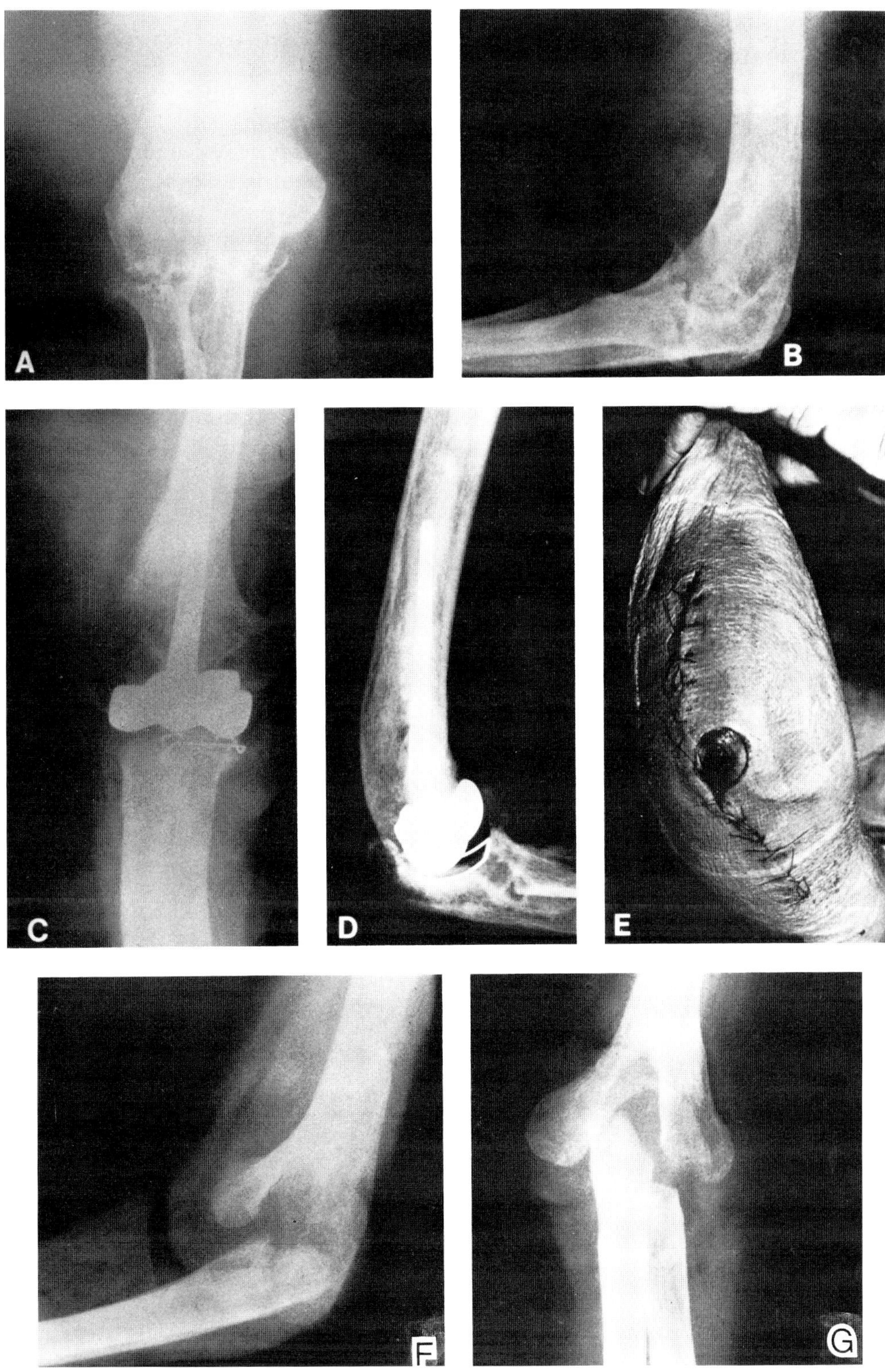

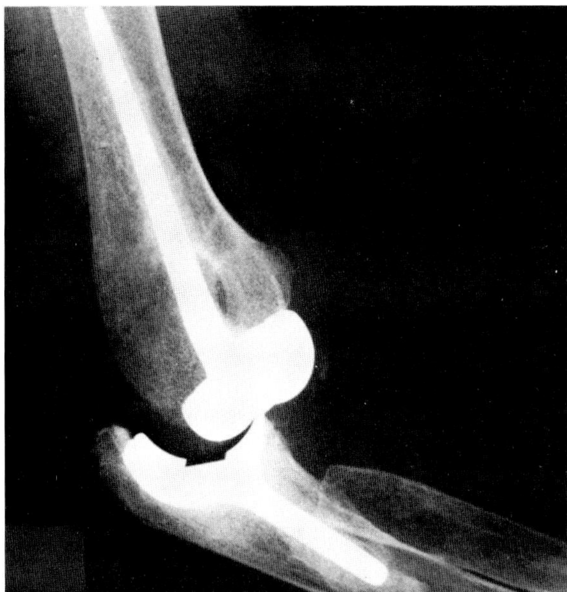

Fig. 10-22. Postoperative subluxation of the Ewald elbow. This patient was pleased with the pain relief from the surgery and has learned to control the subluxation by proper positioning of her arm.

was stable for a long time but then started to subluxate. One patient underwent ligament repair at surgery and is stable; and another patient learned to control the subluxation by properly positioning the elbow. These three elbows are painless, and the patients are pleased. One patient complains of elbow "noises," but the elbow is stable. Two patients experienced skin necrosis over the olecranon, one ending in infection with elbow failure necessitating removal, leaving her with an unstable joint. The other patient had a rotational skin flap that failed, followed by a successful pedicle graft from the abdomen. This patient is the same one who underwent ligament repair for subluxation and who ruptured the triceps tendon attachment to the ulnar, which was repaired by suturing a flap of tendon through drill holes into bone (Fig. 10-23). This patient exercised too vigorously after surgery in an uncontrolled environment, which points out the need for close postoperative supervision. Despite these complications, only one patient claims to be a failure during the period of our study.

Our experience with use of the semiconstrained hinges has shown them to have a low incidence of loosening. Therefore we have restricted the use of the nonconstrained elbow to the under-40-year-old rheumatoid arthritic with adequate bone stock and ligamentous support. For all others and for those with the aseptically failed elbow, we are currently using the semiconstrained Morrey-modified Coonrad device: Morrey and Adams[25] reported on 92 total elbow arthroplasties using the semiconstrained device in rheumatoid arthritis patients. Their results include a 3-year survival rate of 94 percent and no

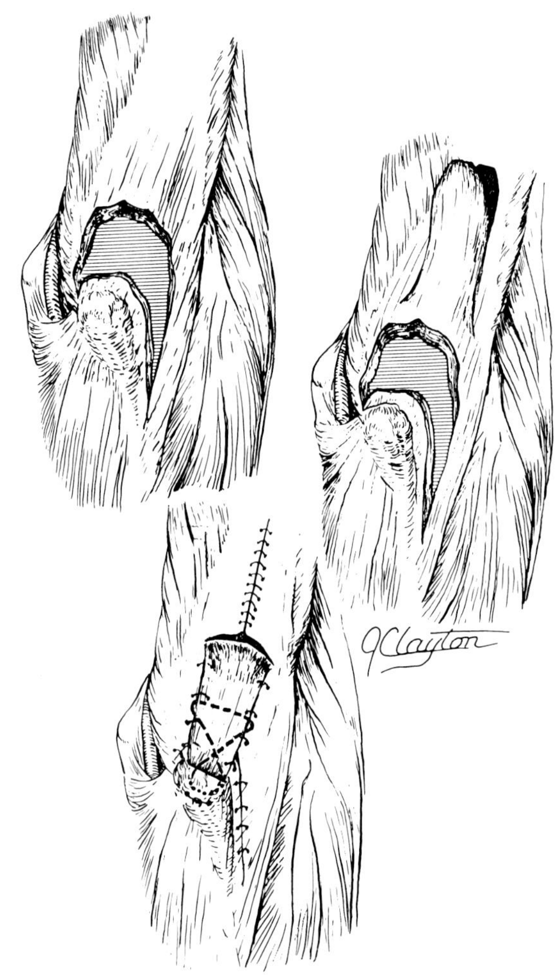

Fig. 10-23. Method for reconstructing the triceps tendon after rupture of its attachment into the olecranon. (From Ferlic,[10a] with permission.)

revisions required for mechanical loosening. They detailed their operative technique in a book on total joint arthroplasty.[25]

Technique for Capitellocondylar (Ewald) Nonconstrained Elbow

Our operative technique has varied throughout this small series. We initially used a posterior incision but switched to a lateral incision because of subluxation problems. The first patient with the lateral approach experienced ulnar neu-ropathy, and we are now making a straight posterolateral skin incision, avoiding the tip of the olecranon.

The ulnar nerve is identified and protected. The triceps is stripped subperiostally off the olecranon and lateral side of the humerus. The strong anterior medial collateral ligament is the key and is preserved. The radial ligaments are divided in such a manner that they can be reattached at the time of closure (Fig. 10-24). The joint is dislocated, the radial head excised, and

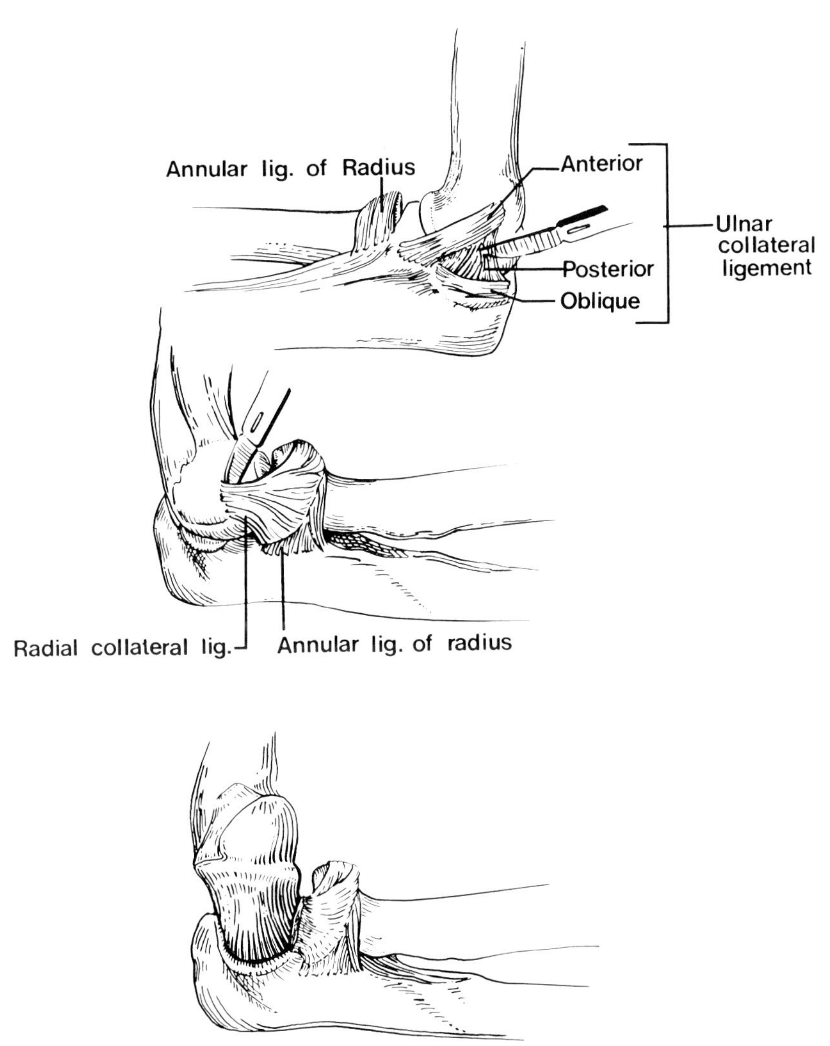

Fig. 10-24. Elbow is hinged open, dividing the radial collateral ligament but preserving the strong anterior medial collateral ligament. The posterior portion of the medial collateral ligament may also be divided.

synovectomy carried out. The medullary canal of the humerus is prepared to accept the prosthesis. The humeral component comes in 5, 10, and 15 degrees valgus prostheses, and the proper one is selected to fit the humerus. Bone is then removed from the semilunar notch of the ulna, with care taken not to weaken and fracture the olecranon by reaming too much bone. The medullary canal of the ulna is then opened with burrs and rasps. Trials are inserted, and the elbow is reduced. Final adjustments are made and the components cemented in place. The tourniquet is lowered after the cement hardens. The ligaments are repaired, a drain is inserted, and the wound is closed. Splints are applied with the elbow in 60 degrees of flexion, which removes some of the pressure from the skin and relaxes the triceps repair. The splints must be well padded, and the surgeon must be aware of possible skin breakdown over the olecranon, particularly in the thin rheumatoid patient who has been on steroids.

Postoperative motion has generally not been as difficult to obtain as in the trauma patient after open reduction and internal fixation, and our series of total elbow replacements reflects this good motion. The problem in the nonlinked elbow prosthesis has been instability, and therefore we do not hesitate to immobilize the elbow for 2 to 3 weeks before beginning motion if necessary; we usually, however, start protected motion at 3 to 5 days if the ligamentous repair is stable.

At the time of surgery the individual's postoperative needs must be considered as well as the integrity of the ligamentous repair. We individualize the patient's rehabilitation to the type of repair that was necessary at surgery and to the type of disease inflicting the patient. For example, the patient with the stiff type of rheumatoid arthritis is mobilized sooner than the patient with the loose type. Moreover, the patient in whom the ligaments were taken down and reattached needs protection for 6 weeks. Close supervision is necessary. We always consider the postoperative therapy while still in the operating room after we have repaired the ligaments, noting the strength of the attachments and the amount of flexion possible before it exerts stress on the triceps repair. This information is useful when the

individualized postoperative program is instituted with the therapist.

In addition, we are constantly aware of the relation of the elbow to the adjacent joints, particularly true in the rheumatoid patient who has a stiff or painful shoulder or wrist. These patients must initially learn to exercise their new elbow in a straight flexion-extension plane without putting torque or angular stress on the elbow, as the latter would cause instability in the nonlinked elbow.

Of all the total joint replacements, the elbow has been the one with the most complications, which has motivated us to think of better methods for managing the rheumatoid patient with stage IV disease. We perform radial head resection and débridement with synovectomy for stage III, hoping to bide time. For late stage III, this treatment may not be successful. Future design modifications may be useful; smaller components that save bone stock may be helpful so stability can be maintained in case of failure. Alternatives to cement fixation may help. Coonrad's long-stemmed humeral component seems to fit tightly in the medullary canal, and perhaps it is not necessary to cement it in place in every case. Porous-surfaced implants are now being used in the lower extremities. The varying sizes of the humeri and the poor quality of bone in many rheumatoid patients are factors that argue against universal use of these implants in the elbow. The goal should be a biologic implant, such as a homograft; the ultimate goal, of course, is eradication of the disease itself.

SUMMARY

Synovectomy of the elbow with radial head resection produces good to excellent results for stage II and early stage III involvement, so relatively few total elbow replacements are necessary. The latter procedure has been associated with a high complication rate, although the overall results of elbow replacement have improved with advances in the surgical technique and component design.

REFERENCES

1. Anderson LD, Heppenstall M: Synovectomy of the elbow and excision of the radial head in rheumatoid arthritis. In Creuss RL, Mitchel N (eds): Surgery of Rheumatoid Arthritis. JB Lippincott, Philadelphia, 1971

2. Clark G, Weiland AJ: Total elbow arthroplasty of the Ewald type. Presented at the midyear meeting of the American Society for Surgery of the Hand. Boyne Mt., MI, July 1979

3. Cofield RH, Morrey EF, Bryon RS: Total shoulder and total elbow arthroplasties: the current state of development. Part 2. JCE Orthop 7:17, 1979

4. Cooney WP III, Bryon RS: Rheumatoid arthritis in the upper extremity: treatment of the elbow and shoulder joints. Instr Course Lect 28:247, 1979

5. Coonrad RP: Results with the Coonrad total elbow arthroplasty. Presented to the Piedmont Orthopaedic Society. Baca Raton, FL, May 1980

6. Coonrad RP: Infection in total elbow arthroplasties. ASSH Correspondence Letter, April 1, 1981

7. Dempster WT: Space requirements of the seated operator: geometrical, kinematic and mechanical aspects of the body with special reference to the limbs. p. 55. Project no. 7214. WADC Technical Reports, Wright-Patterson AFB, OH, 1955

8. Dennis DA, Clayton ML, Ferlic DC et al: Capitello-condylar total elbow arthroplasty for rheumatoid arthritis. J Arthroplasty, suppl., 5:S83, 1990

9. Ewald FC: Total elbow replacement. Orthop Clin North Am 6:685, 1975

10. Ewald FC, Scheinberg RD, Poss et al: Capitello-condylar total elbow arthroplasty. J Bone Joint Surg [Am] 62:1259, 1980

10a. Ferlic DC: Rheumatoid arthritis in the elbow. p. 1767. In Green D (ed): Operative Hand Surgery. 2nd ed. Churchill Livingstone, New York, 1988

11. Ferlic DC, Clayton ML, Parr PL: Synovectomy and arthroplasty of the elbow in rheumatoid arthritis. Orthop Digest 5:11, 1977

12. Ferlic DC, Patchett CE, Clayton ML, Freeman A: Synovectomy of the elbow in rheumatoid arthritis: long term results. Clin Orthop 220:119, 1987

13. Fischer G, cited by Fick, R: Hanbüch der Anatomie und Mechanik du Gelenke unter Berücksichtigung der Bewegenden Muskoln. Vol. 2. p. 299, 1911

14. Inglis AE, Pellicci PN: Total elbow replacement. J Bone Joint Surg [Am] 62:1252, 1980

15. Inglis AE, Ranawat CS, Straub LR: Synovectomy and debridement of the elbow in rheumatoid arthritis. J Bone Joint Surg [Am] 53:652, 1971

16. Knight RA, Van Zandt IL: Arthroplasty of the elbow: an end result study. J Bone Joint Surg [Am] 34:610, 1952

17. Kudo H, Iware K, Watanabe S: Total replacement of the rheumatoid elbow with a hingeless prosthesis. J Bone Joint Surg [Am] 62:277, 1980

18. Laine V, Vainio K: The elbow in rheumatoid arthritis. p. 112. In Hijmans WDP, Herschel H (eds): Early Synovectomy in Rheumatoid Arthritis. Proceedings of the Symposium on Early Synovectomy in Rheumatoid Arthritis, Amsterdam, April 12–15, 1967. Excerpta Medica Foundation, Amsterdam, 1969

19. Lanyi V, Preston R, McEwen C: Synovectomy in rheumatoid arthritis. NY State Med J 68:3135, 1968

20. Linscheid RL: Surgery for rheumatoid arthritis: timing and techniques; the upper extremity. J Bone Joint Surg [Am] 50:605, 1968

21. London JT: Kinematics of the elbow. J Bone Joint Surg [Am] 63:529, 1981

22. London JT, Brumfield RH, Ferlic DC et al: Symposium: total elbow arthroplasty. Contemp Orthop 3:541, 1981

23. Marmor L: Surgery of the rheumatoid elbow. J Bone Joint Surg [Am] 54:573, 1972

24. Moore JR, Weiland AJ: Bilateral attrition rupture of the ulnar nerve at the elbow. J Hand Surg 5:358, 1980

25. Morrey BF, Adams RA: Semiconstrained devices: techniques and results. p. 311. In Morrey BF, Chao EYS, Cooney WP III et al. (eds): Joint Replacement Arthroplasty. Churchill Livingstone, New York, 1990

26. Morrey BF, Chao EYS: Passive motion of the elbow joint: a biomechanical analysis. J Bone Joint Surg [Am] 58:501, 1976

27. Porter BB, Park N, Richardson C, Vainio K: Rheumatoid arthritis of the elbow; the results of synovectomy. J Bone Joint Surg [Br] 56:427, 1974

28. Ray RD, Johnson RJ, Jameson RM: Rotation of the forearm: an experimental study of pronation and supination. J Bone Joint Surg [Am] 33:993, 1951

29. Schuller M: Chirurgische Mittheilungen uber die Chronisch. Rheumatishen Gelerkentzundungen. Arch Klin Chir 45:153, 1893

30. Smith-Petersen MN, Aufranc OE, Larson CB: Useful surgical procedures for rheumatoid arthritis involving joints of the upper extremity. Arch Surg 46:764, 1943

31. Souter WA: Arthroplasty of the elbow. Orthop Clin North Am 4:395, 1973
32. Straub LR: Surgical rehabilitation of the hand and upper extremity in rheumatoid arthritis. Bull Rheum Dis 12:265, 1962
33. Street DM, Stevens PS: A humeral replacement prosthesis for the elbow; results in ten elbows. J Bone Joint Surg [Am] 56:1147, 1974
34. Torgerson WR, Leach RE: Synovectomy of the elbow in rheumatoid arthritis. J Bone Joint Surg [Am] 52:371, 1970
35. Von Meyer H: Kinesiology of the Human Body under Normal and Pathological Conditions. p. 490. Charles C Thomas, Springfield, IL, 1955
36. Walker PS: Human Joints and Their Artificial Replacements. Charles C Thomas, Springfield, IL, 1978
37. Wilkinson MC, Lowry JH: Synovectomy for rheumatoid arthritis. J Bone Joint Surg [Br] 47:482, 1965
38. Wilson DW: Synovectomy of the elbow for rheumatoid arthritis. Proc R Soc Med 64:264, 1971
39. Wilson DW, Arden GP, Ansell BM: Synovectomy of the elbow in rheumatoid arthritis. J Bone Joint Surg [Br] 55:106, 1973

11

Management of the Rheumatoid Wrist

Donald C. Ferlic

The wrist, the key joint of the upper extremity, must be stable, balanced, and pain-free for proper hand function.[50] The wrist joint usually refers to the radiocarpal articulation, but in reality the wrist joint is made up of all the articulations between the metacarpals and distal carpal row, the distal-proximal carpal row and the radiocarpal articulations, and the radioulnar joint. Needless to say, the recorded common wrist motions of flexion, extension, radial and ulnar deviation, and rotation are complex motions involving many joints. All of these joints have synovial linings; and because rheumatoid arthritis is a systemic disease that affects the synovial membranes of joints and tendon sheaths this entire system is under attack in the rheumatoid patient.

The wrist bones are compartmentalized by ligaments, and there may be some normal variation making wrist arthrography difficult to interpret. These ligaments connect the bones of the proximal carpal row, creating a proximal space with the radius. The space between the radius and ulna is blocked off by the articular disc, which attaches to the base of the ulnar styloid on the ulnar side of the radius. A midcarpal space is continuous with the joint cavities between the bones of the distal row, and frequently it connects with the carpometacarpal joints.

The large flexor and extensor tendons cross the wrist going to the hand. These nine flexor tendons and twelve extensor tendons are lined with synovium and are subject to the ravages of rheumatoid disease.

Rotation of the forearm is the most important components for adapting the wrist joint to movements of the hand. Dysfunctions of the distal radioulnar joint in rheumatoid arthritis is commonly characterized by the "caput ulna syndrome."[3] The clinical manifestations of this syndrome are as follows.[52]

1. Increasing weakness of the wrist, crepitation on movement (especially on rotation), and pain, which may be sudden, sharp, severe, and momentarily prevent hand usage
2. Loss of rotation and dorsiflexion of the wrist
3. Dorsal prominence and instability of the head of the ulna
4. Soft tissue swelling over the ulnar dorsal surface of the wrist caused by synovial proliferation
5. Associated descent of the fourth and fifth metacarpals
6. Occasional rupture of the extensor tendons to the digits
7. Loss of normal action of the extensor carpi ulnaris, which produces some of the deformities seen in the rheumatoid hand, including radial rotation of the wrist

With increasing synovial hypertrophy, the ligamentous support of the distal ulna—the so-called distal radio-ulnar-carpal complex formed by the triangular fibrocartilage and its ligaments—and the ulnar collateral ligament and surrounding capsule weaken, allowing the ulnar head to dislocate dorsally. The extensor carpi ulnaris subluxes ulna- and palmarward, losing its stabilizing effect on the distal ulna and allowing increased palmar descent of the fourth and fifth metacarpals, which is a rotary supination deformity of the carpus.[54]

CONSERVATIVE TREATMENT

The wrist is the most commonly involved upper extremity joint in the rheumatoid patient. It is the one part of the hand that can be splinted for long periods with some success; and both static and dynamic splinting may be useful. The position in which the wrist should be splinted is neutral with about 10 degrees ulnar deviation. Lightweight night splints that are simple to use and not too cumbersome for a badly involved arthritic patient to handle are applied (Fig. 11-1). We have found time and again that if a splint is kept simple the patient will wear it. Conversely, the complex, burdensome device is often abandoned.[10] A single steroid injection may be useful, but local steroid injections have been implicated in tendon rupture and joint destruction, so they are used sparingly for dorsal tenosynovitis. Although physical therapy is useful for rheumatoid arthritis, it is of little help with the wrist. We do use joint positioning and joint education techniques, however, and call on the hand therapist to instruct patients in these areas.

INDICATIONS FOR SURGERY

Indications for surgery are progressive pain and deformity in the joints or progression of the syn-

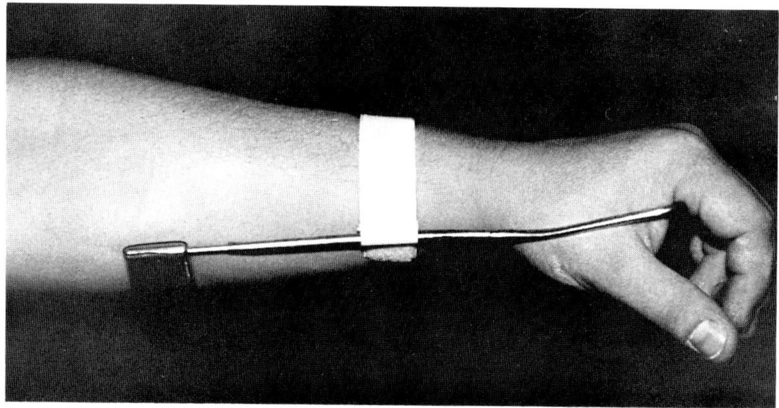

A

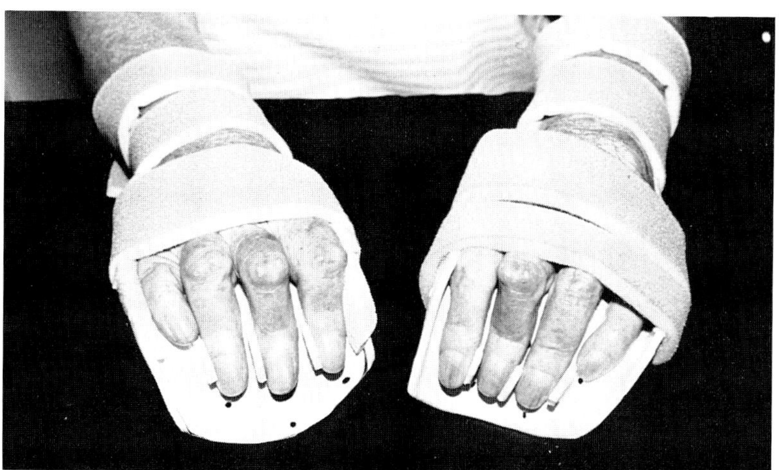

B

Fig. 11-1. (A) Lightweight, plastic-coated wire splint. (B) Molded arthroplasty night splints.

ovial disease in tendon sheaths despite adequate general medical treatment. In general, any patient with rheumatoid arthritis who is selected for surgery should be properly motivated and be willing to cooperate in the pre- and postoperative regimen. Surgery to the wrist, however, may be indicated even in the lackadaisical patient because of the known disastrous natural course of tendon rupture that occurs if surgery is withheld and because a good result may be obtained without a formal postoperative exercise program.

Dorsal Tenosynovitis

Rheumatoid tenosynovitis on the dorsum of the wrist begins underneath the dorsal carpal ligament and extends distally, causing swelling below this rigid ligament.[11] Occasionally, it is misdiagnosed as a ganglion. Ligamentous involvement and instability of the distal radioulnar joint is often present. If the process does not respond to a few weeks of simple splinting and rest, surgical treatment is indicated to prevent tendon damage.

Rupture of the extensor tendons at the wrist level has been blamed solely on the erosive effect of the distal end of the ulna, but tendon rupture has occurred after distal ulnar resection where no other wrist surgery has been performed. Our experience[11] indicated that extensor tendon rupture results from a combination of factors: (1) erosion caused by bone irregularity; (2) compressive effect of the dorsal carpal ligament; and (3) direct rheumatoid invasion of the tendons. Other causes, demonstrated at least in the flexor tendons, are local steroid injections and occlusion by hypertrophic rheumatoid tissue around vincular vessels causing localized infarcts in the tendon.[35]

Extensor tendons may rupture in areas other than the wrist, and we have seen two cases where extensor tendons ruptured over the metacarpal heads as the result of bone spurs at this level. The diagnosis of rupture of the extensor tendons at the wrist usually poses no problem (Fig. 11-2), but two other conditions must be considered in the differential diagnosis in the rheumatoid patient. The first is the result of metacarpophalangeal (MCP) synovitis where the extensor tendons have slipped off the metacarpal heads into the intermetacarpal areas so the extensor tendons are below the axis of rotation, impeding their mechanical advantage (Fig. 11-3). The second is that of posterior interosseous nerve palsy secondary to rheumatoid involvement at the elbow[36,39] (Fig. 11-4).

Tendon rupture of the extensor tendons at the wrist in rheumatoid arthritis is not just an academic issue. There have been many artic-

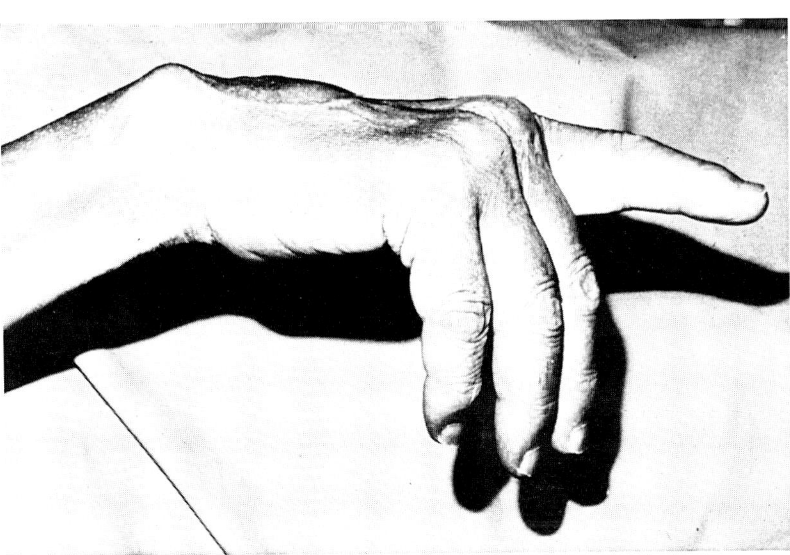

Fig. 11-2. Position of fingers on a hand with rupture of the extensor tendons to the ulnar three digits. (From Ferlic,[18a] with permission.)

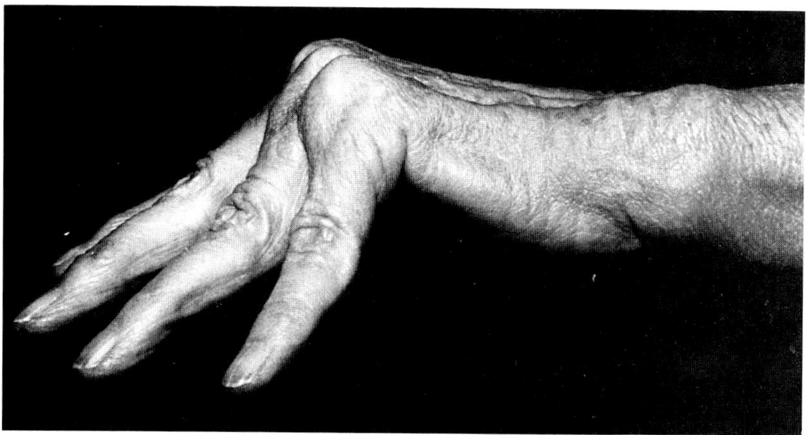

Fig. 11-3. This patient is unable to extend her fingers because of metacarpophalangeal synovitis, which caused the extensor tendons to slip into the intermetacarpal spaces below the axis of rotation. Contracted joints have resulted.

les[11,31,35,40,43,44,50,51] in the literature dealing with spontaneous tendon rupture in the arthritic wrist, beginning with that of Vaughan-Jackson,[58] who reported two cases in 1948.

The most frequently ruptured tendon is the common extensor to the little finger, followed by the tendon to the ring finger. Next, in order of frequency of rupture, is the extensor pollicis longus, extensor digiti minimi, long finger extensor, index extensor, extensor carpi radialis brevis, extensor carpi radialis longus, extensor indicis proprius, and extensor carpiulnaris.[14] Ideal management, of course, is to perform surgery before the tendons rupture. The tendon that is prevented from rupturing always works better than the one that needed reconstruction.

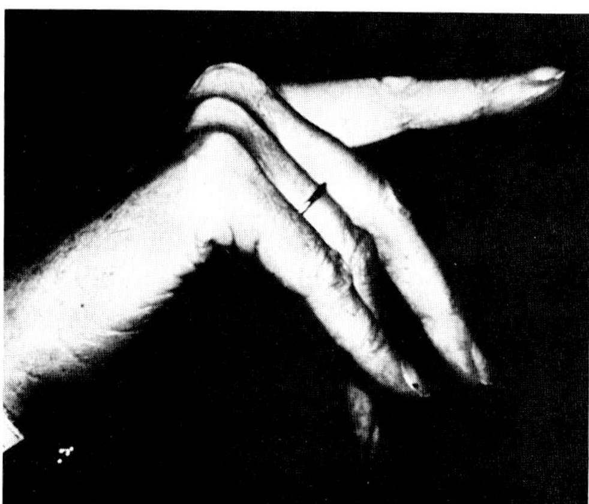

Fig. 11-4. Inability to extend the fingers because of posterior interosseous nerve palsy as a result of elbow synovitis. (From Ferlic,[18a] with permission.)

Early synovectomy is indicated before the extensor tendons rupture.[38] We have reported[14] and others have shown that dorsal wrist surgery, consisting in tenosynovectomy, synovectomy, resection of the distal end of the ulna, and transposition of the dorsal carpal ligament underneath the extensor tendons, indeed prevents tendon rupture.

Surgical Technique

A straight-line or minimally wavy 10- to 14-cm longitudinal dorsal incision is made. It may be diagonal or placed more to the radial or ulnar side, depending on where the tenosynovitis is most severe. The incision is long enough that retraction is gentle (Fig. 11-5). The skin is not undermined, but the subcutaneous fat is left attached to minimize the chance of skin necrosis. Dorsal veins should be preserved as much as possible. Dorsal sensory nerves are easily protected, as the incision is made between them. The dorsal carpal ligament is reflected from the ulnar side, leaving it attached radially. The dorsal carpal ligament is also reflected ulnarward, exposing the extensor carpi ulnaris (Fig. 11-6). All extensor compartments are opened, and each extensor tendon is isolated (Fig. 11-7). A tenosynovectomy is performed. Complete meticulous removal is not necessary, as the tendons rest in a bed of healthy fat and heal in the altered environment. Rheumatoid synovium does not proliferate and invade tendons in healthy fat. Bony spicules are removed from the carpus and distal radius.

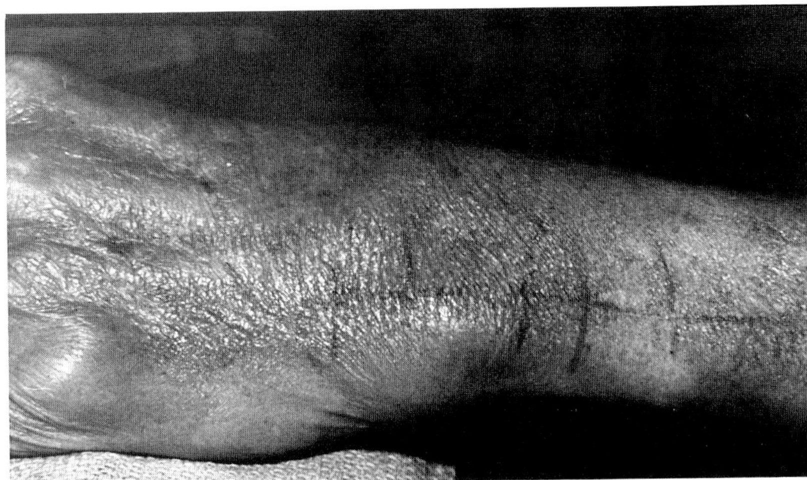

Fig. 11-5. Skin incision for dorsal wrist reconstruction.

The capsule of the distal ulna is opened longitudinally, and the distal 1 to 2 cm of the ulna is resected and smoothed. The radioulnar disc usually is destroyed. Traction on the fingers distracts the wrist. A rongeur is placed in the radiocarpal joint, where a synovectomy is carried out. The

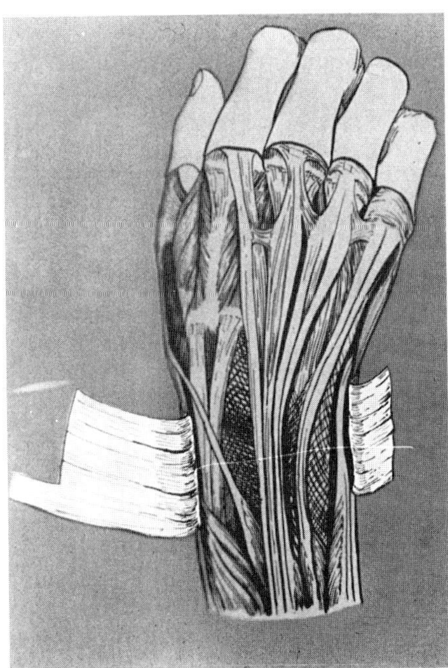

Fig. 11-6. Dorsal carpal ligament is reflected from the extensor compartments. (From Ferlic,[18a] with permission.)

wrist is then reconstructed. The key point of the reconstruction consists in passing the ulnar retinaculum underneath the extensor carpi ulnaris and suturing the retinaculum and ulnar volar capsule to the dorsum of the distal radius. This maneuver reconstructs the radioulnocarpal complex and helps prevent later ulnar sliding and supination deformities. The proximal retinaculum underneath the extensor carpi ulnaris is passed over the distal ulna and sutured to the periosteum along the edge of the radius (Fig. 11-8). The dorsal carpal ligament is then passed underneath the extensor tendons and sutured to its cut edge on the ulnar side, leaving a small strip to be passed around the extensor carpi ulnaris to keep it dorsalized and to help stabilize the distal ulna (Fig. 11-9). Silicone capping of the distal ulna is not necessary. The tourniquet is lowered before wound closure, and drains are inserted. Protective splinting is left in place for 2 to 4 weeks postoperatively.

Using this operative technique before tendons rupture usually prevents this complication in the rheumatoid wrist. Among our first 174 procedures,[14] only one patient subsequently ruptured extensor tendons, and it was due to a technical problem. A rough edge has been left, allowing the ulna to ride dorsalward, and it severed the extensor tendons to the ring and little fingers.

Wound breakdown is another complication encountered with dorsal wrist surgery. It has occurred in about 5 percent of our cases. Most often

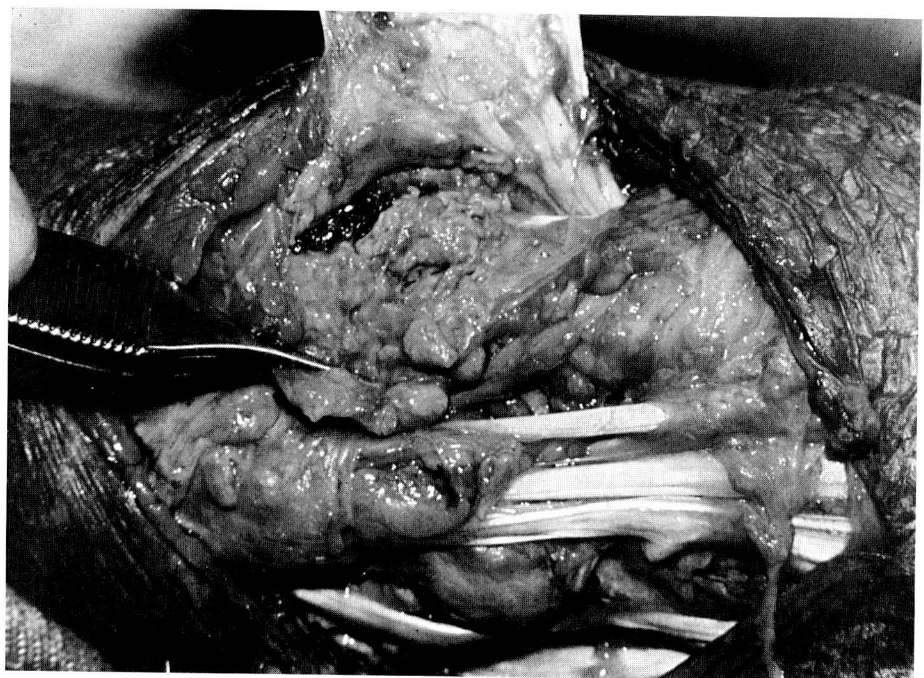

Fig. 11-7. Dorsal tenosynovitis. (From Ferlic,[18a] with permission.)

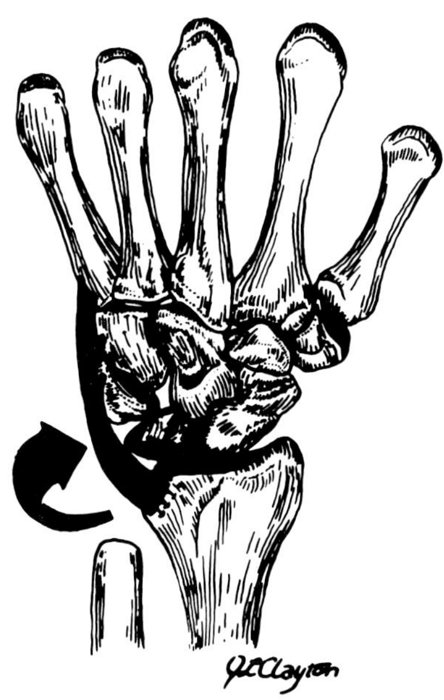

Fig. 11-8. For reconstruction of the wrist, a suture is used to lift up the volar ulnar capsule, placing it into the dorsal capsule. (From Ferlic,[18a] with permission.)

it involves a small area and heals without problem. Rarely, there is a more significant area of the wound that may necessitate débridement or even grafting. This complication can be minimized by (1) making an almost straight, longitudinal, ample incision that does not undermine the skin; (2) leaving all the fat on the skin flaps and preserving all possible dorsal veins; (3) avoiding strong retraction; (4) lowering the tourniquet and obtaining hemostasis; (5) applying wound drainage; (6) apply the dressing to the fingertips with much padding (preferably Dacron batting); and (7) using only light compression and splinting. The splint is applied in the neutral position to avoid tendon bowstringing pressure on the incision. Placing the dorsal retinaculum underneath the extensor tendons decompresses the tendons and places them in the soft subcutaneous tissue.

Abernathy and Bennyson[1] believed that tenosynovectomy is not necessary and found in their series of 54 wrists that the dorsal tenosynovitis resolved in 81.5 percent of the cases after simply transposing the dorsal carpal ligament.

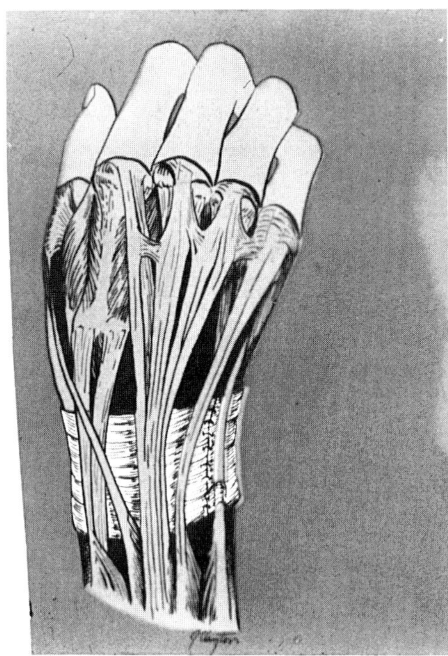

Fig. 11-9. Extensor retinaculum is placed underneath the extensor tendons. Note the loop of retinaculum passing around the extensor carpi ulnaris, keeping this tendon on the dorsum of the wrist. It also helps to stabilize the distal ulna after resection. (From Ferlic,[18a] with permission.)

One possible complication associated with moving the entire retinaculum is bowstringing of the extensor tendons (Fig. 11-10). This problem may be avoided by leaving the dorsal fascia in the forearm proximal to the dorsal carpal ligament. If this fascia must be released, it may become necessary to make a check-rein ligament with a thin strip of dorsal carpal ligament. To prevent the carpus from sliding off the radius, the key suture is made to join the ulnar volar wrist capsule and retinaculum to the dorsal radius.

The use of silicone ulnar cap remains controversial (Fig. 11-11). Swanson[52] stated that the advantages of the implant over simple resection are (1) less bone must be removed; (2) the physiologic length of the ulna is maintained, helping to prevent ulnar carpal shift and provide greater wrist stability; (3) a smooth articular surface in contact with the radius and carpus provides freer movements of the distal radioulnar and carpoulnar joints; (4) there is a smooth surface on which the overlying extensor tendons can glide; (5) the incidence of bone overgrowth is decreased; (6) ligament reconstruction is possible; (7) the important extensor carpi ulnaris tendon may be rerouted over the dorsum of the ulna; and (8) the cosmetic appearance is improved.

Swanson analyzed the results in 73 wrists of 54 patients. He found that all patients were relieved of pain and crepitation and were satisfied with their functional and cosmetic results. All showed improvement in strength of grip and range of motion, especially rotation and dorsiflexion. There was recurrence of the ulnar head subluxation in two, slight distal migration of the implant in five, and bone absorption in two, but it did not affect the clinical results unfavorably. Swanson thought

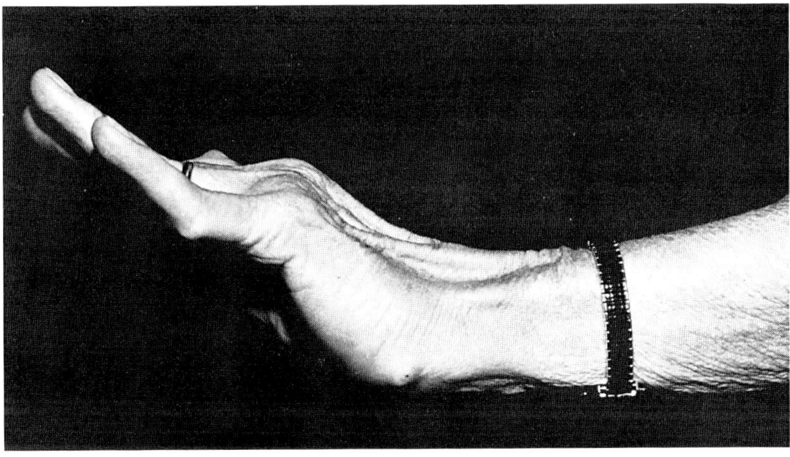

Fig. 11-10. Bowstringing of the extensor tendons.

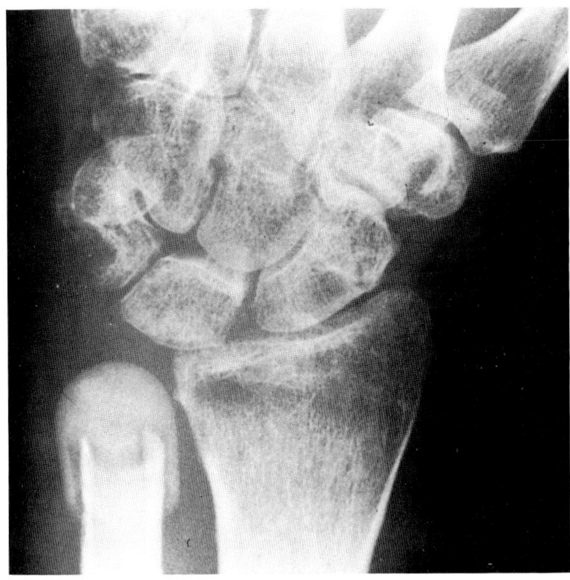

Fig. 11-11. Postoperative wrist roentgenogram after resection of the distal ulnar with a silicone ulnar cap.

that any patient in whom the distal ulna was resected would benefit from the use of the implant for the above reasons. We do not believe that its use prevents the complications it is supposed to avoid; rather, stabilizing the ulnar side of the wrist and the distal ulna by soft tissue reconstruction is the preventative measure one should take in the reconstruction. We have seen several ulnar head implants with bone resorption and implant breakage and do not primarily use this prosthesis (Fig. 11-12).

The last point of emphasis regarding the surgical technique is reconstruction of a flap of retinaculum around the extensor carpi ulnaris, which keeps this tendon on the dorsum of the wrist. It helps stabilize the distal ulna and holds the bases of the fourth and fifth metacarpals from descending and adding to the supination deformity of the hand.

Results

We are confident that dorsal wrist surgery minimizes extensor tendon rupture, but what happens to the wrist joint itself after synovectomy? Does reconstruction on the dorsal side prevent further destruction of the wrist with collapse of the carpus and ulnar translocation? In order to answer these questions, we[55] reviewed our patients after a minimum 5-year follow-up (range 5 to 19 years, average 7.4 years). We found that 95 percent of the patients had excellent relief of

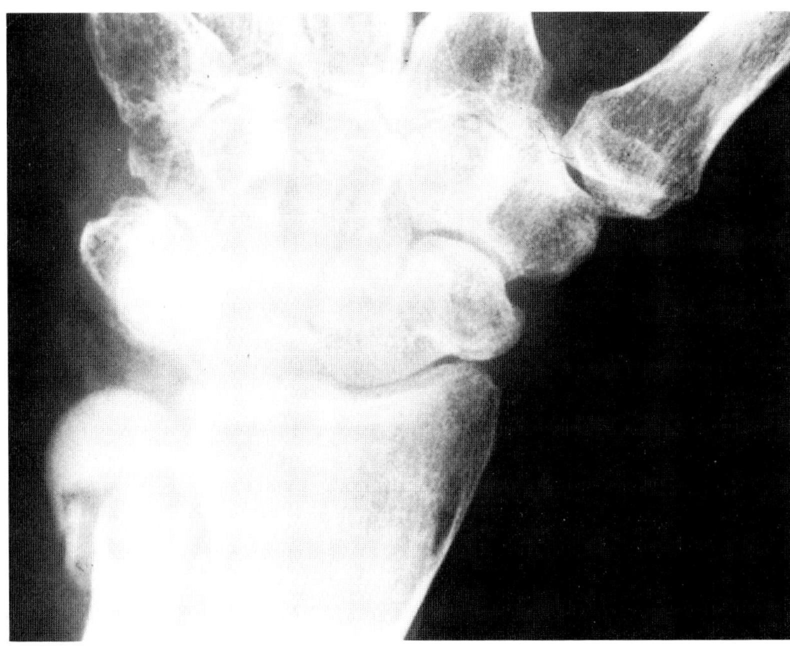

Fig. 11-12. Fractured ulnar head prosthesis with bone resorption.

pain. There was a significant reduction in the arc of wrist motion, but motion was still within a functional range. There was no recurrence of synovitis. The long-term postoperative roentgenograms were compared with preoperative films. Carpal height (the distance from the distal cortex of the capitate and the proximal cortex of the lunate) was measured, as was ulnar deviation of the fingers and ulnar translocation (the change in position of the carpal bones to the ulnar side with reference to a longitudinal line down the radius). The pisiform was chosen as a stable reference for measurement because it is the one carpal bone that is usually unaffected by the rheumatoid process and because this mostly extrasynovial bone has only one small articular surface. Occasionally, a separate joint is formed that is not even connected to the wrist joint. Our findings showed that 70 percent of the patients maintained good carpal height. Those that collapsed more than 5 mm collapsed linearly over a 2-year period, not suddenly. Ulnar translocation of more than 5 mm occurred in 42 percent of the patients and in a linear fashion. Progressive carpal collapse was associated with an increase in ulnar deviation of the fingers. An attempt was made to predict the wrists that would deteriorate with time; this long-term study showed that once collapse and ulnar translocation progressed beyond 5 mm the wrist was likely to continue to change further. Synovectomy does not cure the disease, but it is an effective procedure in the wrist to minimize the destructive effects of the arthritis.

Extensor Tendon Rupture

Many patients with dorsal tenosynovitis experience ruptured tendons, and repair of these structures must be considered at the time of wrist reconstruction. Rarely, if ever, can ruptured extensor tendons in the rheumatoid patient be repaired primarily because they are ruptures of attenuation (Fig. 11-13). In order to reconstruct these tendons, it is necessary to resect a considerable amount of frayed tendon, leaving it too short for end-to-end suture. It results in a contracted digit. The wrist with an acute rupture should, however, be treated with some urgency,[35] the

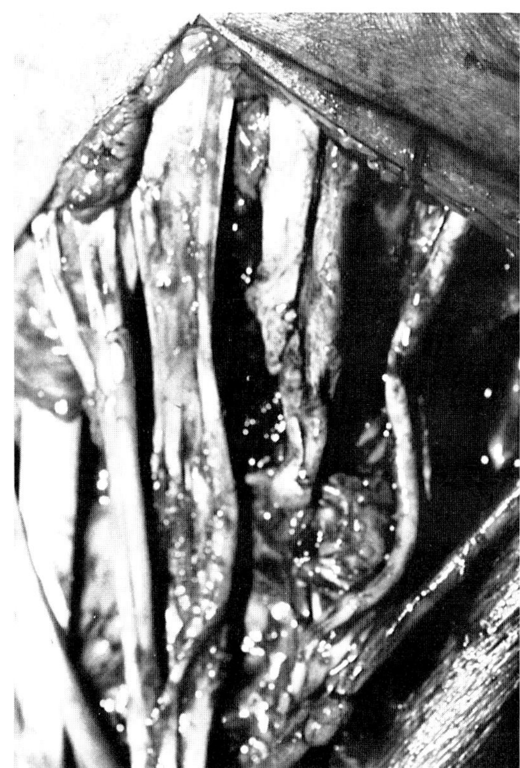

Fig. 11-13. Ruptured extensor tendons showing the frayed and swollen ends.

reason being that a single rupture is often followed by a second rupture; prompt surgery may prevent it. The result of surgery for ruptured tendons is directly proportional to the number of tendons ruptured. A hand with a triple rupture (extensor tendons to the little, ring, and long fingers) cannot be expected to turn out as well as the hand where only the tendons to the little finger were separated. Some of the other general principles of tendon surgery applicable to the traumatically divided tendons may not rigidly apply to the rheumatoid patient. The usual period of tendon immobilization may vary, suture material may be different, silicone rods may be needed, and, lastly, the joint that is being moved by the ruptured tendon may itself need to be sacrificed by arthrodesis or tenodesis rather than attempt a tendon repair. Free grafts are indicated only occasionally in the rheumatoid wrist because the chance of gliding with this devascularized structure is minimal. Other principles of tendon transfer must be appreciated, such as excursion, direction, and power of the transferred muscle, although some bending of these rules may be necessary.

Extensor pollicis longus rupture is common. It is often overlooked because of minimal functional deficit. The extensor pollicis brevis often provides adequate extension of MCP and interphalangeal (IP) joints. It may present as a solitary lesion or be associated with rupture of all the extensor tendons to the digits and wrist, in which case a formidable reconstructive task is obvious. In the isolated case, a number of alternatives are available. Arthrodesis of the IP joint of the thumb may be all that is warranted if the joint is already destroyed or does not have satisfactory passive motion.

Surgical Technique

Goldner[24] reported using a free tendon graft to repair a ruptured extensor pollicis longus tendon and transferred the brachioradialis or extensor carpi radialis longus to the ruptured tendon. In cases where thumb motion must be preserved, our preferred treatment for this rupture is to transfer the indicis proprius. This tendon has excursion similar to that of the extensor pollicis, is easily available, and takes little away from the index finger if the common extensor is present. A separate incision may need to be made over the second MCP joint to detach the indicis proprius. Closure of the extensor hood is necessary to prevent extension lag of the index finger. Usually

the tendon is detached about 1 cm proximal to the MCP joint; traction is exerted on the proximal tendon, and the proprius is then sutured side-to-side to the communis and detached. This move ensures that any pull by the communis is transmitted directly into the hood mechanism, preventing any loss of extension of the MCP joint. The tendon rupture may be far enough proximally that the proprius tendon can be harvested through the original wrist incision.

To treat rupture of the finger extensors, individual transfers work better than mass transfer of one tendon into all that are ruptured. If the extensor tendons to the little finger are gone, transfer of the communis into the adjacent intact ring finger extensor works well. The same principle applies if any single extensor tendon is ruptured, although it is unusual to rupture the extensor to other fingers without also rupturing the little finger extensor (Fig. 11-14). If the extensor to the little and ring fingers have ruptured, the ring finger extensor is sutured into the long finger tendon, and the indicis proprius is used to motor the little finger. The proximal muscles of the ruptured tendon are sutured into the transferred tendon motor. If the adjacent tendon is frayed, it may not be suitable for transfer and should be bypassed to the next tendon. In such a case, a tendon graft is taken to reinforce the weakened area.

In the case of triple rupture, several options are available, but goals are limited. The extensor carpi radialis longus can be transferred into all three ruptured tendons. This method is often

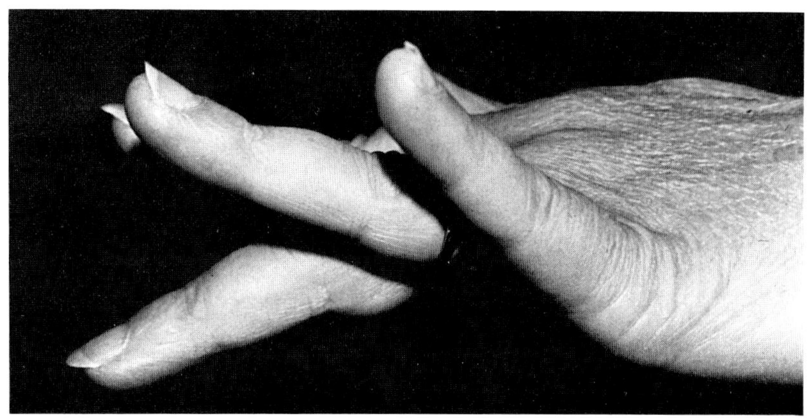

Fig. 11-14. Hand of a patient with rupture of the extensor tendons to the long and ring fingers only, an unusual combination. This hand was successfully treated by transferring the extensor indicis proprius into the long finger and the extensor digiti minimi into the ring finger.

best, considering the extensive pathology involved (Fig. 11-15). Normal finger motion cannot be expected because of the limited excursion of this muscle. If the wrist is supple, a tenodesis effect helps with the motion, but usually the wrist has limited motion in such a case. However, if the wrist has limited motion, the wrist extensors will have enough excursion for full finger motion. Another alternative is to transfer the ruptured long finger tendon into the intact index extensor, transfer the extensor indicis proprius to the little finger, and use a superficialis into the ring finger. One must consider the possibility of using the extensor pollicis longus for transfer if the MCP or IP joints of the thumb are to be arthrodesed at the same time.

Other possibilities of tendon transfer have been expressed by Shannon and Barton,[45] who suggested using the extensor carpi radialis longus for an extensor pollicis longus rupture and saving the indicis proprius. For isolated rupture of the little or ring finger extensors, they recommended use of the extensor indicis proprius or the flexor carpi ulnaris rather than adjacent anastomoses. They also suggested separate transfers for double or triple ruptures, long finger to adjacent tendon, indicis proprius to the ring finger, and flexor carpi ulnaris to the little finger.

In order of preference as the donor muscles, Flatt[23] recommended extensor indicis proprius, extensor carpi radialis longus, extensor carpi ulnaris, and brachioradialis. Harrison et al.[28] recommended the extensor pollicis brevis. Vainio[56] recommended the extensor carpi ulnaris for combined ruptures. Vaughan-Jackson[59] suggested treating the ruptured little finger tendons by splitting the ring finger tendon, detaching the ulnar half of it, and suturing it end-to-end to the distal end of the ruptured little finger tendon. He believed that adjacent end-to-side anastomosis of the distal little finger to the intact ring finger is unsatisfactory. Obviously, there are many possibilities for reconstruction.

In cases where the wrist as well as the finger extensors are ruptured, reconstruction is not possible unless the wrist is fused. The wrist tendons can then be used for transfers. If the wrist is to be fused, the extensor carpi ulnaris makes an excel-

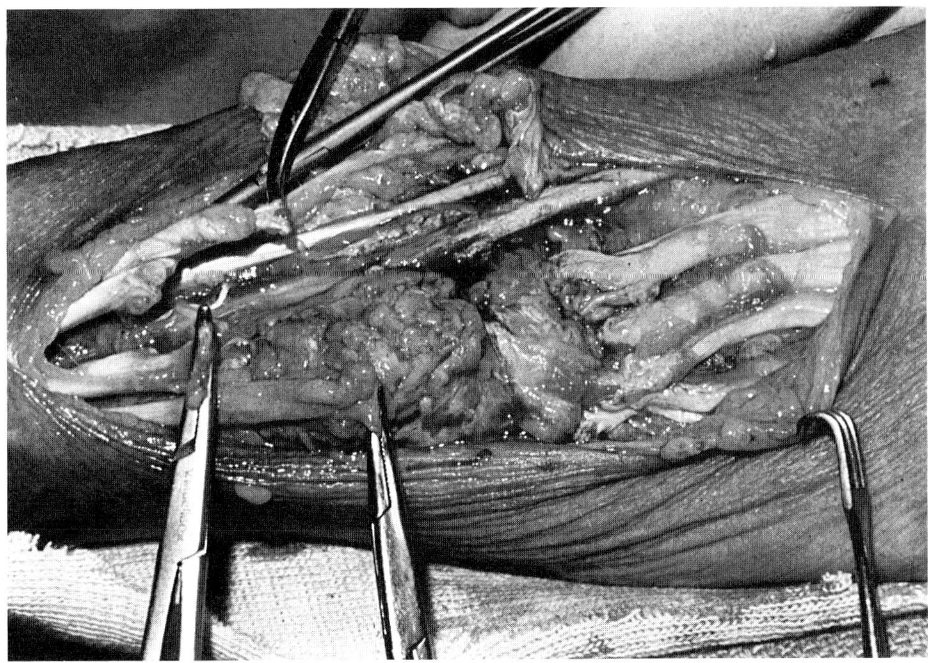

Fig. 11-15. Triple rupture treated with transfer of the extensor carpi radialis longus into all three ruptured tendons.

lent transfer, even for triple ruptures.[12] Surgery to these hands certainly has limited goals, and the patient must be aware of this prognosis before reconstruction is attempted.

The technique of tendon repair is to interweave the tendons, and the technique depends on sufficient length. Suture material should be nonabsorbable. If good fixation is obtained, it may be reasonable to start early protected motion, although it is usually necessary to keep the hand and wrist immobilized 3 to 4 weeks before beginning movement. If adequate length is not available for interweaving or if an interpositional graft is utilized, it is necessary to maintain this extra period of immobilization. When motion is started, dynamic rubberband splints are useful postoperatively.

The hand with ruptured wrist extensors and fixed volar subluxed MCP joints presents a special problem of reconstruction. The MCP joints must be mobilized and the tendon transfers immobilized; thus doing both these procedures together is not advisable. In these cases, the MCP joints should be replaced first and held in extension with dynamic rubberband traction. Motion is started as usual. Wrist surgery and tendon transfers are then performed. This protocol is in contrast to our usual opinion that wrist surgery should be performed first.

Ulnar Drift

It has been hypothesized that radial rotation and deviation of the carpals initiate ulnar drift of the fingers. Ulnar drift begins with a proliferative synovitis of the MCP joints, causing loss of dorsal, radial, and volar support. Thus the fingers may progressively drift toward the ulnar side owing to dynamic influences within the hand,[10,17,49,63] the normal anatomy of the hand,[17,23,27] and external forces acting on the hand.[4,21,22]

In addition, attention has been given to the joints proximal to the MCP level as sites that influence ulnar drift of the fingers. Shapiro[46,47] hypothesized that radial rotation and deviation of the carpals and metacarpals initiates ulnar drift of the fingers. Others have also presented convinc-

ing evidence that these two factors are related. Chaplin et al.[9] have shown statistically that the direction of deviation of the index finger is correlated with deviation of the wrist, but in the opposite direction. Pahle and Raunio[42] reviewed 56 patients with 69 fused wrists and showed a relation between deviation of the wrist and that of the fingers, thus supporting Landsmeer's[33] concept of the "intercalated bone" system, which Shapiro[46] believed is responsible for the deformity. Flatt's[22] clinical observations confirmed Shapiro's views. He further noted that the position and form of the wrist joint may have a direct influence on the posture of the ringers due to the alteration in the line of pull of the extrinsic tendons as in the intercalated bone system.

Although the radial rotation of the metacarpals may not be the sole initiating factor, it is an important one. If radial rotation of the wrist is not corrected, ulnar drift is more prone to occur or recur after ulnar deviation has been corrected. In addition to tenosynovectomy, synovectomy of the wrist, resection of the distal ulna, and transposition of the dorsal carpal ligament, it has been

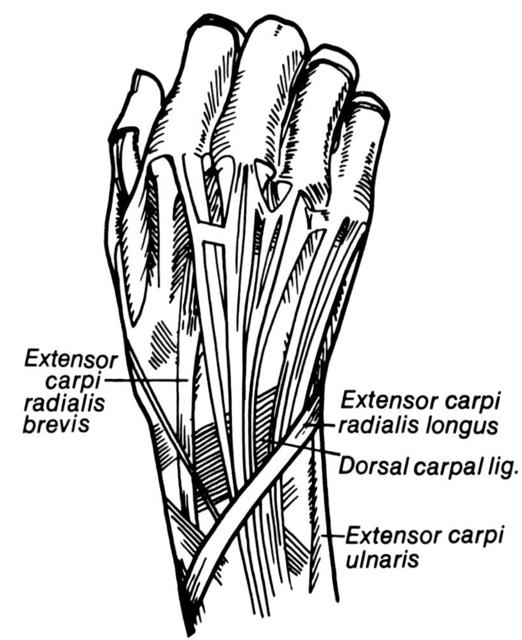

Fig. 11-16. Transfer of the extensor carpi radialis longus into the extensor carpi ulnaris. (From Clayton and Ferlic,[13] with permission.)

our practice to transfer the extensor carpi radialis longus to the extensor carpi ulnaris in patients who do not have the ability to actively ulnar-deviate the wrist or in cases where the extensor carpi ulnaris cannot be properly realigned (owing to attenuation or rupture)[13] (Figs. 11-16, 11-17, 11-18). The rationale of this transfer is enforced by Zancolli's[63] observation of "metacarpal descent" as an important factor in producing ulnar deviation of the fingers and progressive ulnar dislocation of the long extensor tendons. The extensor carpi ulnaris inserts into the base and ulnar side of the fifth metacarpal. With rheumatoid arthritis there is often disintegration of the tendon and its sheath, allowing the tendon to dislocate, which always occurs in an ulnar and palmar direction. It accentuates the dorsal dislocation of

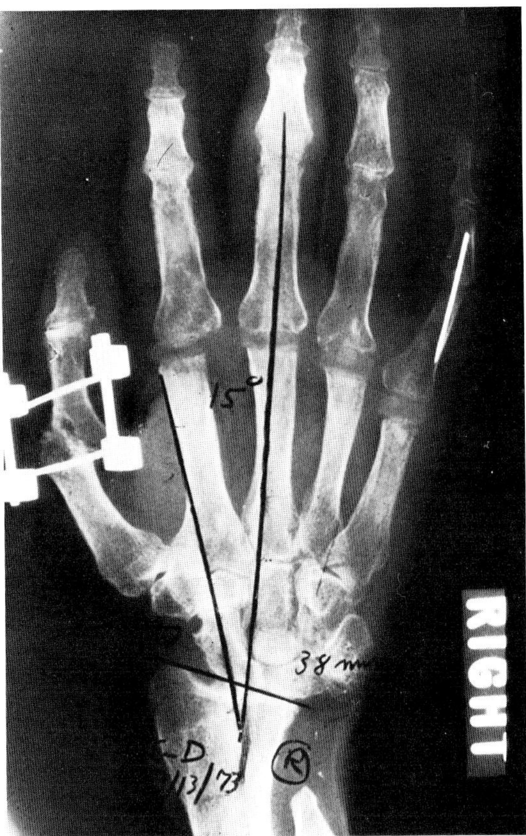

Fig. 11-18. Postoperative appearance of the hand after MCP arthroplasties as well as transfer of the extensor carpi radialis longus into the extensor carpi ulnaris. (From Clayton and Ferlic,[13] with permission.)

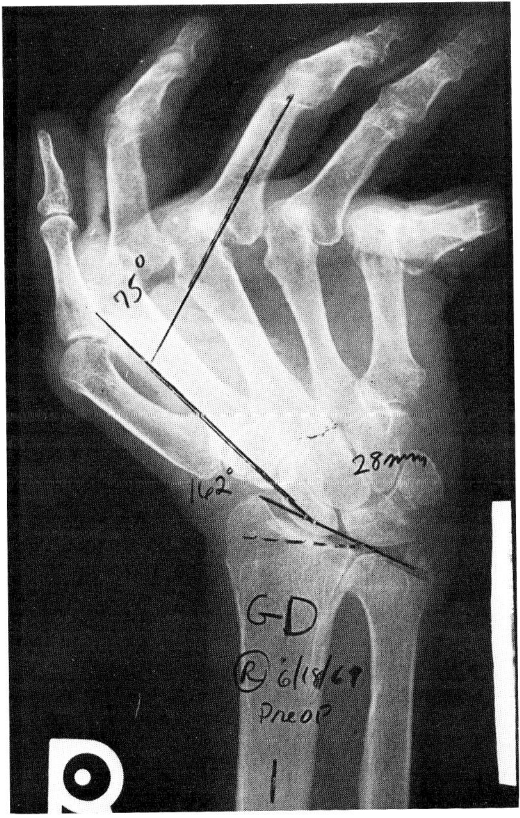

Fig. 11-17. Preoperative roentgenogram of a hand with radial rotation of the wrist and ulnar-deviated fingers. This patient had a rupture of the extensor carpi ulnaris.

the distal ulna and makes the extensor carpi ulnaris a flexor, causing descent of the fifth metacarpal. This descent leads to ulnar deviation of the fingers and progressive ulnar dislocation of the long extensor tendons. The transfer tends to keep the insertion of the extensor carpi ulnaris located on the dorsum of the wrist and prevents or corrects this metacarpal descent.

The extensor carpi radialis longus inserts on the radial side of the second metacarpal so the extensor carpi radialis longus acts as a strong radial deviator but does not extend the wrist past neutral. Therefore using this muscle for a transfer not only provides active ulnar deviation of the metacarpals but also removes a strong deforming force. In addition, the transferred tendon provides a pulley for the finger extensors, keeping them from bowstringing, as the dorsal retinaculum is passed underneath the extensor tendons as part of our dorsal wrist reconstruction.

It is frequently found that the extensor carpi ulnaris is markedly attenuated. Those patients in our series with the most ulnar deviation of the fingers and, correspondingly, the most radial deviation of the wrist have completely ruptured the extensor carpi ulnaris.

Others have contradicted the concept that radial rotation of the wrist effects ulnar deviation of the fingers. Hastings and Evans[29] reported a roentgenographic study of the wrist in rheumatoid patients and refuted the claim that radial rotation is a cause of ulnar deviation of the fingers. Boyce et al.[6] reported their laboratory studies and found that transferring the extensor carpi radialis longus to the extensor carpiulnaris corrected radial rotation of the wrist, but they did not confirm that it affected ulnar deviation of the fingers. Despite these conflicting reports, we continue to perform the transfer and believe we have shown that it favorably affects ulnar deviation of the fingers.

Flexor Tenosynovitis

In many patients, hand pain may be interpreted as arthritic in origin, whereas it is in fact due to carpal tunnel syndrome resulting from swelling caused by rheumatoid tenosynovitis.[30] There may actually be locking or triggering of tendons at the level of the transverse carpal ligament.[11] Initial treatment consists in splinting and perhaps a local injection of steroid into the carpal canal. Failure to respond to this treatment after a single injection is an indication for surgery. Early surgery is advisable, as tendon rupture may occur if the disease process continues.

Wrist flexor tenosynovitis frequently presents as compression of the median nerve, which may be the initial symptom in a new rheumatoid patient. The swollen flexor tenosynovium may not be as apparent as synovitis on the dorsum because it is located deep to the thick volar fascia and transverse carpal ligament. Chamberlain and Corbett[8] have reported that 23 percent of patients

with rheumatoid arthritis have carpal tunnel syndrome, and Nakaro[41] reported that more than 45 percent of all patients with chronic rheumatoid arthritis and severe peripheral joint involvement, as well as subcutaneous nodules, have one or more entrapment neuropathies during the course of their disease.

Carpal tunnel syndrome is common in the rheumatoid patient because the nine flexor tendons pass, along with the median nerve, underneath the rigid, unyielding transverse carpal ligament. There is little extra space in the carpal canal, and any swelling or synovitis of the tendon sheaths compresses the median nerve. The patient characteristically complains of numbness and paresthesias over the thumb, index, long, and radial half of the ring fingers. It starts spontaneously, usually first manifesting at night, awakening the patient from a sound sleep. Weakness and atrophy of the thenar musculature may be apparent several months later. The diagnosis is based on the history and physical findings. A positive Phalen's test, performed by flexing the wrist and extending the elbow, reproduces the symptoms. A positive Tinel sign is also found when the area overlying the median nerve is tapped. Nerve conduction studies and electromyography are occasionally useful. Generally, the diagnosis is not difficult, but the rheumatoid patient may have an entrapment more proximal in the forearm or in the cervical spine. After the volar carpal ligament has been released in what appears to be a typical case of carpal tunnel syndrome and there is no improvement in symptoms, one must look elsewhere for compression.

Surgical Technique

Surgery in the rheumatoid patient may need to be more extensive than in the patient with idiopathic carpal tunnel syndrome. As well as incising the volar carpal ligament to relieve pressure, a flexor tenosynovectomy is carried out when hypertrophic synovium is found. After the transverse carpal ligament is released, it is not necessary to extend the incision, but the operative area is extended by flexing and extending the fingers. In this manner, tenosynovectomy to the lumbrical level and proximal to the musculotendinous juncture can be performed. It is possible because of the excursion of the finger flexor tendons. It is also necessary to inspect the floor of the carpal canal, as we have seen synovium rupture through the volar capsule, resulting in a space-occupying lesion in the carpal tunnel. Bony spicules may also be found in the floor of the canal, and they should be excised and covered. Although less common than entrapment at the elbow, the ulnar nerve may be entrapped at the wrist when it passes through Guyon's canal into the hand. There are no tendons passing through this canal, so there should be no tenosynovium to compress the nerve. The tenosynovium within the carpal tunnel can bulge and compress the ulnar nerve proximal to the canal,[41] or the destruction of the carpal bones may change the relation in Guyon's canal, thereby compressing the nerve. When the ulnar nerve is entrapped, one finds decreased sensation and paresthesias over the little finger and ulnar half of the ring finger. Weakness and atrophy of the intrinsic hand muscles may also be found. Characteristically, entrapment at the wrist can be differentiated from entrapment at the elbow by looking for a Tinel sign and by having normal musculature proximal to the wrist.

Surgical decompression of the nerve in Guyon's canal is the preferred treatment of ulnar nerve compression at the wrist. More common than with the median nerve, the "double crush"[41] phenomenon may compress the ulnar nerve in more than one place; and in the rheumatoid patient involvement at the elbow or cervical radiculopathy may be present as well.

Rupture of the flexor tendons is not nearly as frequent as rupture of the extensor tendons in the rheumatoid patient, but they are more difficult to reconstruct satisfactorily. The most common flexor tendon to rupture is the flexor pollicis longus, followed by the profundus to the index finger (Fig. 11-19). Next, in order of decreasing frequency, are the profundus to the little finger, superficialis to the index fingers, the other profundus tendons, and the remaining superficialis tendons. Ruptured flexor tendons at the wrist can usually be reconstructed, but probably the most important treatment for flexor tendon rupture at the wrist is to prevent additional tendons from rupturing by performing a flexor tenosynovectomy, decompressing the volar carpal ligaments,

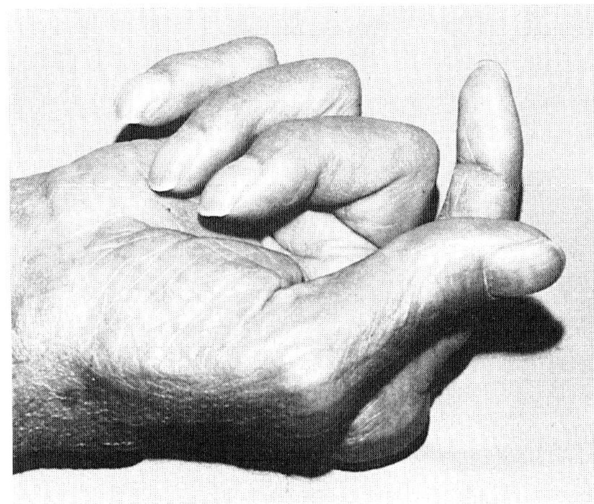

Fig. 11-19. Position of the hand illustrating rupture of the flexor tendons to the index finger and the flexor policis longus.

exploring the carpal canal, and removing bony spicules that could cause additional ruptures. Flexor tendons can rupture in areas other than the wrist: within the digital theca or at their insertion into the phalanges. It may be difficult to determine at which level the rupture occurred. One clue for discovering the area of separation is to note the pattern of rupture of the flexor pollicis longus and the profundus to the index finger. It almost always occurs where the tendons course over the eroded carpal bones at the wrist. In this case, the profundus to the index finger is treated with a tendon transfer, and the IP joint of the thumb is fused.

WRIST ARTHROPLASTY (NONIMPLANT)

A stable, balanced, painless wrist is necessary for optimal hand function. A wrist arthrodesed in a functional (neutral) position with preserved forearm pronation and supination is compatible with useful hand function. To achieve this goal, elimination of wrist motion is not essential and may be objectionable in patients with progressive disease in adjacent joints. Reaching for objects on a shelf, for instance, and personal hygiene may be difficult for the patient with a fused wrist, whereas some motion, especially flexion, facilitates positioning the hand for function. Patients who have had one wrist fused find that certain activities are more difficult if the second wrist is arthrodesed. To be acceptable, an arthroplasty must relieve pain, be stable, correct deformity, provide motion, and leave a reasonable alternative for salvage in case of failure.

Proximal Row Carpectomy

Occasionally, there is destruction and subluxation of the radiocarpal joint in the rheumatoid wrist, and in order to decompress this joint and rebalance the wrist it is useful to remove the proximal carpal row without adding an implant. The capitate then sits in the lunate fossa of the radius. Motion is preserved, and stability is maintained. This procedure may be useful for the non-rheumatoid wrist but has been a failure in the rheumatoid patient.[19]

This procedure is indicated when the distal radius still has good contour, particularly of the lunate fossa, and the capitate has normal contour in the remaining articular cartilage. In the case where there is ligament instability with a volar intercalated segmental instability (VISI) or dorsal intercalated segmental instability (DISI) deformity with gross disorganization of the carpus, an implant is preferred.

Case Report 1
A 54-year-old woman was seen in 1979 with a long history of rheumatoid arthritis. She complained about many of her joints. Her wrists were painful and showed an active dorsal tenosynovitis. Motion of both wrists was 50 degrees dorsiflexion and 50 degrees palmar flexion. A roentgenogram of the left wrist (Fig. 11-20A) showed narrowing and destruction of the radiocarpal joint as well as the intercarpal joints. The patient underwent bilateral wrist synovectomy, tenosynovectomy, and proximal row carpectomy (Fig. 11-20B). The patient did well, and her pain was relieved. However, 9 years later the wrists showed marked deformities with ulnar

translocation, deviation, and pain (Fig. 11-20C & D).

Shelf Arthroplasty

Palmar shelf arthroplasty is another procedure used to decompress and balance the wrist and preserve motion. An implant is not used, and the procedure is similar to proximal row carpectomy in this regard. Instead of removing bone from the carpus, the distal end of the radius is shaped and a volar lip of bone is preserved, giving the wrist stability. If necessary, the wrist and finger tendons may be repaired at the same time. Pins are placed across the wrist and left for 6 weeks. Prolonged splinting may be necessary after the transfixion pins are removed. Albright and Chase[2] reported nine palmar shelf procedures in rheumatoid patients with severe involvement of multiple joints. Preoperatively, all wrists were severely subluxated or dislocated, painful, and markedly disabling. In all of these patients the wrist remained stable, motion was maintained, and function was better than it had been preoperatively. Five were rated excellent, one good, and two fair because of persistent lateral deviation.

Our experience with this procedure is limited; and in one patient some persistent lateral deviation occurred that could possibly have been prevented by a longer period of splinting. We do not use this procedure today.

WRIST ARTHROPLASTY (WITH IMPLANT)

Silicone Arthroplasty

Joint replacement at the wrist level has taken two forms: silicone interpositional arthroplasty and total joint replacement. Swanson has made significant contributions in the field of rheumatoid surgery with his flexible hinges, one of which is used in the wrist (Fig. 11-21). The radiocarpal flexible-hinge implant was designed as an adjunct to resection arthroplasty to maintain an adequate joint space and alignment while supporting the capsuloligamentous system. Constructed

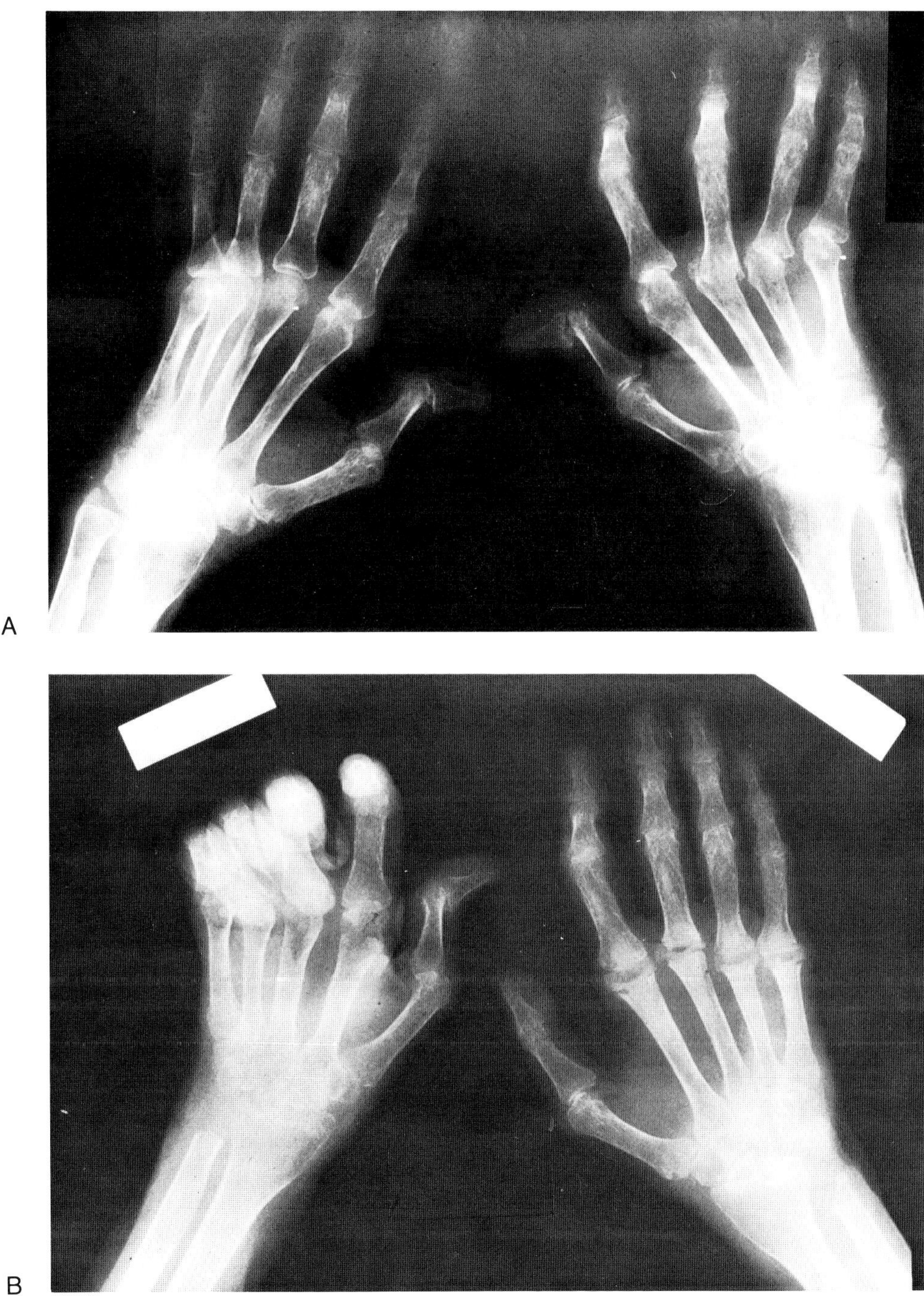

Fig. 11-20. **(A)** Preoperative roentgenogram showing narrowing of the radiocarpal joint and intercarpal joints of both wrists. **(B)** Immediate postoperative roentgenogram showing proximal row carpectomy. (*Figure continues.*)

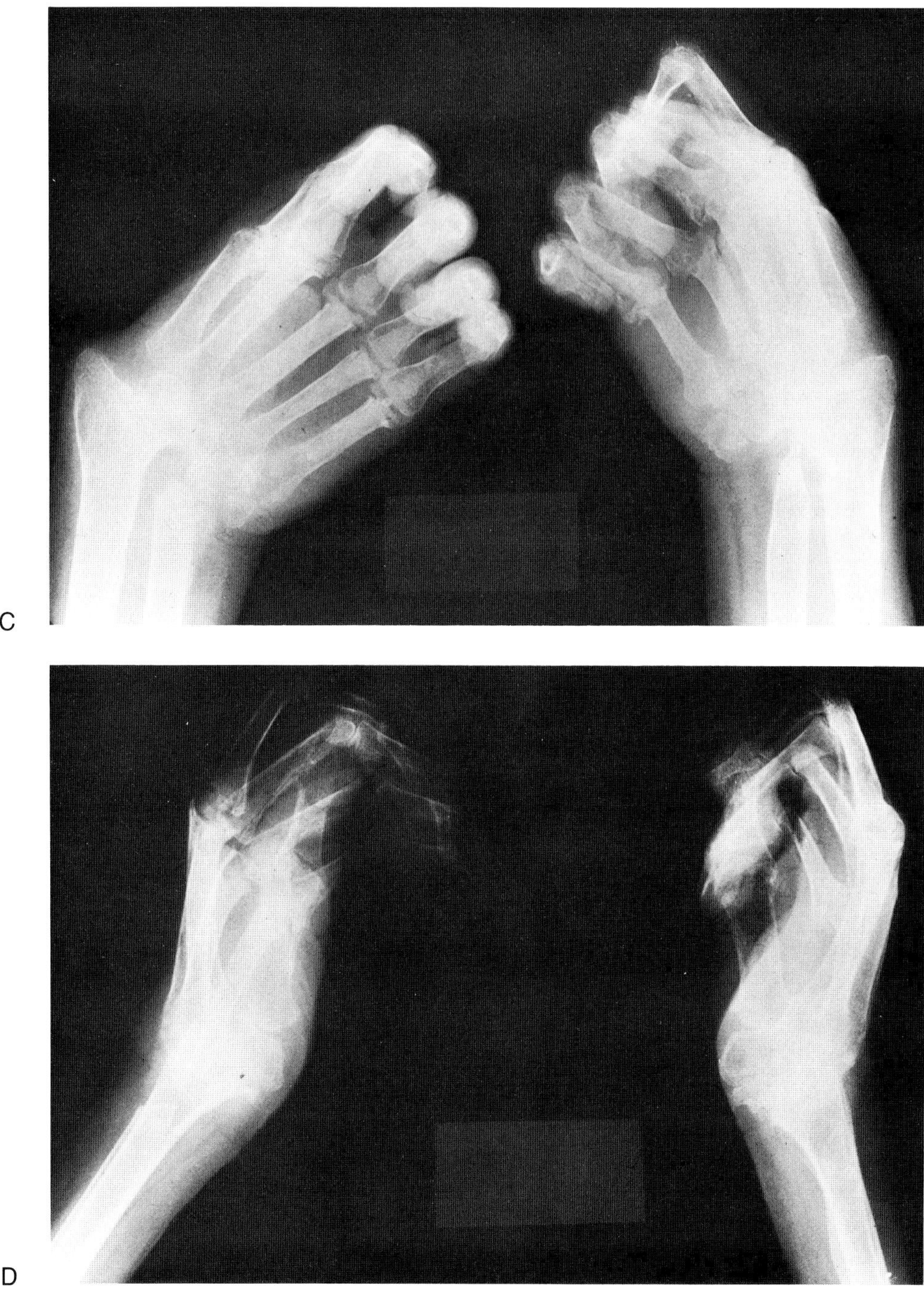

Fig. 11-20 *(Continued)*. **(C & D)** Anteroposterior and lateral roentgenograms of both wrists 9 years after proximal row carpectomy, demonstrating severe deformities of the wrists. (From Ferlic et al.,[19] with permission.)

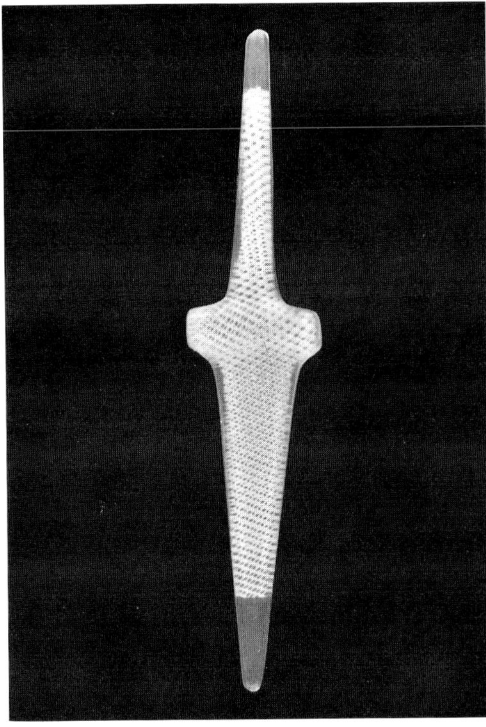

Fig. 11-21. Swanson silicone wrist prosthesis.

as a one-piece hinge with intramedullary stems, it is fabricated from silicone with a Dacron-reinforced core to provide axial stability and resistance to rotary torque. The proximal stem of the implant fits the intramedullary canal of the radius, and the distal stem passes through the capitate and fits the intramedullary canal of the third metacarpal. Swanson and Swanson[53] listed the advantages of the prosthesis as (1) providing reasonable wrist mobility and stability and pain relief for finger function, (2) maintaining joint space, (3) supporting and orienting joint encapsulation, (4) allowing reconstruction and balancing of musculotendinous systems, (5) being well tolerated by bone and soft tissues, and (6) providing high flexural durability and early postoperative motion. Their indications for use of this prosthesis are rheumatoid disabilities of the radiocarpal joint with (1) instability of the wrist due to subluxation or dislocation of the radiocarpal joint, (2) wrist deviation causing digital imbalance, and (3) stiffness where movement is required for hand function. They reported 76 wrists with an adequate pain-free motion averaging from 21 degrees of extension to 41 degrees of flexion. No complications were recorded.

Goodman et al.[25] reviewed 37 silicone wrist arthroplasties in patients with rheumatoid arthritis. Sixteen percent of the patients displayed residual discomfort, 5 percent had recurrent deformity, and 8 percent experienced prosthetic fractures. These patients were followed for a minimum of 6 months. Our experience suggests that further collapse of the carpus over the implant with more loss of motion and a higher rate of implant breakage would occur as time passes; our long-term follow-up indicates a 50 percent failure rate.[20]

Case Report 2

A rheumatoid arthritic woman presented in 1973 with multiple joint complaints. Her wrists had an active dorsal tenosynovitis with instability of the distal ulnae. The tendons were intact. The left wrist was markedly painful with motion, which was limited to 15 degrees dorsiflexion and 30 degrees palmar flexion. Pronation and supination were full but painful. Roentgenograms of both wrists (Fig. 11-22A & B) showed severe destruction.

In April 1975 a wrist synovectomy and tenosynovectomy were carried out, and a silicone implant was inserted on the left. A postoperative roentgenogram (Fig. 11-22C) showed satisfactory seating of the prosthesis with satisfactory alignment. Three months after surgery, she had 40 degrees dorsiflexion and 25 degrees palmar flexion with full rotation. The wrist did well for 2 years, at which time it slipped into ulnar deviation and the prosthesis fractured (Fig. 11-22D).

In February 1978 a Volz total wrist arthroplasty was performed (Fig. 11-22E & F). (She had undergone a Volz wrist replacement on the right in 1977.) Postoperatively she did well. The wrist was balanced, dorsiflexed 45 degrees, and palmar-flexed 15 degrees, but she developed a carpal tunnel syndrome, which was released 4 months after the wrist replacement. Both her wrists have continued to do well.

Note: We have likewise used the silicone prosthesis in the rheumatoid wrist with about the same results as Goodman achieved. It is espe-

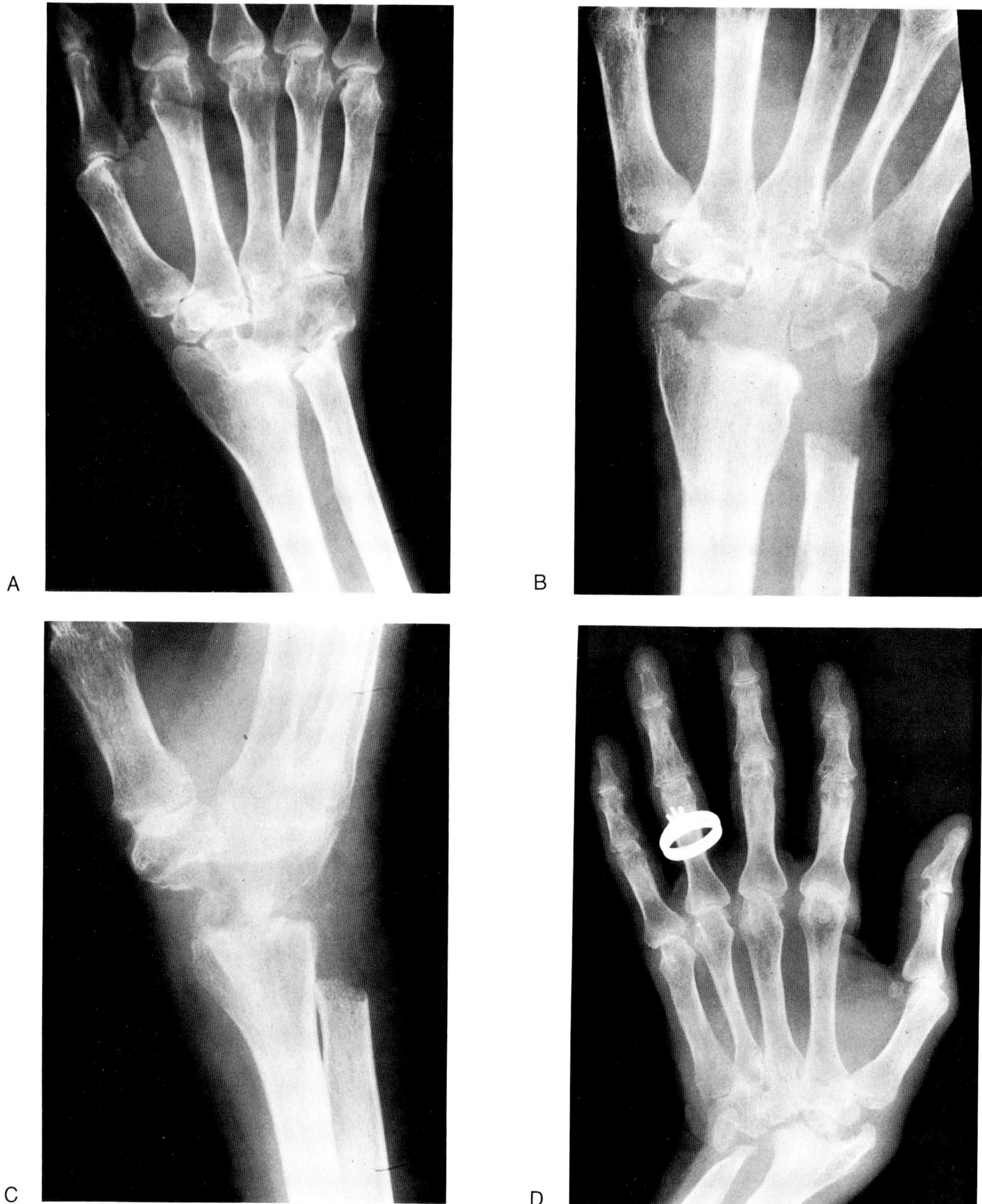

Fig. 11-22. **(A)** Preoperative roentgenogram showing severe destruction of the wrist. **(B & C)** Two weeks after a silicone wrist implant. Note the satisfactory position and alignment. **(D)** Anteroposterior roentgenogram 2.5 years after wrist implant shows that the wrist has slipped into ulnar deviation, and the prosthesis has fractured. (*Figure continues.*)

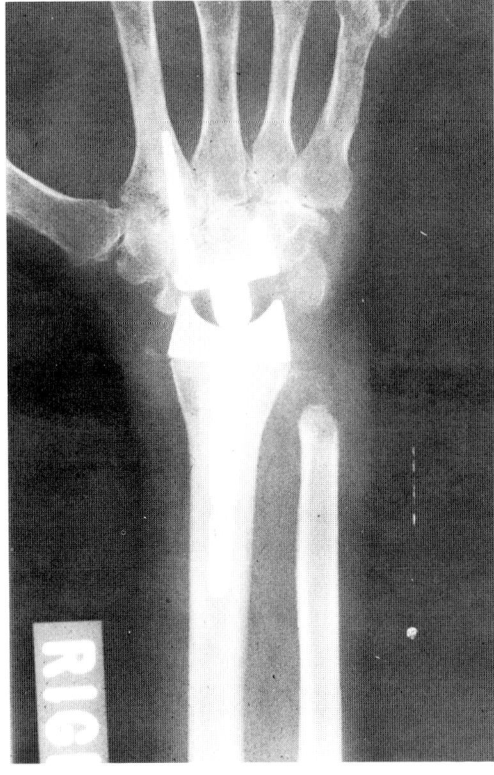
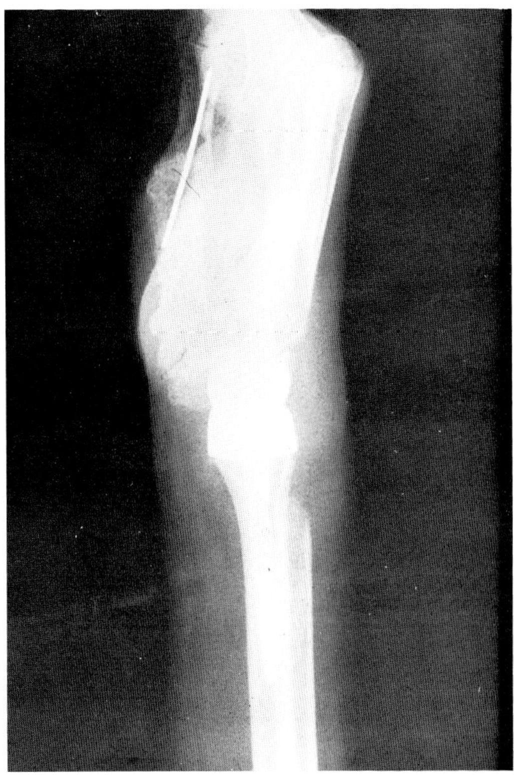

Fig. 11-22 *(Continued)*. **(E & F)** Postoperative roentgenograms show satisfactory alignment following Volz total wrist arthroplasty.

cially useful in the juvenile rheumatoid arthritic with small bones. In this situation, other available total wrist components are too large to be inserted (Fig. 11-23).

Surgical Technique

One basis for silicone replacement arthroplasty must be kept in mind. Silicone prostheses are flexible hinges. They do not and are not supposed to provide stability, and the maintenance of the corrected deformity is dependent on adequate soft tissue releases and bony resection to correct the deformity and restore alignment. The external mechanical forces also need to be balanced to prevent angular deformity.

A dorsal midline straight incision is made. The cutaneous veins and nerves are preserved. The skin is not undermined. Retraction must be gentle in order to minimize the chance of skin necrosis. The dorsal retinaculum is reflected from the ulnar side of the wrist, opening each of the extensor compartments except the first. The tenosynovium is removed from the involved tendons. The dorsal capsule is detached from the radius and reflected distally. The carpus is hyperflexed to expose the wrist joint. The lunate, scaphoid proximal half, and triquetrum are excised; and the distal radius is excised at right angles to the shaft of the bone, removing 1 to 2 cm of bone, which decompresses the wrist and allows the prosthesis to be inserted. An opening is then made into the capitate with a sharp awl and continued into the third metacarpal. A power burr increases the size of the opening. A trial reduction is made. The size of the bones distal to the wrist is the limiting factor for determining the size of the prosthesis, so the distal hole is made before the opening into the radius to avoid excess bone resection from the radius. It is necessary to trim any sharp bone edges. The prosthesis should sit squarely against

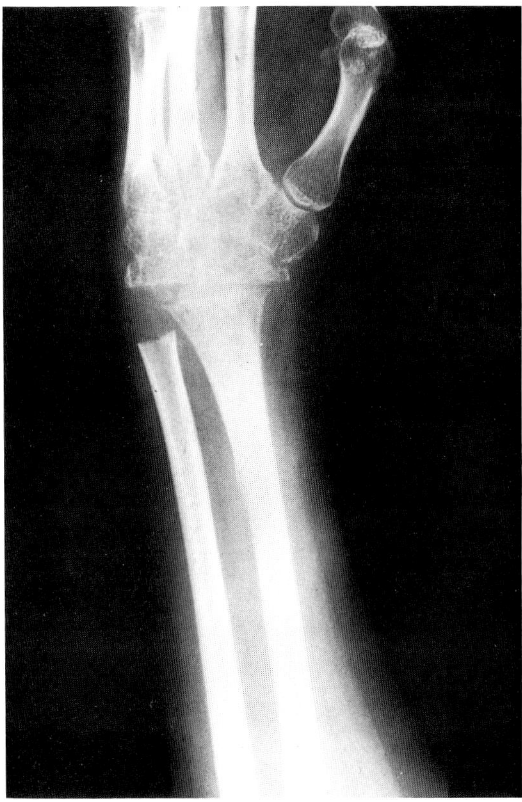

Fig. 11-23. Postoperative roentgenogram shows the silicone prosthesis in place. An attempt was made to implant a total wrist, but the radial shaft was too small to insert the prosthesis. A defect was made in the cortex of the radius when attempting to ream the radial shaft.

the capitate and radius and should not buckle when motion is attempted. The volar capsule can be stripped, if necessary, to avoid excessive bone resection. The distal end of the ulna is resected and the prosthesis inserted in the wrist. The capsule is reattached to the distal radius through drill holes. The radial and ulnar ligaments are tightened, if necessary, and the ulnar-volar capsule is pulled up and sutured to the dorsal capsule. As for wrist synovectomy, the distal radioulnar collateral ligament must be reconstructed. The extensor retinaculum is passed underneath the extensor tendons and sutured to the ulnar side of the wrist, leaving a strip of retinaculum passed around the extensor carpi ulnaris to

keep it on the dorsum of the wrist, thus stabilizing the distal ulna as well as preventing volar migration of the ulnar metacarpals. The tourniquet is lowered, hemostasis achieved, and a suction drain inserted; the subcutaneous tissue and skin are then closed. For the loose type of rheumatoid arthritis, the wrist is splinted for 4 to 6 weeks before motion is started. Motion may be started earlier for the stiff type.

TOTAL WRIST ARTHROPLASTY

Total wrist arthroplasty has gained popularity as total replacement in other joints has progressed. Two types of artificial wrist joint, the Meuli and the Volz, have gained the widest acceptance. In 1977 Beckenbaugh and Linscheid[5] reported their experience at the Mayo Clinic in patients with rheumatoid arthritis. Pain was relieved in 92 percent of these cases. Postoperative motion averaged 32 degrees dorsiflexion, 27 degrees palmar flexion, and 2 degrees radial and 23 degrees ulnar deviation. Complications that required reoperation occurred in 35 percent of this series. Six reoperations were done because of abnormal resting stance of flexion or ulnar deviation: three because of technical errors that resulted in dislocation in one wrist, malpositioned stem in one, and retained radial styloid in the other. Additional complications included temporary subluxation in two, delayed wound healing in two, ulnar nerve paresthesia in one, and extensor tenosynovitis in one.

Volz[60,61] reviewed the first 100 wrists done from 1974 to 1978 by 15 collaborating surgeons; 83 cases had rheumatoid arthritis. The overall results were 86 percent good or excellent and 6 percent failure. The most frequent postoperative problem was wrist motor imbalance, which amounted to 21 percent, with 13 percent exhibiting an ulnar deformity. In addition, 6 percent demonstrated wound healing problems, and all were rheumatoid patients. Four patients experienced a single episode of subluxation, three during the immediate postoperative period. Two patients developed a wound infection, requiring removal of the prosthesis. One patient demonstrated loosening of the distal component. Of the six failures, five had their prostheses removed, resulting in solid ankylosis in three and fibrous ankylosis in two.

Prosthesis Design

The metal radial component has a polyethylene articulating surface, whereas the carpal articulating surface is a highly polished metal hemisphere. The components are designed to be fixed with methylmethacrylate. The prosthesis has a carpal height of 2 cm with a theoretic motion arc of 90 degrees flexion-extension and 50 degrees radioulnar deviation. Some distraction is permitted (Fig. 11-24).

The carpal component was originally constructed with two prongs to be inserted into the second and third metacarpals. In some of his patients' wrists, Volz found a significant problem with motor balancing, and he concluded that the two-pronged component was a design error[60] in that it did not allow insertion of the prosthesis at the instant center of motion, which Youm et al.[62] determined to be at the base of the capitate. The distal component was then modified to a single

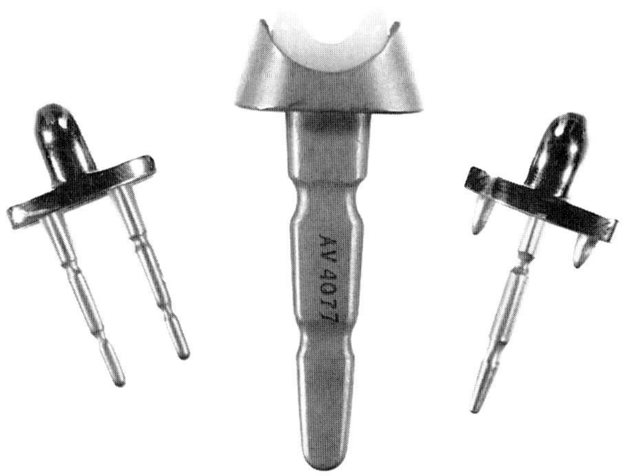

Fig. 11-24. Volz prosthesis. The distal component was introduced with the double prongs, but it was later changed to a single prong because of muscle imbalance.

prong to be inserted through the capitate into the third metacarpal. The proximal component comes in two sizes and is of polyethylene and metal construction.

Surgical Technique

A straight-line dorsal oblique skin incision is made from just proximal to the ulnar head to just proximal to the radial side of the second metacarpal head. Meticulous dissection is used to raise the skin and subcutaneous tissue from the underlying extensor retinaculum, which is then reflected radialward from between the fifth and sixth compartments to the first. The distal ulna is resected. A tenosynovectomy is carried out. The integrity of the extensor carpi radialis brevis is checked carefully. The dorsal capsule is removed subperiosteally from the radius. Synovectomy is performed as necessary. The volar radiocarpal ligament is then released subperiosteally from the radius. The carpus, metacarpals, and distal radius are prepared to accept the two components by cutting the distal radius at a right angle to the longitudinal axis and by removing the lunate, proximal half of the scaphoid, and triquetrum and cutting the distal row off straight. An appropriate amount of bone needs to be resected to allow insertion of the 2 cm prosthesis (Fig. 11-25). The double-prong component is designed to fit into the second and third metacarpals, and the single prong fits into the third. The distal articulating end should be exactly in line with the third metacarpal, corresponding to the resected end of the capitate. Trial reduction is performed and the range of motion checked. There should be no bony or soft tissue projections to prevent the full motion as built into the prosthesis.

Balance is then determined. On the hand table, the wrist should lie in the neutral position in the radioulnar plane. If the wrist has a preoperative contracture into ulnar deviation, an extensive amount of rebalancing may be necessary. It may consist in positioning the radial component further to the ulnar side. In addition, the carpal component can be shifted further ulnarward, which can be done by choosing the double-prong prosthesis and cutting off one of the prongs; this step

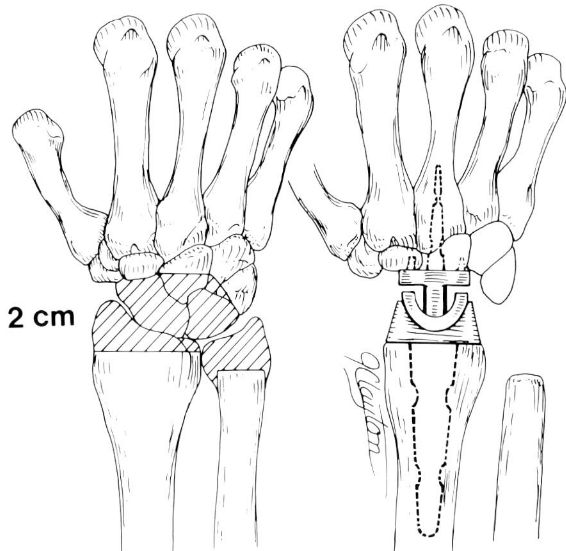

Fig. 11-25. Amount of bone resection necessary for Volz total wrist arthroplasty.

can be accomplished in two ways. If the standard distal prosthesis fits normally into the second and third metacarpals, an ulnar shift can be seen if the small prosthesis is chosen, inserting the ulnar prong into the third metacarpal and the shortened radial prong into the carpus. The other way is just the opposite. If the small prosthesis fits into the metacarpals, the standard is chosen, inserting the radial prong into the third metacarpal and the shortened radial prong into the carpus. The other way is just the opposite. If the small prosthesis fits into the metacarpals, the standard is chosen, inserting the radial prong into the second metacarpal and placing the shortened ulnar prong into the carpus. We have placed one prong into the fourth metacarpal, but this method is not advisable, as loosening is more likely when cementing into one of the mobile metacarpals. The components also have a lateral offset to position the axis more volarward (normal position) and produce better dorsiflexion power. These components must be properly inserted and the real components checked against the trials. If doubtful, an intraoperative roentgenogram should be obtained to ensure the proper location of the distal component before cementing.

The components are then cemented in place with methylmethacrylate. The canals should be plugged and, if feasible, cement injected by syringes with pressurization. The dorsal radiocarpal ligament is sutured into the radius in such a way as to further preserve the balance, keep the wrist from subluxating volarly, and prevent supination of the ulnar metacarpals.

The entire dorsal retinaculum is reattached underneath the extensor tendons. The ulnar aspect of the retinaculum and capsule is secured to the radius so any wrist supination deformity is decreased. The extensor carpi ulnaris is positioned dorsally, utilizing a strip of extensor retinaculum as a sling. The subcutaneous tissue is loosely closed over a drain, and the skin is closed using stitches or staples. After operation, the wrist and forearm are immobilized in a bulky dressing with a volar plaster splint to hold the wrist in neutral. Active motion is started at 2 weeks. The splint is removed for active exercises, which are started after 2 weeks. At 4 weeks the patient may perform light activities without the splint, which is completely discarded at 3 months. Active flexion as well as extension is emphasized.

Results

We prepared a 100-point score sheet to evaluate or judge the results of wrist procedures (Table 11-1). The earliest ratings were done 6 months after operation. Balance, motion, pain relief, and percentage of change in grip strength were measured. Balance was given a relative value of 30 points, with 15 points assessed to the flexion-extension plane and the other 15 points to the ulnar deviation-radial deviation plane. Motion was given a value of 25 points, pain relief 35 points, and grip strength 10 points. Related and developing hand deformities influenced this measurement.

1. *Balance.* Half of the 30 points for balance were given to the active flexion minus extension arc. The other 15 points were given to the active ulnar deviation minus radial deviation plane. Normally, greater ulnar deviation was compen-

Table 11-1.   Wrist Score Sheet (Total 100 Points)

Measurements	Degrees	Score
Balance (30 points)		
Active flexion-extension (15 point)		
Excellent	0–20	15
Good	21–30	10
Fair	31–40	5
Poor	>40	0
Active ulnar deviation-radial deviation (15 points)		
Excellent	20–30	15
Good	0–19	10
Fair	31–40	5
Poor	>40	0
Motion (25 points—sum of flexion and extension)		
Excellent	70–90	25
Good	50–60	20
Fair	15–49	15
Poor	15	0
Pain relief (35 points)		
No pain		35
Mild		30
Moderate		7
Severe		0
Percent of gain in grip strength (10 points)		
Excellent	75	10
Good	50–75	6
Fair	5–49	3
Poor	<5	0

sated by the scoring system. A wrist fused in a neutral position would have a score of 30 but would be downgraded in the motion section to zero. A pre- or postoperative wrist that had a balance rating of poor was considered to be unbalanced.

Wrist balance was more consistently obtained in the flexion-extension plane than in the ulnar-radial deviation plane. The degree of which this ulnar deviation posture compromises function is not known, and in some patients with severe hand involvement it may represent an adaptation for function, especially when flexion is good.

2. *Motion.* Motion was allotted 30 points and was determined by adding the amount of active flexion to active extension. Improvement in wrist motion reflected gain in the useful range in which motion occurred after operation. We were careful to obtain free forearm supination and pronation to supplement wrist function and decrease torsional forces on the prosthesis.

3. *Pain relief.* Pain relief rated 35 points.

4. *Percentage of change in grip strength.* Hand deformities in the rheumatoid patients made grip strength evaluation a less dependable measurement, and so it was rated on only 10 points.

5. *Percentage of change in carpal height ratio.* Carpal height is the distance between the base of the third metacarpal and the distal articular surface of the radius, as measured along the proximal projection of the longitudinal axis of the third metacarpal. The carpal height ratio is the ratio of the carpal height to the length of the third metacarpal, the normal being defined by Youm et al.[62] as 0.54 ± 0.03 mm. In our patients it averaged 0.29 mm before operation. The average increase after operation was 40 percent, ranging from 8 to 70 percent. Although this value could not be used to predict the result, those with low values prior to operation were technically more difficult to fit with a radial component. In order to fit the 2 cm carpal height of the prosthesis, radial bone stock was removed to create space. As a result, the radial component occasionally overhung the radius, which theoretically increased the potential for tendinitis or even tendon rupture.

We have now performed over 50 total wrist replacements in rheumatoid patients using the Volz prosthesis[15,16,32] (Fig. 11-26). Our complications were similar to those reported by Volz, with balance being the greatest problem. Based on the 100-point scale, excellent or good results were obtained in 70 percent. Two patients had poor results. Among the original 20 there were two cases of carpal tunnel syndrome after surgery, and one additional case appeared among the last 30. Of these three patients, two required decompression of the nerve. One postoperative hematoma resolved without surgery. In one case the radius was perforated, and cement leaked into the interosseous membrane. In two patients the prosthesis dislocated immediate postoperatively and was reduced without subsequent problems (Fig. 11-27). One patient had inadequate wrist

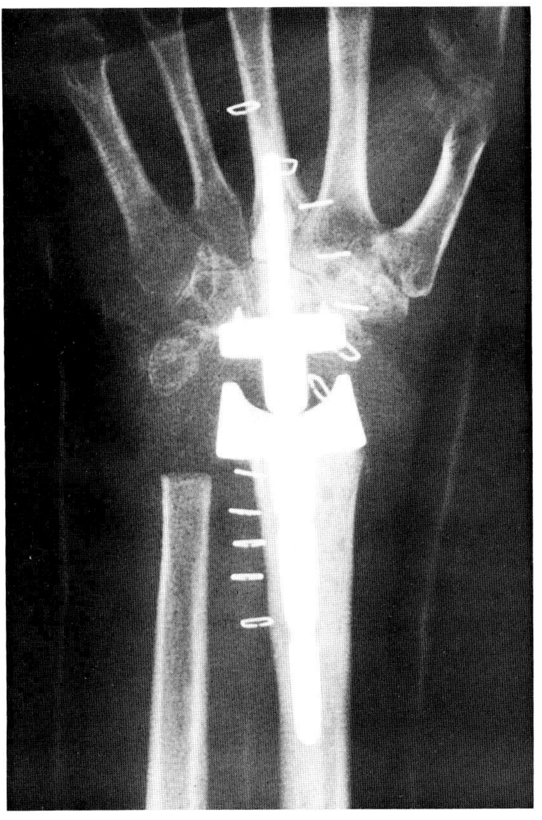 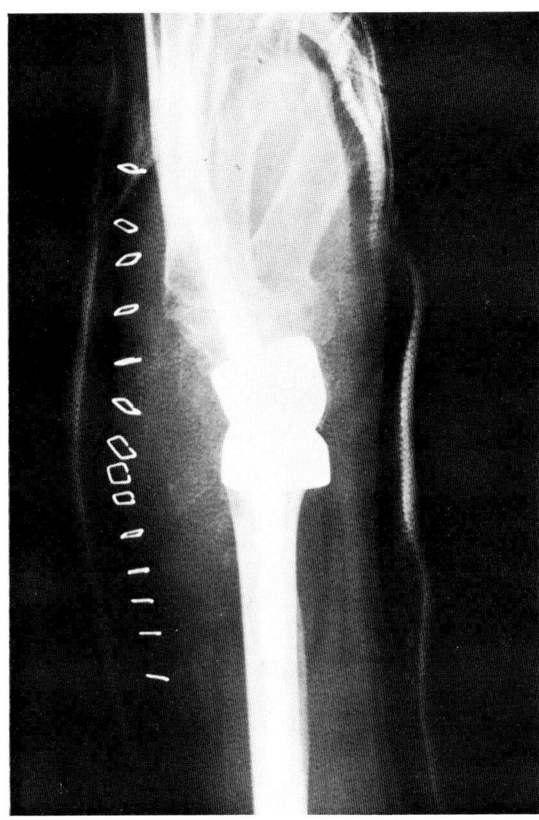

Fig. 11-26. Postoperative anteroposterior (**A**) and lateral (**B**) views of a Volz single stem metacarpal total wrist.

extensors and was reoperated in an attempt to balance these motors, without success.

When we followed these patients for a longer period of time (range 3 to 9 years, average 70 months), we found that 86 percent had no or only mild pain and thought they were better off, but our critical scoring showed 60 percent good and excellent and 13 percent poor results. The roentgenograms of these long-term patients revealed significant number with bone resorption in the radius and radiolucent lines and settling of the distal components[16,18] (Fig. 11-28). We continue to search for a better total wrist and have been using a noncemented device that has been promising in the short term (Fig. 11-29).

Balancing has been the major problem after total wrist arthroplasty. Vaughan-Jackson[57] has said, "The normal alignment and posture of a joint or complex of joints depends upon two kinds of stability: (1) the stability depending upon the intrinsic structure of a joint, and (2) the stability depending upon the balance of the extrinsic forces acting upon the joint, including gravity." Both stabilizing units are undermined in the rheumatoid wrist. Lost bony intrinsic stability is improved by the carpal replacement. Extrinsic stability is not routinely restored by replacement arthroplasty. Multiple extrinsic factors, as well as structural instability, contributed to the deformities seen among the wrists characterized as unbalanced before operation.

The instant center of motion in the normal wrist is located within the proximal pole of the capitate. The original design of the Volz total wrist located the center of motion 4 to 5 mm more radialward, resulting in an increased mechanical advantage to ulnar deviation of the wrist by the flexor and extensor carpi ulnaris muscles.

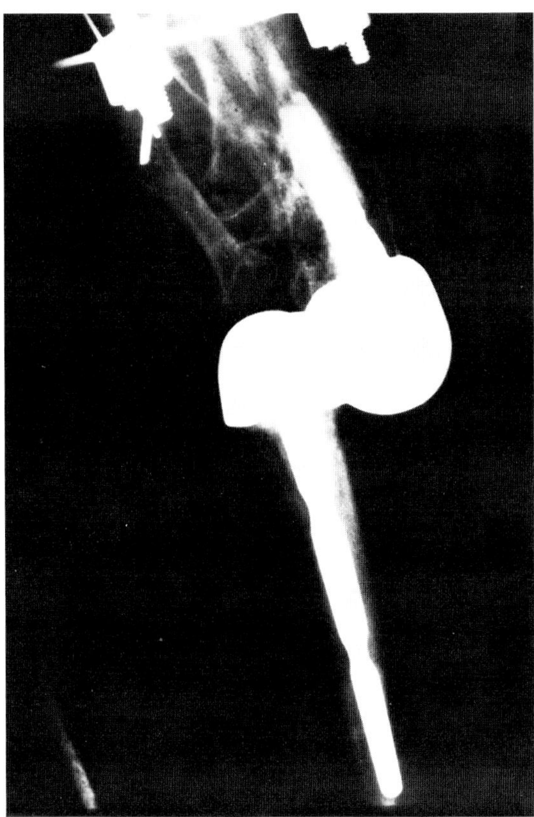

Fig. 11-27. Postoperative dislocation of a Volz total wrist.

Postoperative imbalance was discovered most often in patients who had preoperative roentgenographic evidence of an ulnarly translocated, subluxed, or dislocated carpus, a resting posture of flexion and/or supination of the hand, a grasp pattern of finger flexion and wrist flexion rather than finger flexion and wrist extension, or a loss of voluntary active wrist extension.[32] Initially, the imbalance problems were managed by shifting the center of motion of the distal component by cutting one of the prongs off or by tenotomizing or lengthening the flexor carpi ulnaris and palmaris longus. The redesign of the distal component to one prong has helped alleviate this problem, but some wrists, when contracted, still need release of the wrist flexors. The functional integrity of the extensor carpi radialis brevis, as well as the degree of volar and ulnar contracture, were the most important factors influencing the ultimate result.

Identifying an intact and effective extensor carpi radialis brevis prior to operation may be difficult in a painful, deformed rheumatoid wrist and hand. Reflex inhibition due to pain may be mistaken for a ruptured extensor carpi radialis brevis tendon. Substitution patterns by the common extensor tendons and the extensor carpi radialis longus causing wrist extension may mask an ineffective extensor carpi radialis brevis. In a wrist with ulnar deviation posture, the extensor carpi radialis longus may assume a more dorsal position, acting then to extend the wrist; with improved alignment after operation, it is again more of a radial deviator. If the extensor carpi radialis brevis is destroyed, the wrist would have no effective extensor action. If active extension does not go beyond neutral or if there is significant carpal volar subluxation, the integrity of the extensor carpi radialis brevis must be suspect. In these wrists, an alternate procedure should be

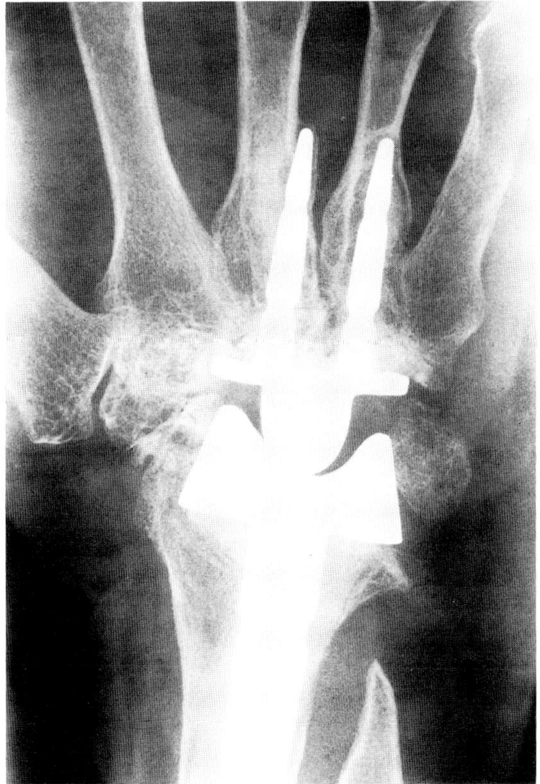

Fig. 11-28. Nine-year follow-up shows marked settling and loosening of the distal components.

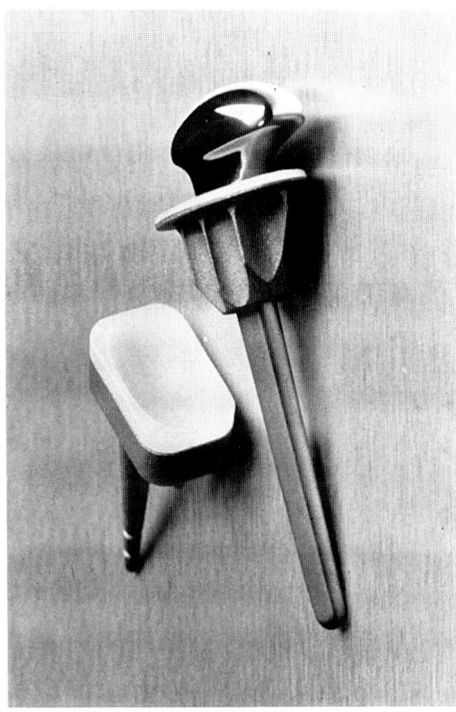

Fig. 11-29. CFV noncemented, press-fit total wrist prosthesis.

considered. All wrist tendons must function for balance.

Component size is another problem we have observed with the total wrist arthroplasties. Even though the radial portion is available in a small and a regular size, it is still large; and we had to change the procedure in a few patients in whom we planned to insert the prosthesis because the radial canal could not be reamed large enough. These patients were adults with juvenile rheumatoid arthritis. In one patient the reamer penetrated the radius, eventually resulting in a fracture through this defect several months later.

The question of when to use a silicone implant and when to use a total wrist is frequently asked. We have had considerable experience with both in rheumatoid patients. We use the total wrist in patients in whom the destruction has been the greatest, with a high degree of deformity, ulnar or volar subluxation, bone erosion, or imbalance, and where the bone structure is not small. We continue to use the silicone prosthesis when the wrist has an intermediate amount of destruction

or deformity, in a patient with small bone structure, or when 2 cm of bone should not be sacrificed. Comparing a "good" silicone arthroplasty to a "good" total wrist is like comparing a "good" cup arthroplasty to a "good" total hip arthroplasty.

Breakage has not been a problem as it has been in the silicone arthroplasties, although the use of grommets around the silicone prosthesis may help solve this problem. Loosening has only rarely been a problem as contrasted to total replacement in other joints (although perhaps in another 5 to 10 years we will start seeing it regularly). There have been collapses and bone growth around the silicone prostheses and recurrence of deformities with the passage of time, and perhaps the total wrists will prevent these problems.

Wrist arthroplasty requires functioning wrist tendons (particularly the extensor carpi radialis brevis) to produce good function. The wrist is one joint where waiting too long may result in it being too late for arthroplasty and necessitate arthrodesis.

ARTHRODESIS

A painless, mobile, stable balanced wrist arthroplasty is to be desired over a wrist fusion, but it cannot always be obtained or maintained. There is still a place for arthrodesis of the wrist in selected patients with rheumatoid arthritis (Fig. 11-30).

Wrist fusion is desirable in certain patients, and occasionally bilateral wrist fusion is necessary. In 1943 Smith-Petersen et al.[48] reported that after fusion of the wrist patients tend to retain better function in the distal joints. This point seemed true for some patients in our series.

Indications for wrist fusion are (1) ankylosis in marked flexion; (2) marked instability as the result of carpal destruction; (3) rupture of the extensor carpi radialis longus and brevis; and (4) moderate changes in the wrist but marked pain when using crutches. (Fortunately, the latter is rare today with good lower extremity joint replacements.)

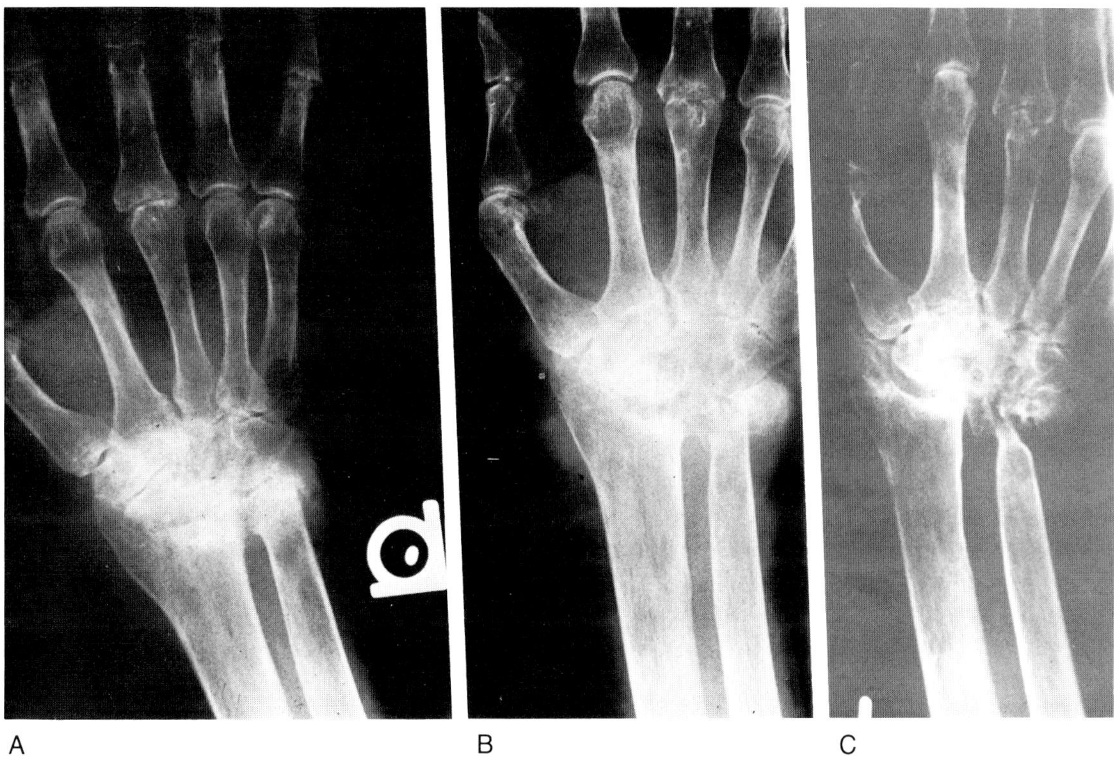

A   B   C

Fig. 11-30. (**A–C**) Roentgenograms of a wrist severely destroyed by rheumatoid arthritis showing the progression of the disease over a 3-year period. (**D**) Postoperative roentgenogram showing arthrodesis of the wrist.

The general recommendation has been fusion in 10 degrees of dorsiflexion[26]; Boyes[7] has recommended 20 to 30 degrees. For bilateral wrist fusions it has sometimes been recommended that one wrist be fused in dorsiflexion and the other in palmar flexion. We recommend fusion in the neutral position for uni- or bilateral cases. Neutral is defined as 0 degrees on the lateral with about 10 degrees ulnar deviation. If one makes a clenched fist and rapidly opens the hand, it is this position that is attained. By placing the wrist at neutral, the arc of motion of pronation and supination substitutes for palmar and dorsiflexion without shoulder or elbow substitution, which is helpful when working at a desk or table top. In this position, the axis of pronation and supination is down the central forearm and along the third

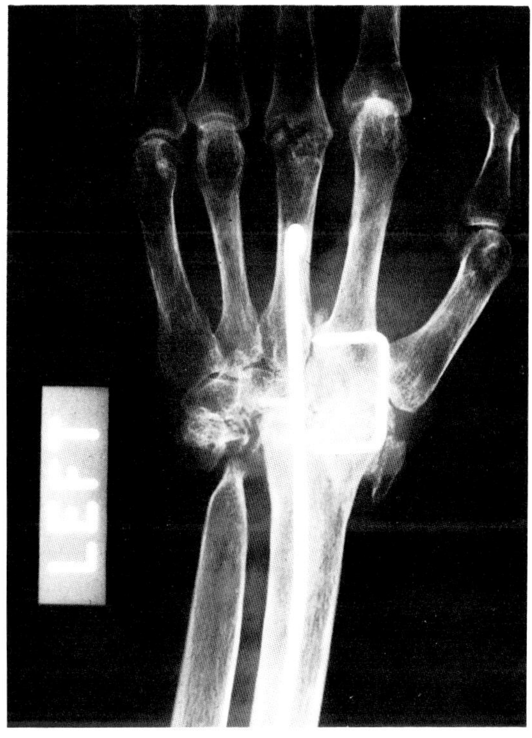

D

metacarpal; the tip pinch of the thumb and index finger is about 7.5 cm below the axis in pronation. Supination gives an arc of elevation 15 cm without awkward movement of the shoulder or elbow. The normal arc of palmar to dorsiflexion in pronation is only about 20 cm; with added supination the arc increased only to 22.5 cm.

With dorsiflexion of 20 to 30 degrees, fingertip pinch is essentially along the axis of forearm rotation and produces a minimal arc of about 5 cm with pronation and supination alone, making desk, table, or bench work much more awkward. One function of the wrist is to position the fingers effectively in space; using a global concept, only about one-third is lost by fusion at neutral compared to two-thirds lost with fusion at 30 degrees dorsiflexion.

Neutral position provides a good gripping position for use of tools and does not cause any distal digital imbalance. A carpenter can still use a hammer. It is also cosmetically pleasing. It allows one to reach in pockets or purse easily and is suited for sanitary toilet function.

Surgical Technique

A method of fusion was devised about 1962 that utilized an intramedullary pin with a local or iliac bone graft. This method has been continued successfully with minor variation.[11,12,34,37] Pronation and supination are essential for good function. If the radioulnar joint is deranged, the distal ulna is excised; conversely, if the radioulnar joint is normal, it is avoided during the fusion. The distal ulna is always excised in the rheumatoid wrist.

The general principles for wrist arthrodesis are as follows.

1. Neutral position
2. Internal fixation
3. Bony contact (bone graft)
4. Compression
5. Obtaining or maintaining rotation of the forearm

The dorsal approach is used, with a long, straight incision extending distally between the second and third metacarpals. As few dorsal veins as possible are ligated, and dissection is carried directly to the dorsal retinaculum. The fat and subcutaneous tissues are carefully reflected with the skin. Wide exposure is necessary. The sensory nerves are protected, and skin must be handled carefully.

The dorsal carpal ligament is reflected, incised directly over the ulna, and reflected radialward like the page of a book in about 5 cm width. The distal 1.5 to 2.0 cm of the ulna is resected subperiosteally. A longitudinal incision is made in the capsule of the wrist, exposing the bases of the second and third metacarpals and distal radius. A good bony bed must be prepared to connect these areas. Some bone may have to be removed to gain satisfactory contact and position; in many cases excellent bony contact is obtained. In other cases local bone graft from the ulnar head or an iliac graft is used. A slot is sawed dorsally in the carpus from the base of the second and third metacarpals to the radius at a depth of 1.0 to 1.2 cm and a width of 2.5 cm. An opening is undercut into the radius and the bones of the second and third metacarpals. A unicortical inner table iliac graft or the sliding distal radius graft is removed, shaped to fit the prepared bed, and tightly wedged proximally and distally. Local bone suffices in nearly all cases. Often such good contact is obtained that no formal graft is necessary. Fixation is obtained with a ⅛ inch Rush pin introduced at the distal end of the third metacarpal from the radial side into the radius for about 15 to 20 cm.[34] If a bone graft has been utilized, it is shaped and placed either through or volar to the Rush pin so the pin holds it in position. Manual compression is then applied and a staple or a Kirschner (K)-wire can be driven into the second metacarpal and radius to maintain contact-compression and prevent rotation. Special-length staples can be made from small pins and used for compression. Postoperatively, a short arm cast or a removable splint is the only external fixation necessary.

With this technique, the position of the wrist is automatically at neutral. If a few degrees alteration is desired, the intramedullary pin can be bent manually after insertion. The dorsal wrist capsule is closed, the dorsal carpal ligament is passed underneath the long thumb and finger extensors, and the dorsal carpal ligament is repaired snugly to stabilize the distal end of the resected ulna.

The tourniquet is released, hemostasis obtained, and a drain inserted. The wound is closed with skin staples. Using a conforming bulky, light compression dressing with nonadherent gauze over the incision, the hand is immobilized in a position of function for a few days. Drains are removed at 48 hours. Finger motion is allowed with 3 to 10 days according to the status of the wound. Proximal IP motion is allowed at 2 to 3 days, as it gives minimal long extensor tendon motion at the incision. Sutures remain in place for at least 2 weeks. A short arm cast or a simple volar splint is then utilized as protection if the internal fixation is rigid; but if a large graft was necessary or if there is no cross fixation, a long arm cast is necessary for about 6 weeks. Union is obtained between 2 and 3 months.

The fusion should extend to the metacarpals in the rheumatoid patient. We have seen patients in whom it was not done, resulting in instability, destructive changes developing in the metacarpocarpal joints, or a flexion deformity in this joint.

Wrist arthrodesis has proved to be a reliable procedure in the rheumatoid patient who is beyond the stage at which wrist arthroplasty would be advised.

SUMMARY

The wrist is the key joint of the upper extremity; and a stable, balanced, pain-free wrist is necessary for proper hand function. Indications for surgery are progressive pain and deformity in the joints or progression of the synovial disease in tendo sheaths despite adequate general medical treatment.

Dorsal wrist surgery can prevent extensor tendon rupture and should be performed early in the patient with chronic tenosynovitis. Ruptured extensor tendons can be repaired, but function is not as good as in the wrist where the tendons have been prevented from tearing.

Ulnar drift of the fingers may be contributed to by radial deviation of the wrist, which should be corrected by transfer of the extensor carpi radialis longus into the extensor carpi ulnaris in patients who are unable to ulnar-deviate their wrists actively or in patients in whom the extensor carpi ulnaris is not functioning.

Flexor tenosynovitis may present as a carpal tunnel syndrome. Decompression of the median nerve and volar tenosynovectomy may be necessary to prevent ruptured flexor tendons and to relieve symptoms of median nerve entrapment.

Wrist arthroplasty has been shown to be effective. Proximal row carpectomy is not advised in the rheumatoid patient; silicone replacement is used for wrists with more extensive destruction; and a total wrist is implanted in cases with severe destruction, a high degree of deformity, subluxation, erosion, or imbalance. Wrist arthrodesis in the neutral position is reliable and useful in the patient whose wrist is beyond the stage at which arthroplasty is advisable.

REFERENCES

1. Abernathy PJ, Bennyson WG: Decompression of the extensor tendons at the wrist in rheumatoid arthritis. J Bone Joint Surg [Br] 61:64, 1979

2. Albright JA, Chase RA: Palmar-shelf arthroplasty of the wrist in rheumatoid arthritis. J Bone Joint Surg [Am] 52:896, 1970

3. Backdahl M: The caput ulna syndrome in rheumatoid arthritis. Acta Rheumatol Scand [Suppl] 5:1, 1963

4. Backhouse KM: The mechanics of normal digital control in the hand and an analysis of the ulnar drift of rheumatoid arthritis. Ann R Coll Surg 43:154, 1968

5. Beckenbaugh RD, Linscheid RL: Total wrist arthroplasty: a preliminary report. J Hand Surg 2:339, 1977

6. Boyce T, Youm Y, Sprague BL, Flatt AE: Clinical and experimental studies on the effect of extensor carpi radialis longus transfer in the rheumatoid hand. J Hand Surg 3:390, 1978

7. Boyes JH: Bunnell's Surgery of the Hand. p. 296. JB Lippincott, Philadelphia, 1970

8. Chamberlain MA, Corbett M: Carpal tunnel syndrome in early rheumatoid arthritis. Ann Rheum Dis 29:149, 1970

9. Chaplin D, Pulkki T, Saarimaa A, Vainio L: Wrist and finger deformities in juvenile rheumatoid arthritis. Acta Rheumatol Scand 15:206, 1969

10. Clayton ML: Surgery of the rheumatoid hand. Clin Orthop 36:47, 1964

11. Clayton ML: Surgical treatment at the wrist in rheumatoid arthritis. J Bone Joint Surg [Am] 47:741, 1965

12. Clayton ML: Wrist arthrodesis and tendon reconstruction in rheumatoid arthritis. American Academy of Orthopaedic Surgery Film Library, 1966 (movie)

13. Clayton ML, Ferlic DC: Tendon transfer for radial rotation of the wrist in rheumatoid arthritis. Clin Orthop 100:176, 1974

14. Clayton ML, Ferlic DC: The wrist in rheumatoid arthritis. Clin Orthop 106:182, 1975

15. Dennis DA, Clayton ML, Ferlic DC, Patchett CE: Bilateral traumatic dislocation of Volz total wrist arthroplasties: a case report. J Hand Surg [Am] 10:503, 1985

16. Dennis DA, Ferlic DC, Clayton ML: Volz total wrist arthroplasty: long term results. J Hand Surg [Am] 11:483, 1986

17. Ellison M, Flatt AE, Kelly KJ: Ulnar drift of the fingers in rheumatoid disease. J Bone Joint Surg [Am] 53:1061, 1971

18. Ferlic DC: Implant arthroplasty of the rheumatoid wrist. Hand Clin North Am 3:169, 1987

18a. Ferlic DC: The rheumatoid wrist. p. 345. In Lichtman D (ed): The Wrist and Its Disorders. WB Saunders, Philadelphia, 1987

19. Ferlic DC, Clayton ML, Mills MF: Proximal row carpectomy: a review of rheumatoid and non-rheumatoid patients. J Hand Surg 16A:420, 1991

20. Ferlic DC, Jolly SL, Clayton ML et al: Swanson silicone arthroplasty of the wrist in rheumatoid arthritis: a long term follow-up. J Hand Surg 17A, 1992

21. Flatt AE: Some pathomechanics of ulnar drift. Plast Reconstr Surg 37:295, 1966

22. Flatt AE: The pathomechanics of ulnar drift. Final Report, Social and Rehabilitation Services. Grant RD 2226M, 1971

23. Flatt EA: The Care of the Rheumatoid Hand. 3rd Ed. CV Mosby, St. Louis, 1974

24. Goldner JL: Tendon transfers in rheumatoid arthritis. Orthop Clin North Am 5:425, 1974

25. Goodman MJ, Millender LH, Nalebuff EA, Philips GA: Arthroplasty of the rheumatoid wrist with silicone rubber: an early evaluation. J Hand Surg 5:114, 1980

26. Haddad RJ Jr, Riordan DC: Arthrodesis of the wrist. J Bone Joint Surg [Am] 49:950, 1967

27. Hakstian RW, Butiana R: Ulnar deviation of the fingers (Proceedings of the American Society for Surgery of the Hand). J Bone Joint Surg [Am] 48:608, 1966

28. Harrison S, Swannell AJ, Ansell BM: Repair of extensor pollicis longus using extensor pollicis brevis in rheumatoid arthritis. Ann Rheum Dis 31:490, 1972

29. Hastings DE, Evans JA: Rheumatoid wrist deformities and their relation to ulnar drift. J Bone Joint Surg [Am] 57:930, 1975

30. Henderson ED, Lipscomb P: Surgical treatment of the rheumatoid hand. JAMA 175:431, 1961

31. Laine VAI, Vainio KJ: Spontaneous rupture of tendons of rheumatoid arthritis. Acta Orthop Scand 24:250, 1955

32. Lamberta FJ, Ferlic DC, Clayton ML: Volz total wrist arthroplasty in rheumatoid arthritis; a preliminary report. J Hand Surg 5:245, 1980

33. Landsmeer JMF: Studies in the anatomy of articulation. II. Patterns of movement of bimuscular biarticular systems. Acta Morphol Neerl Scand 3:304, 1960

34. Mannerfeldt L, Malmsten M: Arthrodesis of the wrist in rheumatoid arthritis; a technique without external fixation. Scand J Plast Reconstr Surg 5:124, 1971

35. Mannerfeldt L, Norman O: Attrition ruptures of flexor tendons in rheumatoid arthritis caused by bony spurs in the carpal tunnel. J Bone Joint Surg [Br] 51:270, 1969

36. Marmor L, Lawrence JF, Dubois EL: Posterior interosseous nerve palsy due to rheumatoid arthritis. J Bone Joint Surg [Am] 49:381, 1967

37. Millender LH, Halebuff EA: Arthrodesis of the rheumatoid wrist. J Bone Joint Surg [Am] 55:1026, 1973

38. Millender LH, Nalebuff EA: Preventive surgery: tenosynovectomy and synovectomy. Orthop Clin North Am 6:765, 1975

39. Millender LH, Nalebuff EA, Holdsworth DE: Posterior interosseous nerve syndrome secondary to rheumatoid arthritis. J Bone Joint Surg [Am] 55:753, 1973

40. Moberg E: Tendon grafting and tendon suture in rheumatoid arthritis. Am J Surg 109:375, 1965

41. Nakaro KK: The entrapment neuropathy of rheumatoid arthritis. Orthop Clin North Am 6:837, 1975

42. Pahle I, Raunio P: The influence of wrist position in finger deviation in the rheumatoid hand. J Bone Joint Surg [Br] 51:664, 1969

43. Rana NA, Taylor AR: Excision of the distal end of the ulna in rheumatoid arthritis. J Bone Joint Surg [Br] 55:96, 1973

44. Rasmussen KB, Sneppen O: Operativ behandlung of polyarthritis. Nord Med 77:433, 1967

45. Shannon FT, Barton NJ: Surgery for rupture of extensor tendons in rheumatoid arthritis. Hand 8:279, 1976

46. Shapiro JS: A new factor in the etiology of ulnar drift. Clin Orthop 68:32, 1970

47. Shapiro JS: The etiology of ulnar drift (Proceedings of the American Society for Surgery of the Hand). J Bone Joint Surg 48:634, 1968

48. Smith-Petersen MM, Aufranc OE, Larson CB: Useful surgical procedures for rheumatoid arthritis involving joints of the upper extremity. Arch Surg 36:764, 1943

49. Straub LR: Surgical rehabilitation of the hand and upper extremity in rheumatoid arthritis. Bull Rheum Dis 12:265, 1962

50. Straub LR, Ranawat CS: The wrist in rheumatoid arthritis. J Bone Joint Surg [Am] 51:1, 1969

51. Straub LR, Wilson EH: Spontaneous rupture of extensor tendons in the hand associated with rheumatoid arthritis. J Bone Joint Surg [Am] 38:1208, 1956

52. Swanson AB: The ulnar head syndrome and its treatment by implant resection arthroplasty (Proceedings of the American Society for Surgery of the Hand). J Bone Joint Surg [Am] 54:906, 1972

53. Swanson AB, Swanson G: Flexible implant resection arthroplasty: a method for reconstruction of small joints in the extremities. Instruct Course Lect 27:27, 1978

54. Swanson AB, Swanson GdeG: Pathogenesis and pathomechanics of rheumatoid deformities in the hand and wrist. Orthop Clin North Am 4:1039, 1973

55. Thirupathi R, Ferlic DC, Clayton ML: Dorsal wrist synovectomy in rheumatoid arthritis: a long term study. J Hand Surg 8:848, 1983

56. Vainio KJ: Hand p. 130. In Milch RA (ed): Surgery of Arthritis. Williams & Wilkins, Baltimore, 1964

57. Vaughan-Jackson OJ: Rheumatoid hand deformities in the light of tendon imbalance. J Bone Joint Surg [Br] 44:764, 1962

58. Vaughan-Jackson OJ: Rupture of extensor tendons by attrition of the inferior radioulnar joint. J Bone Joint Surg [Br] 30:528, 1948

59. Vaughan-Jackson OJ: Tendon ruptures in the hand. Hand 1:122, 1969

60. Volz RG: Total wrist arthroplasty. Clin Orthop 128:180, 1978

61. Volz RG: Total wrist arthroplasty: a review of 100 patients. Orthop Trans 3:268, 1979

62. Youm Y, McMurty RV, Flatt AE, Gillespie TE: Kinematics of the wrist. J Bone Joint Surg [Am] 60:423, 1978

63. Zancolli E: Structural and Dynamic Basis of Hand Surgery. JB Lippincott, Philadelphia, 1972

12

Management of the Rheumatoid Hand

Donald C. Ferlic

Many rheumatoid patients are seen in our office for consideration of surgery to their hands. Some are referred by other patients, some by rheumatologists, and others just come to ask what can be done for their hands now that we have helped their feet or hips. All these patients have some deformity or disability, and some procedure should theoretically improve the hand. Certainly not all of these patients should undergo a surgical procedure. The risks, the average result that can be expected, the lasting effects, the need to repeat the procedure at a later time, and the willingness of the patient to rehabilitate him- or herself, wear splints, and undergo some discomfort during therapy are issues that must be addressed beforehand. In addition, the question of whether function will be improved must be addressed.

Patients with chronic hand deformities are often able to perform all activities of daily living through trick or substitution motions; and although one can make the digit straighter or look better, will function be improved? Occasionally, the patient who has a severely deformed thumb can pinch because the index finger is also angulated but conforms to the thumb deformity; and, in fact, if this thumb is operated on with one of the acceptable surgical techniques, function may be decreased. The patient with a metacarpophalangeal (MCP) joint stiff in extension and a boutonnière deformity of the proximal interphalangeal (IP) joint may have decreased function if the MCP joint is flexed or the proximal IP joint is straightened. Many patients ask for increased function, but on close questioning their problem is found to be a decrease in strength that may not be helped with surgery. The surgeon should beware of promising something with surgery to the patient who claims to have no pain and can do everything just as well as the patient with hand deformities who claims to be unable to do anything at all. This type of patient is often poorly motivated and may well be just as disappointed with the hand afterward, even though it may be better aligned and improved cosmetically. Many patients have had hips, feet, or wrists operated on already and may not need extensive postoperative therapy to obtain a good result. Before undergoing hand surgery, these patients require counseling regarding the postoperative rehabilitation program. A patient who refuses to engage in the therapy afterward usually does not have a good result. We do not insist that patients stay in town for prolonged periods after the surgery, but they must return for frequent check-ups, even if travel is inconvenient. A hand therapist is important, but a husband, wife, other family member, or the patients themselves can be trained to help with specific exercises if a competent therapist is not available within a reasonable distance. This area, of course, needs to be discussed before the surgery is scheduled so that there are no surprises afterward.

Souter[62] presented his thoughts on the planning of treatment of the rheumatoid hand. They bear mentioning, as they run current to our philosophy.

1. The surgeon must exercise wisdom and possess a profound understanding of the natural history of the disease together with a detailed assessment of the individual patient's physical requirements, aspirations, intelligence, and personality.
2. The mere existence of deformity is not necessarily an indication for surgery.
3. The surgical program must be tailored to the individual patient.
4. The aims of surgery must be established, considering relief of pain, restoration of function, prevention of further damage, and cosmetic improvement, in decreasing order of importance.

There are a number of surgical procedures for the rheumatoid hand that are more certain to produce a good result or require less patient effort postoperatively. If a series of operative procedures on the hand are proposed, start with a more reliable one, such as arthrodesis of the MCP joint of the thumb or dorsal wrist synovectomy, instead of proximal IP arthroplasties or correction of boutonnière deformities. Lastly, as pointed out by Souter, surgeons should at all times be completely realistic and severely self-critical with regard to what they can personally achieve and what is required of the patient during the postoperative period. The surgeon needs to convey what an ''average result'' may be, showing patients the arc of motion that can be reasonably expected if they follow the rehabilitation regimen and how it will improve function or prevent further deterioration, or how the hand will look better. Given such information, the patient can then decide whether to choose the surgery.

FLEXOR TENOSYNOVITIS

Flexor tenosynovitis in the rheumatoid finger may cause pain, triggering, or limitation of motion. The swelling is usually palpable over the proximal phalanx: Crepitus and catching are present with active motion. A classic diagnostic test is that passive flexion exceeds active flexion

of the finger. In the presence of a stiff proximal IP joint, the diagnosis may be difficult. If conservative measures fail, surgery is indicated. The usual procedure for stenosing tenosynovitis in the nonrheumatoid finger is decompressing the digital theca by dividing the proximal pulley. This procedure may not be proper in the rheumatoid hand because motion may still be limited by the thickened synovium in the area of one of the more distal pulleys, and there is also a greater chance that ulnar drift will result after the tendons are released from the proximal pulley system.

The pathomechanics of ulnar drift in rheumatoid arthritis are not completely understood. Most agree that MCP synovitis[17] initially causes loss of dorsal, radial, and volar support. The digit is then left vulnerable to the potentially deforming forces acting on the hand. One of these forces is the flexor tendons. Smith et al.[57–59] outlined a

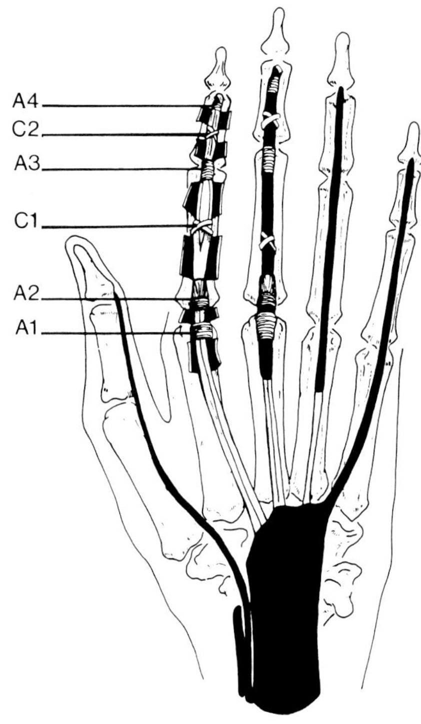

Fig. 12-1. Ulnar bend of the flexor tendons as they enter the digital theca. (From Ferlic and Clayton,[19] with permission.)

convincing case of flexor tendon involvement combined with synovitis of the MCP joints as the prime factor in the production of ulnar drift.

The key to the destructive effect of the flexor tendons at the MCP joint is the large force they transfer to the collateral ligaments of the joint. During pinch or grasp, the tendons make a volar and ulnar bend at the mouth of the flexor tunnel. They are prevented from "bowstringing" by the sling arrangement of the collateral system[2] (Fig. 12-1).

Another effect of the flexor tendons was reported by Flatt,[27] who found that a definite increase in ulnar torque occurred when the proximal tendon sheath was cut and the flexor tendons were allowed to shift in an ulnar direction. The operation for trigger finger or tenosynovitis that releases the flexor tendons from their sheath increases the chance of creating ulnar drift in the rheumatoid hand (Fig. 12-2). Riordan (personal communication, 1960) warned against resection of the pulley system in the rheumatoid hand for this reason.

We have developed a different approach to flexor tenosynovitis and trigger finger in the rheumatoid patient because of these observations. The pulley mechanism should be left intact Tenosynovectomy is accomplished by excising the sheath between the pulleys, and the content of the flexor sheath is further decreased by resecting the ulnar slip of the superficialis. The finger should be explored up to the distal IP joint because of the possibility of triggering in this area (Fig. 12-3).

Surgical Technique

Wrist block or intravenous lidocaine anesthesia is used to allow assessment of active flexion after the tourniquet is lowered. A volar zigzag incision is made from the middle phalanx into the palm, and a tenosynovectomy is carried out. The pulleys are trimmed but left as far proximal as possible. A pulley over the proximal IP joint is preserved, although the remainder of the sheath is usually excised. The ulnar slip of the superficialis is then detached from its insertion and removed as far as the palm, being certain that the cut end does not catch on the proximal pulley. Before the skin is closed, the digit is checked to see that the remaining content of the sheath glides smoothly. Motion is started on the second or third day.

This procedure has been rewarding in our series of patients.[19] Postoperative stiffness can be prevented by starting motion early and encouraging motion by having these patients work regularly with a hand therapist. We had to perform a tenolysis in one patient because motion was not begun until 2 weeks after surgery. In another patient, minimal motion was presented 11 days after surgery. A wrist block was performed in the office, and the hand was seen through both active and passive range of motion. The adhesions could be felt to give with this maneuver. The patient maintained active motion equal to passive motion. If this procedure was done later than 2 weeks postoperatively, there would be a risk of

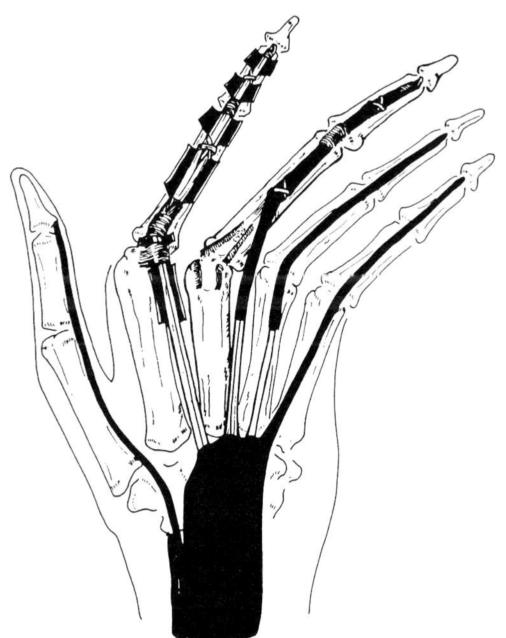

Fig. 12-2. When the proximal pulley system has been cut, the flexor tendons exert an even greater ulnar-deforming force. (From Ferlic and Clayton,[19] with permission.)

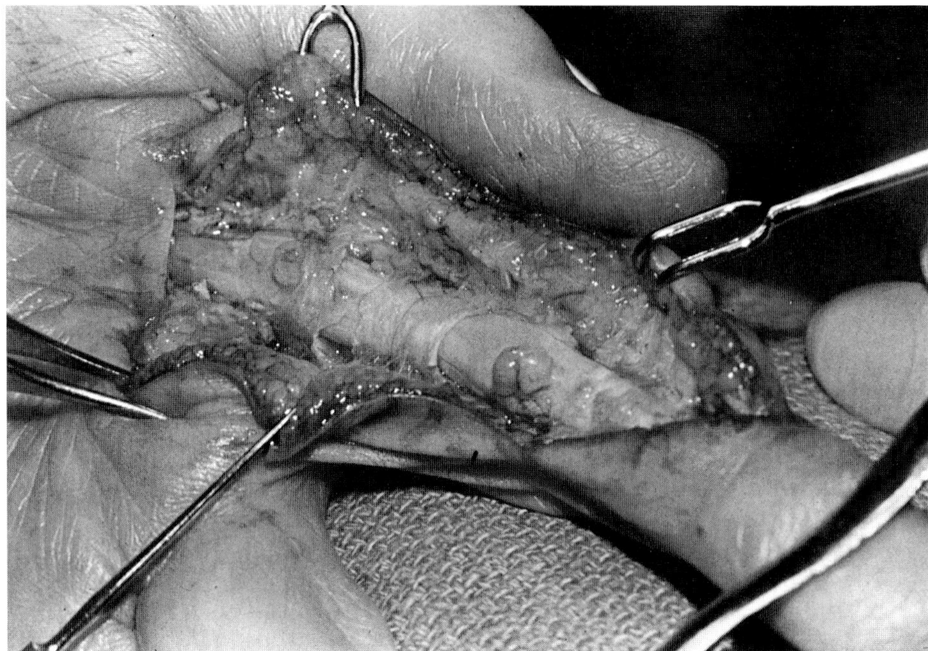

Fig. 12-3. Triggering caused by flexor tenosynovitis in the midfinger. Release of the proximal pulley would not have stopped it. (From Ferlic and Clayton,[19] with permission.)

tendon rupture. In another patient a proliferative tenosynovitis occurred in all fingers, necessitating tenosynovectomy; one of the fingers was a repeat procedure. The immediate problems of limitation of motion and locking were solved by this procedure; and except for one patient in whom the tenosynovitis recurred, the effect of tenosynovectomy seems to have some lasting value.

We prefer to leave half of the superficialis to prevent the development of swan-neck deformity, which may be caused or accelerated by lack of function of this tendon. If a patient has a mild flexion contracture of the proximal IP joint, the entire superficialis may be excised if it is invaded by tenosynovium.

Whether ulnar drift of the fingers is influenced by this procedure is impossible to prove because of the variable nature of the disease. In our original series of patient,[19] more than half had MCP arthroplasty or synovectomy either before or after the flexor tendon surgery. Extensive flexor tenosynovitis must be controlled before arthroplasty of the finger joints is performed.

THUMB

Anatomy

The detailed anatomy of the thumb, particularly the extensor mechanism, must be appreciated to understand the pathology of many thumb deformities. The abductor pollicis brevis and flexor pollicis brevis on the radial side and the adductor pollicis on the ulnar side contribute fibers to the extensor mechanism through the transverse hood and oblique fibers. These muscles insert on the sesamoid bones and the base of the proximal phalanx. The combined action of these three muscles is to flex the MCP and extend the IP joints. The short extensor inserts into the base of the proximal phalanx and into the extensor hood. In a large percentage of cases this muscle does not have a firm insertion on bone but blends into the capsule of the MCP joint and the hood. It then extends the IP as well as the MCP joint. At the wrist the long extensor of the thumb courses through a separate fibrous sheath, arcs sharply around Lister's tubercle, and inserts on the distal phalanx through the medium of the extensor mechanism overlying the dorsum of the proximal phalanx. This muscle extends the MCP and IP joints, but its unique action is to draw the thumb back into the plane of the palm. There are four, and in many cases five, tendons that can extend the distal phalanx of the thumb: the long extensor, the three intrinsic muscles through the hood mechanism, and in many cases the short extensor. The flexor pollicis longus courses through the carpal tunnel along the tendon sheath on the flexor aspect of the thumb and through a thickened pulley over the MCP joint to finally insert in the distal phalanx.

Rheumatoid arthritis can involve destruction in any of the three joints of the thumb—IP, MCP, or basal joints—and the resulting deformities may be caused by the disease starting in an adjacent joint, as demonstrated by swan-neck or boutonnière deformity with basal joint arthritis. Millender and Nalebuff[50] classified rheumatoid thumb deformities into four types; and although it is occasionally useful to characterize these deformities, rheumatoid arthritis is such a variable disease that rigid classification may be cumbersome and confuse an examiner who tries to put each thumb into a specific category.

Type I: It is a boutonnière deformity with MCP flexion and IP extension. It starts with synovitis of the MCP joint (Fig. 12-4).

Type II: This type also results in a boutonnière deformity but is a result of carpometacarpal synovitis (Fig. 12-5).

Type III: It starts with carpometacarpal synovitis and results in a swan-neck deformity characterized by MCP extension and IP flexion (Fig. 12-6).

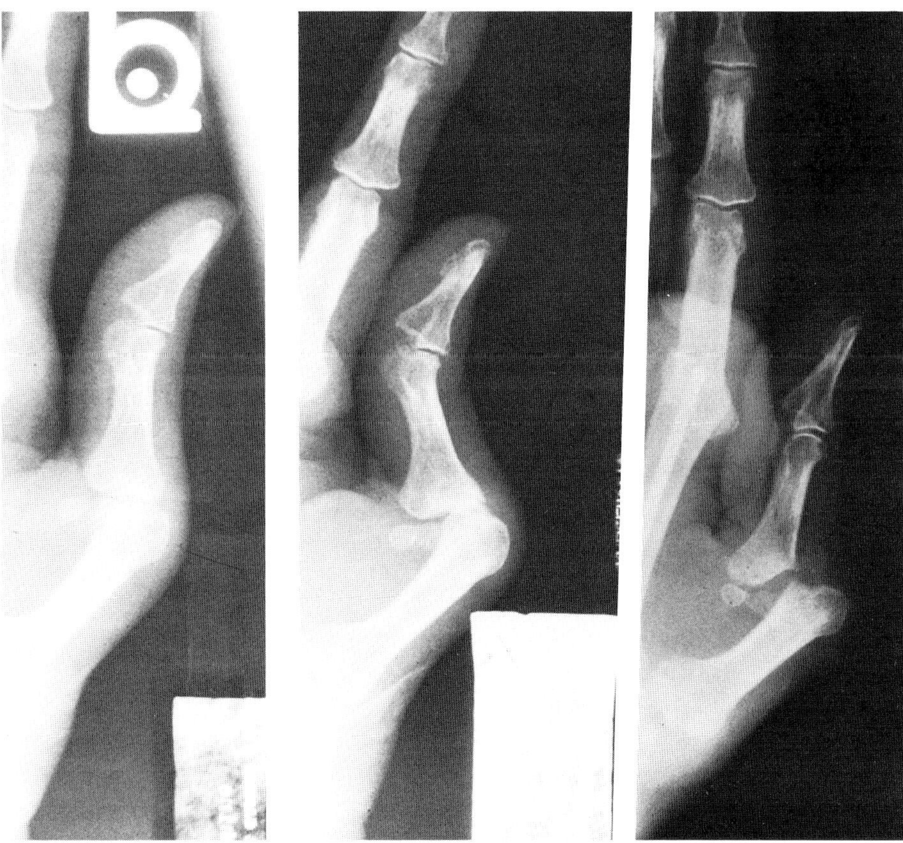

Fig. 12-4. Type I thumb deformity showing progression over a 5-year period.

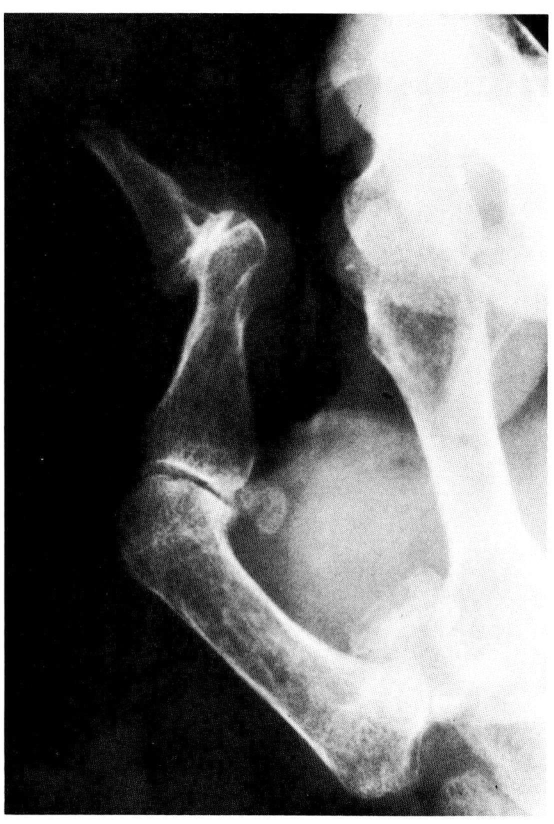

Fig. 12-5. Type II thumb deformity.

Type IV: It starts with MCP synovitis and results in a swan-neck deformity as in type III but also has an adduction contracture of the metacarpal (Fig. 12-7).

The most common deformity in the rheumatoid patient is the "collapse type," type I, deformity (Fig. 12-4). It is initially due to a synovitis of the MCP joint with stretching of the capsule, the hood fibers, and the short extensor tendon insertion. The MCP joint actually moves forward volarly, then loses extension when the hood slips distally. Hyperextension of the IP joint results. Active pinching accentuates the deformity. Lateral instability may develop in either joint but more commonly in the IP joint.

For the conservative treatment of thumb deformities, we have not found long-term splinting to be practical or useful, but we do use a splint or even a steroid injection intra-articularly for a temporary painful exacerbation. In an occasional early case that is passively correctable, we have performed a synovectomy of the MCP joint and reconstructed the extensor mechanism by transferring the short extensor or long extensor tendon to the base of the proximal phalanx or the capsule. Another method is to treat the early boutonnière thumb deformity similar to treatment for a

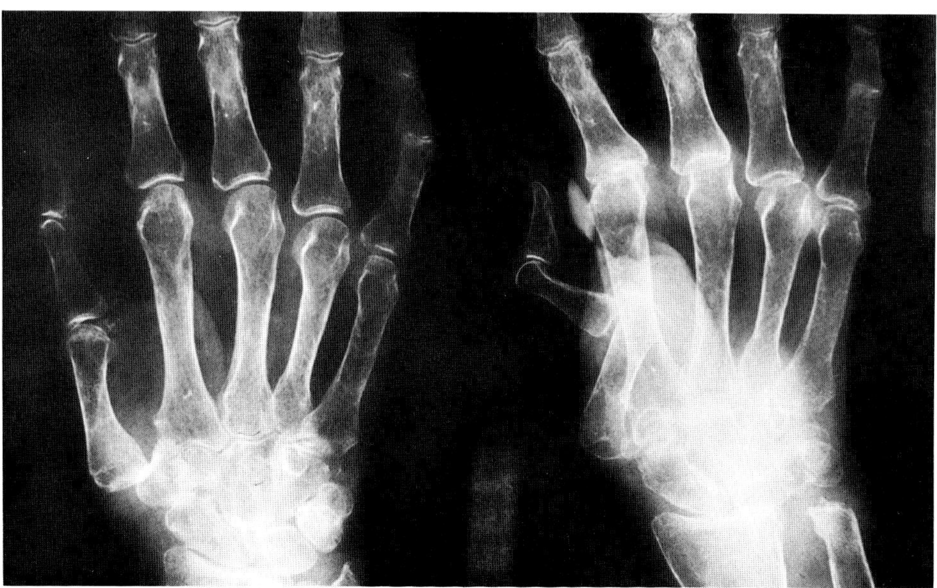

Fig. 12-6. Type III thumb deformity showing progression over a 2-year period.

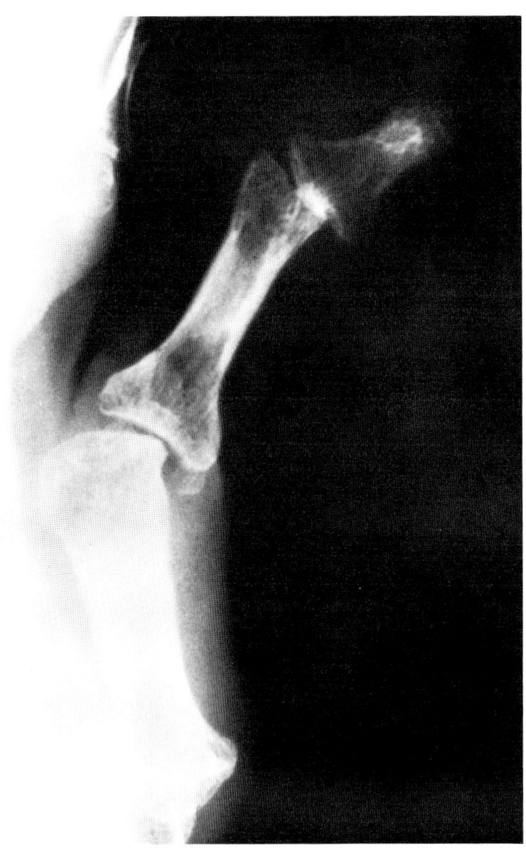

Fig. 12-7. Type IV thumb deformity.

The MCP joint is of less functional importance than the IP joint and is the joint of choice for fusion, provided the IP joint has lateral stability. Many people normally have less than 40 degrees of flexion of the MCP joint, and most activities require little or no motion of this joint.

If the metacarpal is adducted, a release may be indicated. The adductor muscle may be contracted to such an extent that the first metacarpal is drawn into the palm so tightly that the carpometacarpal joint is dislocated and the MCP joint is subluxated and hyperextended to the extent that the thumb can neither pinch nor grasp. In such cases it may be useful to excise the trapezium to reduce the carpometacarpal dislocation, shorten the bone, and restore the metacarpalcarpal hinge. If the thumb is rotated or angulated, the position of the fusion may need to be adjusted so the tip of the thumb can approach the index finger, making pinch possible. If the IP joint is laterally unstable, fusion of this joint in extension produces improved function. Fusion of just the MCP joint, when the IP joint is laterally unstable, only places more stress on the deformed IP joint. Fusion of both joints, when markedly involved, may be necessary.

Fusion

finger boutonnière: advancing and plicating the short extensor tendon and dorsal capsule followed by releasing the lateral bands and relocating them on the dorsum of the joint. A Kirschner (K)-wire is inserted across the joint for 3 weeks. Motion is then started in the MCP joint, although IP flexion is encouraged immediately. These procedures have been useful during the early flexible stages, but because of the nature of the progressive destructive effects of the rheumatoid disease and the forces on the thumb they have not held up over a long period of time. Most cases of MCP or IP thumb deformity in the rheumatoid are best treated by arthrodesis.[15]

Fusion of one thumb joint often results in increased control and stability of the other joint. It is easily demonstrated by temporarily immobilizing the joint and having the patient demonstrate the effect of this maneuver on thumb function.

There is the general impression that arthrodesis is easily obtained in the rheumatoid patient. It is not necessarily true in the patient with the loose type of the disease or in one in whom there has been a considerable amount of bone absorption.

The multiplicity of methods used to obtain thumb fusion indicate the lack of an ideal operation. Several authors[14,46,52] have reported 91 to 100 percent successful bony fusion rates regardless of the method employed. Lister[46] reported a 100 percent fusion rate in five IP and four MCP arthrodeses using an interosseous wiring technique. Brumfield and Conaty[11] reported an 80 percent fusion rate (74 of 92) at the MCP joint using crossed K-wires for fixation, and Beckenbaugh[4] reported a 100 percent fusion rate in 367 MCP arthrodeses using the same technique. Harrison et al.[37] used polypropylene peg fixation and reported an 85 percent fusion rate (85 of 100) in the thumb MCP joint and a 57 percent fusion rate (8 of 14) in the thumb IP joint; the arthrodeses that did not form bony union proceeded to stable, pain-free fibrous union.

Other methods have been employed in an attempt to gain solid bony fusion. Moberg[52] and Potenza[56] used bone grafts. Wexler et al.[75] used rubber band compression with antero-posteriorly placed K-wires. In 1972 Tupper[71] developed a small compression arthrodesis device designed to be implanted underneath the skin.

In 1968 Micks and Hager[49] demonstrated the Micks External Compression Fixator (MECF), a small compression device that accelerates small joint fusion. In 1979 Leonard and Capen[45] reported on 21 thumb joint arthrodeses (14 MCP and 7 IP) using the MECF. Twenty of these arthrodeses proceeded to bony union, which was usually attained in 6 weeks.

The MECF is a reliable method of obtaining arthrodesis (Fig. 12-8). In 1982 we reviewed the patients on whom we performed this procedure and reported on 82 arthrodeses in 66 patients, 55 being rheumatoid arthritics.[22] All of the joints in the rheumatoid patients fused except one, although one patient needed a secondary procedure when the position was lost. Generally, crossed K-wires provide adequate fixation for thumb fusion. If the bone stock is inadequate, our present method of fixation is with a tension band wire technique.[41]

Surgical Technique

A longitudinal skin incision is made directly over the dorsum of the joint. In the case of the MCP joint, the extensor pollicis longus is separated from the extensor pollicis brevis. The joint is then entered, and the soft tissue attachments are released about the joint surfaces, including the collateral ligament origins. The reciprocating power saw is used to resect the joint surfaces at the desired angle. Number 0.065 K-wires are then passed perpendicularly across the shafts of both bones with a mini power driver. Care is taken to pass the wire at a point midway from volar to dorsal at the interface so the compression force does not tend to angulate the fusion site. The compression clamp is then applied. A longitudinal K-wire is usually passed across the joint to prevent volar or dorsal angulation, as it is difficult to measure the exact center in these small bones (Fig. 12-9).

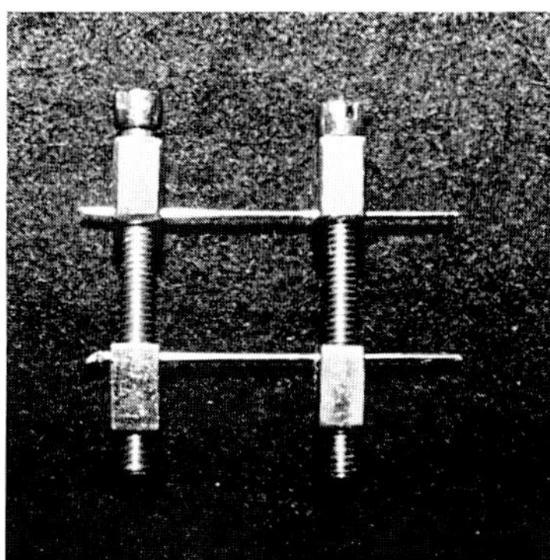

Fig. 12-8. Micks external compression device. (From Ferlic et al.,[22] with permission.)

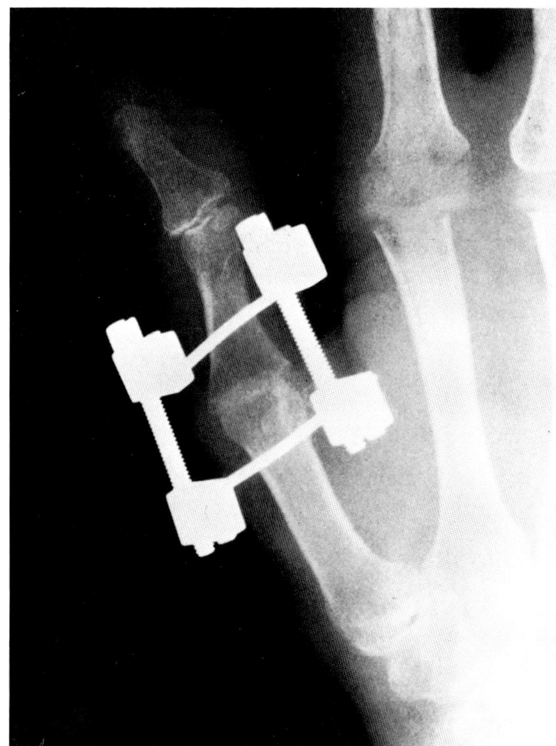

Fig. 12-9. Micks device in place fusing the MCP joint. (From Ferlic et al.,[22] with permission.)

Proper pin placement is critical to prevent bowing and flexion deformities at the arthrodesis site. On the lateral view, the line formed between the two pin sites should be placed so it falls in line with the axis of the arthrodesis (Fig. 12-10). Proper pin placement may preclude the need for a longitudinal K-wire for stabilization. However, in the small bones and in rheumatoid arthritics, it may be difficult to get the exact pin placement, and a longitudinal K-wire is an effective method for preventing angulation. Furthermore, correct pin placement ensures that equal compressive forces are exerted on all portions of the resected articulating surfaces. Soft tissues and skin are closed. No other postoperative immobilization is necessary, and the compression clamp is removed when bony union is present, which is usually at 6 weeks.

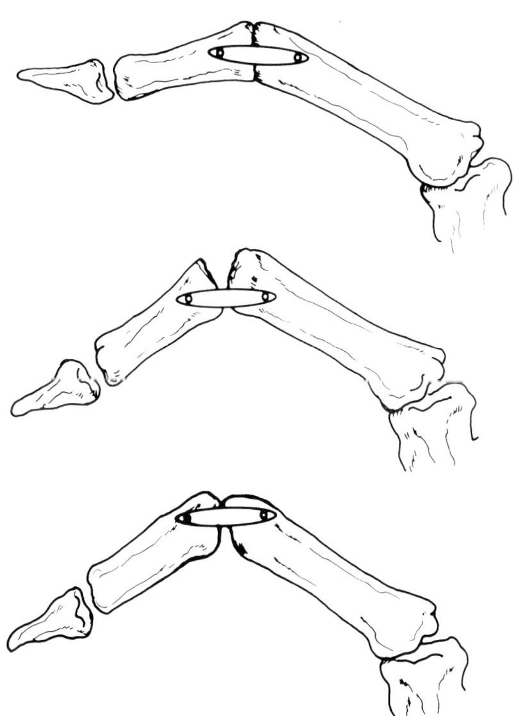

Fig. 12-10. Proper pin placement is shown in the top diagram. If wires are placed too far volarly, the bones open dorsally, as shown in the middle figure. If the pins are placed above the axis of rotation, the fusion site opens volarly, as in the lower illustration.

The recommended position of the fusion is 15 degrees of flexion with slight internal rotation and abduction. Full extension produces a functional fusion if the sesamoids are not too prominent. One needs just enough flexion so there is not a prominence in front of the MCP joint with gripping. Another important point is that some type of immobilization of the fusion is needed so the IP joint can be kept moving during the fusion. The best results of MCP joint fusion in a thumb are with a mobile IP joint with 50 to 90 degrees of motion so the patient can still have a good fingernail type of fine pinch. If the IP joint must be fused, the patient loses part of this fine pinch; but if a good distal IP joint of the index finger is present, this finger can substitute for part of this loss.

The patient who has the most trouble with fine pinch has a fused IP thumb joint and a stiff or poorly controlled distal IP joint of the index finger. Generally, the IP fusion alone gives a fine result, but not as good as MCP fusion alone. We avoid performing an arthrodesis on both the MCP and IP joints, but occasionally it is necessary after a failed arthroplasty or when no other alternatives are available. These thumbs are satisfactory considering the limited established goals.

Arthroplasty

Rheumatoid patients with severe deformities in the remainder of their hand and wrist need as much functional motion in their thumbs as possible. Interpositional arthroplasty has been popular in the MCP joints of the fingers, and the procedure has also been applied to the thumb. The capability of prosthetic joint arthroplasty of the hand began in 1959 when Brannon and Klein[8] described their experiences with a finger joint prosthesis in an injured joint. Flatt[24,29] modified Brannon's prosthesis to a two-pronged prosthesis (Fig. 12-11). Others worked with different materials, but it was Swanson[66,67] who first described a silicone rubber implant with the advent of methylmethacrylate. The concept of metal articulating with high density polyethylene has been adapted for finger and hand joint prostheses.

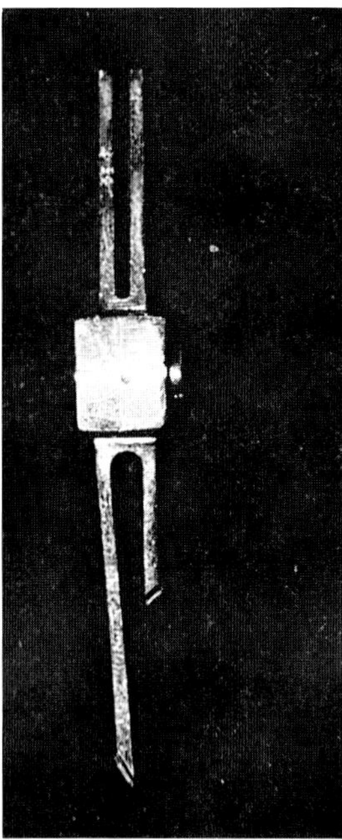

Fig. 12-11. Flatt digit prosthesis. One of the proximal prongs has been cut off for a better fit in the metacarpal.

These joints have not been generally as successful in the thumbs, although Swanson and Herndon[68] reported 44 thumb MCP arthroplasties, with a minimum follow-up of 2 years and good to excellent results in 42 thumbs. These thumbs were pain-free, gained an increased arc of motion of the MCP joint in a more functional range, and functioned more effectively in the activities of daily living.

For the implant to work satisfactorily, an adequate extensor mechanism must be restored by suturing the extensor pollicis brevis and longus, if needed, into the proximal phalanx and the extensor expansion. The medial and lateral intrinsic muscles are brought over the brevis tendon and sutured to each other to increase the extensor power and enhance the stability of the joint. In addition, the IP joint must be stabilized by either arthrodesis or tenodesis if there is a hyperextension deformity.

We have performed a few of these procedures in the thumb where both the MCP and IP joints were destroyed. The IP joints were fused and the prosthesis inserted into the MCP joint. Limited range of motion has resulted, and they have been reasonably stable. Beckenbaugh and Steffee[6] presented a preliminary report on 42 cemented metal-polyethylene prostheses inserted into the MCP joint of thumbs. Follow-up of 12 to 40 months revealed an average motion of 16 degrees. There were no infections and no necessary reoperations. Two patients had radiologic evidence of loosening, but both were asymptomatic. Although a number of these types of prosthesis have been introduced, usage has declined because range of motion has deteriorated with time, loosening has developed, and there seemed to be no advantage over the more easily inserted silicone prostheses. We have not used a cemented prosthesis in the thumb but have had experience with the Flatt prosthesis in a number of cases.[21,32] All patients were candidates for arthrodesis of both distal and MCP joints. Indications for use of the Flatt prosthesis were (1) gross joint destruction of the IP joint with subluxation or dislocation of the MCP joint or instability of the IP and MCP joints; (2) a functional, stable finger to pinch against; and (3) intact muscle tendon units capable of flexing and extending the MCP joint. The Flatt prosthesis withstands the forces applied to it in the thumb functions much better here than in the ring fingers. It provides satisfactory range of motion of the MCP joint with stability and simultaneously stabilizes the IP joint for arthrodesis. Flatt noted the problems with the prosthesis as being bony resorption and fatigue with failure of the prosthesis due to prong breakage or loosening of the screw. This prosthesis has been generally abandoned for these reasons, but in our patients in whom there have been limited goals for the thumb the prosthesis has occasionally been useful. Of the nine thumbs we reported in 1978, eight have been satisfactory with an average 20 degrees of motion[21] (Fig. 12-12). (The prosthesis is no longer available.)

Basal Joint

Surgical treatment of arthritis of the carpometacarpal joint of the thumb has consisted of arthrodesis, excisional arthroplasty, and replacement

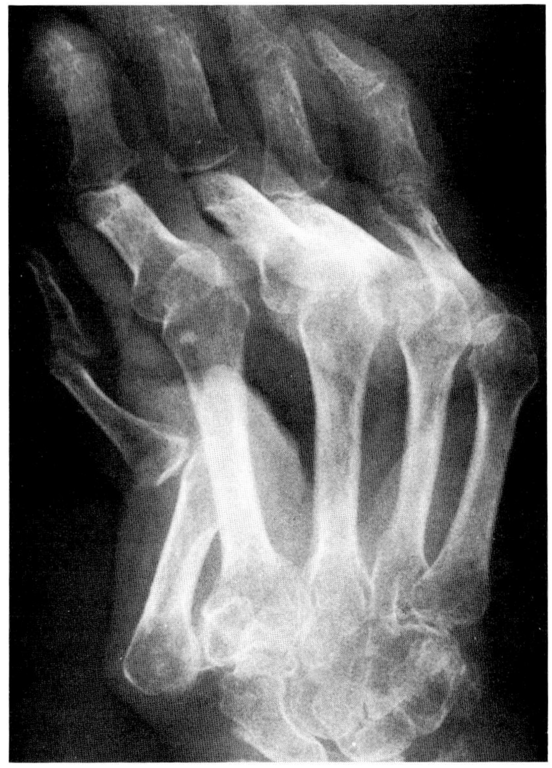

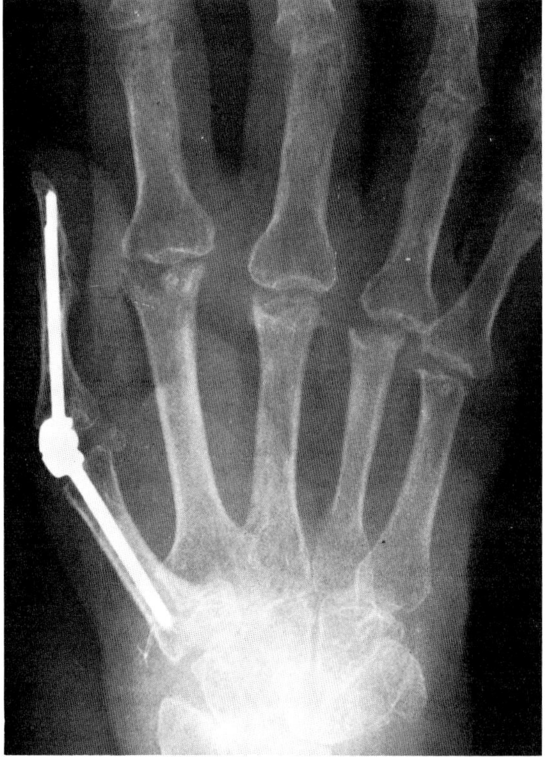

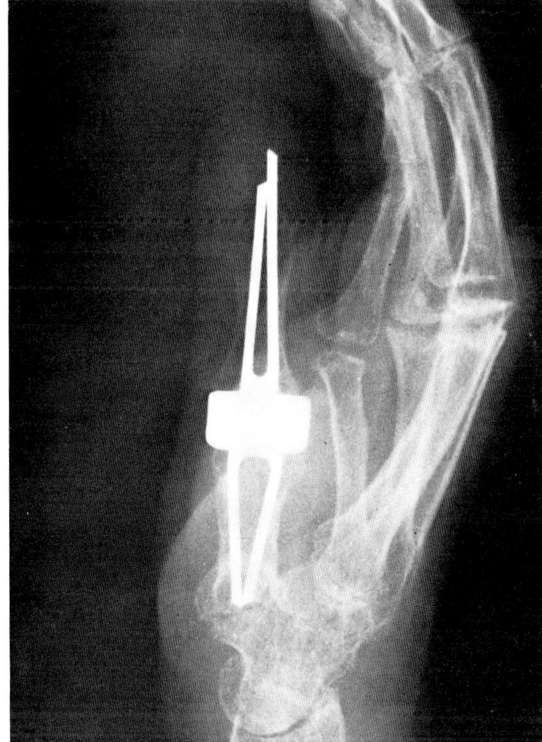

Fig. 12-12. (**A**) Preoperative roentgenogram of a thumb with MCP and IP joint destruction, as well as basal joint dislocation. (**B & C**) Postoperative roentgenograms of the thumb treated with a Flatt prosthesis. The device has been reversed so the long prongs go across the IP joint. This method stabilizes the joint, which is to be fused. The MCP joint has 30 degrees of motion and is painless and stable. (From Ferlic et al.,[21] with permission.)

Table 12-1.   Advantages and Disadvantages of Various Procedures

Procedure	*Advantages*	*Disadvantages*
Arthrodesis	Pain relief Stability	Decreased dexterity with age as MCP joint motion decreases Cannot flatten hand to pick up objects Thumb protrudes when placed in a confined space With trapezium arthritis, other sides of articulations might cause pain Difficulty gaining fusion with prolonged immobilization
Resectional arthroplasty	Pain relief Mobility Relatively simple procedure	Lacks stability for busy tasks Decreased strength Shortens thumb
Implant arthroplasty	Pain relief Maintains mobility No shortening of thumb Allows normal positioning thumb Strength increase	Dislocation Fracture of implant Reaction to implant

arthroplasty. The advantages and disadvantages of each type of procedure are summarized in Table 12-1.[20,21,33,40,43,44,65,67,74] All procedures attempt to relieve pain, with mobility and stability being secondary goals.

All three thumb joints are sometimes affected, and occasionally the basal joint is so far destroyed that there is no stability as well as a marked adduction contracture. We originally used a resection arthroplasty in these cases. It decompresses the thumb, releases the contracture, and improves the patient. We now use an interposition arthroplasty, with either a silicone implant or a tendon interposition, and believe that a better thumb results with these methods. If bony shortening is part of the procedure or the trapezium must be removed, we use the Swanson trapezium prosthesis or an interposition with a strip of flexor carpi radialis tendon (Fig. 12-13). Basal joint replacement arthroplasty is most frequently performed for osteoarthritis, and most reports are for that disease; however, there are a certain number of cases where this procedure is indicated for rheumatoid arthritis. Simple excision arthroplasty without tendon interposition, though, is the most common procedure for rheumatoid arthritis.

Replacement arthroplasty of the trapezium is a

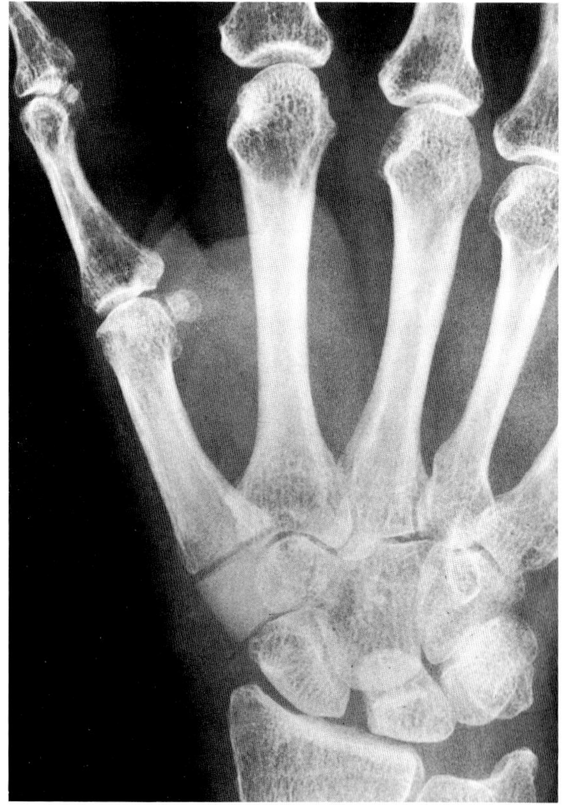

Fig. 12-13. Swanson silicone trapezium implant inserted into the base of the thumb.

logical approach for treating arthritis at the base of the thumb. This operation does not have the disadvantage of arthrodesis, which results in decreased dexterity with inability to flatten the hand, nor does it have the disadvantage of resectional arthroplasty, which results in a lack of stability. In rheumatoid hands where there is marked bony destruction, a regular trapezium implant does not fit properly, and we usually use a tendon interposition arthroplasty.

Operative Procedures

Utilizing general or regional anesthesia and a pneumatic tourniquet, a transverse incision is made over the radial aspect of the base of the thumb, extending from the flexor carpi radialis to the extensor carpi radialis longus. The incision is then curved proximally to run along the flexor carpi radialis (Fig. 12-14A). The branches of the superficial radial nerve are identified and preserved (Fig. 12-14B). The abductor pollicis longus is dissected from its insertion in the base of the first metacarpal, and the capsule overlying the trapezium is incised and preserved. The trapezium is resected with a rongeur as either one piece or in piecemeal fashion, and a small amount of the trapezoid is excised. This maneuver allows a better fit and more prosthetic stability. The base of the first metacarpal is trimmed off flat, and the shaft is reamed to accept the prosthesis before insertion. We now use the Swanson, high performance silicone prosthesis. The joint capsule is closed tightly with nonabsorbable suture. The distal 7 cm of the tendon of the flexor carpi radialis is then exposed, and half of this tendon is divided proximally, leaving its insertion intact. This distal tendon section is passed across the dorsum of the metacarpal at the joint and sutured onto the extensor carpi radialis longus and the capsule, thus making a check rein and preventing dislocation of the implant (Fig. 12-14C). The palmaris longus tendon may also be used, leaving it attached distally. This move may be especially useful if the carpal tunnel needs to be decompressed, as the distal part of the dissection is already open. The abductor pollicis longus is advanced distally on the metacarpal and sutured in place. If there is any suggestion of insta-

bility, the prosthesis is sutured in place with a 3–0 Dexon suture. If the MCP joint hyperextends, it is corrected by simply pinning with a K-wire in mild cases, capsulodesis in more severe cases, and arthrodesis if the joint is stiff, painful, or destroyed. The wound is closed, and the thumb and wrist are immobilized for 4 to 5 weeks, at which time the plaster dressing and K-wires are removed and range of motion exercises begun.

The most frequent complication after replacement arthroplasty is implant subluxation (Fig. 12-15). Our series[18] of 11 prosthetic arthroplasties did not reveal any subluxations after a tendon graft was used to reinforce the capsule. These procedures were all done for osteoarthritis. Swanson[65] reviewed 46 thumbs treated with replacement arthroplasty, 13 for rheumatoid arthritis. A review 6 months to 5.5 years later showed no evidence of bony absorption or reactive bone formation and no evidence of change in implant contour. Radial subluxation of the implant occurred in eight cases. There were no cases of infection and no fractures. In 1981 Swanson et al.[70] reported on 150 thumbs treated by flexible implant arthroplasty, with 147 of them having a mobile, stable, pain-free, durable arthroplasty.

The subluxation problem can be minimized or obliterated by emphasizing several points in the operative procedure. First is the hyperextension of the MCP joint, which must be corrected by pinning, capsulodesis, or fusion. Second is excision of enough bone from the base of the metacarpal, the area between the bases of the first and second metacarpals and the radial side of the trapezoid, and lastly by providing adequate capsular support by closing the capsule, advancing the abductor, and using a sling of flexor carpi radialis or palmaris longus (Fig. 12-16).

Not everyone agrees that a silicone spacer need be inserted. Carroll,[13] Froimson,[30] Buck-Gramcko,[12] and Monon et al.[48] published a series of patients utilizing the flexor carpi radialis tendon, fascia lata, or other tendinous material as an interpositional material. They all reported satisfactory results.

Amadio et al.[1] reported on their comparison study of basal joint arthritis after trapezium resection. All were done for osteoarthritis. Half the

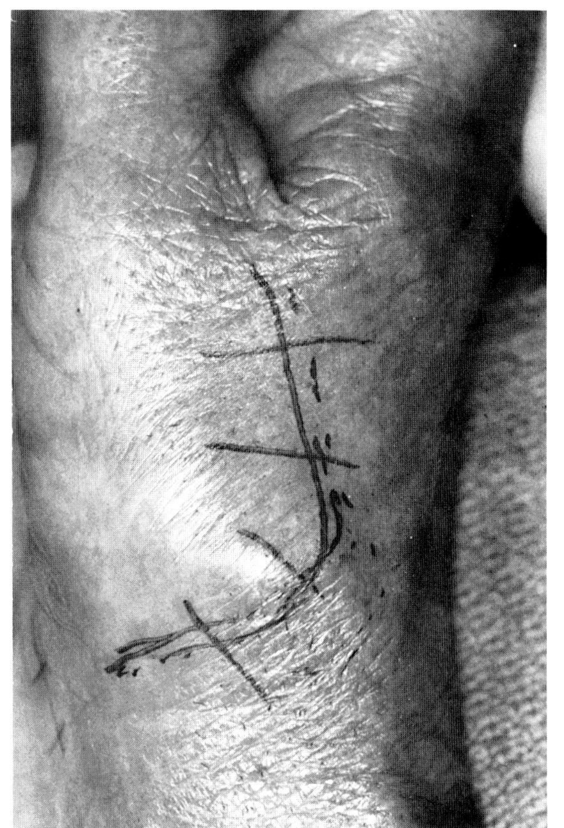
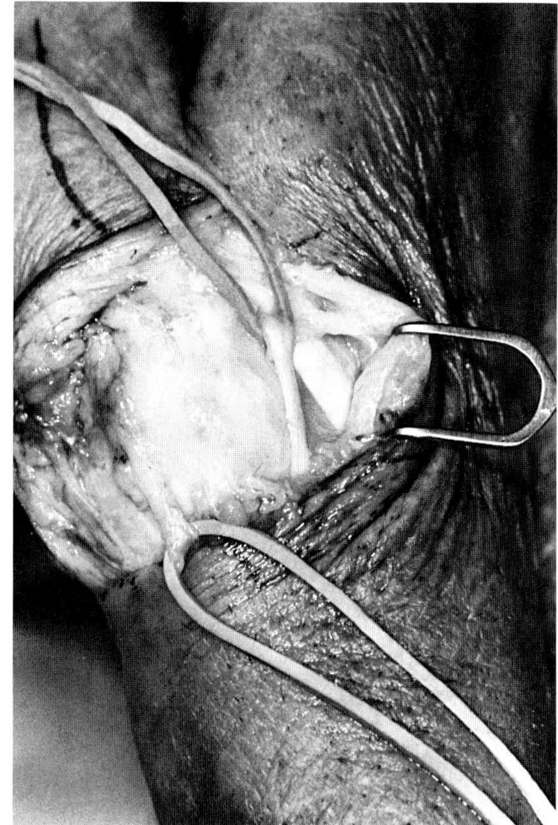
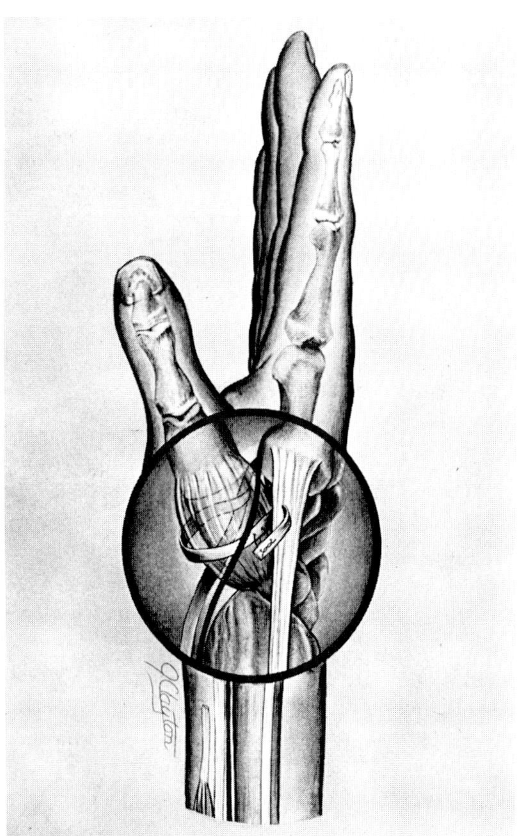

Fig. 12-14. Operative procedure for basal joint replacement arthroplasty. (A) Skin incision. (B) Superficial radial nerve branches are protected by the rubber bands. (C) Tendon graft is used to reinforce the capsular closure. One-half of the distal 6 cm of the flexor carpi radialis is passed across the prosthesis and sutured into the capsule and the extensor carpi radialis longus.

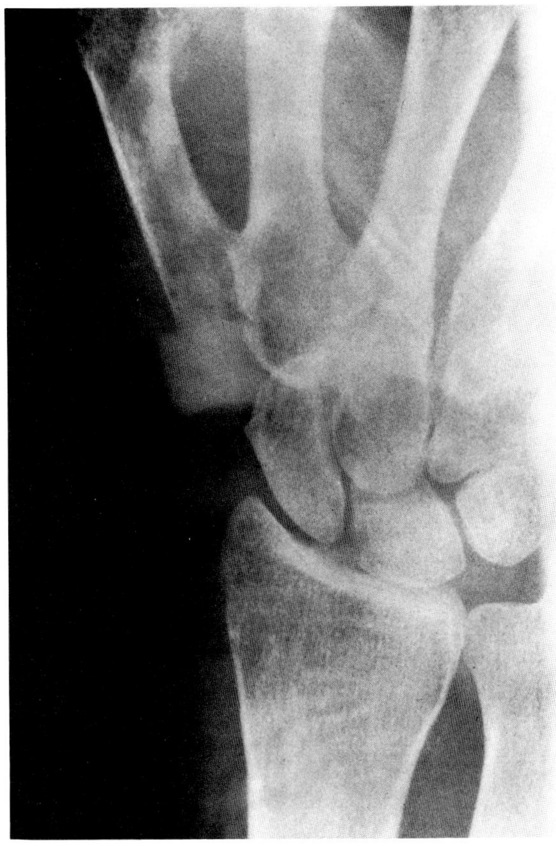

Fig. 12-15. Subluxation of a trapezium silicone implant that was not reinforced with a tendon graft.

patients were treated with silicone replacements and the other half with tendon or Gelfoam interposition arthroplasty. Results were similar in the two groups.

Total joint replacement with cemented metalpolyethylene components has also been advocated. Braun[9] reported on 29 patients, 8 with rheumatoid arthritis. There were three cases of prosthetic loosening, all in the osteoarthritic group. Hamlin,[35] using the "caffiniere" prosthesis on 40 patients, reported 10 percent loosening. This complication concerns us the most, and only time will tell whether the cemented arthroplasties in the base of the thumb will hold up or be abandoned as they have been for the most part in the other small joints of the hand.

Others believe that a simple resection arthroplasty is as satisfactory as one where some material is inserted.[16,31,53] The opponents of this procedure claim that pinch strength is diminished.

Although most basal joint problems are due to osteoarthritis, many patients with rheumatoid arthritis have a disability at the base of the thumb. There may be differences in the deformities in these two types of arthritis. In the rheumatoid patient there may be destruction of other carpal bones or of the trapezium itself, so if it were resected there may be no place to insert a prosthesis or allow the prosthesis to articulate with the distal radius. In these cases, the thin condylar implant may be useful (Fig. 12-17). This prosthesis may also be used where only the metacarpotrapezoid joint is affected and one does not want to resect the entire trapezoid.

With the most severe type of deformity, where there is no bony stability of the carpals left at all and the thumb metacarpal is unstable and painful, we occasionally have suspended the metacarpal on a slip of the abductor or flexor carpiradialis, bypassing this tendon through a drill hole in the base of the bone. This method restores stability, allows motion, relieves pain, and has been satisfactory in these "limited goals" thumbs. These thumbs also have an adduction contracture that requires release as well as an MCP joint deformity that requires correction.

FINGER

The emphasis on rheumatoid hand surgery has been on the MCP joints, specifically replacement arthroplasty. Results are more predictable, and the deformity for which this procedure is carried out is a common one. Enough similar cases can be gathered so conclusions can be reached and the deformed MCP joints can be classified into specific patterns, making discussion of these joints easier. Lastly, many rheumatoid hands have the MCP joint as their only significant deformity.

The MCP joints of the fingers are not simply hinge joints acting in one plane but have abduction, adduction, and rotational movements. The MCP joint is subjected to great stress by the constant movements required during functional ad-

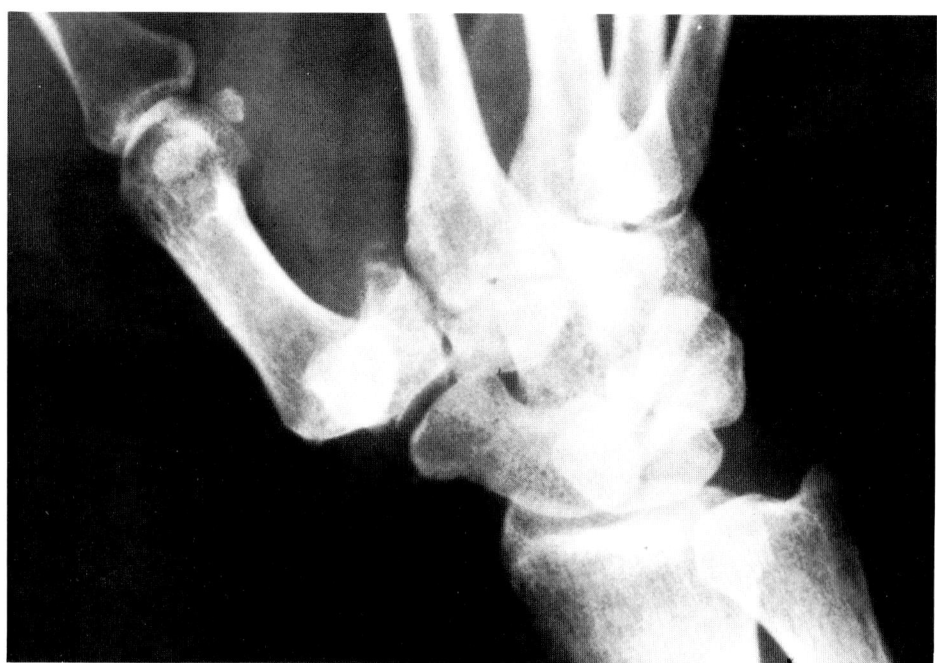

A

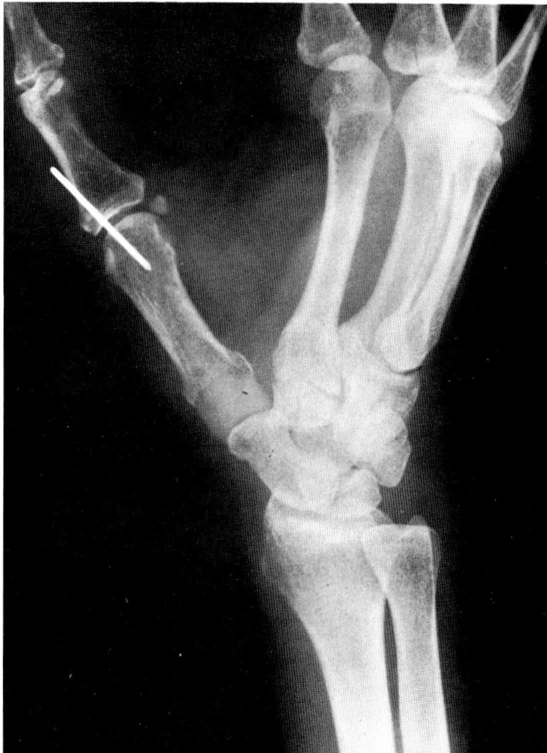

B

Fig. 12-16. (**A**) Preoperative roentgenogram of a hand with severe basal joint arthritis. This patient complained of pain, instability, and weakness of the thumb. (**B**) Postoperative roentgenogram shows good position of the trapezium implant. Pain has been relieved, and strength is improved. The joint is stable and has excellent motion.

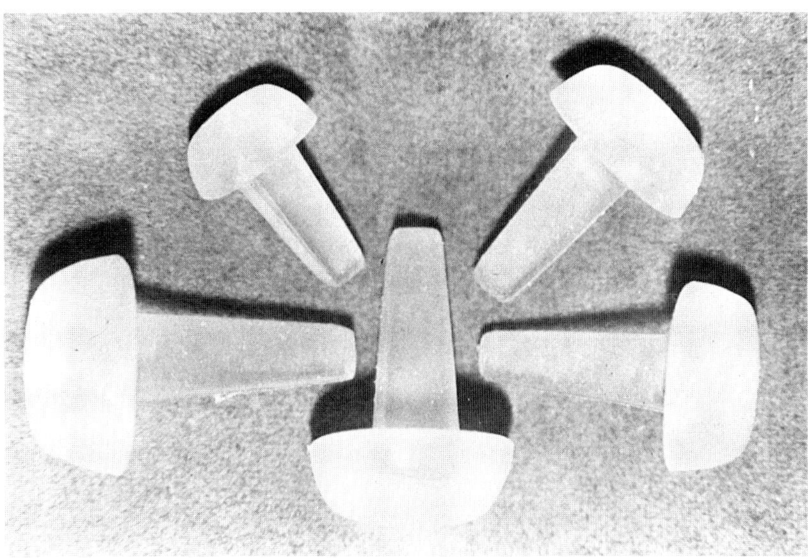

Fig. 12-17. Thin condylar silicone prosthesis to be used for severe rheumatoid destruction.

aptation, and it is potentially unstable if normal muscle balance is lost or if the restraining structure of the ligament system is destroyed by the rheumatoid disease.[60]

Common Deformities

The most common deformities of the MCP joints in rheumatoid arthritis are ulnar drift of the fingers and volar subluxation of the proximal phalanges. Most agree that ulnar drift starts with synovitis of the MCP joints, which weakens the collateral ligaments and capsular support. It leaves the joints subject to all the forces acting on them. Wise[76] summarized the possible causes of ulnar drift as follows.

1. *Shape of the metacarpal heads.* There is some slope of the metacarpal heads to the ulnar side, thus allowing greater ulnar than radial deviation. The dorsum of the ulnar side of the metacarpal head is more pronounced than on the radial side, restricting movement of the ulnar collateral ligament, whereas the radial collateral ligament is free to glide over its side of the head.[34] Lansmeer[42] and Smith and Kaplan[60] noted that the ulnar collateral ligament is nearly

parallel to the axis of the finger, whereas the radial collateral ligament is more oblique, allowing greater ulnar deviating "unwinding" (supination).

2. *Gravity.* The influence of gravity has been implicated in the production of ulnar drift, but it does not act consistently in the hand, which assumes many different positions.[76]

3. *Activities of daily living.* Thumb pressure, cutting food, and leaning the head against the hand are activities we try to eliminate in the rheumatoid patient through counseling and therapy. These activities may play a role in ulnar drift, but certainly seem to be secondary, as they are present for such short periods of time.

4. *Interosseous spasm.* Backhouse[3] found that ulnar deviation and rotation are stronger than radial deviation. Brewerton[10] found that intrinsic spasm was more common during the first 3 years of the disease but thought that intrinsic contracture was more important. Boyes[7] believed interosseous spasm to be one of the causes of ulnar deviation.

5. *Variations in the extensor apparatus.* Backhouse[3] believed that the ulnar-sided interosseous muscles had a strong connection through the transverse fibers to the extensor tendon, whereas the radial-sided interossei sent most of its fibers

in the line of the finger and had a smaller number of transverse fibers, producing a weak triangular area proximally in the hood. He suggested that an area of inflamed synovium was prone to herniate through this area, thus impairing the abductor pull of the radial interosseous and deviating the extensor tendon to the ulnar side of the joint. Snorrason[61] suggested that ulnar dislocation of the long extensor tendon was the cause of ulnar deviation, but we believe that it is the result of the deformity, not the cause, although we have seen an acute traumatic dislocation of an extensor tendon result in ulnar deviation of the finger.

6. *Pull of the long flexor tendons.* We believe that if this pull is not the prime cause of ulnar drift, it certainly is an important contributing factor.

Many of these forces are at work simultaneously. When ulnar drift is corrected, all of these points must be kept in mind to prevent recurrence of deformity.

Because ulnar drift begins with synovitis of the MCP joints, it seems logical to remove the offending synovium before it has a chance to destroy the joint and its surrounding capsular support. Occasionally, synovectomy of the MCP or IP joints is performed chemically with intra-articular injections of steroid, thiotepa,[23] or nitrogen mustard.[73] Clinical evidence suggests that joint motion aggravates inflammation. If joints are injected, they should be rested by splinting; but during this same period of time, the splints should be removed daily and the joints put through a full range of motion.[47]

We perform surgical synovectomy on the MCP or IP joints when the roentgenograms indicate no destruction, motion is near normal, and the disease has not responded to adequate medical treatment. Joint motion may be decreased after this surgical procedure, and postoperative therapy is imperative. Soft tissue reconstruction must be performed with synovectomy in the hand with ulnar drift of the phalanges. It consists in division of the ulnar collateral ligaments and lateral bands and centralization of the extensor mechanism with plication of the radial collateral ligaments. Although results may be temporary, joint de-struction is delayed, and pain is almost always relieved until the synovitis recurs.

Does joint synovectomy really have any lasting effect on joint destruction? This question is difficult to answer because of the variable course of the disease. To be truly prophylactic, the synovectomy must be done early, perhaps after only a few months of persistent synovitis that does not respond to medical management. How often have we gone into the joints to perform a synovectomy and seen articular changes? It becomes obvious during synovectomy that all the inflamed tissue cannot be removed, further emphasizing the fact that rheumatoid arthritis must be a medical disease, not a surgical one, and that its control or eradication must come from our medical colleagues.

Metacarpophalangeal Joint Replacements

Digital replacement arthroplasty started in 1959 when Brannon and Klein[8] introduced their metal prosthesis, which was subsequently modified by Flatt.[24,26,29] The silicone prosthesis was later introduced by Swanson.[66–68] With the advent of the total hip, metal-polyethylene prostheses fixed with methylmethacrylate were introduced for the small joints of the hand (Fig. 12-18). These cemented implants have been a disappointment, and when Steffee[63] presented his material in Denver in 1981, he recommended that these cemented prostheses not be used in the hinge joints of the hand because of a high failure rate. The new biometric prosthesis has had encouraging, early short-term results.[77]

Our experience with prosthetic arthroplasty started with the Flatt prosthesis (Fig. 12-19); and although it was a failure in the fingers, we were encouraged with its use in the thumb, where the alternative would be arthrodesis of both MCP and IP joints.[21] We have had some experience with the cemented Steffee and Schultz prosthesis in the MCP joints. Our early results were excellent, producing stable, well-aligned joints with good motion; but as time went by, motion was lost and components loosened or failed (Fig.

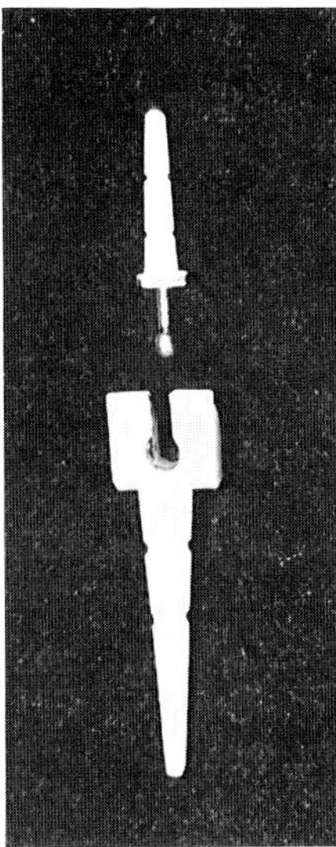

Fig. 12-18. Schultz finger joint prosthesis. It is a metal-polyethylene device designed to be cemented in the bone.

12-20). These prostheses have essentially disappeared from use. Except for this limited experience, we have used the Swanson prosthesis in the MCP joints and have generally been satisfied with this device (Fig. 12-21). We have found, as others, that it has some limitations. There is a certain failure rate, and meticulous soft tissue reconstruction is necessary to obtain satisfactory motion, prevent angulation, and avoid breakage. There is certainly a place for the more rigid finger joint prosthesis that can restrain the heavy deforming forces that work on the rheumatoid hand; but as of this date we have failed to see one with satisfactory long-term results.

The question of what should be operated on first is often asked with a hand with severe deformities involving the thumb, MCP joints, and wrist. In most cases, the wrist, being the key joint of the upper extremity, should be corrected initially, and the thumb can be done at the same time. The MCP arthroplasties should be done as the second stage of the procedure. The one exception to this protocol is if the wrist is destroyed and there are extensor tendon ruptures. In this case, the MCP joints should be corrected first.

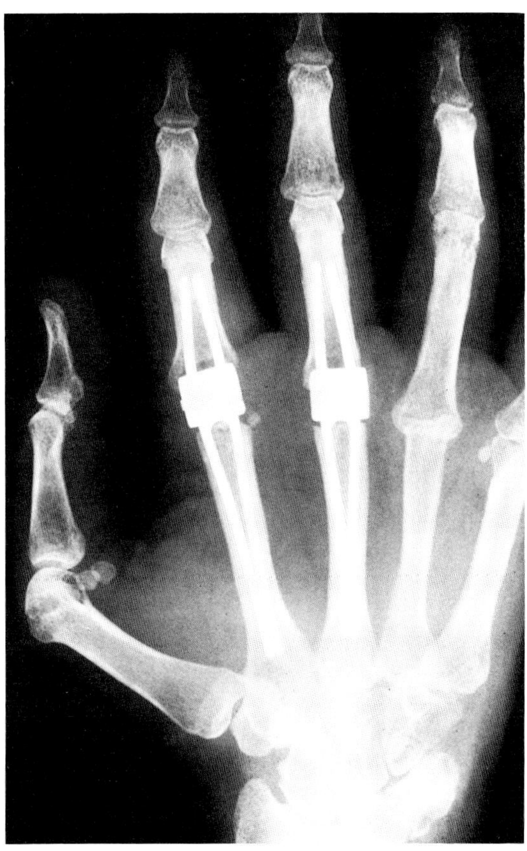

Fig. 12-19. Flatt prosthesis in the finger of a patient with severe destruction of the proximal IP joint. This prosthesis failed, as did most of them eventually.

They can be maintained in an extended position with extensor rubber band splints while waiting for the second stage where the wrist is operated on and the extensor tendons repaired. Proper tension for these repaired extensor tendons can then be determined more easily. One can obtain adequate correction with the silicone arthroplasties if attention is paid to detail. Although these fingers gain motion rapidly, they may lose some of it as time passes, and they may develop some flexion contracture with extensor lag after the splinting is discontinued and the therapy stops.

Surgical Technique

Our surgical procedure for inserting silicone prostheses is similar to that described by Swan-

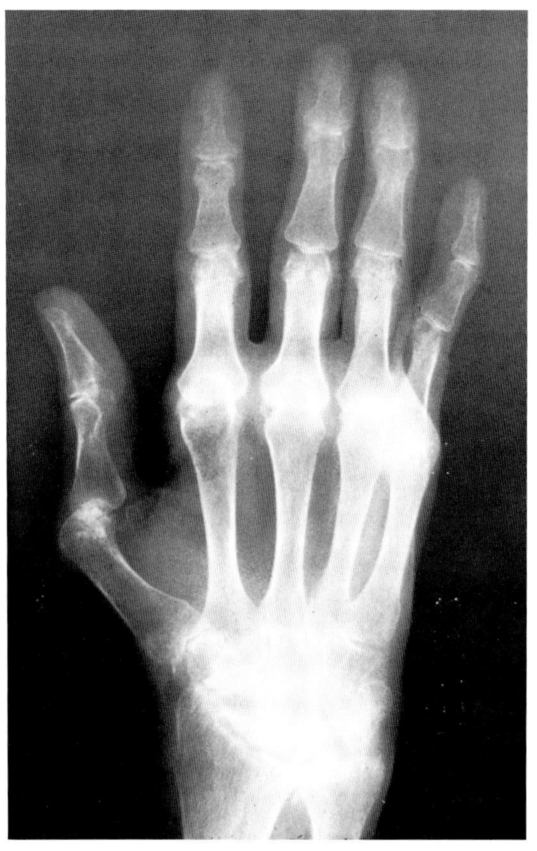
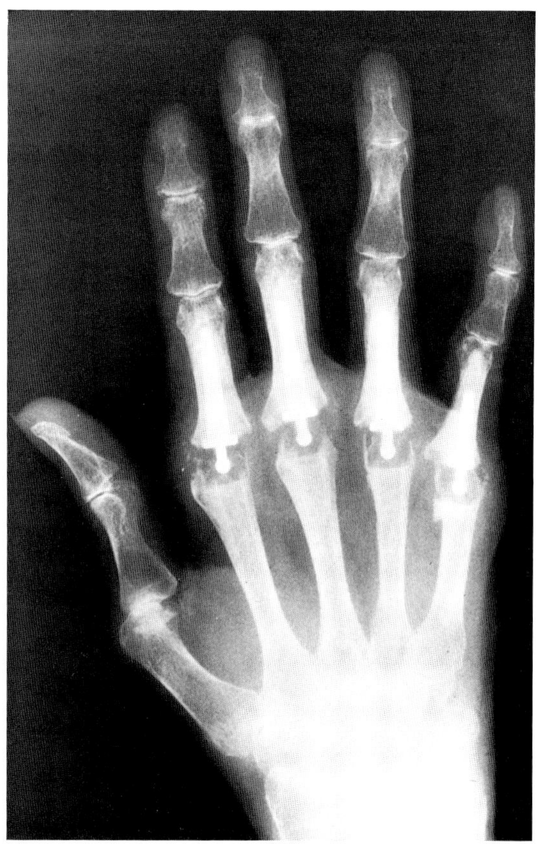

Fig. 12-20. **(A)** Preoperative roentgenogram of a hand with severe deformities of the MCP joints treated with a cemented Schultz prosthesis. **(B)** Postoperative roentgenogram showing the digits well aligned.

son.[66,67] A straight or slightly wavey transverse incision is made over the dorsum of the MCP joints (Fig. 12-22). The skin and subcutaneous fat are reflected in one layer, and care is taken not to undermine the skin. The most likely area of skin necrosis is generally the proximal skin, and one must be extra cautious to avoid skin traction in that area. As many dorsal veins as possible are left intact. Longitudinal incisions between the metacarpals may also be used. These incisions can be lengthened to include the IP joints if necessary. Proponents say that there is less chance of skin breakdown, but others believe that a more contracting scar may develop and exposure is not as good. We have not had problems with the transverse incision.

The extensor tendons are often dislocated off the mountain of the MCP joints into the valleys of the intermetacarpal spaces on the ulnar side (Fig. 12-23). The extensor mechanism overlying each joint is opened on the radial side and retracted to the ulnar side (Fig. 12-24). The ulnar collateral ligaments are divided, and a synovectomy is carried out using a small rongeur. Occasionally, the synovium can be dissected from the dorsal capsule, which is preserved for lateral closure and tightening over the joints. The heads of the metacarpals are then excised (Fig. 12-25).

In order to take off a sufficient amount of bone to insert the prosthesis in a badly deformed hand, the radial collateral ligament must also be detached from its metacarpal attachment. This collateral ligament is tagged for later attachment into the neck of the metacarpal (Fig. 12-26). There is always a radial collateral ligament, even in the badly deformed hand, although it may be

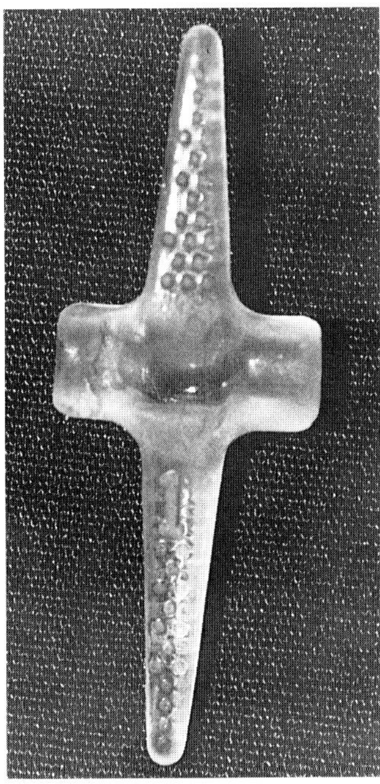

Fig. 12-21. Swanson silicone prosthesis.

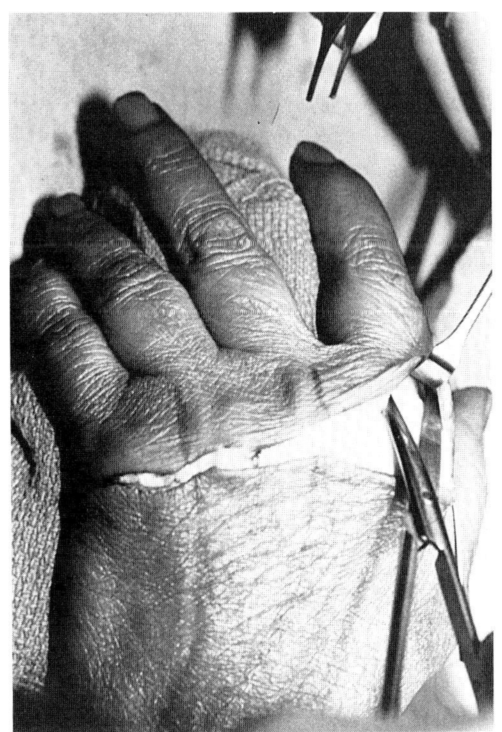

Fig. 12-22. Incision used for MCP arthroplasty.

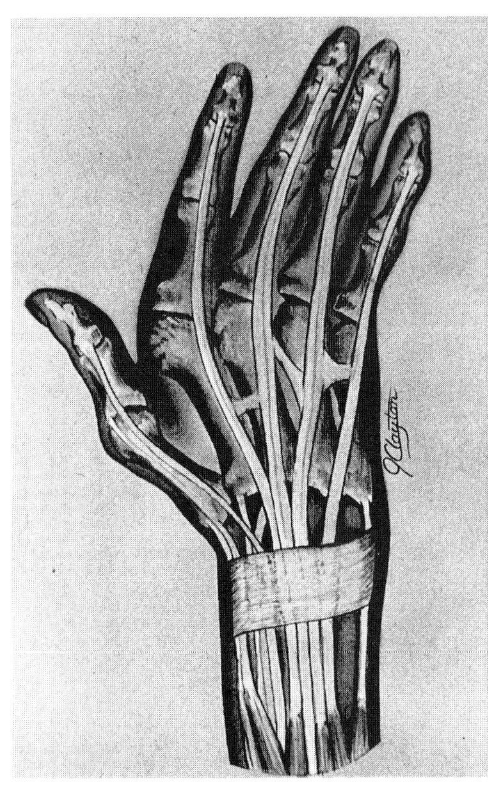

Fig. 12-23. Extensor tendon dislocation in the case of ulnar drift.

subluxed far to the volar side and difficult to find. In a hand that has been previously operated on, if an adequate radial collateral ligament is not present a portion of the volar capsule can be swung up over the side to act as the radial collateral ligament. It is important to have some restraining structure on the radial side, particularly the index and long fingers.

The abductor digit quinti is divided at its bony attachment on the proximal phalanx. The other ulnar intrinsics are also divided from their bony attachments, as are the ulnar lateral bands if there is any intrinsic contracture present. The articular surface of the proximal phalanges are trimmed off so they are flat. The volar plate may be freed from the metacarpal and the proximal phalanx with a small curved osteotome so the proximal phalanx can be brought up out of its subluxed position without removing any excess bone. A longitudinal incision may be made

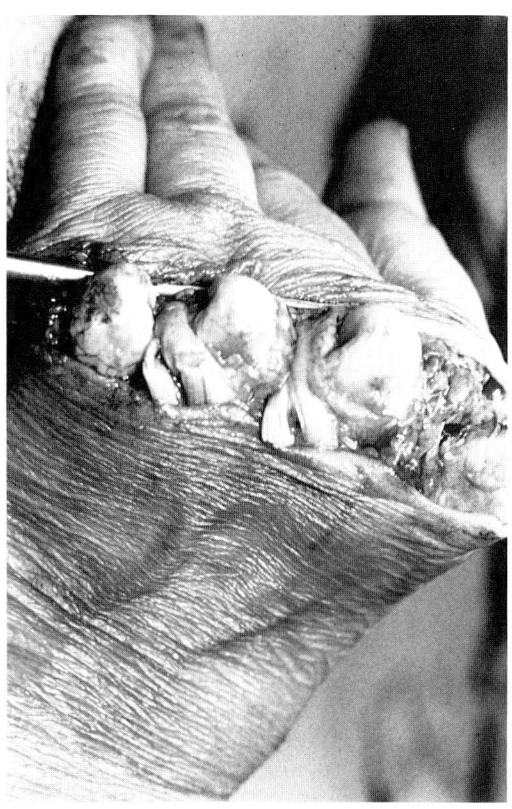

Fig. 12-24. Surgical exposure of the joints.

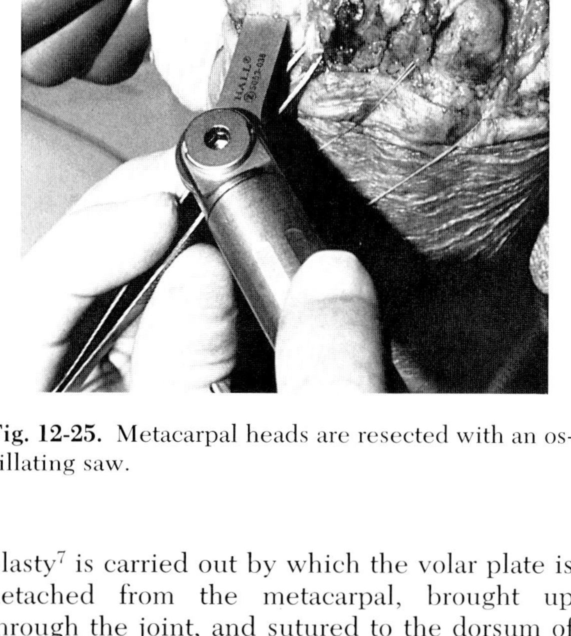

Fig. 12-25. Metacarpal heads are resected with an oscillating saw.

through the volar plate to expose the flexor tendons. They can be drawn up into the incision to relieve a mild flexor tenosynovitis and allow independent superficialis and profundus action.

The medullary canals are reamed with power burrs and rasps (Fig. 12-27). Drill holes are placed on the radial side of the metacarpal neck, through which sutures are placed for reattachment of the radial collateral ligament (Fig. 12-28). The proper sized prosthesis is selected: It is the largest one that can be inserted into the medullary canal. The prosthesis is kept in an antibiotic solution until it is inserted and is not handled with sharp instruments or by hand.

There is an occasional phalanx that is so flat in the anteroposterior diameter that the medullary canal has been obliterated to the extent that it is not possible to fit any prosthesis, no matter how small. In these cases, Tupper volar plate arthro-

plasty[7] is carried out by which the volar plate is detached from the metacarpal, brought up through the joint, and sutured to the dorsum of the metacarpal. The radial and ulnar collateral ligaments are attached using the same suture as in the volar plate (Figs. 12-29 and 12-30). This procedure may also be useful in a finger where use of a prosthesis is not desirable, e.g., one with infection or where the patient might have a sensitivity to silicone.

The prostheses are inserted, placing the longer stem in the metacarpal first. At this point, it is necessary to look at the hand and see that it is balanced on the table. The fingers should lie in a neutral position at this stage. The joints are then reconstructed. The radial collateral ligaments are sewn to the drill holes in the metacarpal neck with 3–0 white nonabsorbable suture. Tension on the ligaments is adjusted to prevent volar sub-

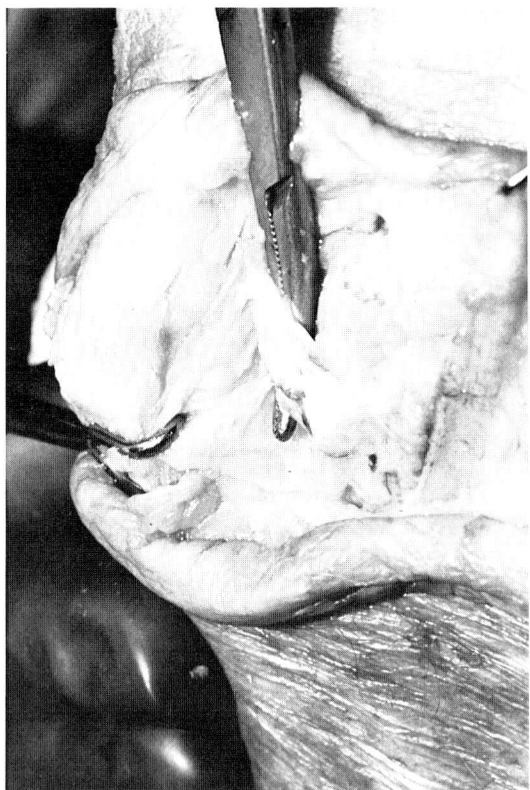

Fig. 12-26. Collateral ligaments are exposed. Both are released from the metacarpal head, and the radial one is tagged for reattachment later. The hemostat is underneath the collateral ligament. The hook is retracting the extensor mechanism.

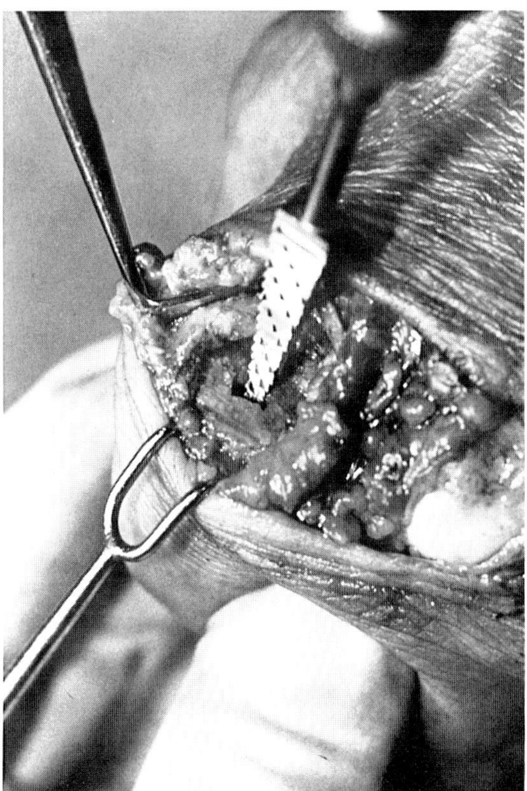

Fig. 12-27. Medullary canals are reamed with a power rasp.

luxation, realign and centralize the flexor tendons, and correct a rotational deformity. This step is most important in the index finger. If the radial collateral ligament is not adequate, the radial half of the volar plate can be detached proximally and swung up to substitute for this ligament. The extensor mechanism is centralized over the joint. It may be necessary to divide the ulnar attachments of the extensor hood, releasing the contracture of these structures from the intermetacarpal areas. In a hand that is difficult to correct or to centralize the extensor tendon, a tongue of capsule may be left at the base of the proximal phalanx, which is sutured to the extensor tendon with the distal joints flexed.[72] In addition, the ul-

nar extensors may be transferred into the radial side of the adjacent extensor tendon proximal to the MCP joint to act as a tenodesis to prevent ulnar sliding of the tendon but not to act on intrinsic transfer. The fingers are tested for range of motion, stability, and alignment; and tension adjustments are made if necessary. The tourniquet is lowered. The wound is drained with a suction or Penrose drain, the skin closed, and splints applied with the MCP joints in gentle extension. Motion is started on the fourth or fifth day.

Two splints are then made for each patient. For daytime the fingers are supported in rubber band dynamic extensor splints (Fig. 12-31), and for nighttime a resting splint with the MCP joints in neutral is applied (Fig. 12-32). This splint is not so bulky that it interferes with sleeping. The splints are removed twice a day for exercises.

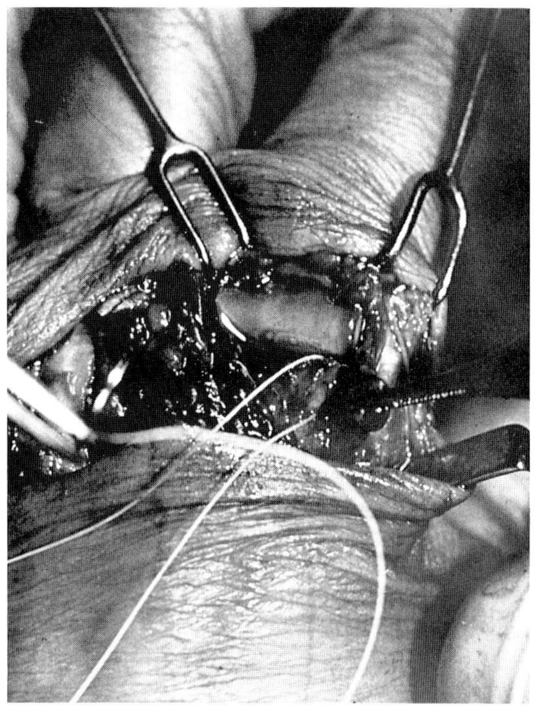

Fig. 12-28. Drill holes are placed in the metacarpal for attachment of the radial collateral ligament. The suture is through the bone.

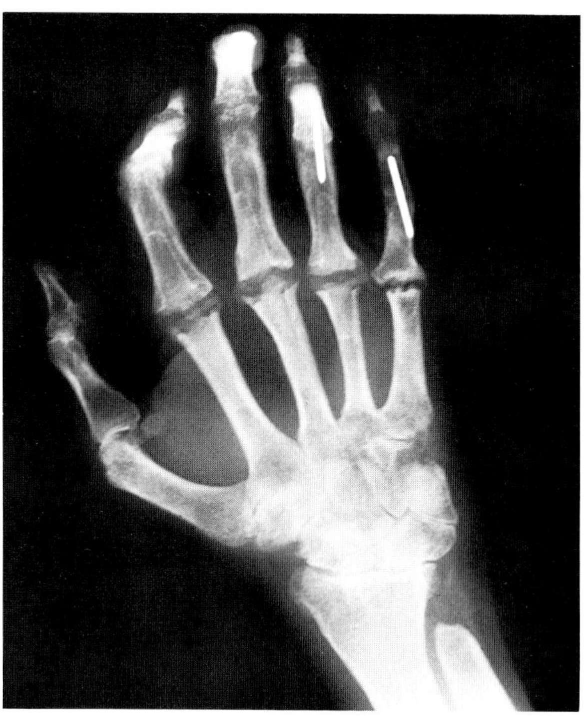

Fig. 12-29. Volar plate arthroplasty was performed in the little finger. Silicone prostheses were inserted in the other MCP joints.

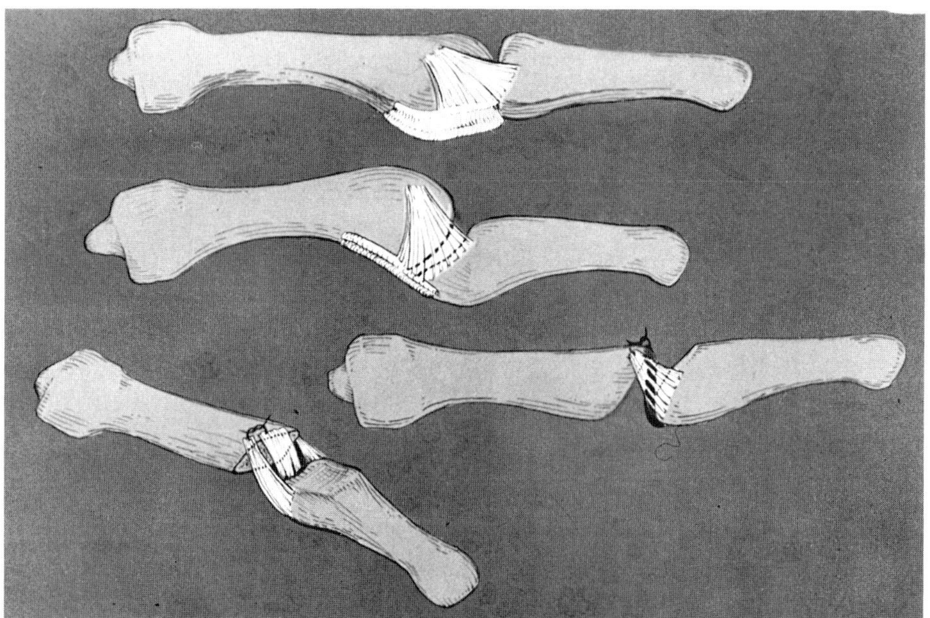

Fig. 12-30. Volar plate arthroplasty.

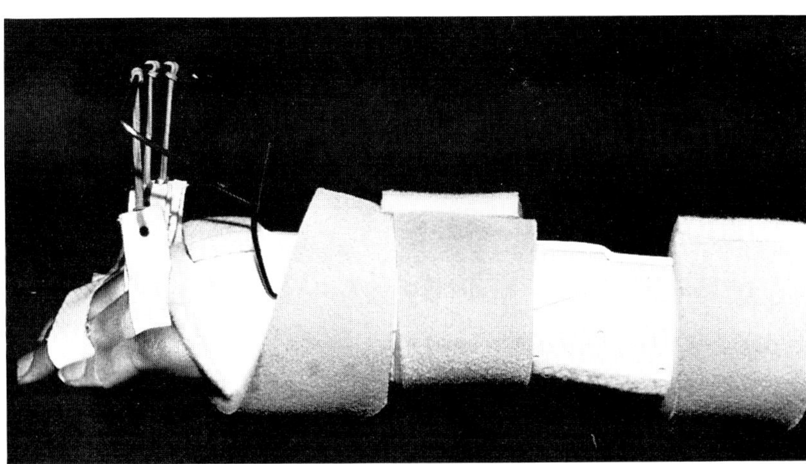

Fig. 12-31. Daytime dynamic splint is made for each patient.

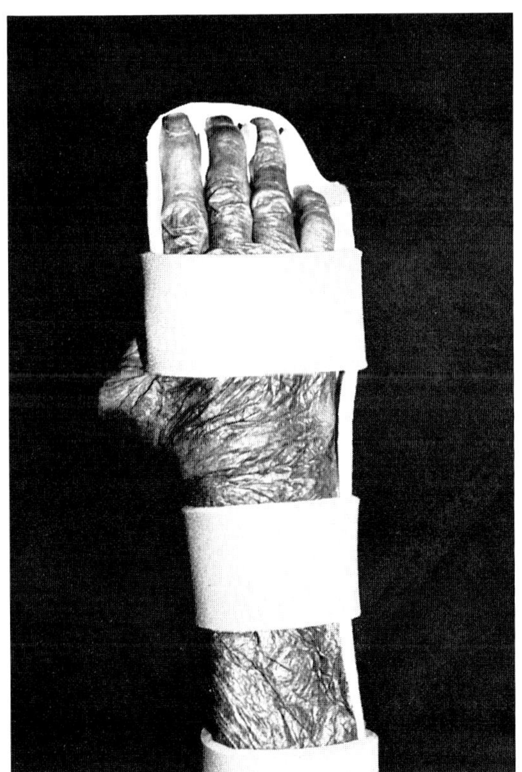

Fig. 12-32. Nighttime splint keeps the MCP joints extended in a resting position. This splint is less cumbersome than the daytime dynamic splint and is not as apt to interfere with sleep.

Our postoperative range of motion has ranged from 90 degrees to only a few degrees. Generally, the little finger has the least amount of motion, and we often do not splint the little finger in extension for this reason. Our results have gotten consistently better over the years. We believe that it is partly due to surgical technique and familiarity with the procedure but also that some of the improvement has been in our postoperative management and the expertise of our hand therapist. We carefully go over the rehabilitation program before surgery, ensuring that the patient is aware of what will be involved after the surgical procedure, and we occasionally refuse to do rheumatoid hand surgery in a patient in whom no adequate therapy can be worked out. It is not to say that all patients need a hand therapist; many patients can manage their own therapy or have their spouse work with them. In the nonchalant patient with no introspection and little determination, the result is predictably discouraging.

The hand that has been a failure after previous MCP arthroplasties (Fig. 12-33) requires particular care and skill during reconstruction. These hands have tremendous deformity and are markedly disabled; often the patient has lost trust and confidence in the rheumatoid hand surgery. However, because there is such severe deformity, patients often wish another attempt at reconstruction. Sometimes an attempt at a more pre-

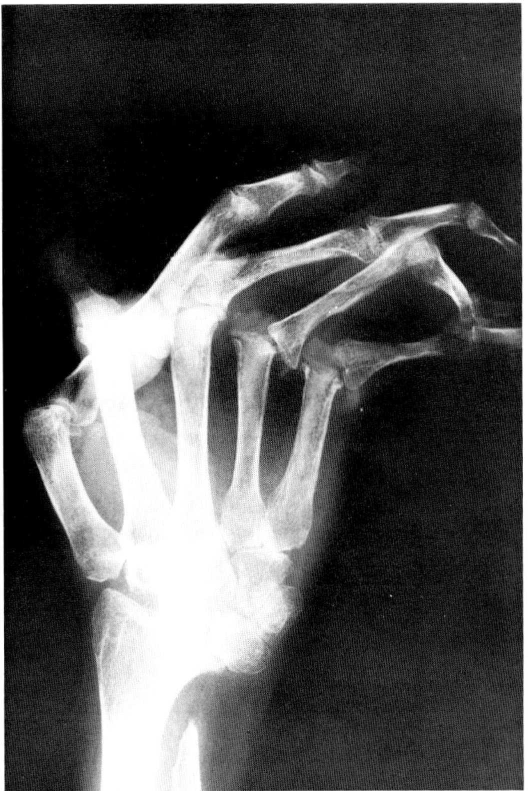
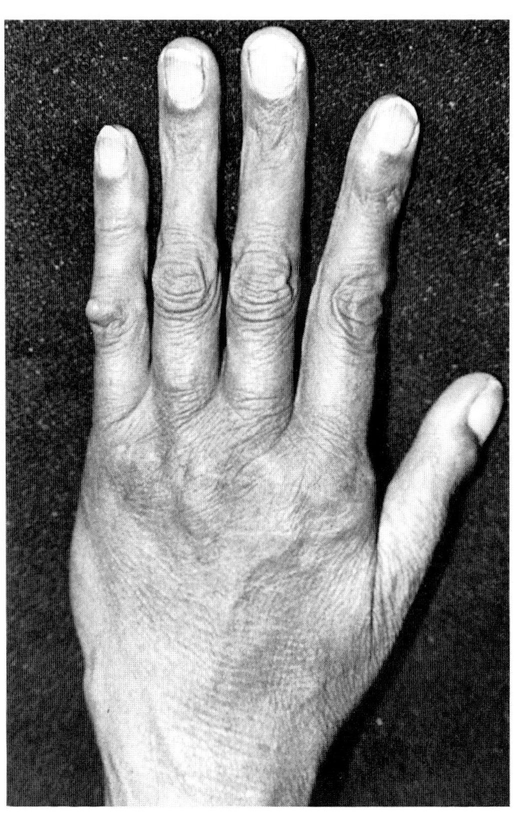

A   B

Fig. 12-33. (**A**) Hand of a patient who had previously undergone silicone arthroplasty with breakage of the prosthesis and recurrence of deformity. (**B**) After reconstruction of the arthroplasty; digits have been realigned and function well.

dictable procedure should be done first with this patient. If the procedure that has a better chance for a good result does work out well, the trust can be re-established and another attempt made to reconstruct the hand. For many of these failed hands there is no therapy or splinting past the immediate postoperative period. These patients are usually surprised at how much they are going to have to go through after this second surgical procedure. Rewarding results can often be obtained, but these hands require a longer period of splinting and exercises.

Complications of silicone implant surgery have been numerous. Swanson[66] reported 3,915 MCP arthroplasties that resulted in 0.94 percent fracture, 0.69 percent infection, and 0.81 percent dislocation. Niebauer[55] reported no breakage in 178 MCP and IP prostheses, with 2.2 percent infec-

tion and 1.1 percent subluxation. Urbaniak et al.[72] reported one infection in 26 patients in whom MCP and IP implant surgery was carried out. Aptekar et al.[2] reported one case of foreign body reaction, and Flatt[25] reported a 10.7 percent breakage rate with silicone MCP prostheses. We presented our complication rate with 162 silicone MCP prostheses and found 15 fractured implants, with one case of a significant foreign body reaction that necessitated removal[20] (Fig. 12-34). There were two infections, and four hands had a significant recurrence of ulnar drift. Our study was a rather short one, ranging from 1.5 to 63 months; certainly as more time passes one would expect to see more breakage.

Millender et al.[51] reported on 2,105 silicone prosthetic arthroplasties in hands of 631 patients, with infection occurring in 10. The prostheses

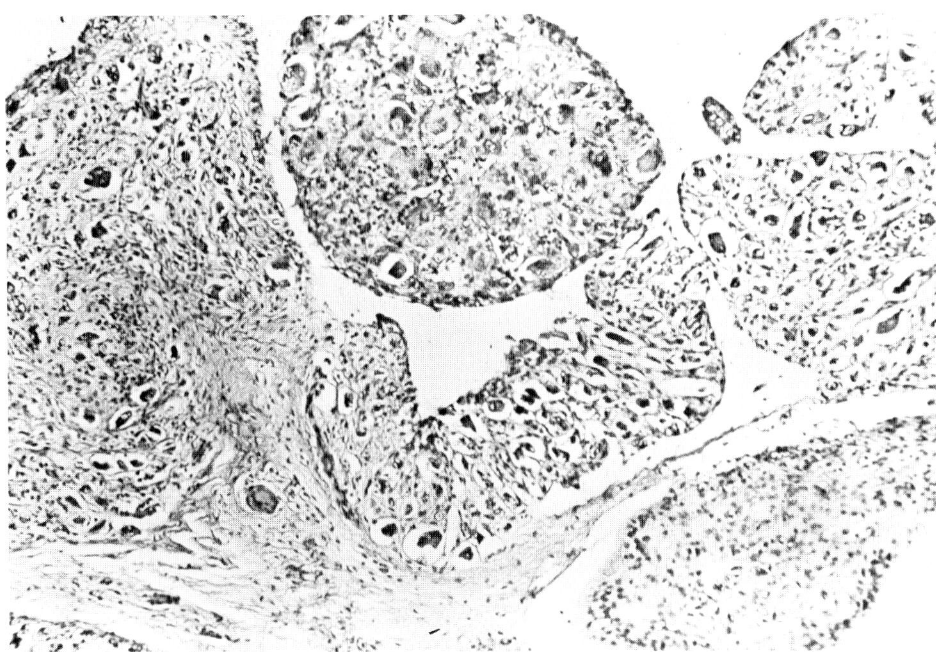

Fig. 12-34. Microscopic section of a foreign body reaction in a wrist with synovitis after breakage of a silicone prosthesis. Particles of silicone can be identified within the inflammatory reaction, as can foreign body giant cells.

were removed in seven patients. Beckenbaugh et al.[5] reported a 26.2 percent fracture rate of the Swanson prostheses and 11.3 percent recurrence of clinical deformity. For the silicone Dacron prostheses the fracture rate was 38.2 percent with a 44.17 percent recurrence of clinical deformity (total study of 530 arthroplasties in 119 patients). We have been impressed with the newer high performance silicone elastomer prosthesis. This material is stronger, and failure is less apt to occur. A prosthesis that can withstand the forces of the rheumatoid hand and promote inherent stability instead of relying on the stability of the poor rheumatoid tissues will be an important development in the future.

One type of hand in which motion is particularly difficult to obtain after MCP arthroplasty is the hand that started off with stiff MCP joints but supple proximal IP joints or proximal IP joints that are fixed in 90 degrees of flexion. The natural tendency in these joints is flexion through the proximal IP joints without motion of the MCP joints. It is difficult to apply an extension splint to

these fingers and often useful to block the proximal IP joints before attaching the MCP joints to the rubber band splints, so all flexion motion is concentrated on the MCP joints (Fig. 12-35). It can be done with a small cast, a small figure-of-eight orthoplast splint, or even K-wires across the proximal IP joints at the time of surgery. Rubber bands may be attached to the fingernails for traction, using a glove or wrist band when flexion is desired. In a patient with a mobile wrist, these devices work poorly because the mobile wrist then goes into flexion and takes the tension off the rubber bands, leaving the MCP joints with less motion than desired. A wrist band, however, is useful in a patient who has limited or no motion of the wrist.

Fingernail traction has been useful for obtaining flexion, but hooks placed on the fingernails with Superglue often pull out. We have had better success with gluing artificial fingernails onto the real fingernails, then drilling holes in the artificial fingernails and placing the hooks through the holes (Fig. 12-36). This method provides a

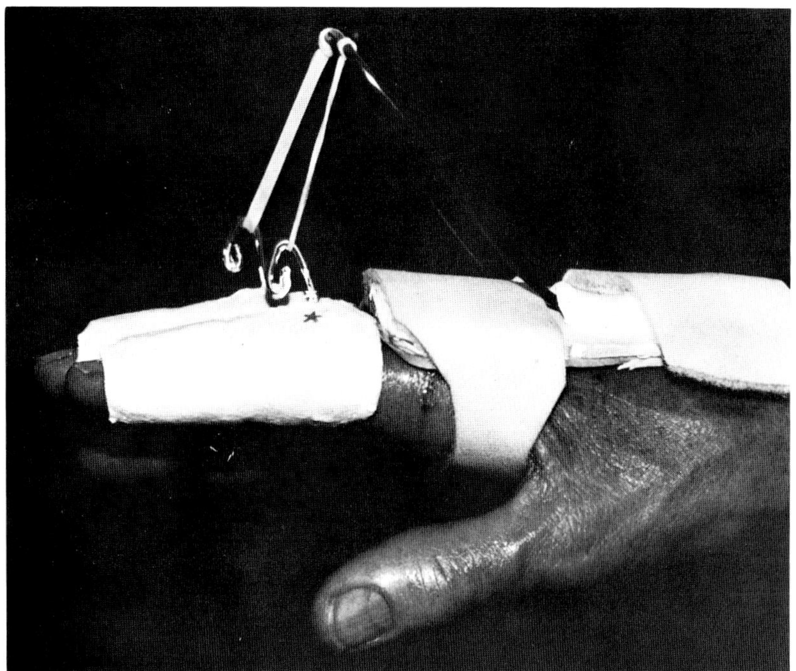

Fig. 12-35. Splints used to block the IP joints while attempting to regain motion of the MCP joints after arthroplasty.

larger surface for the glue to hold. Exercises done by squeezing foam rubber balls or Silly Putty are used extensively. We also apply electrical stimulation to the extensor muscles to help with motion. Patients are given extensive home programs.

Replacement arthroplasty of the MCP joint is a useful procedure. Although we have continued to use the Swanson silicone prostheses, we are aware of their limitations and of the exact surgical procedure necessary to obtain satisfactory results with these devices.

Interphalangeal Joints

The longitudinal arch of the finger is often disrupted in the rheumatoid patient and requires restoration. The zigzag deformity of the hand is commonplace in rheumatoid arthritis, with radial rotation of the wrist and ulnar deviation of the finger being a frequent finding. In the digits these compensating angular deformities are demonstrated by the swan-neck deformity (with flexion of the distal IP joint, extension of the proximal IP joint, and flexion of the MCP joint) and the boutonnière deformity (with extension of the distal IP joint, flexion of the proximal IP joint, and MCP extension).

The emphasis has always been on the MCP joint, but if we look carefully at these markedly

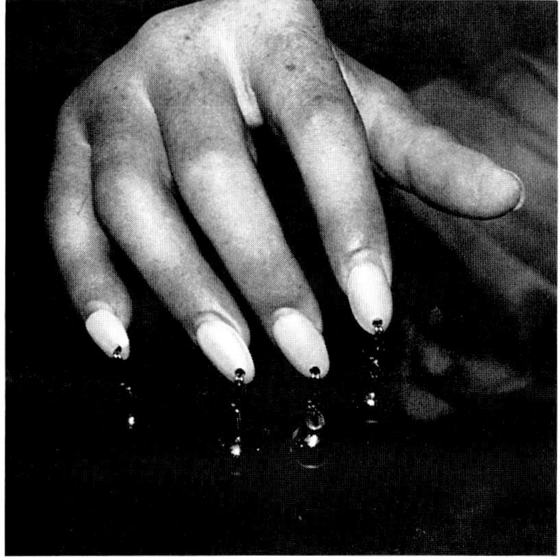

Fig. 12-36. Fingernail traction. Artificial fingernails with holes punched in them have been glued onto the nails.

deformed hands with severe MCP joint deformities we often see 90 degree contractures of the proximal IP joints with boutonnière deformities, severe swan-neck deformities, or sometimes disabling swan-neck and boutonnière deformities in the same hand.

The restoration of function in the IP joints has been ignored in favor of arthrodesis because the function is either not appreciated or other alternatives were not explored. There are a number of procedures that may be useful for the IP joints, including synovectomy, tenosynovectomy, joint releases, tendon reconstruction, arthroplasty, and arthrodesis, all of which must be considered.

The isolated mallet finger can sometimes be a significant deformity in the rheumatoid patient by being painful or interfering with function. It is most often secondary to a swan-neck deformity, but sometimes the mallet finger with its acute rupture of the extensor mechanism over the distal IP joint causes a secondary swan-neck malformation. Treatment may be simple manipulation and pinning of the distal joint in extension, causing enough fibrosis to adequately correct the deformity. Tenodermodesis, as described by Iselin et al.,[39] takes a flap of skin and extensor tendon and holds it in a pinned position for 4 to 5 weeks; it is satisfactory in the rheumatoid finger (Fig. 12-37). We often use this method in cases where many other procedures are planned for the hand, and the patient asks at the last minute, "I know my little finger's joint is not important, but it is in the way and can something simple be done to help it?" Arthrodesis is well understood and is a frequent operation for the destroyed joint. The rate of bony nonunion is high, but most patients

obtain a satisfactory fibroarthrosis that prevents a recurrence of the deformity and relieves the pain.

The last procedure to be considered is silicone arthroplasty: a hinged arthroplasty of the Swanson type or a unicondylar prosthesis that is inserted (Fig. 12-38). Many of these procedures maintain motion, relieve pain, and prevent recurrence of deformity. These fingers must be splinted in extension for 6 weeks after this procedure.

A useful method for arthrodesing the small finger joints has been the use of the Harrison-Nickol polypropylene pegs.[36,37] Harrison stated that no other internal fixation was necessary, but we add one or two K-wires for stabilization. We find these pegs useful because their predetermined angle more easily determines the desired angle of arthrodesis. The recommended angle for the distal IP joint is 25 to 30 degrees. Many of these IP joints in the rheumatoid have poor bone stock and are still unstable after being fixed with K-wires. A tension band technique has proved satisfactory in these cases.[41]

Rheumatoid arthritis commonly affects the IP joints, creating swan-neck or boutonnière deformities and stiffness in either flexion or extension. Limited motion of the proximal IP joint can result from articular, periarticular, or tendinous pathology. One must remember that the proximal IP joint that is stiff in extension may have started as a result of flexor tenosynovitis. It may not be the usual triggering at the A-1 pulley but the result of intratendinous nodules or synovitis well out into the finger. After correcting a proximal IP joint deformity, one must make certain that the

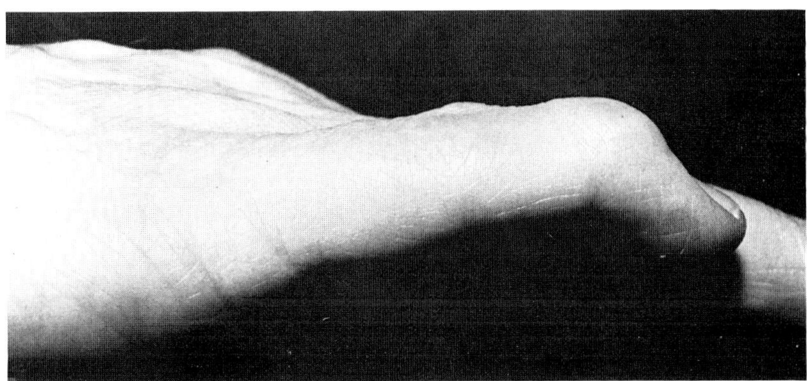

Fig. 12-37. Tenodermodesis was performed for this mallet finger. Roentgenograms showed that the joint space was well preserved. The finger had full passive extension. A full-thickness section of skin and extensor tendon was resected, and a full-thickness suture was used to close the gap; the joint was pinned in extension for 6 weeks.

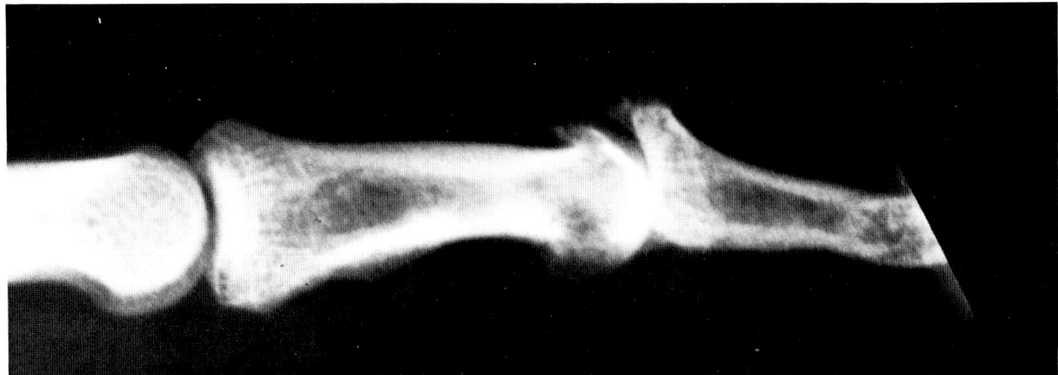

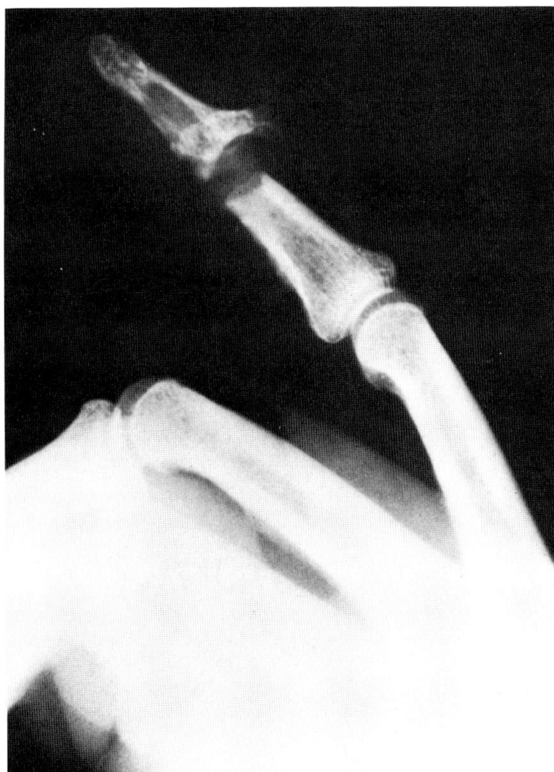

Fig. 12-38. (**A**) Preoperative finger with distal IP joint destruction. (**B**) Postoperative joint treated with a silicone prosthesis.

flexor tendon is gliding. Occasionally, it is necessary to look at the flexor tendon and test it at the wrist or to awaken the patient and have him show that active motion is now equal to passive motion.

Boutonnière Deformity

The pathology of the boutonnière deformity starts with synovitis of the proximal IP joint. The central slip then elongates, and the lateral bands sublux below the axis of rotation. The retinacular ligaments contract, and a stiff joint results. The intrinsic–intrinsic-plus deformity is a useful test to determine if a true boutonnière deformity is developing. This determination is useful for both an acute injury and a chronic situation. It is similar to the Bunnell test for intrinsic tightness but is done with the proximal IP joint held in extension and passive flexion put on the distal IP joint. The test is positive when distal IP joint motion is limited (in contrast to much easier distal IP joint motion being obtained when the proximal IP joint is left-flexed) (Fig. 12-39).

For the impending boutonnière deformity with synovitis of the proximal IP joint, a chemical synovectomy is occasionally useful, with cortisone, nitrogen mustard, or thiotepa being injected into the joint followed by splinting of the joint in extension. Synovectomy of this joint with repositioning of the lateral bands may be useful. For the flexible proximal IP joint, synovectomy and reconstruction of the central tendon and lateral

bands with a distal tenotomy to relieve the extension contracture of the distal joint sometimes corrects the deformity. There are many methods for correcting a flexible boutonnière deformity, including an anatomic repair and variations thereof, substitution procedures, and tendon transfers. Several choices are available for the late stage boutonnière deformity with a fixed contracture. One is correction of the contracture by releasing the capsule and collateral ligaments followed by reconstruction of the extensor mechanism by freeing the lateral bands from the contracted retinacular ligaments and reconstructing the central tendon by plication or substitution.

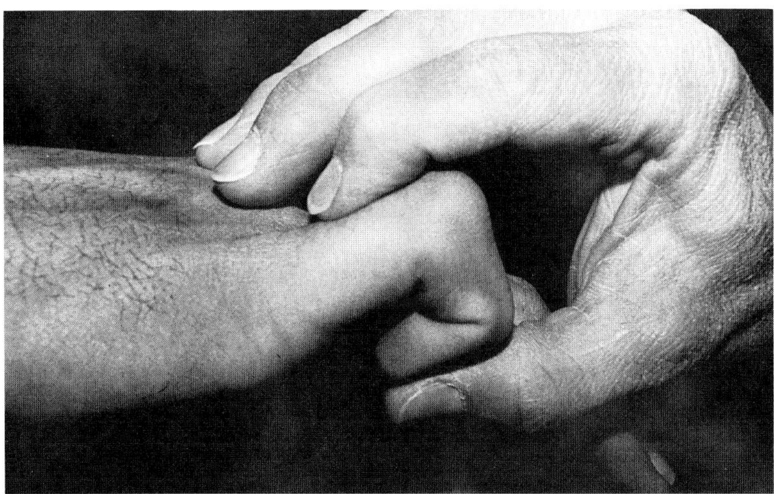

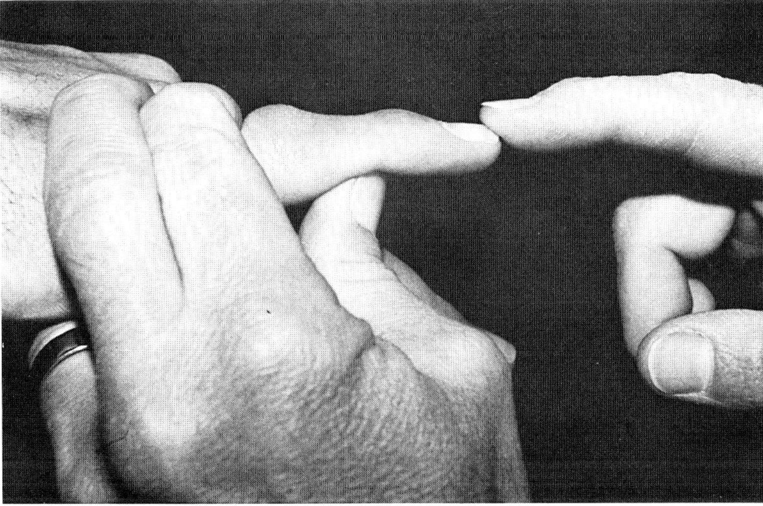

Fig.   12-39. Intrinsic–intrinsic-plus test for boutonnière deformity. The test is positive if there is more passive motion of the distal IP joint when the proximal joint is held in flexion (**A**) than when it is held in extension (**B**).

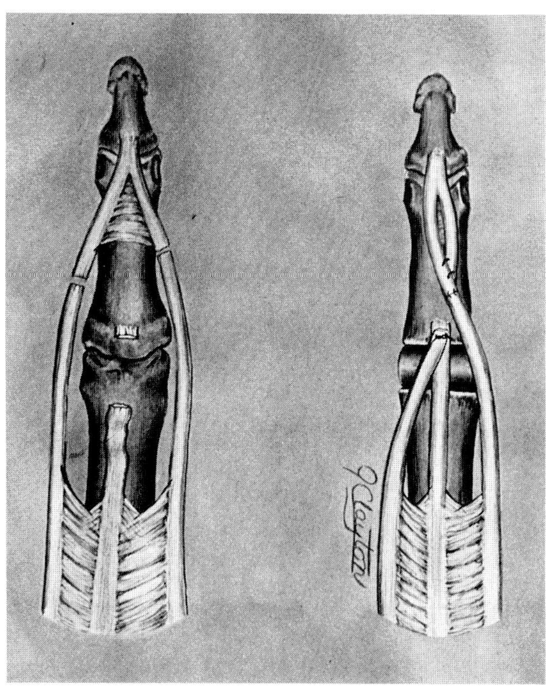

Fig. 12-40. Matev procedure for reconstructing the extensor mechanism of a finger.

For the severely destroyed joint in the rheumatoid patient in whom soft tissues are of poor quality, the Matev procedure (Fig. 12-40) is useful for reconstructing the central tendon, as the lateral bands are always present and can be used for dynamic structures. A distal tenotomy is done in addition if the distal joint is tight when the proximal joint is held in extension. In the rheumatoid joint with poor roentgenographic appearance, soft tissue reconstruction is doomed to fail and should not be done (Fig. 12-41). In such cases there are two possibilities; one is implant arthroplasty and the other arthrodesis. There is a place for both procedures in the rheumatoid hand. We have found implant arthroplasty to be successful in the single central digit and the index or little fingers, as well as in fingers that have both severe MCP and distal IP joint deformities. This procedure certainly does not leave the fingers with perfect motion, but stable motion can be obtained.

Implant Arthroplasty. A dorsal midline incision is made over the proximal IP joint. Subcuta-

neous dissection is carried out on both sides to where the lateral bands are held in a volar direction by the contracted retinacular ligaments, which are freed, allowing the lateral bands to resume their more normal dorsal location. A longitudinal incision is then made between the ulnar lateral band and central slip. The capsule is incised and the joint opened. The distal end of the proximal phalanx is excised, releasing the collateral ligaments. The proximal end of the middle phalanx is trimmed so a flat base is formed. The contracted joint is thus released. The central tendon may be freed completely from its bony attachment in the middle phalanx. The medullary canals are reamed with Swanson burrs and the Riordan rasp. Drill holes are placed in the dorsum of the middle phalanx for attachment of the central tendon and on the radial side of the proximal phalanx for reconstruction of the radial collateral ligament.

This step is especially important in the index and little fingers. Nonabsorbable sutures are put through these drill holes, the prosthesis inserted, and the central slip advanced and sutured. The radial collateral ligament is then reattached. The joint should be fully extended now but should passively flex to 50 degrees without stress on the sutures. Rarely can the central slip reinsertion stand 90 degrees flexion and be tight enough for good extension. When there is little central tendon with which to work, the lateral bands are used to reconstruct the central tendon. One band is divided, putting it into the central tendon attachment in the middle phalanx, and the other is divided and the proximal end crossed over the distal end of the first one (Matev procedure). The wound is closed and the finger splinted in extension.

The splint is removed on the third to fifth day to start active and passive flexion exercises to the extent the surgical repair allows, but the splint is otherwise worn for 4 weeks. It is then removed during the daytime but kept on at night if there is any extensor lag. In some fingers with a severe flexion contracture, it may be necessary to maintain the splinting at night for many months.

Patients have generally been pleased with this procedure, but it is demanding on the patient's postoperative time. Complete cooperation must

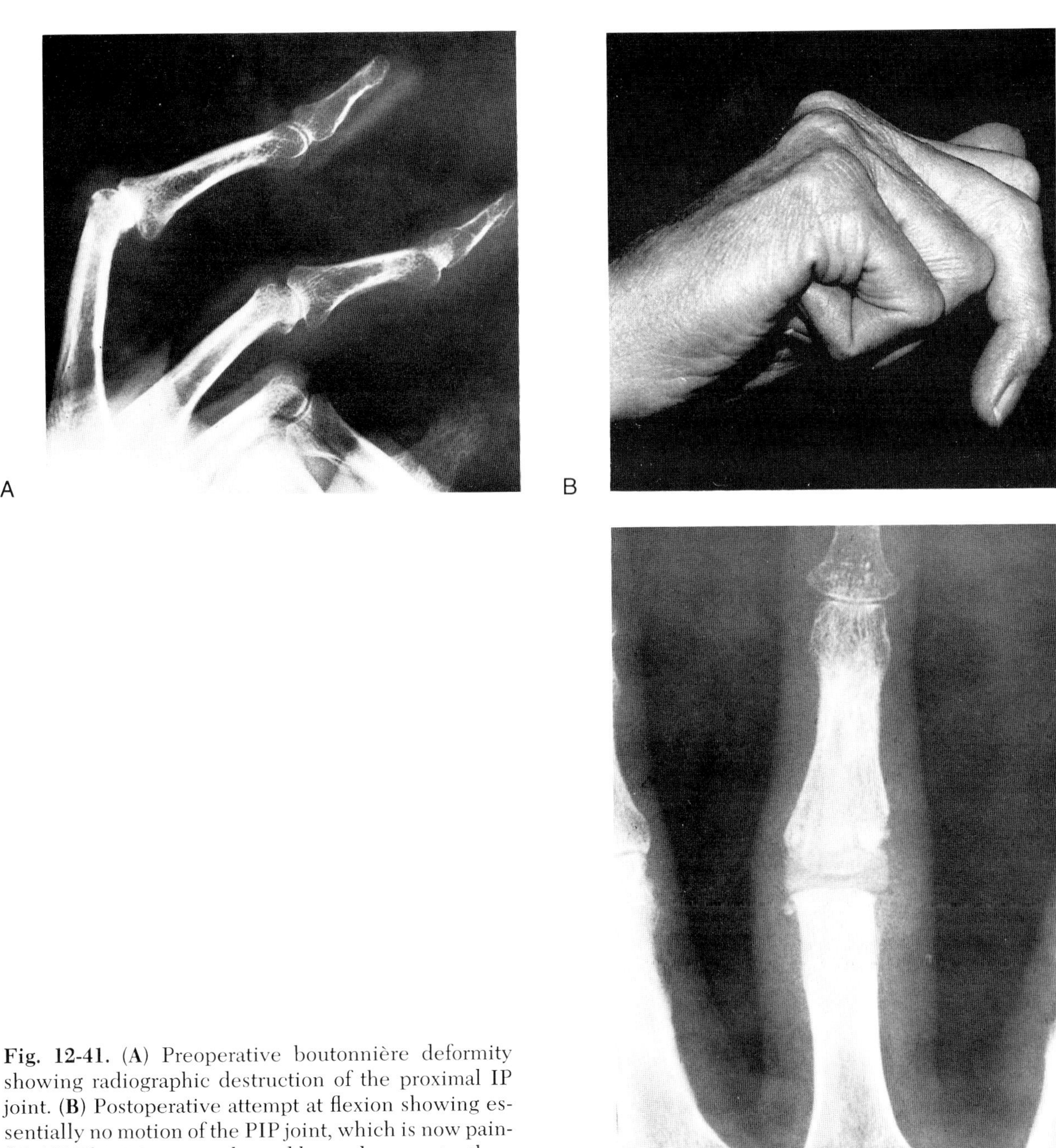

Fig. 12-41. (**A**) Preoperative boutonnière deformity showing radiographic destruction of the proximal IP joint. (**B**) Postoperative attempt at flexion showing essentially no motion of the PIP joint, which is now painful. (**C**) This joint was salvaged by replacement arthroplasty. There are 45 degrees of motion, and the joint is stable and pain-free.

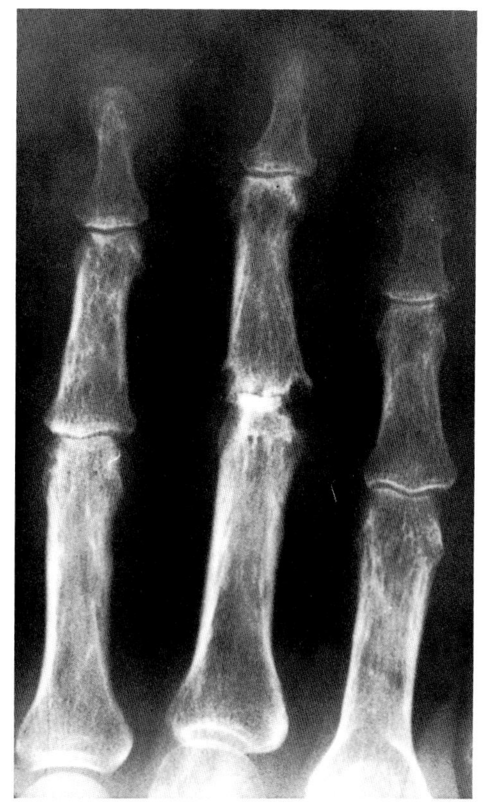

A

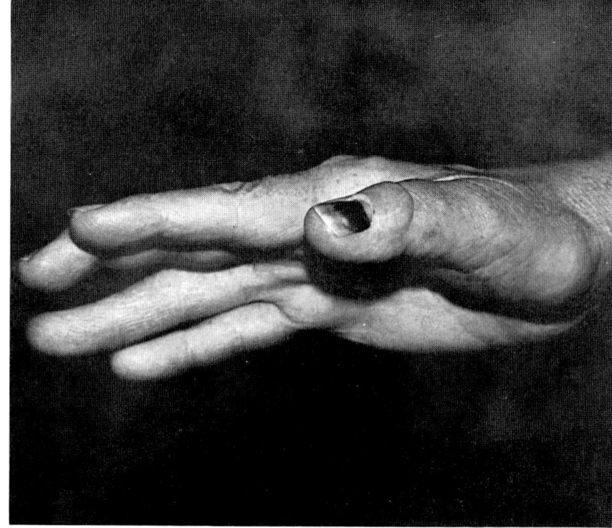

B

C

Fig. 12-42. (A) Preoperative appearance of the proximal IP joint of the long finger showing severe destruction. (B & C) Postoperative silicone replacement arthroplasty of the proximal IP joint showing range of motion in extension (B) and flexion (C).

be ensured regarding both therapy and splinting before undertaking this procedure (Fig. 12-42).

Arthrodesis.   The second procedure that can be done for the patient with the fixed boutonnière of the finger and a fixed flexion contracture, is arthrodesis of the middle joint. This technique provides a stable, painless joint, but the finger may be cumbersome because of its lack of motion. It is especially true if three of the fingers have supple middle joints and only one is fused or in the patient in whom the MCP joints have markedly limited motion. The proximal IP joints should be fused between 30 and 50 degrees, with the index finger straighter than the little finger. Harrison pegs have been useful for determining the desired angle of arthrodesis. The finger should be placed in the position that allows the greatest function. Specific indications may dictate in what position the joint should be fused, such as the condition of the adjacent joints or according to the patient's preference. The position and function of the thumb may dictate rotation or angle of the index finger arthrodesis.

Swan-Neck Deformity

The second type of deformity is the swan-neck deformity or the joint that is stiff in extension. The prime cause is often a flexor tenosynovitis. The flexor tendon is unable to flex the IP joint, which concentrates all the flexion forces on the MCP joint. The intrinsic muscles then contract. The synovitis of the proximal IP joint adds to the deformity, stretching out the capsule with dorsal migration of the lateral bands. The swan-neck deformity may be secondary to a mallet finger deformity when the extensor mechanism retracts after division of the terminal tendon. For the early swan-neck deformity, chemical synovectomy may be useful, followed by splinting in flexion.

Nalebuff and Millender[54] have conveniently classified swan-neck deformities in the rheumatoid patient and have presented a useful treatment plan for the various types. Type I deformity is the finger that is flexible in all positions. A flexor dermodesis may be all that is necessary in mild cases; but in one that is more severe, a flexor tenodesis using one slip of the superficialis sutured into bone or into the tendon sheath around

a pulley may be necessary. In addition, fusion of the distal IP joint may be indicated if it is stiff or in an unacceptable position.

The type II deformity, which is flexible when the MCP joint is flexed but limited when the MCP joint is held in extension (positive Bunnell test), has a contracture of the intrinsic muscles (Fig. 12-43). The Bunnell test shows the lateral bands to be contracted, and with this deformity it is necessary to release the intrinsic tendon as well as perform a flexor superficialis tenodesis. Additionally, it may be necessary to correct subluxation and flexion contracture of the MCP joints because it may contribute to the intrinsic contracture.

The type III deformity, defined as limited flexion in all positions, has two treatment options. The first is to manipulate and pin the joint into flexion. After this step the tourniquet must be lowered because the skin on the dorsum of the fingers may be ischemic. The pins may need to be taken out and the fingers pinned in less flexion, but first a relaxing skin incision on the dorsum of the finger is made (Fig. 12-44). It is a diagonal incision through the skin that allows some separation and relaxation of the edges. Circulation may be seen returning to the edges. The skin is left open; rapid healing results with thin scars despite this seemingly large gap.

The second option is to completely reconstruct the joint by lengthening the central tendons and separating them from the lateral bands, releasing the joint capsule and collateral ligaments, and volarly repositioning the lateral bands. The flexor tendons must be assessed. They can be exposed at the wrist and pulled to see that they are gliding; or if the surgery is performed under wrist block anesthesia, the tourniquet can be lowered and the patient can actively flex the fingers. If necessary, flexor tenosynovectomy is performed. The joint is pinned into flexion. The skin incision we use is a long chevron incision centered over the proximal IP joint so the distal leg of the incision is left open for relaxation. Generally, for these stiff fingers we prefer the simpler first option, as the long-term results are about the same.

For the type IV joint, which is a stiff proximal IP joint with a poor roentgenographic appear-

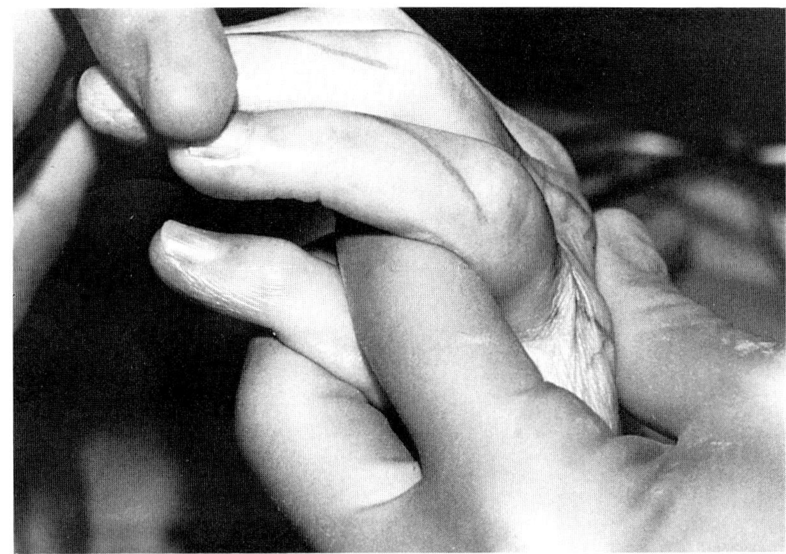

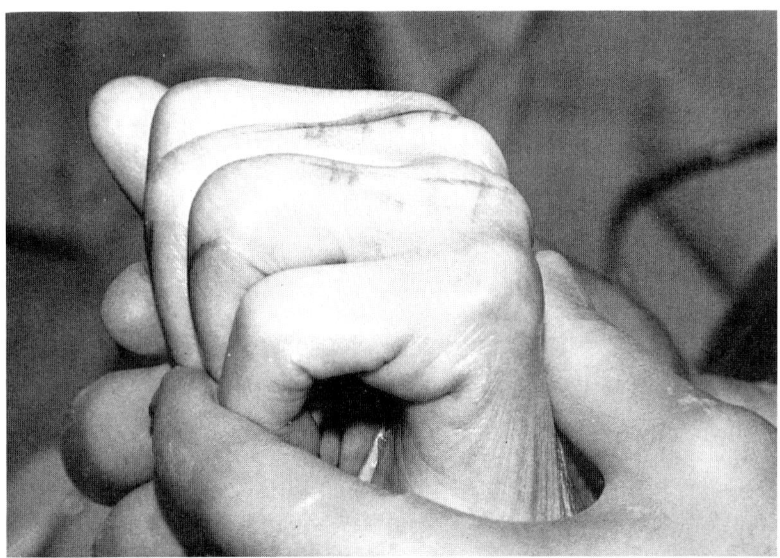

Fig. 12-43. Positive Bunnell test for intrinsic tightness. There is less passive flexion of the proximal IP joint possible when the MCP joint is held in extension (**A**) than when the MCP joint is allowed to flex (**B**).

ance, the two alternatives are arthrodesis and arthroplasty. Another reconstruction is doomed to failure. Implant arthroplasty works well for this type of joint, but soft tissue reconstruction must be part of this procedure. The central tendon is lengthened and separated from the lateral bands, which are allowed to migrate in a volar direction. The distal IP joint is fixed in extension by either pinning or arthrodesis. The finger is splinted in a few degrees of flexion. Motion is started on the third to fifth day. The joint is then splinted con-

tinuously for 1 month except for exercise. Night splints are used until the repair is stable.

We have been satisfied with proximal IP joint arthroplasties and will continue to use them. There have been few specific reports of the results of proximal IP joint arthroplasties in the literature despite numerous instructional course lectures and symposia on the subject. Urbaniak et al.[72] reported on four proximal IP joints in 1970. Although there was a short follow-up, all had satisfactory results. In 1975 Iselin[38] reported

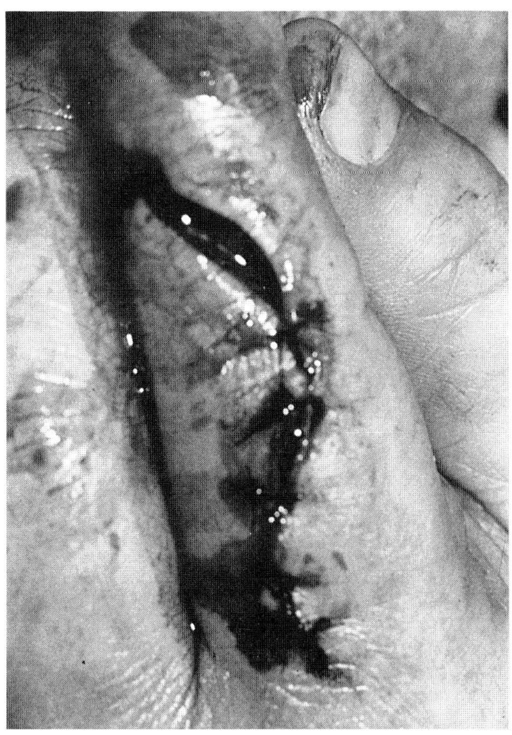

Fig. 12-44. Relaxing skin incision on the dorsum of the middle phalanx when correcting an extension contracture of a finger. The proximal end of the excision is closed; the distal end is left open and will heal uneventfully.

45 proximal IP joint replacements performed because of trauma. Nine failed. Range of motion ranged from 8 to 48 degrees. In 1972 Swanson[66] reported on 148 joints in 77 hands with an average range of motion of 65.5 degrees, and in 1983 he reviewed 424 joints.[69] Ninety-eight percent were relieved of pain, but there was a 30 percent revision rate over 10 years. The rheumatoid joints gained an average of 11 degrees and had 50 degrees average flexion. The best results were seen in rheumatoid arthritics. In 1982 Strickland et al.[64] reported 100 silicone proximal IP arthroplasties in 91 patients with posttraumatic disabilities. The average arc of motion increased 23 degrees. Complications included two infections, one patient with persistent pain, two with instability sufficient to require revision, three fracture implants, and one case of severe bone erosion that required fusion.

Our series of patients with silicone arthroplasties of the proximal IP joints consisted of 30 patients with 50 joints. Indications were pain and deformity in 40 and deformity in 10. Nineteen of the 30 patients had rheumatoid arthritis, five osteoarthritis, four trauma, one ankylosing spondylolysis, and one mixed connective tissue disease. Follow-up was admittedly short, averaging only 11 months. Preoperative motion was 26 degrees and postoperative motion 47 degrees. Pain had been relieved and the deformities corrected. We had only one failure, which was due to breakage and angulation, and we have redone this arthroplasty (Fig. 12-45). We have found proximal IP joint silicone arthroplasty useful even in the isolated index finger or other single digits, as well as in a hand where all proximal IP joints are destroyed. More of them will undoubtedly fail with the passage of time, but at this time we believe that this procedure is a reasonable choice and will continue to recommend it.

Proximal IP joint arthroplasties must be splinted for a prolonged period, and in a case where there has been 90 to 100 degrees of flexion contracture of the proximal IP joints with stiff MCP joints it may be necessary to keep patients in night splints for months to maintain correction and useful function. We believe that silicone arthroplasty has been a reliable method to correct deformity, relieve pain, and maintain mobility in the arthritic proximal IP joint in selected cases.

Arthrodesis has been a predictable method for reducing deformity and relieving pain, but there has been a significant rate of nonunion after this procedure. In a rheumatoid hand where MCP joint motion is limited even after arthroplasty, some motion of the proximal IP joints is useful.

Complex Hand

The last type of hand that must be considered independently of the others is the hand with deformed and contracted MCP and IP joints. The MCP joints may be stiff in flexion and the proximal IP joints fixed in extension, or vice versa. In these hands the MCP joints should be replaced first; if the proximal IP joints are stiff in extension, they can be manipulated and pinned in flex-

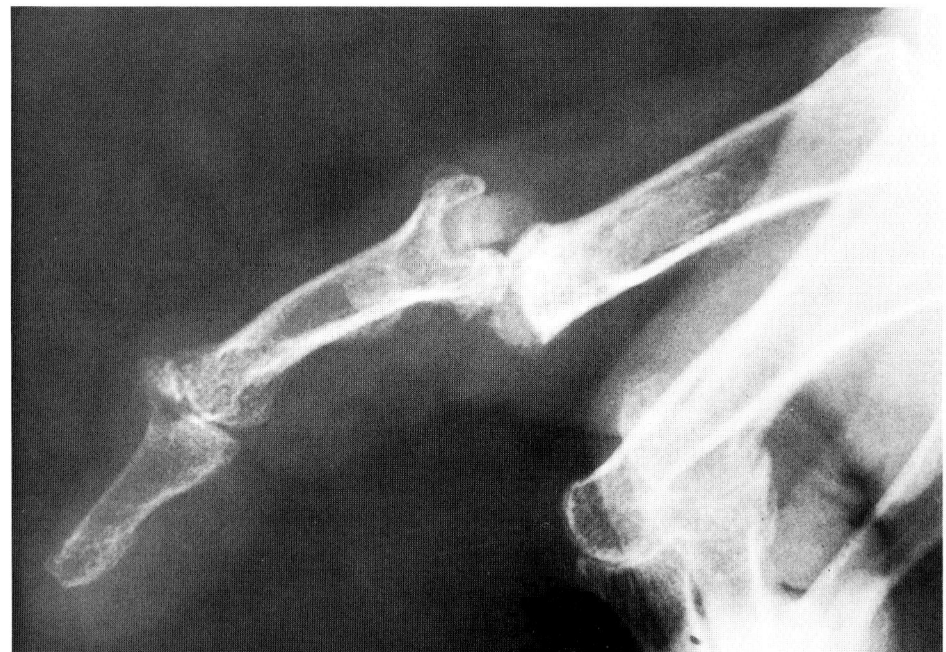

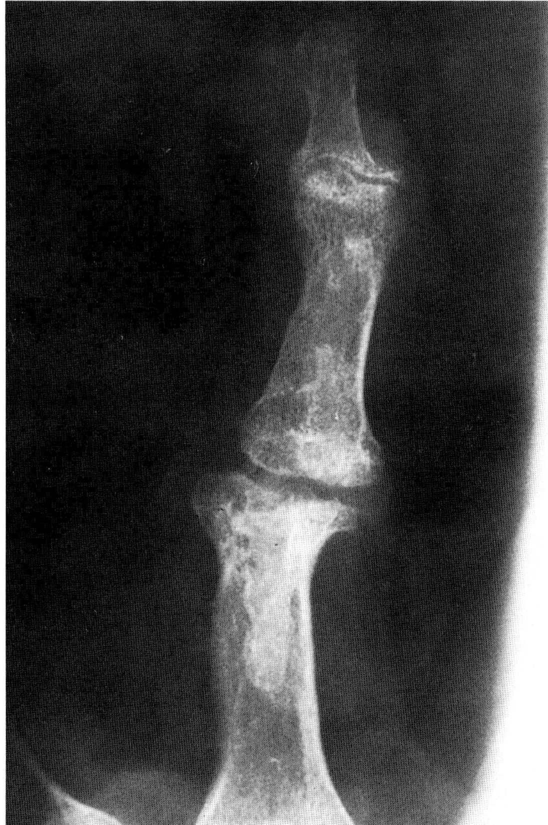

Fig. 12-45. Breakage of the proximal IP silicone arthroplasty with recurrence of deformity.

ion at the same time. When an MCP arthroplasty is performed in the presence of swan-neck deformity, the volar plate can be opened after resecting the metacarpal heads and the flexor tendons pulled through the opening to free them and to test motion after manipulation (or open release) of the proximal IP joints before pinning. It is important to obtain full extension of the MCP joints to prevent recurrence of the swan-neck deformities. We frequently suture the extensor tendon to the base of the proximal phalanx (or dorsal capsule), being sure the distal joints are flexed at the time of suture. In the hand with new MCP joints and an arc of motion between 0 to 50 degrees and fixed swan-neck contractures, functions poorly. If there are boutonnière deformities with marked flexion contractures of the proximal IP joints and the MCPs are allowed to flex, poor opening for grasp results. In these hands the decision to perform an arthrodesis of the proximal IP joints for a better functional position must be weighed against replacement arthroplasty. Arthrodesis is easier to obtain in these hyperflexed joints. The joint capsule is opened, the articular cartilage removed, and the joints then manipulated to the desired position. This method compresses the joint surfaces, allowing more rapid and dependable fusion. Pins and Harrison pegs are inserted to hold the position. Double row arthroplasty (Fig. 12-46) occasionally is performed with satisfying results, but it must be done at a second operative procedure for two reasons: (1) Too much time is involved for replacement and reconstruction of all eight joints (perhaps the distal joints need to have an arthrodesis as well); and (2) trying to splint and gain motion of two joints in the same finger at the same time is not likely to gain satisfactory motion in either joint. This situation is analogous to the hand in which one replaces the MCP joints alone. Motion is usually easier to obtain if the fingers are stiff in extension than if they are supple because these joints flex instead of the newly inserted joints.

In the same category is the hand with the MCP joints stiff in extension after replacement arthroplasty, when there are boutonnière deformities with severe flexion contractures of the proximal

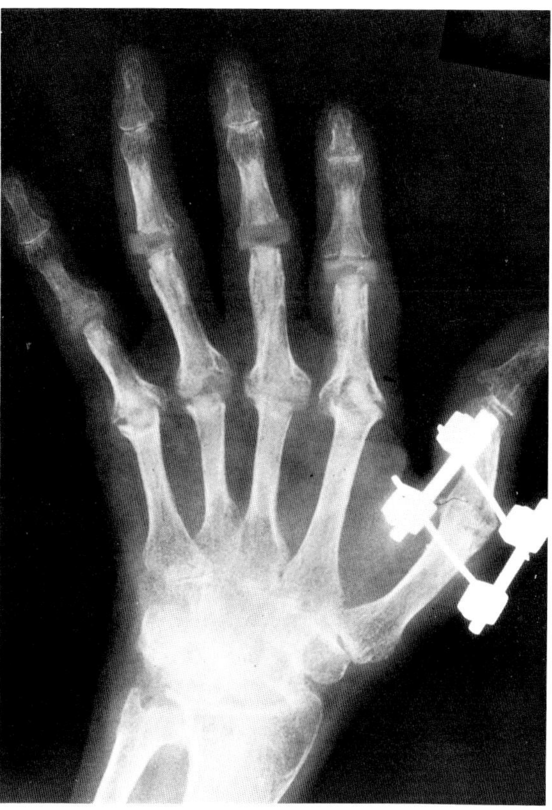

Fig. 12-46. Postoperative roentgenogram with double row silicone arthroplasties.

IP joints. These hands may function poorly. If an arthrodesis is performed on the proximal IP joints, a rigid hand results, and double row arthroplasty is recommended. Some motion is useful to these patients, but these hands certainly fit into a limited goals category. The patient's expectations of the surgery must be heavily weighed against what can reasonably be achieved and then a decision made whether to proceed with the surgical procedure.

SUMMARY

Careful selection must be undertaken before subjecting a rheumatoid patient to hand surgery. The presence of deformity is not a sufficient indication for operation. The patient must be motivated and willing to undergo prolonged postoperative splinting and therapy.

Flexor tenosynovitis may cause pain, triggering, or limitation of motion of the digit. The usual surgical procedure of releasing the proximal pulley is not satisfactory in the rheumatoid finger because of the chance of contributing to the ulnar drift of the digits. Instead, the pulleys should be preserved and the contents of the tendon sheath reduced.

The most common thumb deformity in rheumatoid arthritis is the collapse-type of boutonnière deformity. In the early stages, it may be treated by synovectomy and tendon reconstruction, but usually arthrodesis of the MCP joint is the preferred method of treatment. If the IP joint is destroyed as well as the MCP joint, the distal joint is fused and an arthroplasty performed on the proximal one. Occasionally, these thumbs are treated by arthrodesing both joints.

Rheumatoid patients develop deformities at the thumb basal joints also. Most often, a resection arthroplasty is preferred to the silicone replacement that is so common with osteoarthritic joints. Occasionally, a soft tissue interposition is added to the resection arthroplasty.

Rheumatoid hand surgery has focused on MCP joint replacement. Early synovectomy and tendon balancing are occasionally useful before the joints are destroyed. Silicone replacements have been the mainstay, however, in later stages of the disease. This procedure is predictable and reliable.

Interphalangeal joints have received little attention in rheumatoid arthritis. They can be stiff in extension or flexion, or they may develop swan-neck or boutonnière deformities. If the joints have a good roentgenographic appearance, soft tissue reconstruction may be satisfactory; but if they have been destroyed, arthrodesis or arthroplasty is indicated.

REFERENCES

1. Amadio PC, Millender LH, Smith RJ: Silicone spacer or tendon spacer for trapezium resection: comparison of results. J Hand Surg 7:237, 1982

2. Aptekar RG, Davie JM, Cattell HS: Foreign body reaction to silicone rubber: complication of a finger joint implant. Clin Orthop 98:231, 1974

3. Backhouse KM: The mechanics of normal digit control in the hand and analysis of the ulnar drift of rheumatoid arthritis. Ann R Coll Surg Engl 43:154, 1968

4. Beckenbaugh RD: Arthrodesis of the metacarpophalangeal joint of the thumb. Orthop Trans 4:291, 1980

5. Beckenbaugh RD, Dobyns JH, Bryon RS: Review and analyses of 532 silastic metacarpophalangeal implants. J Bone Joint Surg [Am] 58:483, 1976

6. Beckenbaugh RD, Steffee A: Total joint arthroplasty for the metacarpophalangeal joint of the thumb: a preliminary report. Orthopedics 4:295, 1981

7. Boyes JH: Bunnell's Surgery of the Hand. 5th Ed. JB Lippincott, Philadelphia, 1970

8. Brannon EW, Klein G: Experience with a finger joint prosthesis. J Bone Joint Surg [Am] 41:87, 1959

9. Braun RM: Total joint replacement at the base of the thumb: preliminary report. J Hand Surg 7:245, 1982

10. Brewerton DA: Hand deformities in rheumatoid disease. Ann Rheum Dis 16:183, 1957

11. Brumfield RH, Conaty JP: Reconstructive surgery of the thumb in rheumatoid arthritis. Orthopedics 3:529, 1980

12. Buck-Gramcko D: Operative bekandling der Sallelgelenksartrose des Daumens. Handchirugie 4:105, 1972

13. Carroll RE: Fascial arthroplasty for carpometacarpal joint of the thumb. Orthop Trans 1:15, 1977

14. Carroll RE, Hill NA: Small joint arthrodesis in hand reconstruction. J Bone Joint Surg 51:1219, 1969

15. Clayton ML: Surgery of the thumb in rheumatoid arthritis. J Bone Joint Surg [Am] 44:1376, 1962

16. Dell P, Brushart TM, Smith RJ: Treatment of trapeziometacarpal arthritis: results of resection arthroplasty. J Hand Surg 3:243, 1978

17. Ellison M, Flatt AE, Kelly KJ: Ulnar drift of the fingers in rheumatoid disease. J Bone Joint Surg [Am] 53:1061, 1971

18. Ferlic DC, Busbee GA, Clayton, ML: Degenerative arthritis of the carpometacarpal joint of the thumb: a clinical follow-up of eleven Niebauer prostheses. J Hand Surg 2:212, 1977

19. Ferlic DC, Clayton ML: Flexor tenosynovectomy in the rheumatoid finger. J Hand Surg 3:364, 1978

20. Ferlic DC, Clayton ML, Holloway M: Complications of silicone implant surgery in the metacarpo-

phalangeal joint. J Bone Joint Surg [Am] 57:991, 1975

21. Ferlic DC, Serot DI, Clayton ML: The use of the Flatt hinge prosthesis in the rheumatoid thumb. Hand 10:94, 1978

22. Ferlic DC, Turner BD, Clayton ML: Compression arthrodesis of the thumb. J Hand Surg 8:207, 1983

23. Flatt AE: Intra-articular thiotepa in rheumatoid disease of the hands. Rheumatology 18:70, 1960

24. Flatt AE: Restoration of rheumatoid finger joint function. J Bone Joint Surg [Am] 43:753, 1961

25. Flatt AE: Rheumatic and arthritic conditions in the upper extremity. Presented at the American Society for Surgery of the Hand Symposium. Vail, CO, 1974

26. Flatt AE: Salvage of the rheumatoid hand. Clin Orthop 23:207, 1961

27. Flatt AE: Some pathomechanics of ulnar drift. Plast Reconstr Surg 37:295, 1966

28. Flatt AE: The Care of the Rheumatoid Hand. CV Mosby, St. Louis, 1963

29. Flatt AE: The surgical rehabilitation of the rheumatoid hand. Ann R Coll Surg Engl 31:279, 1962

30. Froimson A: Tendon arthroplasty of the trapeziometacarpal joint. Clin Orthop 71:191, 1970

31. Gerris WH: Excision of the trapezium for osteoarthritis of the trapeziometacarpal joint. J Bone Joint Surg [Br] 31:537, 1949

32. Girzadas DV, Clayton ML: Limitations of the use of metallic prostheses in the rheumatoid hand. Clin Orthop 67:127, 1969

33. Goldner JL, Clippinger FW: Excision of the greater multiangular bone as an adjunct to mobilization of the thumb. J Bone Joint Surg [Am] 41:690, 1959

34. Hakstian RW, Tubiana R: Ulnar deviation of the fingers. J Bone Joint Surg [Am] 49:299, 1967

35. Hamlin C: Total joint replacement of the thumb carpo-metacarpal joint. Orthop Trans 5:107, 1981

36. Harrison SH: The Harrison-Nickol intramedullary peg: follow-up study of 100 cases. Hand 6:304, 1974

37. Harrison SH, Smith P, Maxwell D: Stabilization of the first metacarpophalangeal and terminal joints of the thumb. Hand 9:242, 1977

38. Iselin F: Arthroplasty of the proximal interphalangeal joint after trauma. Hand 7:41, 1975

39. Iselin F, Levame J, Godoy J: A simplified technique for treating mallet fingers: tenodermodesis. J Hand Surg 2:118, 1977

40. Kessler I, Axer A: Arthroplasty of first carpometacarpal joint with a silicone implant. Plast Reconstr Surg 47:252, 1971

41. Khuri SM: Tension band arthrodesis in the hand. J Hand Surg [Am] 11:41, 1986

42. Landsmeer JMF: Anatomical and functional investigation on the articulation of human fingers. Acta Anat (Basel), suppl., 25:24, 1955

43. Lasserre C, Pauzat D, Derennes R: Osteoarthritis of the trapeziometacarpal joint. J Bone Joint Surg [Br] 31:534, 1949

44. Leach RE, Bolton PE: Arthritis of the carpo-metacarpal joint of the thumb. J Bone Joint Surg [Am] 50:1171, 1968

45. Leonard MH, Capen DA: Compression arthrodesis of finger joints. Clin Orthop 145:193, 1979

46. Lister G: Interosseous wiring of the digital skeleton. J Hand Surg 3:427, 1978

47. McCarty DJ: Treatment of rheumatoid joint inflammation with triamanolone hexacetonide arthritis. Rheumatology 15:157, 1972

48. Menon J, Schoene HR, Hohl JC: Trapeziometacarpal arthritis: results of tendon interpositional arthroplasty. J Hand Surg 6:442, 1981

49. Micks JE, Hager DL: A method of accelerating fusion of small joints. J Bone Joint Surg [Am] 50:1269, 1968 (exhibit)

50. Millender, LH, Nalebuff, EA: Reconstructive surgery in the rheumatoid hand. Orthop Clin North Am 6:709, 1975

51. Millender LH, Nalebuff EA, Hawkins RE, Ennis R: Infections after silicone prosthetic arthroplasty of the hand. J Bone Joint Surg [Am] 57:825, 1975

52. Moberg E: Arthrodesis of finger joints. Surg Clin North Am 40:465, 1960

53. Murley AHG: Excision of the trapezium in osteoarthritis of the first carpometacarpal joint. J Bone Joint Surg [Br] 42:402, 1960

54. Nalebuff EA, Millender LH: Surgical repair of the swan-neck deformity in rheumatoid arthritis. Orthop Clin North Am 6:733, 1975

55. Neibauer JJ: Dacron silicone prosthesis for the metacarpophalangeal and interphalangeal joints. p. 96. In Cramer LM, Chase RA (eds): Symposium on the Hand. CV Mosby, St. Louis, 1981

56. Potenza AD: A technique for arthrodesis of finger joints. J Bone Joint Surg 55:1534, 1973

57. Smith EM: Mechanical factors in rheumatoid hand deformities. Univ Michigan Med Center J (Special Arthritis Issue) December: 274, 1968

58. Smith EM, Juvinall RC, Bender LF, Pearson JR: Flexor forces and rheumatoid metacarpophalangeal deformity. JAMA 198:130, 1966

59. Smith EM, Juvinall RC, Bender LF, Pearson JR: Role of the finger flexors in rheumatoid deformities of the metacarpophalangeal joints. Arthritis Rheum 7:467, 1964

60. Smith RJ, Kaplan EB: Rheumatoid deformities of the metacarpophalangeal joints of the fingers. J Bone Joint Surg [Am] 49:31, 1967

61. Snorrason E: The problem of ulnar deviation of the finger in rheumatoid arthritis. Acta Med Scand 140:359, 1951

62. Souter WA: Planning treatment of the rheumatoid hand. Hand 11:3, 1979

63. Steffee A: Cemented finger prosthesis. Presented to the Symposium on Total Joint Arthroplasties in the Upper Extremity. American Academy of Orthopaedic Surgeons, Denver, June 1981

64. Strickland JW, Dustman JA, Stelzer L et al: Management of post-traumatic arthritis of the proximal interphalangeal joint with silicone implant arthroplasty. p. 173. In Strickland JW, Steichen JB (eds): Difficult Problems in Hand Surgery. CV Mosby, St. Louis, 1982

65. Swanson AB: Disabling arthritis at the base of the thumb. J Bone Joint Surg [Am] 54:456, 1972

66. Swanson AB: Flexible implant arthroplasty for arthritic finger joints. J Bone Joint Surg [Am] 54:435, 1972

67. Swanson AB: Silicone rubber implants for replacement of arthritic or destroyed joints in the hand. Surg Clin North Am 48:1113, 1968

68. Swanson AB, Herndon JH: Flexible (silicone) implant arthroplasty of the metacarpophalangeal joint of the thumb. J Bone Joint Surg [Am] 59:362, 1977

69. Swanson AB, Maupin BK, Gajjan NV: Long term review of flexible implant arthroplasty in the proximal interphalangeal joint of the hand. Presented to the Annual Meeting, American Society for Surgery of the Hand, March 1983

70. Swanson AB, Swanson GdeG, Watermeier JJ: Trapezium implant arthroplasty: long-term evaluation of 150 cases. J Hand Surg 6:125, 1981

71. Tupper JW: A compression arthrodesis device for small joints of the hand. Hand 4:62, 1972

72. Urbaniak JR, MacCollum MS, Goldner JL: Metacarpophalangeal and interphalangeal joint reconstruction; use of silicone rubber dacron prostheses for irreparable joints of the hand. South Med J 63:1281, 1970

73. Vainio K, Julkenen H: Intra-articular nitrogen mustard treatment of rheumatoid arthritis. Acta Rheumatol Scand 6:25, 1960

74. Weinman DT, Lipscomb PR: Degenerative arthritis of the trapezio-metacarpal joint: arthrodesis or excision. Mayo Clin Proc 42:276, 1967

75. Wexler MR, Rousso M, Weinberg H: Arthrodesis of finger joints by dynamic external compression. Plast Reconstr Surg 60:882, 1977

76. Wise KS: The anatomy of the metacarpophalangeal joints with observation of the aetiology of ulnar drift. J Bone Joint Surg [Br] 57:485, 1975

77. Wood KE: Early experience with biomeric finger implants. Orthop Trans 6:506, 1982

13

Management of the Rheumatoid Hip

Morris H. Susman
Mack L. Clayton

Although the success of present-day treatment of arthritic disease of the hips has attracted considerable medical and public attention, it may come as a surprise that, with rheumatoid arthritis, hip disease is substantially less common than that of other major lower extremity joints. Vainio and Pulkki[30] reported a 10 percent incidence of hip disease in their rheumatoid population. Predictably, the female group of patients showed three times the incidence as did the male group. Gschwend[15] studied 300 rheumatoid patients with an average duration of disease of 10 years. Demonstrable hip lesions were present in only 17 percent of this group, whereas 74 percent showed knee lesions, 52 percent hindfoot involvement, and 79 percent forefoot disease.

Additional evidence as to the incidence of hip disease in rheumatoid arthritis patients can be found in a review of arthroplasty procedures on the hip. Only 6 to 15 percent of hip arthroplasties at two large referral centers were for rheumatoid disease.[10,24] In another report, the total knee arthroplasty procedures exceeded total hip replacements in rheumatoid disease patients by a ratio of nearly 2 : 1 at an institution known for its large rheumatoid population.[25]

With this information as background, it would be a serious error to conclude that hip disease in rheumatoid arthritis poses a less difficult problem for the patient than does the more common involvement of other major weight-bearing lower extremity joints. Indeed, the painful rheumatoid hip can be and often is the single most disabling joint in a rheumatoid patient. Pain can be so severe as to require narcotic and analgesic medication despite reduced activity, supported walking, and increased rest time. Usually the hip pain is of gradually increasing severity, but at times the progression of hip pain is rapid, requiring surgical consideration within several weeks of the apparent increase in the severity of pain. Pain at rest—first sitting and then at night—heralds the progression of hip disease. Painful and inhibited activities of daily living are more common with hip disease than with involvement of other lower extremity joints. Sexual activity is frequently compromised.

The impact of hip disease on the rheumatoid patient can therefore be devastating. Painful, and perhaps impossible, ambulation markedly limits activities of personal hygiene, dressing, and caring for oneself; and the continued presence of hip pain affects the rheumatoid patient physically as well as mentally, reflecting clearly the profound impact rheumatoid hip disease can have on the patient.

ANATOMY AND PHYSIOLOGY

Unlike the smaller joints affected by rheumatoid disease, the hip joint, a deeply situated "ball and socket" joint, depends on its shape and the large muscles surrounding it for stability. Contractures in these muscles result from the intra-articular synovial disease of this large synovial joint, which in turn causes pain and early loss of motion. Hip disease is typified by rather early loss of motion in contrast to a less rapid loss of motion in other large weight-bearing and non-weight-bearing joints in rheumatoid arthritis. With contracture goes the development of flexion, abduction, and external rotation deformities, most often seen in the latter stages of the disease as it involves the hip. There is an abundant vascular and nerve supply to the hip joint as well as to the periarticular soft tissue structures. The nature and location of "hip pain" can be explained by the contributing branches from the sciatic, femoral, and obturator nerves, which supply the hip joint and surrounding supportive tissues.

The inherent congruence of the femoral acetabular articular surfaces is augmented by the fibrocartilaginous acetabular labrum and the transverse acetabular ligament. The labrum provides greater acetabular depth, and the transverse ligament provides additional inferior femoral head coverage as it courses across the acetabular notch (Fig. 13-1). It is thought that the hip joint may be most congruous under loaded conditions owing to the compliance of the combined femoral ace-

tabular cartilage, both articular and labral, and the ligamentous complex that comprises the joint.

The blood supply to the femoral head and neck is found in the capsular retinaculum, a collagenous layer underneath the fibrous sleeve or capsular ligament that surrounds the hip joint. The capsule is thinnest posteriorly and thickest anteriorly, although there is a relatively weak area anteriorly where direct communication between the hip joint and the iliopsoas bursa may exist. Chronic inflammation, as in rheumatoid hip disease, may lead to substantial bursal enlargement and subsequent, at times baffling, clinical symptoms and signs (Fig. 13-2).

PATHOLOGY

The synovium from a rheumatoid hip demonstrates diffuse inflammatory changes, with lymphocytes and plasma cells, and focal chronic inflammation with lymphoid follicles. The severe

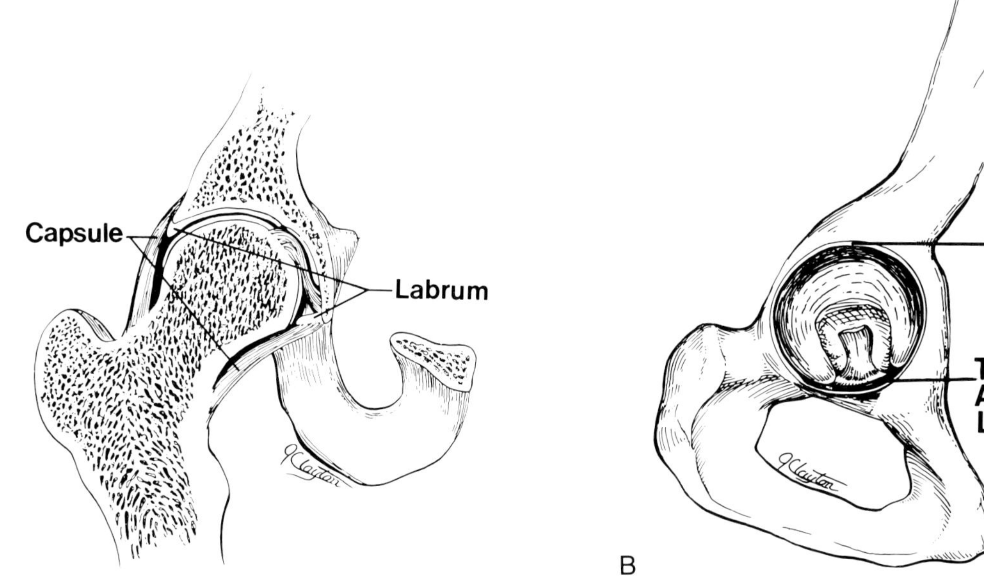

Fig. 13-1. Acetabulum is surrounded by the labrum and transverse acetabular ligament, each of which increases femoral head coverage.

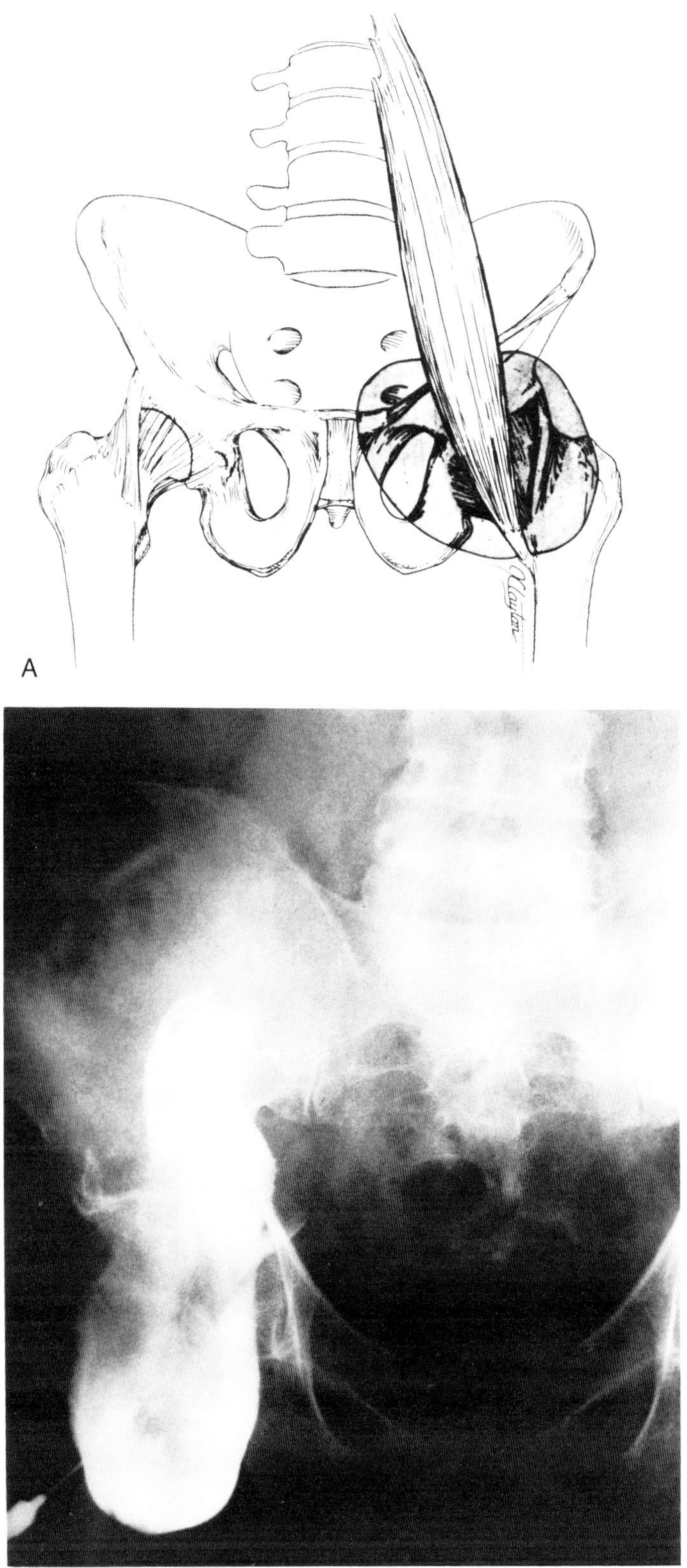

Fig. 13-2. (**A**) Iliopsoas bursa is enlarged at times, causing a symptomatic inguinal or groin mass. (**B**) Radiopaque injection of the bursa. Note proximal extension into the abdomen.

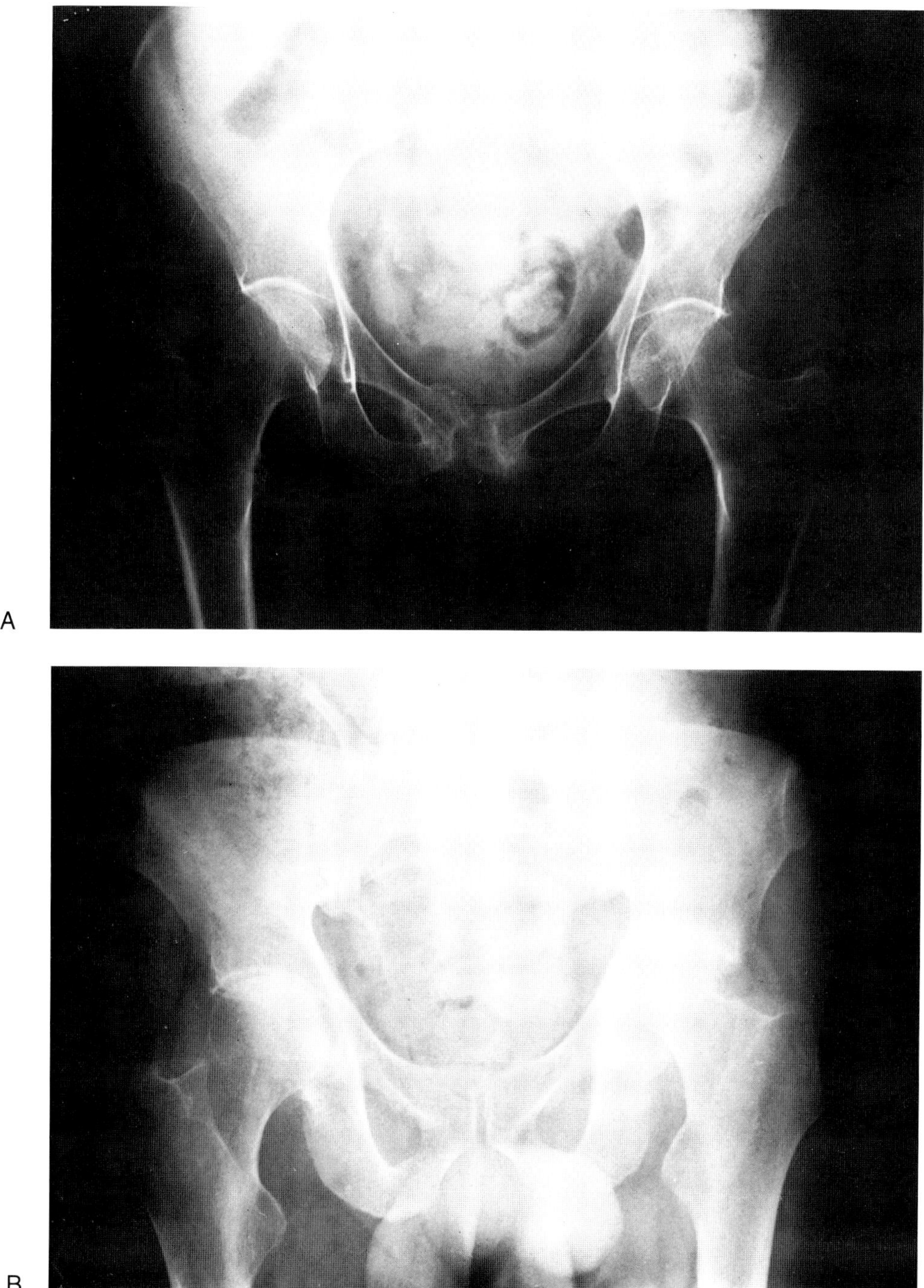

Fig. 13-3. **(A)** This 57-year-old woman has bilateral stage I rheumatoid hip disease, osteoporosis, and no joint narrowing. An old fracture symphysis is not due to rheumatoid arthritis. **(B)** Left hip of a 53-year-old man is stage II, with mild joint narrowing but no erosions. Right hip is stage IV with complete narrowing and marked bony destruction with ankylosis. (*Figure continues.*)

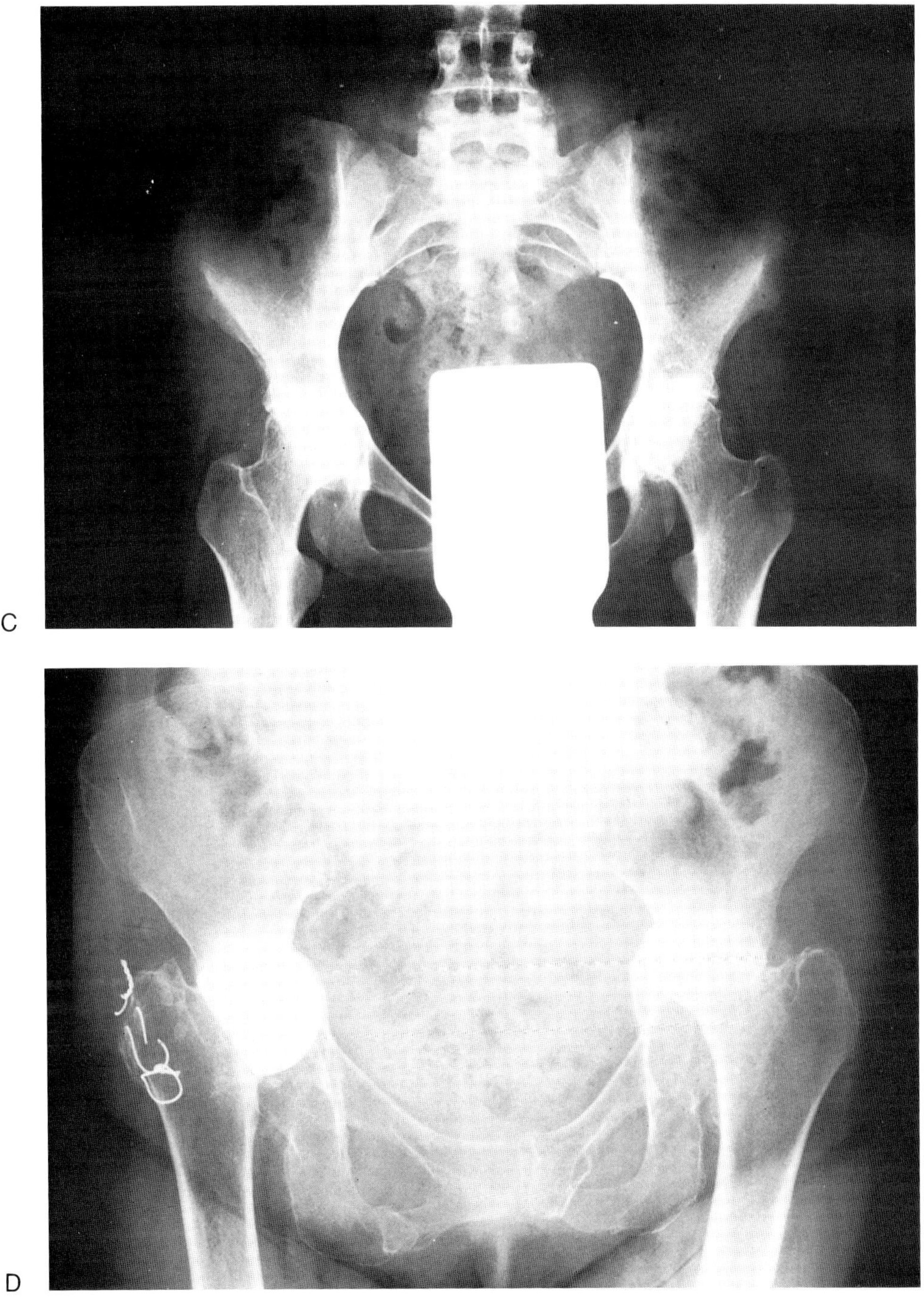

Fig. 13-3 (*Continued*). (**C**) Juvenile rheumatoid patient with bilateral stage III disease; note the moderate to marked narrowing and erosions. (**D**) This 63-year-old woman with chronic rheumatoid arthritis, demonstrates severe stage IV hip disease with marked protrusio acetabula of the left hip. A cup arthroplasty was done on the right hip 11 years earlier and now shows moderate protrusion, although it functions well.

inflammation of rheumatoid synovium is associated with microvascular disturbances, notably venous dilatation and stasis. The increased volume of synovial fluid within the confines of the tough, inelastic fibrous capsule of the hip produces increased intra-articular pressure. A proliferative synovitis develops early in the evolution of rheumatoid hip disease, but later this proliferative process with pannus formation gives way to fibrous transformation of the synovium. Clinically, it is often seen as a "dry," or "burned out," hip joint (in contrast to a "wet," or actively inflamed, hip joint seen during the relatively early phase of the proliferative synovitis).

Hip joint involvement is usually bilateral and characterized by symmetric cartilage loss and osteoporosis on both sides of the joint (Fig. 13-3). The condition of protrusio acetabuli is seen in 15 to 20 percent of patients with rheumatoid arthritis or ankylosing spondylitis. A possible explanation of this condition is osteoporosis with medial acetabular wall softening and deformation due to the stress of continued weight-bearing. Protrusio is most common in women with rheumatoid disease of 10 years or more and who have had long-term systemic steroid treatment; it is often bilateral.

PREOPERATIVE EVALUATION

Evaluation of Pain and Function

The clearest indication for surgical intervention in rheumatoid hip disease is pain not responsive to reasonable medical control, i.e., pain not controlled by the prudent use of analgesic and anti-inflammatory medication, rest and limitation of activity, and supported weight-bearing. Pain managed during the daytime but so severe as to disturb sleep on a regular basis often justifies surgery. At times, pain is less dominant than is stiffness and deformity; and when independent mobility is compromised, surgery should be considered. Because hip disease in the rheumatoid patient is commonly bilateral, the physician

is usually aware of the patient's loss of ability to perform certain activities of daily living. Ambulation, sitting, toilet and hygienic functions, and dressing oneself (i.e., shoes and socks) are progressively limited and frustrating for the patient. The physician must assess this functional loss as well as the degree of pain when evaluating the patient for possible reconstructive hip surgery.

Physical Findings

Careful examination of the rheumatoid patient is an essential part of the evaluation for hip surgery. An antalgic gait is often present with a painful hip. In some cases, particularly in those so severely disabled as to not ambulate, observing transfer abilities discloses important information about both hips and knee joints as well as the status of the upper extremities. Range of hip motion, the presence of contractures, and leg length measurements are noted. Crepitation usually means bone-on-bone contact, consistent with severe articular cartilage loss. It is essential to observe the circulatory status, both arterial and venous, of the lower extremities.

After assessing pain and functional loss and after examining the patient, the roentgenograms are reviewed (Fig. 13-4). Not only can they provide definitive confirmation of hip disease that justifies surgery, it is with this step that initial planning of the technical aspects of surgery can begin. At this point, if the decision to proceed with hip surgery has been made, additional preoperative evaluation remains.

Therapeutic goals must be established. Usually, it is simply restoration of painless hip function so the patient can ambulate, undertake personal hygiene, and engage in sexual activity. Rarely, the goal of surgical treatment is simply more comfortable and functional sitting and transfer activities. The latter situation prevails in the severely disabled, bedridden rheumatoid patient who may have upper and lower extremity involvement, spinal problems, marked generalized weakness, and other systemic effects of the rheumatoid disease.

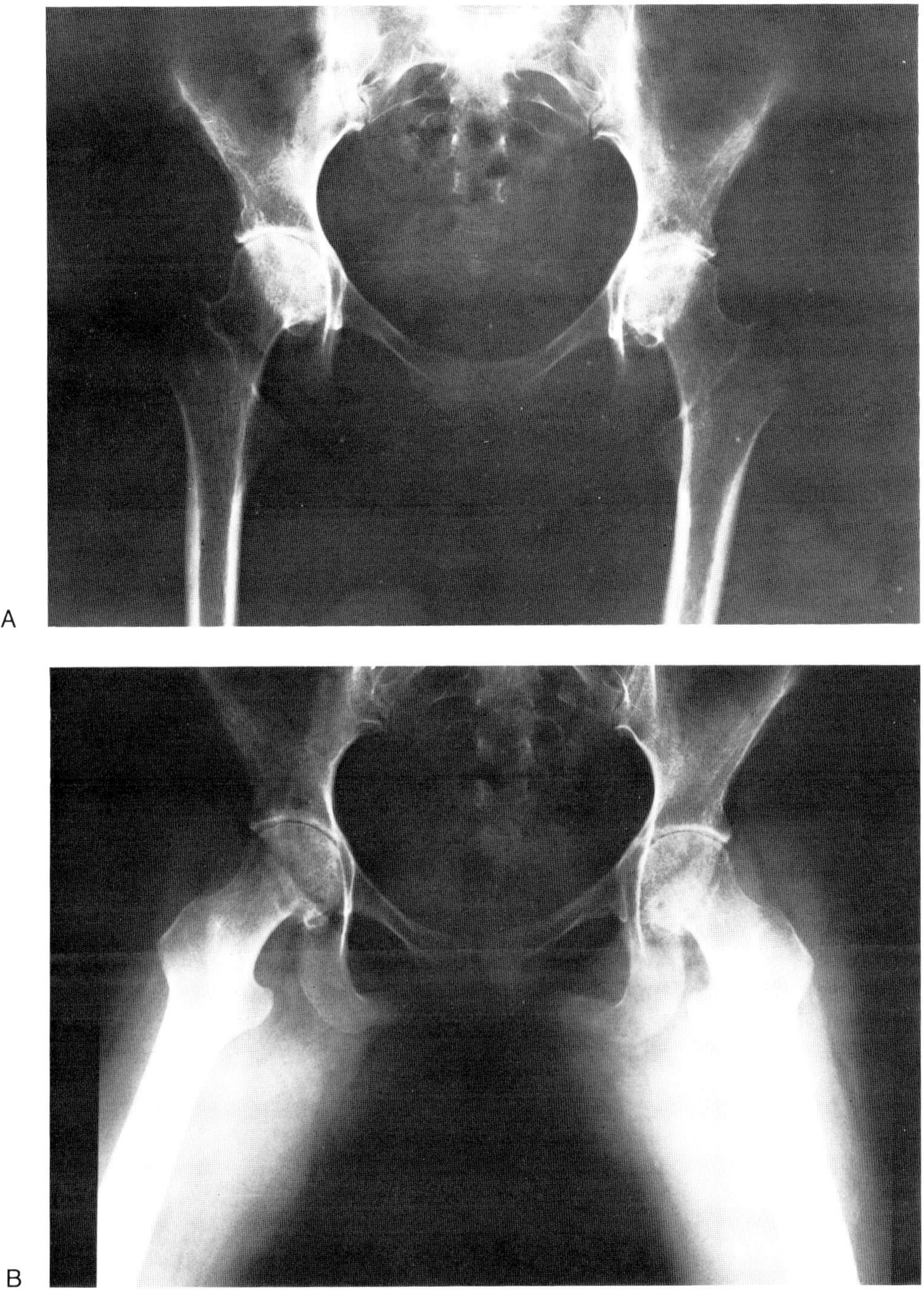

Fig. 13-4. Standard anteroposterior (**A**) and "frog-leg" lateral (**B**) views used for assessing rheumatoid hip disease. A lateral view of the involved hip is helpful, and an anteroposterior view of both hips (pelvis) is necessary. Other views may be necessary when planning surgery.

Evaluation of Other Joints

The status of upper extremity disease often dictates special considerations in postoperative support. Platform crutches, platform rolling walkers, canes with special hand grips, custom-made splints, and other modified equipment can assist the rheumatoid with upper extremity disease, postoperative activity, and gait training. In general, hip reconstruction should precede upper extremity procedures in order to avoid stressing the reconstructed upper extremity joints excessively. Appropriate protection of previously reconstructed upper extremity joints is indicated when hip surgery follows the upper extremity surgery. For example, it may be necessary to protect the wrist that has previously undergone a total wrist arthroplasty by splinting it or by using forearm bearing (platform) crutches. Each situation must be individualized but always with the goal of either avoiding damage to reconstructed upper extremity joints or accommodating coexisting upper extremity deformity and functional limitation.

With the success of hip replacement surgery, it may no longer be correct to speak of forefoot reconstruction in the rheumatoid as the most consistently pain-alleviating operative procedure. One must still be aware of foot disease when considering hip surgery. The painful forefoot may compromise the ipsilateral hip procedure. More importantly, the presence of skin breakdown and low grade infection precludes proceeding with hip surgery. Indeed, in the presence of severe deformity with potential skin breakdown, it is probably best to consider forefoot surgery prior to either hip or knee reconstruction, be it ipsilateral or contralateral.

When both hip and knee disease are present, the problem may arise as to which area warrants surgical treatment first. The degree of pain can be the determining factor; that is, if pain from the hip or knee is clearly dominant in terms of the patient's disability, that joint should be treated first. If severe pain is not localized, the advantages of hip arthroplasty as the initial treatment are the rapid functional gain and the dramatic, often immediate relief of hip pain. Rehabilitation after hip arthroplasty is also much simpler and certainly less demanding for the patient. These additional considerations strengthen the recommendation to select hip reconstruction as the initial procedure.

A patient who has seen the positive effects of hip replacement will be encouraged during subsequent difficult times regarding the treatment of his or her disease. There are instances, however, when knee arthroplasty is best done initially. The presence of severe flexion contracture or an equally severe valgus, external rotation deformity of the knee may make rehabilitation after hip arthroplasty difficult if not impossible. Such changes may make it necessary to do the initial surgery on the arthritic knee. (See Figs. 17-1 and 17-2).

Advances of the Team Approach

At times the component members of the "arthritis team" combine their thoughts to arrive at a decision regarding the initial therapeutic goals for the rheumatoid patient with untreated multiple joint disease. Although the above principles are generally valid, input from the orthopaedic surgeon, rheumatologist, physical and occupational therapists, and social worker can result in justifiably altered goals of treatment to be obtained by deviating from the principles previously described.

The degree of pain and disability due to rheumatoid hip disease can be quantitated using one of several rating systems. Although helpful for assessing results of surgical treatment, the numerical systems do not consider the complex interactions of multiple diseased joints as in rheumatoid arthritis. Progression of upper and lower extremity disease can compromise the results of hip arthroplasty by altering the requirements for support and causing new and increased lower extremity pain. What is clear, therefore, is the critical importance of looking at the rheumatoid patient with a broad prospective aimed at total musculoskeletal and systemic function interaction. For example, a successful hip arthroplasty can be less successful by far in the patient's mind if rheumatoid vasculitis, mononeuritis, and footdrop should ensue. Severe hindfoot disease may cause painful, limited ambulation despite the painless hip arthroplasty proximally. Acquired inability to arise from a sitting position can tarnish the glowing initial results of hip arthroplasty. Thus hip surgery is but one step in the total care of the rheumatoid patient. Although dramatic in its relief of pain and improvement in function, hip arthroplasty must always be evaluated with close awareness of the generalized progressive nature of the rheumatoid disease process.

Available Reconstructive Procedures

Reconstructive surgery on the rheumatoid hip has evolved to that of total joint arthroplasty. There are special situations in which femoral and acetabular replacements are not necessary. Certain problems involving the rheumatoid hip with fracture, avascular necrosis, or failed prior arthroplasty may require or justify surgical procedures other than total replacement. For the most part, however, surgery of the hip in rheumatoid arthri-

tis patients today is that of total replacement surgery.

In the past, only cup arthroplasty, as defined and advocated by Aufranc,[1] gained recognition and acceptance in the treatment of rheumatoid hip disease (Fig. 13-5). Cup arthroplasty, however, required much more of both the patient and the surgeon. Success in large numbers was confined to a few centers. Postoperative therapy was demanding; muscle strengthening and education were deliberate; and protected weight-bearing was necessary for several months to a year or more. Yet the necessity for revision (or "supplementary") surgery was high, being required in nearly one-third of the rheumatoid group. The infection rate was higher than that for comparable numbers of total hip replacements today,[1] and the need for indefinite use of support with a cane or crutches was common.

Other surgical procedures, for the most part, are no longer used for primary treatment of rheumatoid hip disease. Synovectomy of the hip, based on the same principles as for synovectomy

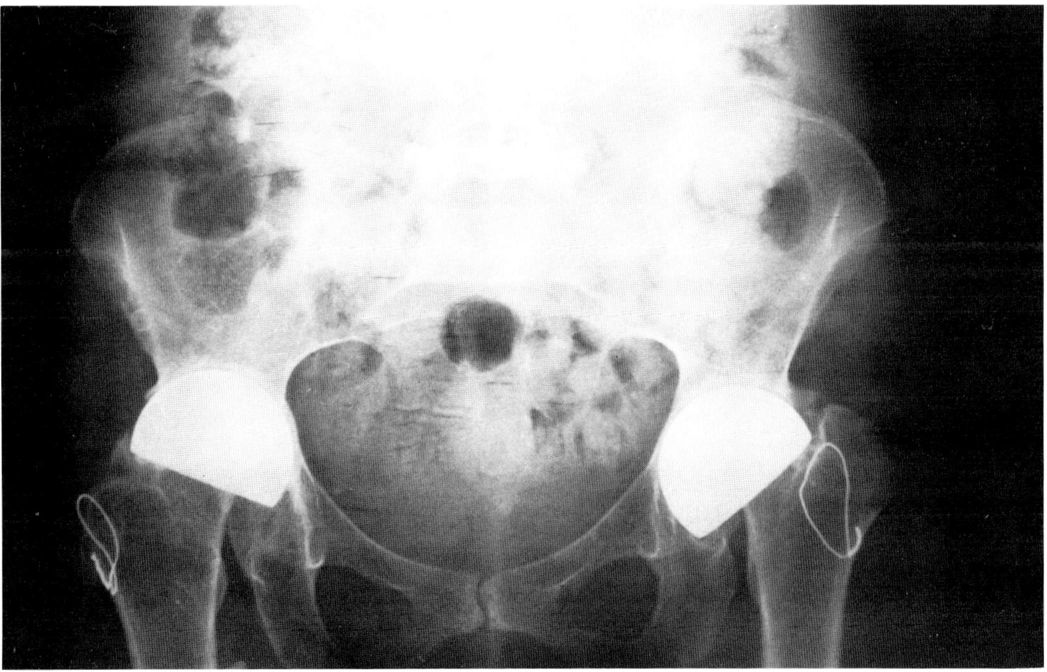

Fig. 13-5. Bilateral cup arthroplasties, 25 years postoperatively, in a woman with chronic ankylosing spondylitis (formerly called rheumatoid spondylitis). She had bony ankylosis of both hips. She now has no pain, walks without support and has 80 to 90 degrees of flexion in each hip.

of the rheumatoid knee, has been used by some, notably Cruess,[11] but long-term reports of good results are not available. Generally, this procedure is not done today unless in the rare instance in which iliopsoas bursal cyst excision is combined with synovectomy of the adjacent hip joint. Intertrochanteric osteotomy, still utilized by a small number of surgeons for management of osteoarthritis of the hip, is occasionally done. It may be indicated in the rare "burned-out" rheumatoid hip with mild to moderate superimposed degenerative arthritis in a young patient without significant rheumatoid disease elsewhere or in patients who, for other reasons, do not fulfill the criteria for implant arthroplasty.

Arthrodesis of the hip and endoprosthetic arthroplasty are not being utilized for rheumatoid hip disease. Of the former, it can be stated that the current state of implant arthroplasty, including that done for prior septic arthritis, dictates against its use. Endoprosthetic (hemi) arthroplasty for rheumatoid hip disease has been abandoned owing to the persistent pain often associated with it, as well as the many occurrences of prosthetic migration into the softened acetabulum, at times progressing to frank protrusion into the pelvis.

The development of bipolar hemiarthroplasty has provided a procedure applicable to certain situations involving the rheumatoid hip. This operation may be satisfactory for a femoral neck fracture in a previously asymptomatic rheumatoid hip (Fig. 13-6).

Finally, excisional arthroplasty, often referred to as a girdlestone procedure, has limited application for primary treatment of rheumatoid hip disease. Its use is limited to the severely disabled patient confined to a chair in whom hip pain, even in this limited activity, is disabling. For a combination of reasons, i.e., profound weakness and other systemic manifestations of rheumatoid disease, such a patient should not be considered a candidate for replacement arthroplasty with its associated functional advantages.

STATUS OF TOTAL HIP REPLACEMENT ARTHROPLASTY

Today, total hip replacement is the definitive surgical treatment of rheumatoid hip disease and is the operation of choice.[6] The noted European arthritis surgeon Gschwend has described total hip replacement as "the symbol of progress" in orthopaedic surgery.[15] The modern era of total hip arthroplasty was pioneered by Charnley, who reported his procedure and prosthetic components during the early 1960s.[4,5,31] The polyethylene acetabular and metal femoral components he introduced were much like those in use today. The mechanical anchoring of the components with acrylic cement (the method of fixation introduced by Charnley) remains a standard and widely accepted practice today. The "low-friction" concept advocated by Charnley continues as a basic principle in total joint arthroplasty. Other innovative prosthetic systems using cementless fixation, such as that of McKee and Watson-Farrar[21] and Ring,[27] were destined to failure owing to wear, production of friction-related debris, and poor fixation associated with metal-on-metal prosthetic systems.[13]

The enthusiasm for surface replacement hip arthroplasty has essentially vanished owing to recurrent problems associated with this procedure.[18] Referred to as the "conservative" total hip procedure, this operation may be considered conservative on the femoral side but rather radical on the acetabular side, where the large acetabular component requires considerable reaming and sacrifice of bone stock, thus making revision of the acetabular component even more difficult than after conventional hip replacement. Femoral side failures have been related to femoral neck fractures, loosening, and avascular necrosis of the femoral head bone under the femoral metallic cup. Acetabular loosening has been reported, and wear of the thin acetabular polyethylene cups has been a concern. Metal backing of the acetabular components has been provided

Fig. 13-6. (**A**) Displaced right femoral neck fracture in a 66-year-old woman with chronic rheumatoid arthritis. Note the "normal" hip joint preoperatively. (**B**) Postoperative bipolar arthroplasty in place.

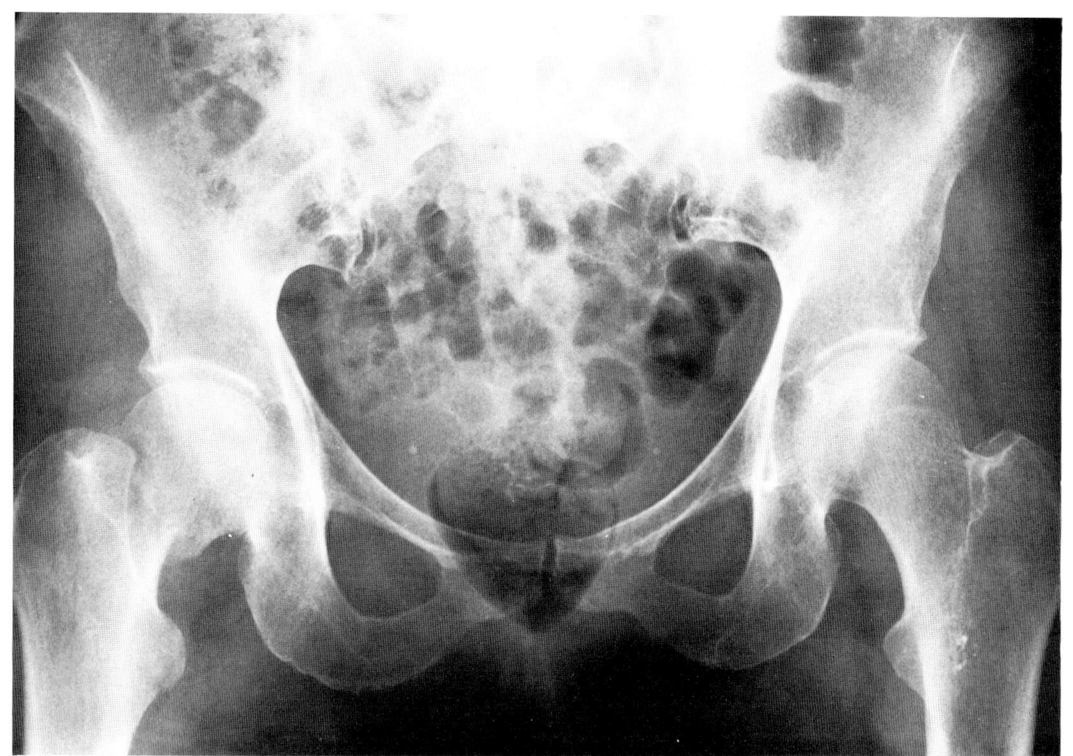

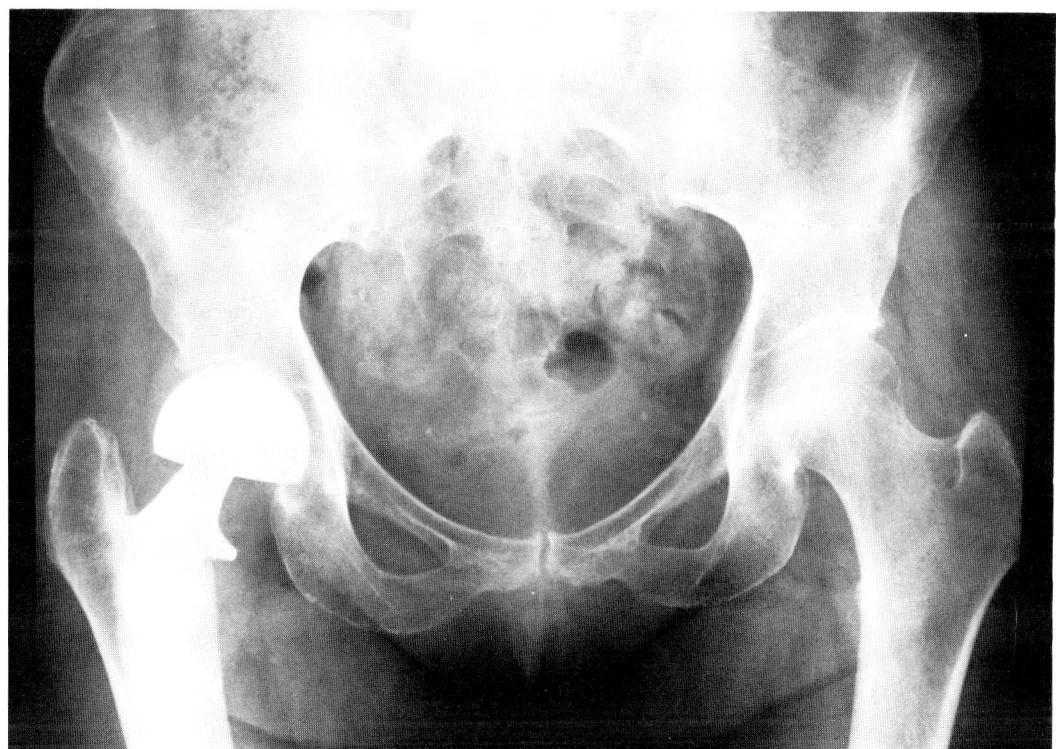

to increase acetabular rigidity and lessen the incidence of loosening or the potential for frank breakage in young, active people. This procedure has not yet excited any of the enthusiasm with which it was regarded in the past, particularly in rheumatoid arthritis with its concomitant osteoporosis; surface replacement arthroplasty is no longer recommended.

At present, important refinements in the use of methylmethacrylate cement (bone preparation, pressurization, medullary canal plugging, and most recently centrifugation of cement) have made prosthetic fixation by cement the standard to which other methods of arthroplasty are compared. Improved polyethylene acetabular components strengthened by metal backing with roughened or porous surfaces are now better anchored to bone and resist the stresses of weight-bearing more effectively (Fig. 13-7). Femoral component design changes have also improved the quality of cemented hip systems.

Cementless hip arthroplasty is gaining rapidly in both recognition and application. Impetus for the development and acceptance of cementless fixation has come from the difficulties encountered when treating the eventual failures of cemented systems due to mechanical loosening (occurring in increasing numbers), as well as from substantial improvements in techniques of cementless fixation.

Two general types of cementless fixation are currently available. The first is a microfixation method (Fig. 13-8) that depends on biologic fixation,[2,14] or bone ingrowth into the specially prepared surfaces of the femoral and acetabular prostheses. Such surfaces are called porous for the obvious reason of surface porosity; bone ingrowth for microfixation definitely can occur given the proper close apposition of implant surface to "good quality" bone with osteogenic potential. Biologic fixation, as evidenced by histologic proof of bone ingrowth, occurs at about 4 to 6 weeks after operation with progressive matura-

tion of this process up to 4 to 6 months after surgery. During this interval, it is thought that biologic fixation becomes as strong as that utilizing cement fixation methods. One system of titanium employs a dense wire mesh coating, which also seems to be an effective surface for microfixation. Yet questions remain to be answered as to optimum pore size, the choice of metals, and the effect of surface preparation on the strength of the implant, potential metal toxicity associated with noncemented application of prostheses with markedly increased surface area, and, most importantly, long-term success.

The second type of cementless fixation is a macrofixation method. Press-fit femoral components, without true pores or mesh, provide macrofixation. Such stems may have surface modifications such as fenestrations, fins, or scalloped recesses to enhance purchase of the implant in the femoral canal. As with microfixation methods, many questions remain to be answered in order to accurately assess macrofixation techniques. We do not recommend its use in rheumatoid arthritis patients.

Clinical data are emerging in support of cementless hip systems. One of the early "cementless" hip surgeons is Lord,[19] who reported favorable results after cementless hip arthroplasty, including that done for the primary treatment of rheumatoid hip disease. Despite some reports of short-term success with cementless arthroplasty for rheumatoid hip disease, concern about component fixation and stability in softened rheumatoid bone, particularly on the acetabular side, is well founded. There is little disagreement that cementless application of any system of hip arthroplasty in the rheumatoid patient with severe osteopenia, regardless of whether associated with steroid administration, is not prudent. It is in the young rheumatoid patient with reasonably good bone quality, perhaps even in the presence of corticosteroid use, that there is the most promise for success with cementless hip arthroplasty.

Fig. 13-7. This 66-year-old woman has disabling pain in the right hip due to rheumatoid arthritis. She underwent total hip replacement with cement fixation of the prosthetic components. (Numbers in the pelvic opening are preoperative measurements for the prosthetic components.)

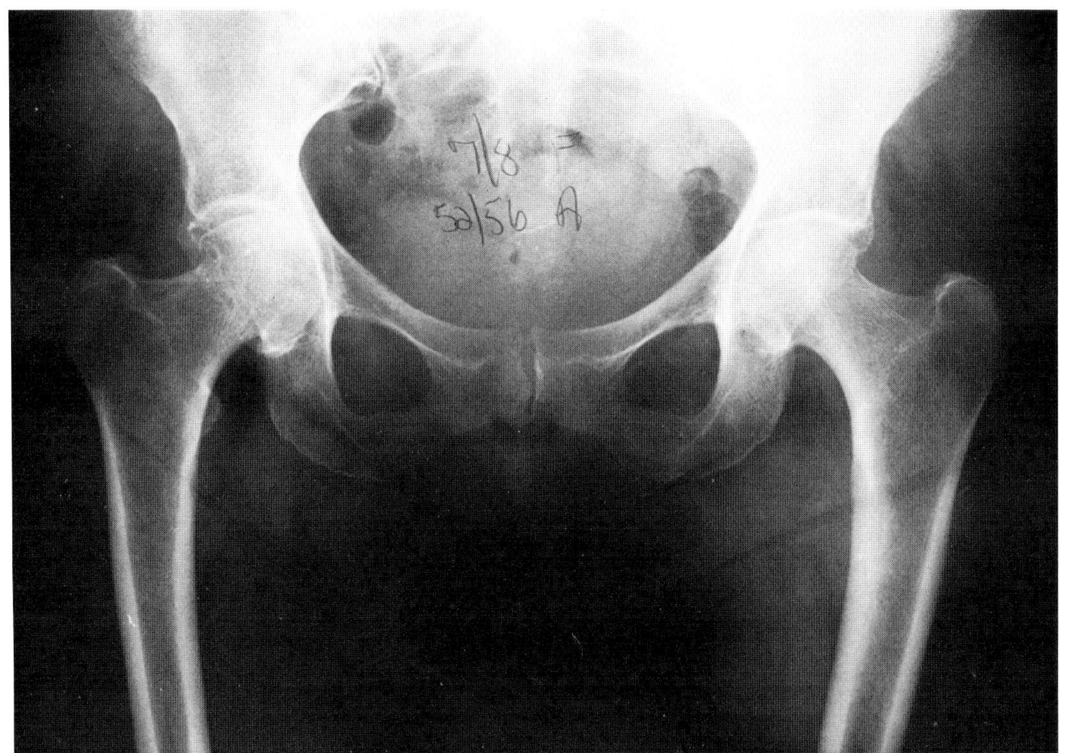

A

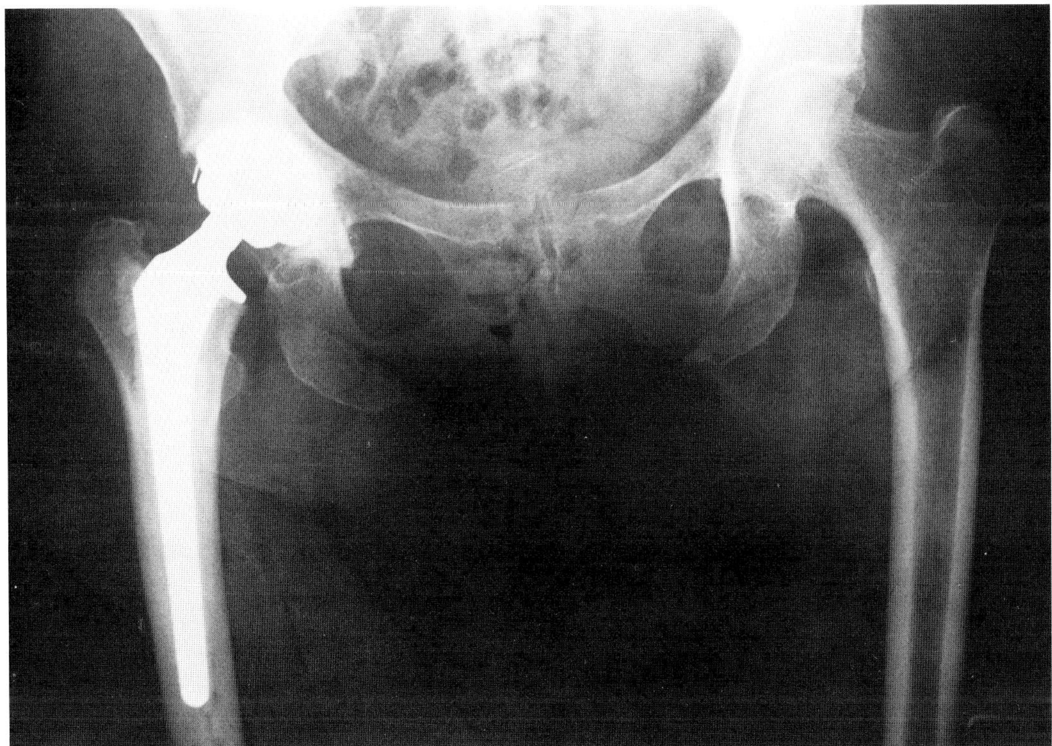

B

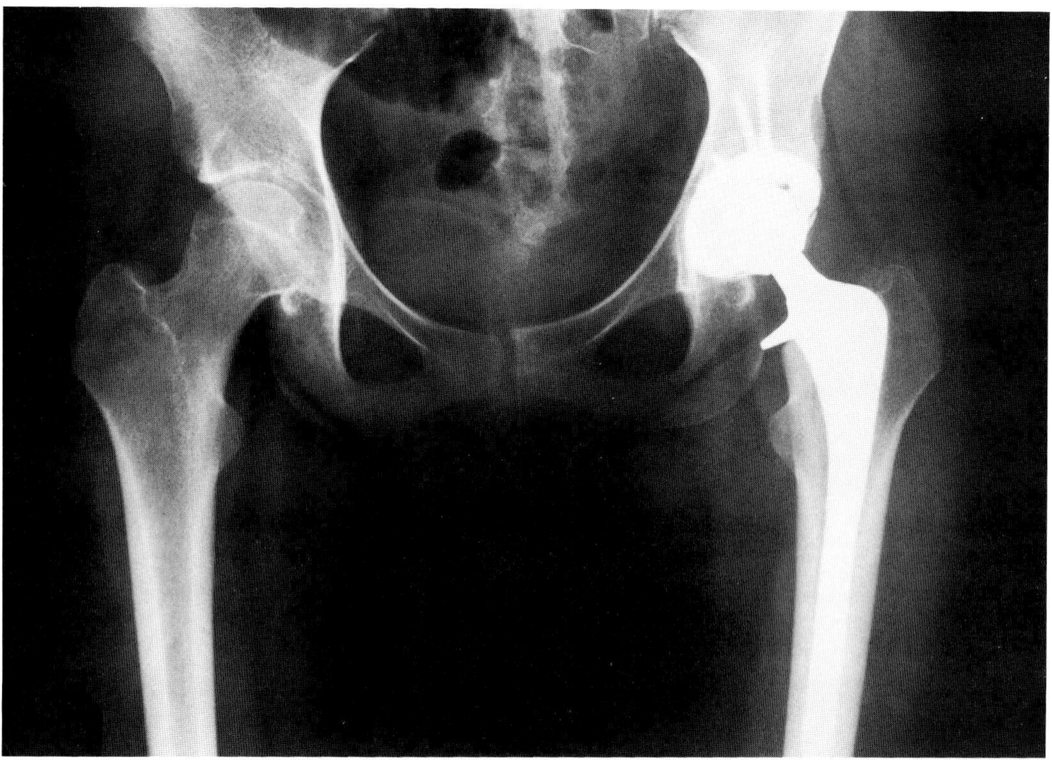

Fig. 13-8. This 19-year-old woman with juvenile rheumatoid arthritis underwent cementless total hip replacement. This particular system, a microfixation prosthetic system, is dependent on bone ingrowth into the porous surfaces of the prosthetic components with initial fixation, augmented by the acetabular screws.

Elimination of the technical problems of acrylic cement and prosthesis removal in revision situations, e.g., in the presence of mechanical loosening, also encourages further study of cementless systems in rheumatoid hip surgery. One report[24] confirmed a higher rate (1.8 times) of infection associated with total hip replacement for rheumatoid arthritis than with osteoarthritis. These statistics provide additional impetus to the emerging trend toward cementless arthroplasty. At present, however, the choice of a cementless system in the surgical management of rheumatoid hip disease should be made only if one is convinced that, for a particular patient, cementless application offers definite, predictable, and reproducible advantages over cemented arthroplasty. Even in the young rheumatoid patient, total hip replacement is and has been the surgical treatment of choice for symptomatic hip disease.

The juvenile rheumatoid arthritic in the late teen years or early twenties, the young woman in her thirties, or the male patient in his middle twenties are best treated with femoral and acetabular replacement given the presence of significant rheumatoid hip disease. We[6] have stressed this point, emphasizing that the benefits of total hip arthroplasty far outweigh the potential future problems, e.g., aseptic or mechanical loosening, that would necessitate revision. A period of 10 to 25 years of painless improved hip function justifies the potential risk and problems associated with revisional hip surgery. In addition, the present refinements in surgical technique permit optimism that, even in the young patient, the initial reconstructive procedure may be the final and definitive one. In this regard it is important to recognize again the generalized nature of the rheumatoid process. Approximately 60 percent of patients with rheumatoid hip disease have knee involvement; functional demand and stress on prosthetic joints are thereby reduced. Thus the extent of the disease and the concomitant reduced stress on weight-bearing joints combine to improve significantly the outlook for long-term success with total hip replacement arthroplasty in both the young and the older rheumatoid patient. Cementless acetabulum is often combined with a cemented femoral component (hybrid); cementless acetabula have a low loosening rate, but longer follow-up is needed.

When bilateral symptomatic hip disease exists, the question arises as to the timing of bilateral procedures. The usual recommendation is an interval of at least 6 weeks to 3 months between operative procedures, with a period of time at home during this interval. When the degree of contralateral hip disease is such that postoperative rehabilitation or nursing care is particularly difficult and restricted, it is reasonable and perhaps necessary to perform the second procedure 7 to 10 days after the first. For example, painful bilateral stage III hip disease with contractures could be best approached in this manner, assuming that the medicorheumatologic condition of the patient would permit two major operations within this short span of time. Another example is the unusual bilateral stage IV disease with ankylosis, where postoperative gait training would be impossible in the presence of contralateral ankylosis. Bilateral procedures at one operation are done infrequently. The presence of advanced bilateral hip and knee disease and concern about the difficulty of anesthesia, as in a juvenile rheumatoid arthritic with cervical and temporomandibular disease, might justify bilateral hip operations during one anesthesia session. Unlike the knee, simultaneous bilateral hip replacements are not usually performed.

TOTAL HIP ARTHROPLASTY: SURGICAL TECHNIQUE

The technique described here can be used for both cemented and cementless total hip arthroplasty. Only the former is discussed. Today's methods of hip arthroplasty differ markedly from those of earlier years, yet many principles of reconstructive surgery of the hip are those of Aufranc.[1] Meticulous surgery with great respect for the delicacy of tissue, careful hemostasis, and exceptionally attentive care remain as some of the hallmarks of his "constructive" hip surgery.

Preoperative Preparation

Preparation of the rheumatoid patient for hip surgery does not differ appreciably from that for other procedures. For example, the use of steroid preparation prior to the procedure is a common requirement for preparation of a patient with rheumatoid arthritis for a major surgical procedure. Autologous blood for transfusion should be used when possible, and blood should be available through the hospital blood bank. Perioperative systemic antibiotics alone or in conjunction with a "clean-air" surgical environment in the operating room are used, commencing either just before or shortly after induction of anesthetic.

Generally, antibiotics, usually a cephalosporin, are continued for 48 hours postoperatively. In the operating room an indwelling urinary catheter is generally inserted before starting and remains for 24 to 48 hours. Intermittent compression air boots are utilized on both legs during surgery; patients are also required to walk before receiving their preoperative medications. If urinary catheterization has been continued, or if other postoperative complications such as atelectasis or pneumonitis should ensue, oral antibiotic coverage is generally continued for several more days.

Choice of Anesthesia

General anesthesia has been used in most cases. When possible, hypotensive techniques are of value. Spinal or epidural anesthesia can also be used. Special situations are commonly encountered with rheumatoid arthritis patients, requiring specialized techniques such as nasotracheal intubation utilizing fiberoptic instrumentation in the presence of temporomandibular joint disease or severe cervical spine involvement. When concern about a particularly difficult anesthesia exists, it is important that the anesthesiologist be so notified in order to facilitate the preoperative evaluation.

Operative Procedure

A posterolateral approach to the hip is routinely utilized (Fig. 13-9). Trochanteric osteotomy is rarely done, except for some difficult protrusio problems and for selected revision arthroplasties. Release of the short external rotators from the piriformis superiorly to the upper part of the quadratus femoris inferiorly is followed by capsulotomy for posterior femoral head dislocation. Occasionally it is helpful to release all of the quadratus and part of the gluteus maximus tendon. When necessary, the anterior capsule is easily exposed by hip flexion and external rotation and by locating the landmark pericapsular fat over the anterior capsule under the anterior gluteus medius. Careful deep retraction is essential to avoid sciatic nerve injury, always a concern when

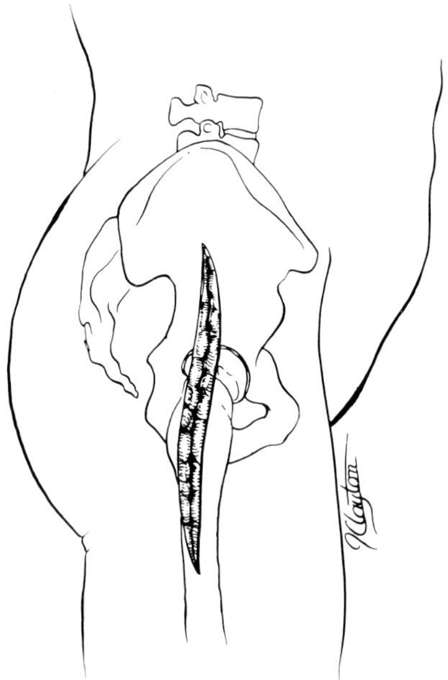

Fig. 13-9. Skin incision for a posterolateral approach to the hip.

using the posterior approach. Leg length measurement is carried out prior to dislocating the hip; two fixed points are used: a fixed retractor pin in the ilium well above the lateral acetabular margin, and a mark or pin in the trochanter itself. When the actual measurement is done, the operated extremity is placed on and parallel to the opposite down-lying extremity in the straight side-lying position in which surgery is carried out. This position can be reproduced later for assessing leg length after prosthetic insertion.

Once dislocated, the femoral head and neck are amputated, and acetabular reaming is carried out. Exposure for this procedure need not be compromised; when properly executed, this approach provides exposure equal to that employing trochanteric osteotomy or abductor release from the trochanter. After limited capsulectomy and, at times, anterior capsular release, the proximal femur is translocated anteriorly with a "cobra" retractor placed over the anteroinferior iliac spine. A wide-pointed retractor is placed inferiorly after resecting the transverse acetabular ligament. An ischial pin retractor provides posterior retraction and sciatic nerve protection (Fig. 13-10). When possible, subchondral bone is preserved. In general, the largest acetabular component that can be used without excessive reaming is recommended. Cement anchoring holes are made in the ischium, ilium, and pubis, at times making additional holes or "furrowing" sclerotic acetabular bone with a high speed burr (Fig. 13-11A). Vigorous irrigation of acetabular bone and prepared holes using a mechanical lavage instrument is followed by drying and packing the anchoring holes with a hemostatic material such as Surgicel or peroxide-soaked gauze. Acrylic cement, in the low viscosity phase, is pressure-injected into the anchoring holes with a cement gun fitted with a small appropriately sized nozzle. The remaining cement mass is also pressurized with a simple instrument that essentially occludes the acetabular mouth while compacting the cement mass. Acetabular component insertion follows with the desired position of 20 degrees forward flexion and 30 to 40 degrees abduction (Fig. 13-11B).

When protrusio acetabuli is mild to moderate, a larger acetabular component is used to take ad-

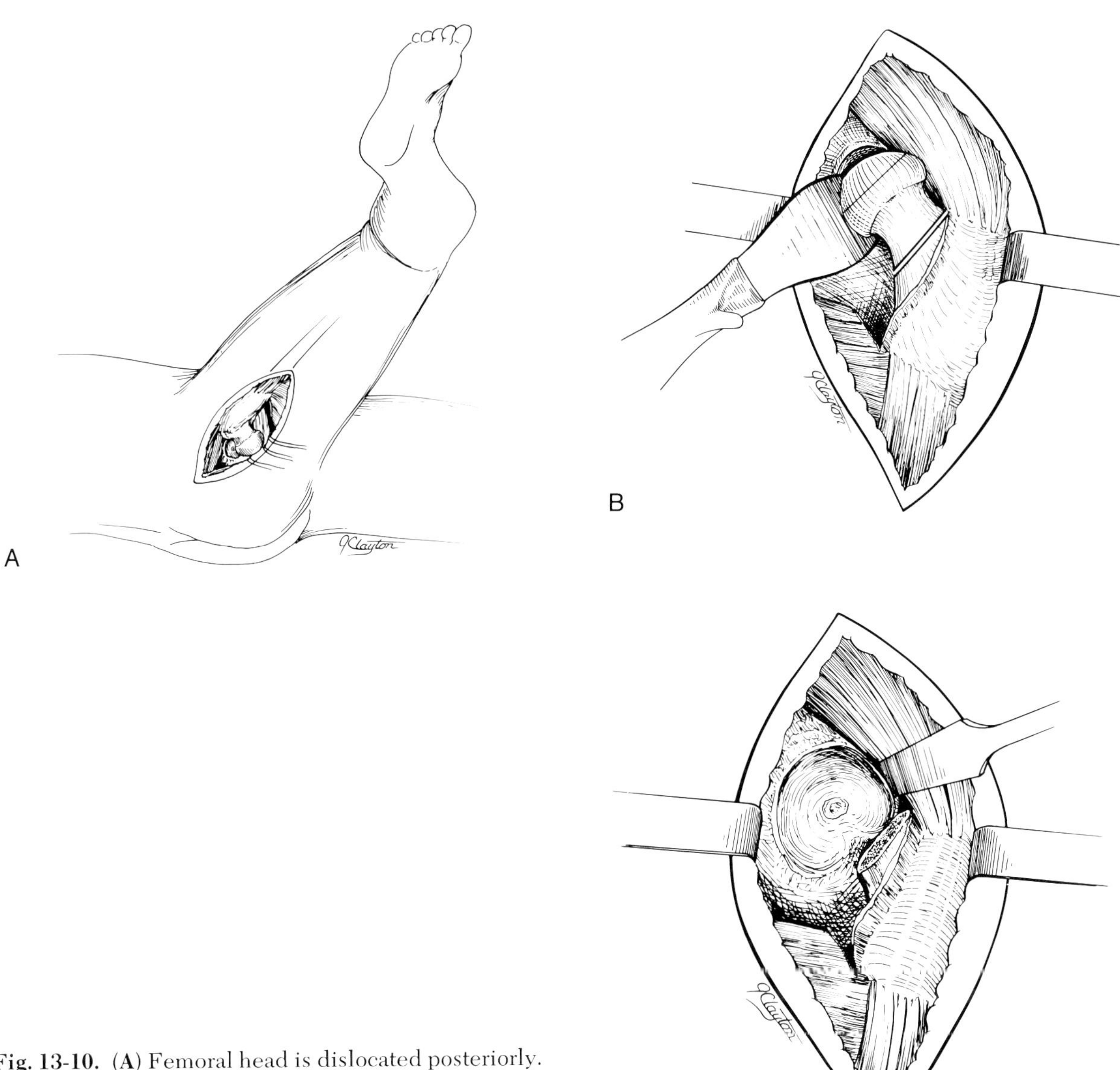

Fig. 13-10. (**A**) Femoral head is dislocated posteriorly. (**B**) Femoral head and neck are amputated. (**C**) Acetabular exposure prior to preparation for the acetabular component.

vantage of its size not only for wider stress distribution on the protruded medial wall but also for better support of this component by the important lateral or iliac column of bone (Fig. 13-12). For severe protrusion, the superior end of the femoral head is amputated after being reamed (as for "conservative" hip arthroplasty) prior to transection of the femoral neck. This bone is then used, as described by Heywood,[17] for medial

bone grafting followed by prosthetic insertion (Fig. 13-13). Metallic shells, rings, and mesh are less satisfactory and are not favored. Occasionally, severe protrusio requires in situ femoral neck amputation when posterior dislocation of the femoral head is not possible; anterior retraction then allows the femoral head to be extracted. Protrusio acetabula, in other than a primary surgical situation (i.e., failed prior arthroplasty), is

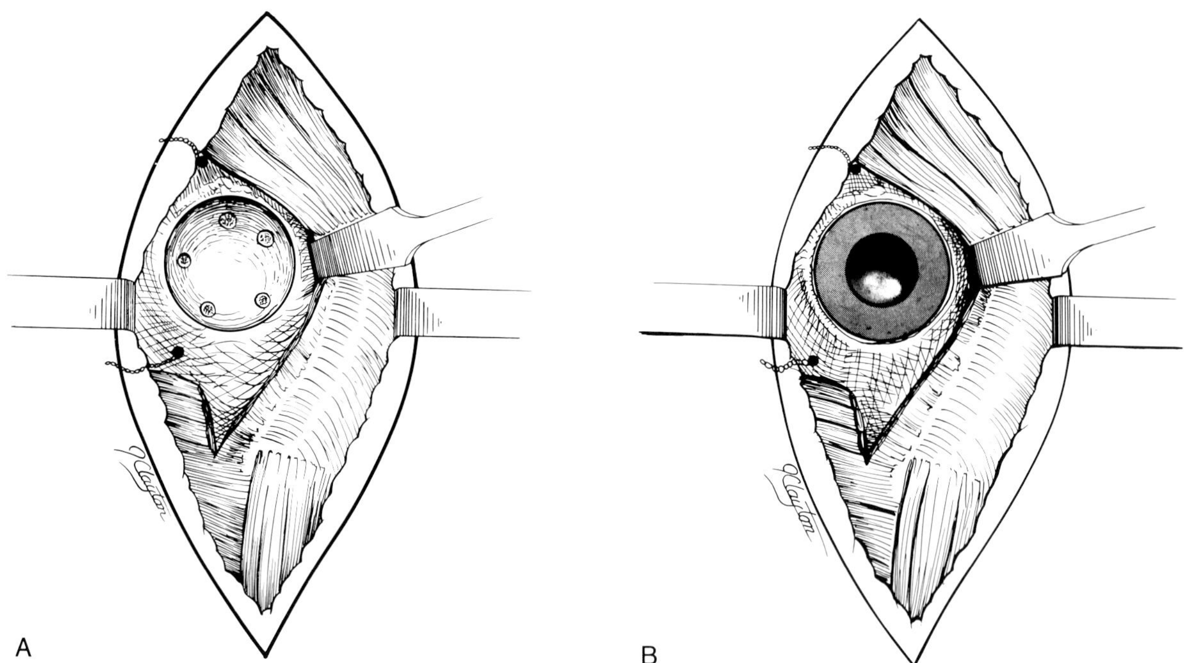

Fig. 13-11. (**A**) Prepared acetabulum prior to component insertion. (**B**) Acetabular component in place.

managed in a similar fashion, but an allograft femoral head is used for grafting.

It should be stressed that the osteopenic bone of the rheumatoid hip can be so soft that acetabular reaming may be hazardous if not done slowly and with great care. Periacetabular cysts, not utilized for cement fixation, should be packed with bone graft from the acetabular reamings or local cancellous bone.

A well-placed posterolateral incision access to the proximal femur, given proper retraction, is excellent (Fig. 13-14). Prior external rotator and quadratus release and, at times, partial release of the gluteus maximus tendon, allows the femur to be pistoned up out of the depths of the surgical wound. Usually the soft bone of the rheumatoid proximal femur is easy to prepare using a femoral rasp and reamers for insertion of the trial femoral

component. Femoral anteversion of 0 to 10 degrees is desired. Trial reduction follows, and stability and leg length measurements are determined. The largest femoral component that best fills the medullary canal should be used.

Femoral preparation should always be done with flexion of the ipsilateral knee to avoid sciatic nerve traction injuries; this rule also applies to the acetabular portion of the procedure. The rheumatoid knee must be handled with care during manipulation of the hip. Intraoperative fracture in the severe rheumatoid hip, though uncommon, can occur with overly vigorous manipulation of the osteopenic femur. One situation is recalled in which a subtrochanteric fracture occurred during skin preparation prior to surgery. The position of hip adduction combined with protrusio and advanced osteopenia led to this

Fig. 13-12. (**A**) This 65-year-old woman demonstrates mild protrusio acetabuli with superior femoral head migration. (**B**) Relatively large actabular component (without bone graft) was used to reconstruct the acetabulum. Acetabular component is well supported by the lateral or iliac column of bone and is well fixed by methacrylate cement.

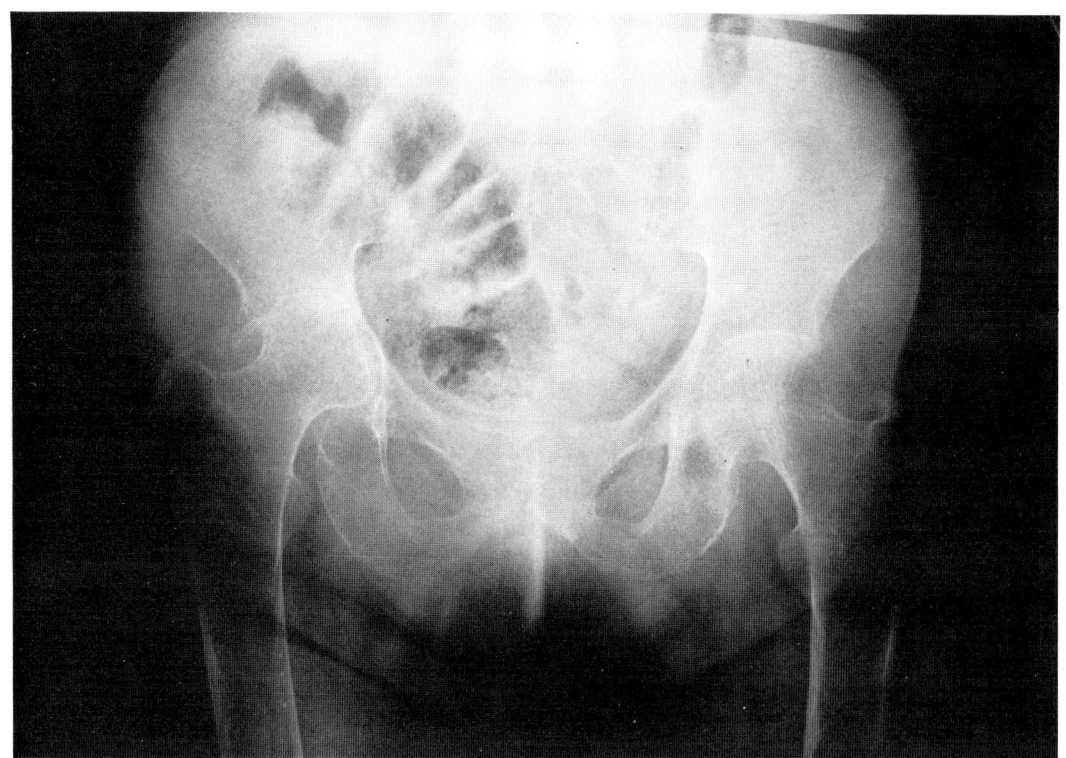

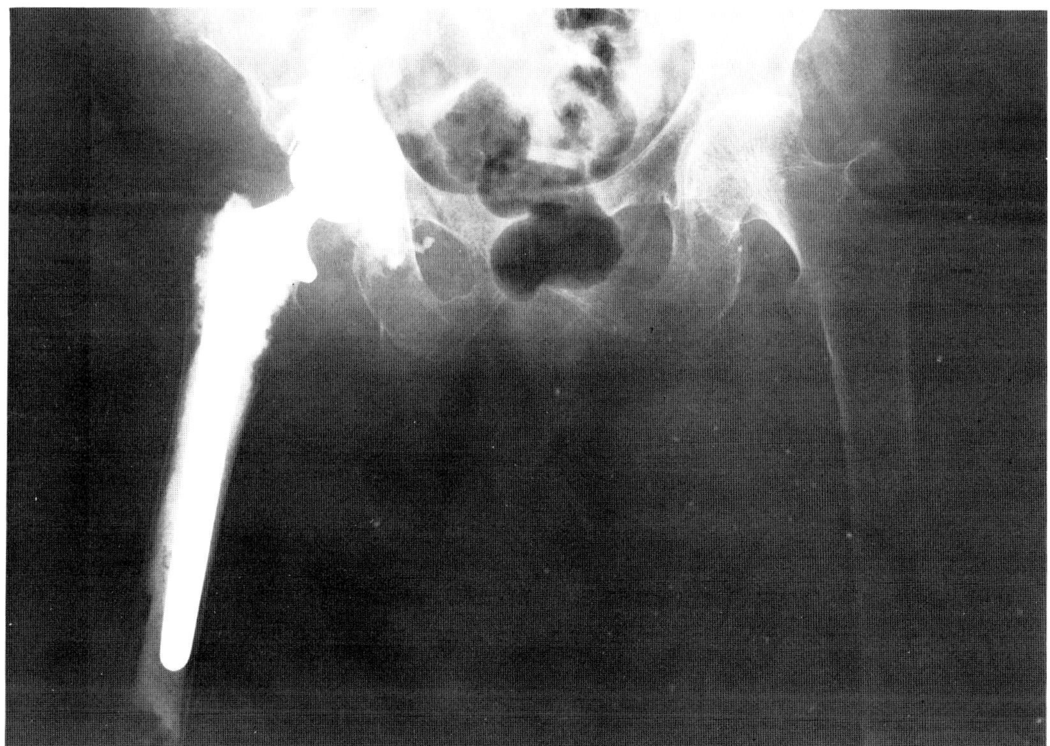

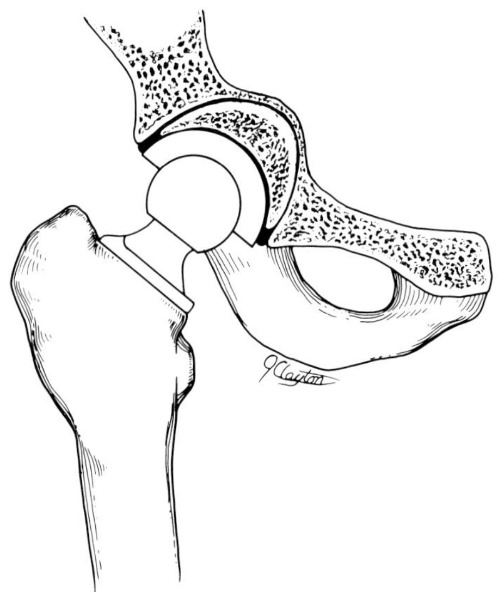

Fig. 13-13. Medial bone grafting (Heywood) for protrusio. Acetabular component is "lateralized" by the central bone graft.

preoperative problem. (The arthroplasty was carried out with open reduction and internal fixation of the fracture, accomplished with a longer-stem femoral component and acrylic cement.)

Loose cancellous bone is removed from the medullary canal with a medullary brush. The canal is plugged with an appropriately sized bone, plastic, or silicone plug inserted up to 2 cm distal to the point were the tip of the femoral component will reside. The canal is subjected to mechanical lavage and then dried. Acrylic cement in a low viscosity phase is injected from distal to proximal and pressurized using a device to occlude the opening in the femoral neck while injecting the remaining cement under pressure. The femoral implant is then introduced without toggling, and excess cement is removed during maturation of the cement itself (Fig. 13-15). It is essential to avoid varus positioning of the femoral component; proper technique and longer-stem components facilitate component positioning in the desired relative valgus orientation. Final reduction follows. At this point, assessing the stability of the implanted system is important, as a stable hip permits a less cautious postoperative activity program; marginal stability necessitates a more carefully controlled, supervised postoperative program. Wound closure is carried out over two large suction tubes. The external

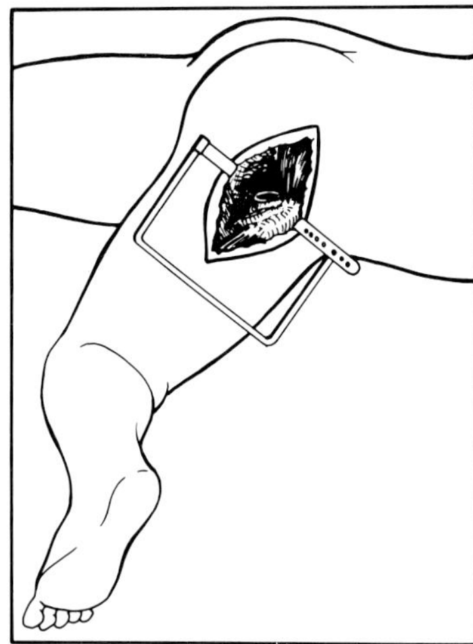

Fig. 13-14. Proximal femoral exposure with the extremity in internal rotation and proper placement of retractors.

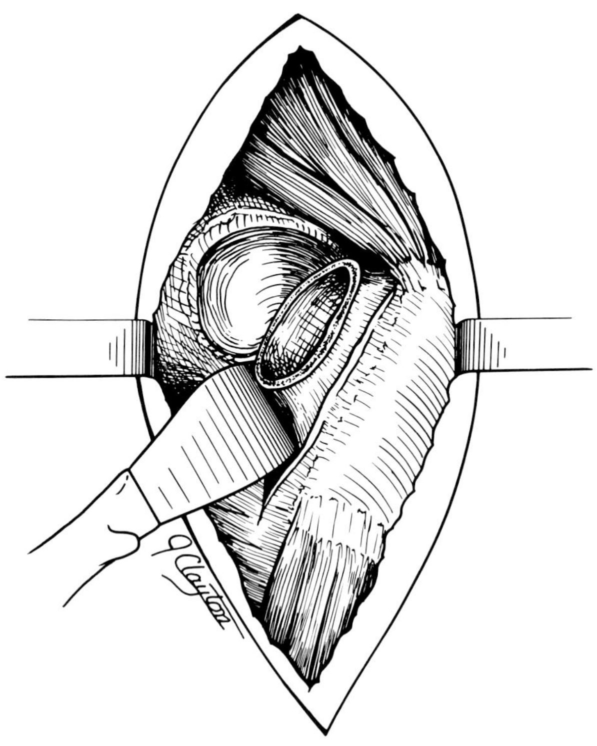

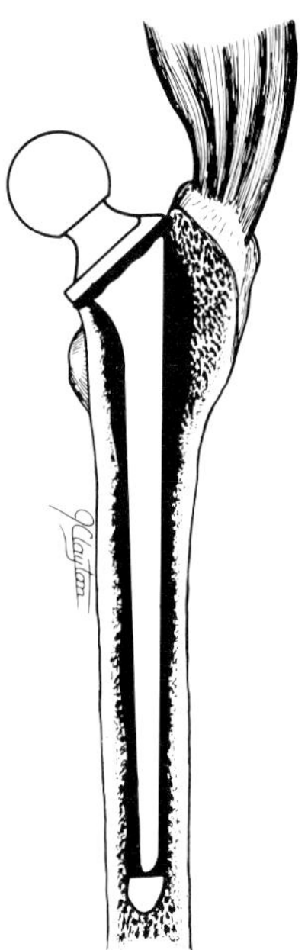

Fig. 13-15. Femoral component cemented in place with prior plugging of the medullary canal.

rotators are repaired to both the posterior trochanter (through drill holes in bone) and the posterior tendinous portion of the abductors. Such a repair augments posterior stability.[8]

Postoperative Care

An electric circle or tilting bed has been used postoperatively (Fig. 13-16); it facilitates the patient's return to the erect position and allows ambulation directly out of bed. Postural hypotension is well managed in this way, and the need for transport to the physical therapy department and use of a tilt table is eliminated. The circle bed allows the patient's feet to be higher than his or her head without breaking or gatching the bed in the middle. Such measures as elastic surgical stockings and pulsatile air boots are used intraoperatively and postoperatively. Early isometric exercise and intentional ambulation of the patient on the day of surgery, prior to operation, lessen the chance of postoperative venous thrombosis. Chemical prophylaxis is also used: Salicylates, so prevalent in the management of rheumatoid arthritis, are most often used. Warfarin (Coumadin) can also be of considerable value, particularly in the patient thought to be at risk for thromboembolic disease, i.e., the patient who has had prior venous thrombosis or pulmonary embolization. Systemic antibiotics are administered for 48 hours, and the surgical drains are removed 48 hours postoperatively.

Intraoperative and postoperative bleeding

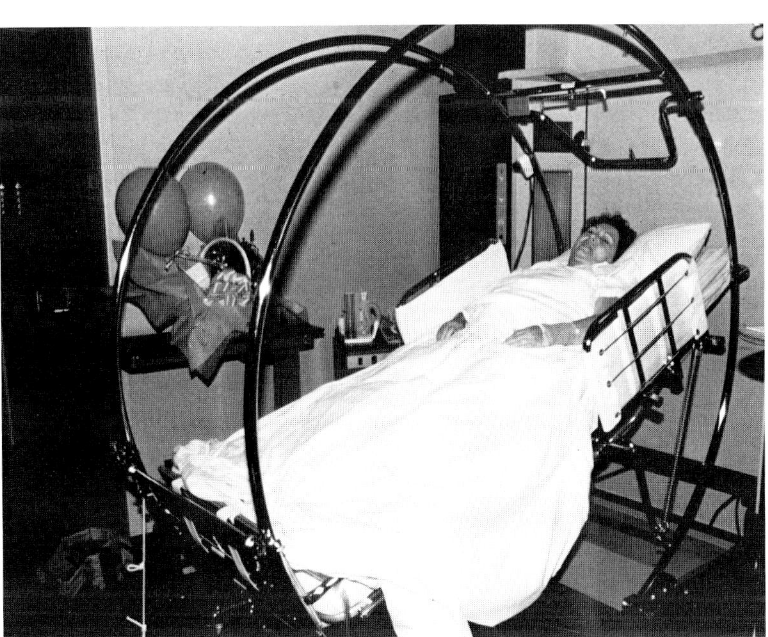

Fig. 13-16. Electric circle bed is routinely used to facilitate initial resumption of ambulation.

have not proved to be a problem despite rheumatoid patients' widespread use of salicylates and other anti-inflammatory medications that affect blood clotting mechanisms. The use of platelet transfusions can be helpful should the occasional instance of bleeding so warrant. Close monitoring of the postoperative hemoglobin and hematocrit is important as with any major surgery.

Postoperatively, the patient stands in the electric tilting or circle bed, partially weight-bearing on the operated side at 24 to 48 hours, and ambulates out of bed with appropriate support the following day. A regular bed is then used when the patient is comfortable, has begun ambulation, and begins to gain some muscle control of the operated lower extremity. Total hip precautions such as avoiding hip adduction and excessive flexion are stressed by the physician, nursing staff, and physical therapist as part of the postoperative education of the patient. Partial weight-bearing is continued for 4 to 6 weeks in the ambulatory patient, with a single cane or crutch recommended for 6 to 12 weeks thereafter. It is important to stress, however, that many modifications in the "usual routine" are necessary for the rheumatoid patient, unlike the osteoarthritic, because of the generalized nature of the disease and the wide difference in severity from patient to patient.

Discharge Planning

Prior to discharge, the occupational and physical therapists combine their efforts to prepare the patient for the transition from hospital to home. Evaluation of the patient's abilities and limitations in activities of daily living is essential. Certain aids, e.g., "grabbers" for putting on stockings and shoes, can be of great assistance to patients who not only have upper extremity disease but have been carefully instructed in total hip precautions regarding hip motions. A high toilet seat, often equipped with side rails or handles, is essential, as total hip dislocations are an unfortunate, yet common, occurrence in the narrow confines of the bathroom during toilet function. Informed practical advice is an indispensable part of preparation for home; it includes advice about kitchen activities, bathing, sleeping, and other aspects of home life. An extra mattress on top of the regular mattress converts a "low" bed to one of acceptable height. A bath shower fitted with a nonslip bench and handrails and a secure single platform step allows the postoperative hip patient to step into the tub with little risk and to sit down comfortably for showering. Home exercises are outlined, which are simple prone and isometric strengthening exercises when flexion contracture persists, as well as a limited range of motion program. Later, use of a stationary bicycle with appropriate seat height adjustment is allowed. Similarly, a program of walking or water exercises can be started as the patient's strength permits, usually after the initial period of supported gait with two crutches or a walker. Obviously, a large percentage of rheumatoid patients are either not able or do not desire to participate in such intentional exercises; for those who can, exercise is highly desirable.

Finally, the surgeon must take time to review all of the patient's questions and concerns prior to discharge. Issues should be clearly addressed, such as those concerning sexual activity, driving, exercise and activity limitations, and even how long the patient should wear the antiembolism elastic stockings provided in the hospital. Warning regarding the potential for prosthetic joint infection and ways to avoid this ultimate tragedy are the responsibility of the surgeon. Metal detection devices in airports often concern the patient. A letter and wallet card are provided to assist with these often confusing matters (Fig. 13-17).

Complications Following Total Hip Arthroplasty

Three potential problems are of particular concern following total hip arthroplasty. The first, and perhaps the most difficult and costly to treat, is that of infection.[22] The second is the problem of mechanical (aseptic) loosening of one or both prosthetic components. The third problem is dislocation of the total hip arthroplasty. Fortunately, the incidence of any one of these postoperative complications is low. One other complication peculiar to hip arthroplasty should be noted, i.e., the problem of postoperative leg length inequal-

---

DENVER ORTHOPEDIC CLINIC, P.C.
2005 Franklin Street
Denver, Colorado 80205
303-839-5383

Patient ______________________________________

Operation(s) 1) ____________________________

2) ____________________________

IMPORTANT INFORMATION — SEE OVER

---

1. The named operation involves implantation of metal into the body which may activate a metal detection device.
2. The doctors in the Denver Orthopedic Clinic have given this patient permission to travel.
3. It is recommended that protective antibiotic drug therapy be initiated should this patient develop any serious infection or undergo tooth extraction(s) or prophylactic teeth cleaning, urologic manipulation, or any other potentially bacteremia-producing procedures.

Patient Drug Allergies: ____________________________

____

Fig. 13-17. Wallet card provided for patients with total joint replacements. (Courtesy of Denver Orthopedic Clinic.)

ity. Despite intraoperative efforts to equalize leg length measurements, inequality can occur. In the rheumatoid patient with other lower extremity joint involvement, leg length inequality is less bothersome than it would be in the case of a patient with isolated osteoarthritis of a single hip. Nevertheless, this complication deserves recognition. Treatment, when necessary, usually consists in appropriate shoe modifications.

Thromboembolic disease is always a concern following reconstructive lower extremity surgery. Venography and lung scans are the principal diagnostic methods used to confirm clinical impressions. Early postoperative ambulation and

use of pulsatile boots, elastic stockings, chemical prophylaxis (usually salicylates or low dose warfarin), and active muscle exercise have made thromboembolic disease an uncommon problem following total hip arthroplasty. One report noted a 1.5 percent incidence of deep vein thrombosis and a 1 percent incidence of pulmonary embolization.[24]

Other complications of hip arthroplasty in rheumatoid arthritis patients certainly can occur, and they parallel those that follow hip reconstruction done for other conditions. Postoperative nerve palsies are infrequent and usually recover spontaneously, either partially or completely; an increased susceptibility to traction injury at the level of the hip, in contrast to that at the level of the valgus, externally rotated rheumatoid knee, is not the case. Peroneal nerve palsy due to postoperative traction may be related to traction on the leg with forced knee extension and peroneal nerve stretch, or to direct pressure of the traction boot on the proximal peroneal nerve itself. Fragile rheumatoid skin can cause problems with blistering and breakdown postoperatively, particularly when adhesive dressings are applied directly to the skin. The osteopenic rheumatoid bone must be carefully respected. Intraoperative fractures during manipulation of the hip or femoral perforation and fracture during femoral canal preparation are uncommon but do pose somewhat greater risks than in the osteoarthritic femur.

Infection

The generalized disease process of rheumatoid arthritis with its disturbed immunologic mechanisms and the physical debilitation of the patients seems to predispose the rheumatoid patient to infection. The use of corticosteroids, immunosuppressive and cytotoxic drugs, and other medications for the medical management of rheumatoid arthritis has always raised particular concern about infections, as well as wound healing, following surgery in these patients. This concern persists but has not been proved. Nevertheless, it now appears that the rate of infection in rheumatoid patients who have undergone total hip arthroplasty is greater than that for hip arthroplasty in osteoarthritis.[24] This difference is attributed to the appearance of late (more than 2 years postoperative) infection in the susceptible rheumatoid group. The potential for hematogenous seeding of the prosthetic hip joint is real, from the frequent sites of skin breakdown in many rheumatoid arthritics as well as from other sources, e.g., the respiratory tract. For example, areas of broken-down skin are commonly seen in

the rheumatoid patient over rheumatoid nodules of considerable size as well as on contiguous severe hand or foot deformities with marked bony prominences.

Treatment of the infected total hip joint depends on factors such as the duration of infection prior to recognition, the causative organism, and the state of the prosthetic joint, i.e., whether there is associated component loosening. Surgical alternatives range from drainage and débridement with component retention and intensive systemic antibiotic therapy to resection arthroplasty, component and cement removal, débridement, and antibiotics. Subsequent revision hip arthroplasty can be considered when suitable conditions for implantation exist. "Direct exchanges," or removal of the infected hip components and immediate reimplantation of new components after débridement, have been successfully accomplished in the presence of sepsis. This procedure requires careful patient selection on the basis of the organism and its antibiotic sensitivity, the patient's condition, and findings in and about the hip joint at surgery. Acrylic cement impregnated with antibiotic powder is being used effectively for direct exchanges as well as for delayed revision arthroplasties after prior component removal for sepsis.

Dislocation

Patients with rheumatoid arthritis sustain postoperative total hip dislocation for the same reasons osteoarthritic and other patients do (Fig. 13-18). The incidence of dislocation is between 1.0 and 2.5 percent.[12] One cause of dislocation—retroversion or excessive anteversion of the femoral component—is more likely to occur in the rheumatoid arthritic owing to the intraoperative difficulty of assessing femoral anteversion in the presence of ipsilateral valgus knee deformity and associated ligamentous laxity. These conditions commonly coexist in the rheumatoid knee. To avoid this problem, it is recommended that the

---

Fig. 13-18. (A) Superior (and posterior) dislocation of total hip replacement in a patient with long-standing rheumatoid arthritis who failed to heal an intertrochanteric hip fracture and underwent total hip replacement utilizing a femoral component with an elongated neck. In this case abductor muscular insufficiency predisposed to dislocation. **(B)** Postreduction roentgenogram. Previously operated hip remained asymptomatic.

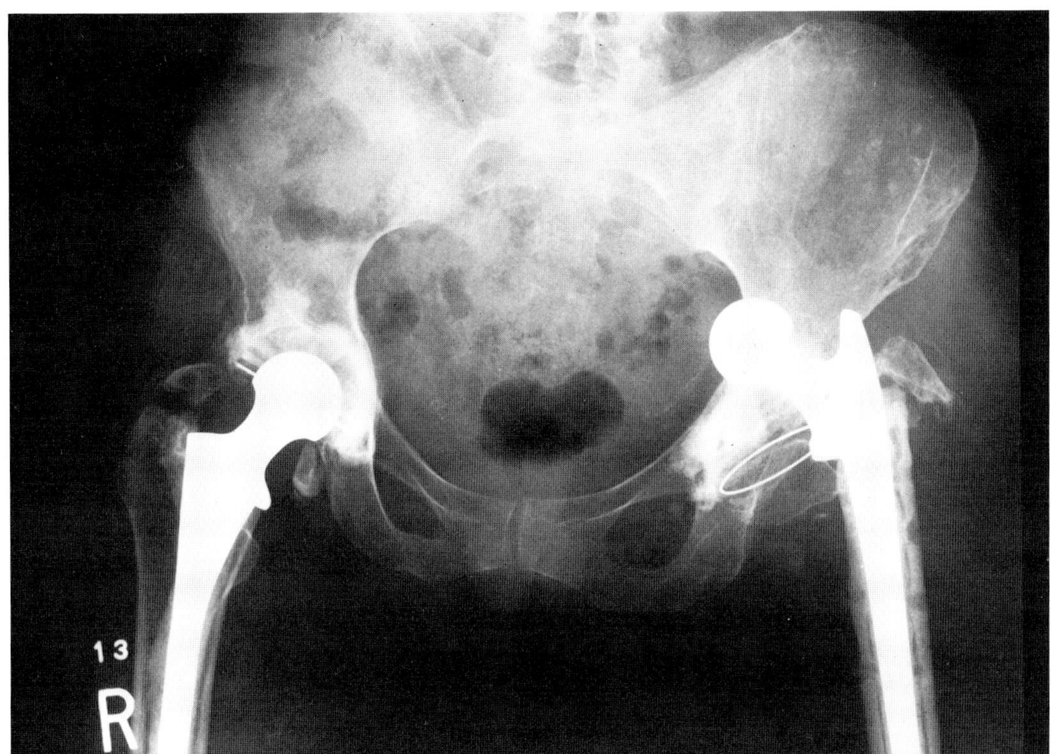

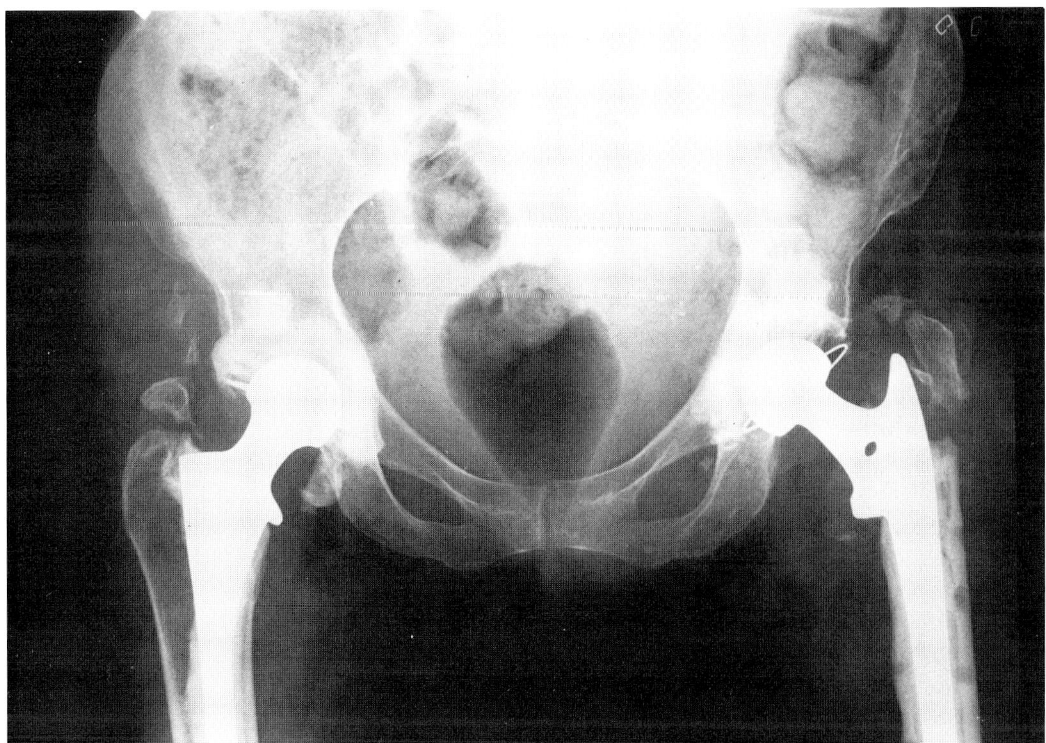

femoral condyles and patellae distally and, when possible, the remaining femoral neck proximally be used to assess anteversion for component placement. Myofascial tension problems, e.g., abductor muscles' quality and length, may cause dislocation. Dislocation after trochanteric osteotomy, in contrast to arthroplasty done with trochanteric retention, may be less frequent.[24] Nevertheless, unless conditions requiring abductor advancement exist, primary hip replacement is best done with trochanteric retention. Careful intraoperative technique results in a stable total hip system and avoids the problems associated with trochanteric reattachment (nonunion, broken wires—when used, and painful trochanteric bursae) in the osteopenic rheumatoid bone. Acetabular component malposition is another cause of dislocation. Retroversion, excessive lateral tilt or abduction, or superior positioning are errors common to unstable total hip replacement arthroplasties.

Again, the postoperative education of the patient is stressed. Excessive motion during the postoperative hospital stay and the first several months after surgery can cause dislocation. The rheumatoid patient, indeed all patients, must be instructed carefully about allowed hip motions, particularly during exercise, sitting, getting in and out of bed, automobile transfers, and toilet and hygiene activities.

Treatment of recurring hip dislocation is difficult and at times immensely frustrating for both patient and surgeon. Isolated dislocations, if due to patient error, may be avoided in the future by reeducating the patient. When recurrent dislocation not due to patient error occurs, a brace that limits hip flexion and adduction is used[9]; 6 months of continuous usage of this brace may convert an unstable hip to one with less motion but more stability. When it fails or when definite component error is identified, revision surgery is considered. When component error is not clear and impaired myofascial tension is suspected, abductor advancement—with or without component change—may be of value. It is important to emphasize that revision surgery, whether for dislocation or aseptic loosening, or after prior hip surgery and certainly after prior sepsis, is associated with a higher incidence of infection than is primary hip surgery.[26]

Mechanical (Aseptic) Loosening

Improvements in prosthetic design, e.g., longer, larger femoral components and metal backing of acetabular components, will lead to diminished rates of mechanical failure.[20] Refinement of fixation methods using acrylic cement will similarly reduce the incidence of mechanical failure. Future data may support cementless systems as even more effective in terms of long-term successful fixation. What is known now is that femoral failures occur more frequently and earlier than do acetabular failures.[28,29] A review of mechanical failures of total hip arthroplasties in rheumatoid arthritis patients confirmed this finding; the required revision surgery was for femoral side failures only.[24]

It is essential to distinguish clinical failure from roentgenographic failure. The former is symptomatic loosening, perhaps requiring revision surgery. The latter refers to the common roentgenographic presence of widening demarcation zones or radiolucencies, calcar resorption, femoral subsidence, and acetabular component migration (Fig. 13-19). Obviously, clinical failure implies roentgenographic failure, but the reverse is not the case. The incidence of nonprogressive acetabular radiolucencies is high; one report, for a relatively small number of patients, showed a higher roentgenographic incidence of acetabular loosening than femoral loosening in rheumatoid arthritis patients.[28] The incidence of femoral subsidence or calcar resorption is also high in rheumatoid arthritis, a finding consistent with the early clinical failures on the femoral side that required revision arthroplasty.[24]

It does appear that rheumatoid total hip replacement patients are less likely to experience clinical failure caused by aseptic loosening than are their osteoarthritic counterparts. A 1.6 percent revision rate with rheumatoid arthritis in contrast to a 3.4 percent revision rate with osteoarthritis, during the same period of time, has been reported.[24] It most likely relates to the lessened functional demands on the prosthetic hip system in the rheumatoid patient with multiple

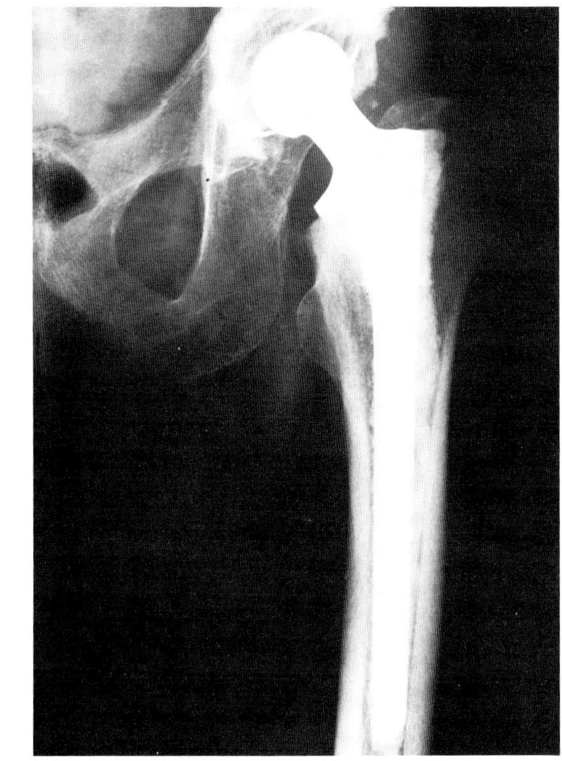

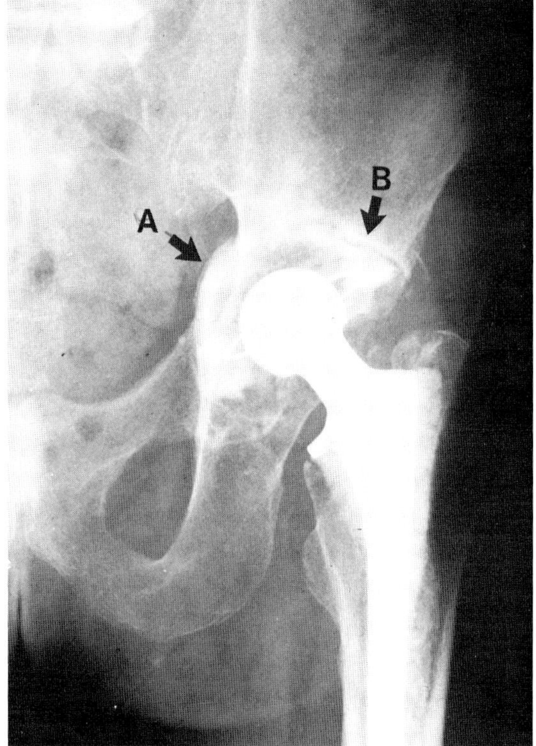

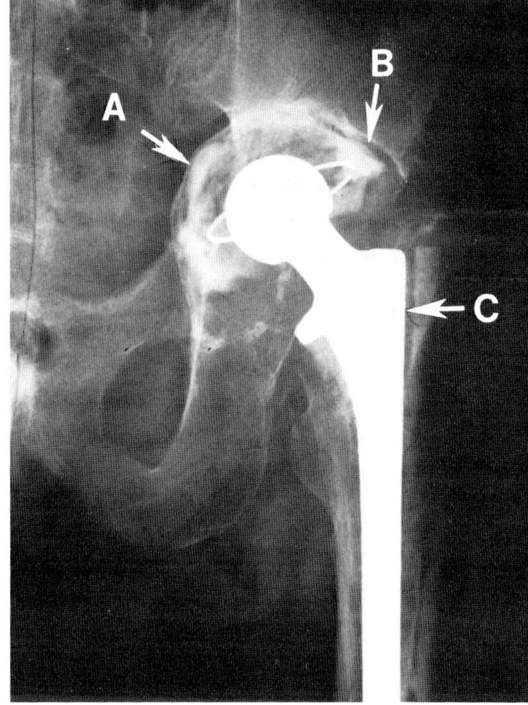

Fig. 13-19. (**A**) Roentgenographic failure is not apparent. The minimal acetabular radiolucent zone is not a sign of failure. (**B**) Seven years later, two examples of roentgenographic failure can be seen: central acetabular component migration (*A*); and a large, widened acetabular radiolucent zone consistent with acetabular component loosening (*B*). Surprisingly, symptoms were minimal at this time. (**C**) Three years later the symptoms are much increased, and a clearly seen radiolucent zone adjacent to the femoral component is indicative of femoral component loosening (*C*). Further central acetabular migration (*A*) has occurred, and the superior actabular radiolucent zone has widened (*B*).

joint involvement and to the usually smaller size of the patients with the generalized rheumatoid disease process.

The problem of acetabular component migration is particularly important in the rheumatoid hip. Preoperative protrusio acetabuli predisposes the acetabular component to recurrent migration, usually in an axial direction.[24] In addition to the roles of osteopenia and the stresses of weight-bearing, it has been suggested that a medially inclined weight-bearing acetabular surface predisposes to protrusio.[3] Proper initial acetabular reconstruction avoids recurrent axial (and medial) acetabular component migration. This reconstruction should restore both anatomic position and orientation, and it is best done with medial bone grafting—not acrylic cement—to translocate the acetabular component laterally, placing it under the support of the iliac column of bone. A large acetabular component should also be used as previously indicated. Cementless acetabula (see Fig. 13-21B & C, below) may reduce the late loosening and migration if the bone stock is adequate and good peripheral rim support is obtained. This procedure is recommended at this time.

RESULTS

Despite the ominous potential complications after total hip arthroplasty, most rheumatoid patients consider their hip arthroplasties highly satisfactory. Many patients who have had upper and lower extremity prosthetic joints implanted regard the hip arthroplasty as the "best" of their joint replacements. Pain relief is excellent and function improved, at times even to the point of eliminating the need for support during gait.

We (Papenfus et al.[23]) reported on a rheumatoid group whose average preoperative Harris[16] hip rating was 50 (of a possible 100). This same group of patients had average postoperative ratings of 89 and 84 at 5 and 10 years, respectively. The rheumatoid arthritis patients did as well as the osteoarthritis group (Tables 13-1 and 13-2). The differential magnitude of 5 postoperative points remains constant. It is important to note

Table 13-1. Mean Harris Hip Scores

		Postoperative Scores	
Diagnosis	Preoperative Score	5 Years	10 Years
Osteoarthritis	53	95	89
Rheumatoid arthritis	50	90	84
Mean score		93	87

Table 13-2. Comparison of Harris Hip Scores

		Postoperative Scores (%)	
Category	Rating	5 Years	10 Years
Excellent	90–100	82 ($n = 55$)	59 ($n = 29$)
Good	80–90	14 ($n = 9$)	31 ($n = 15$)
Fair	70–80	0 ($n = 0$)	0 ($n = 0$)
Poor	<70	4 ($n = 3$)	10 ($n = 5$)
Total		100 ($n = 67$)	100 ($n = 49$)

the difference between the pre- and postoperative ratings. Between 5 and 10 years, slight deterioration was expected; but the mean result still qualified for a good or excellent result. Not only can the use of support during gait be eliminated or modified, but some patients, few as the number may be, who were confined to bed-to-chair activity prior to hip reconstruction either are able to ambulate after arthroplasty or have begun the series of reconstructive procedures that will return them to a more functional, active, pain-free existence.

CASE REPORT 1

A 63-year-old woman with chronic rheumatoid arthritis presented with an impacted right femoral neck fracture (Fig. 13-20A). The hip had not been symptomatic and had normal joint spacing. Treatment consisted in internal fixation using multiple peripheral pins and side plate, which allowed "sliding" (Fig. 13-20B). This type of fixation is ideal in a "good" rheumatoid arthritic hip because the central bone of the neck is generally poor for internal fixation purposes, and the side plate gives added support for possible subsi-

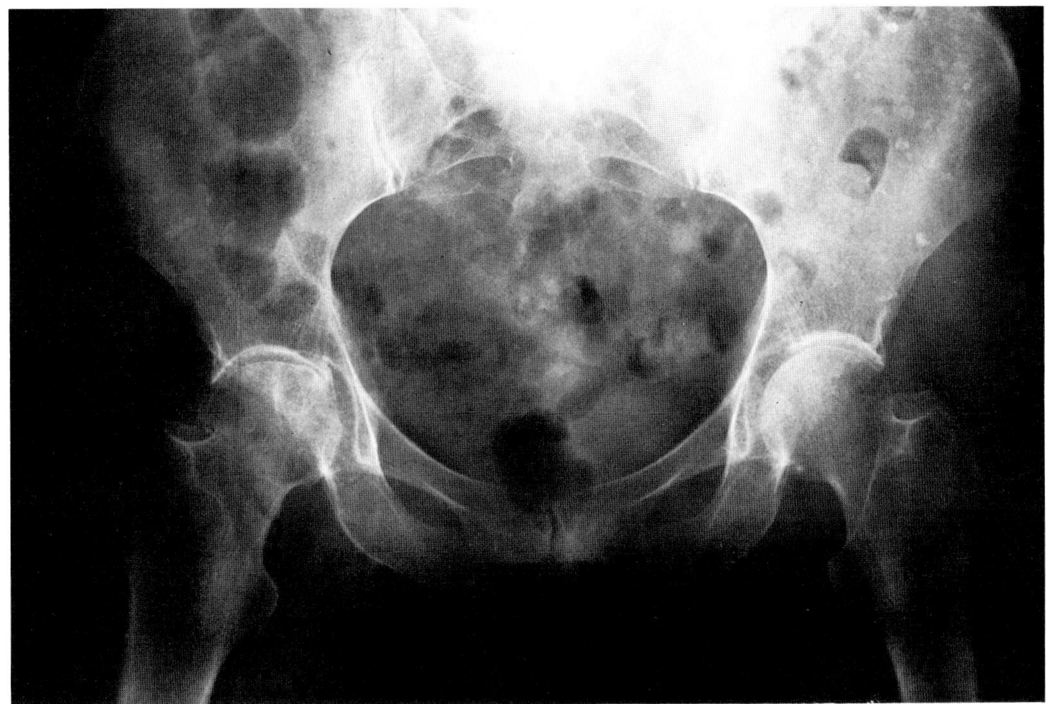

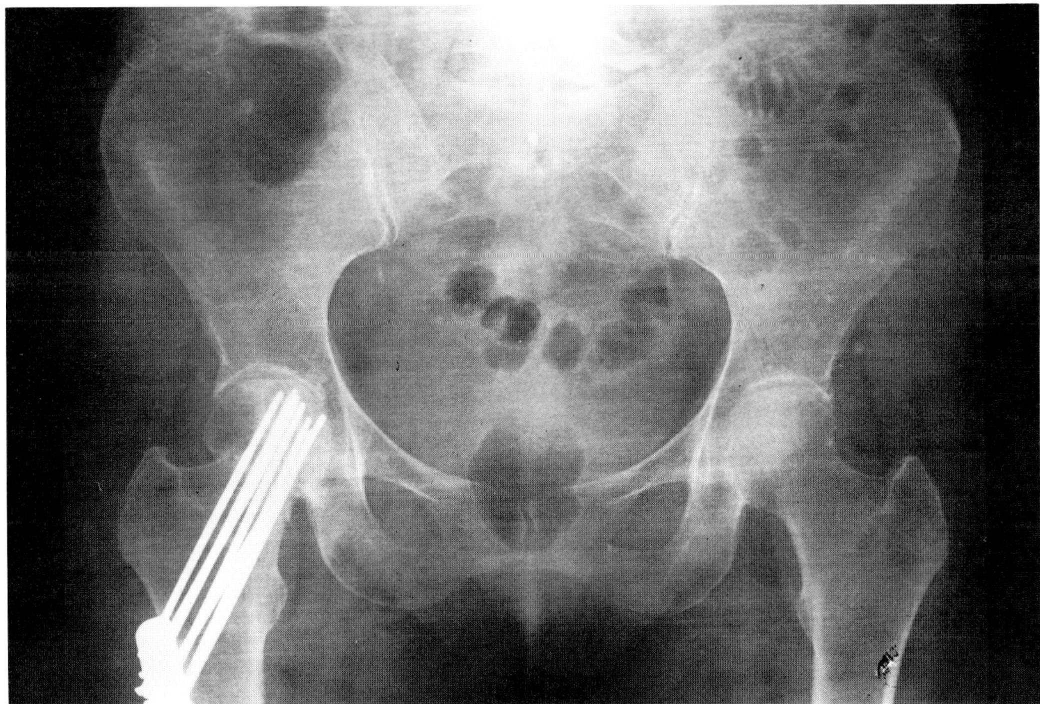

Fig. 13-20. (**A**) Nondisplaced right neck femoral fracture. (**B**) Multiple pin fixation of right femoral neck fracture. (*Figures continues.*)

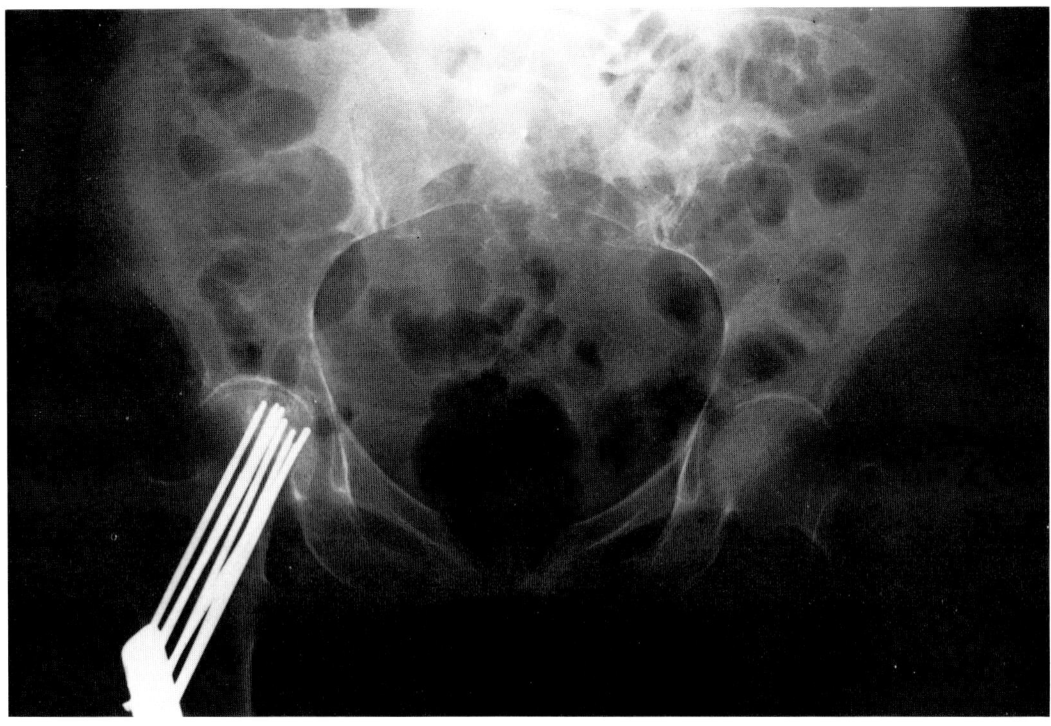

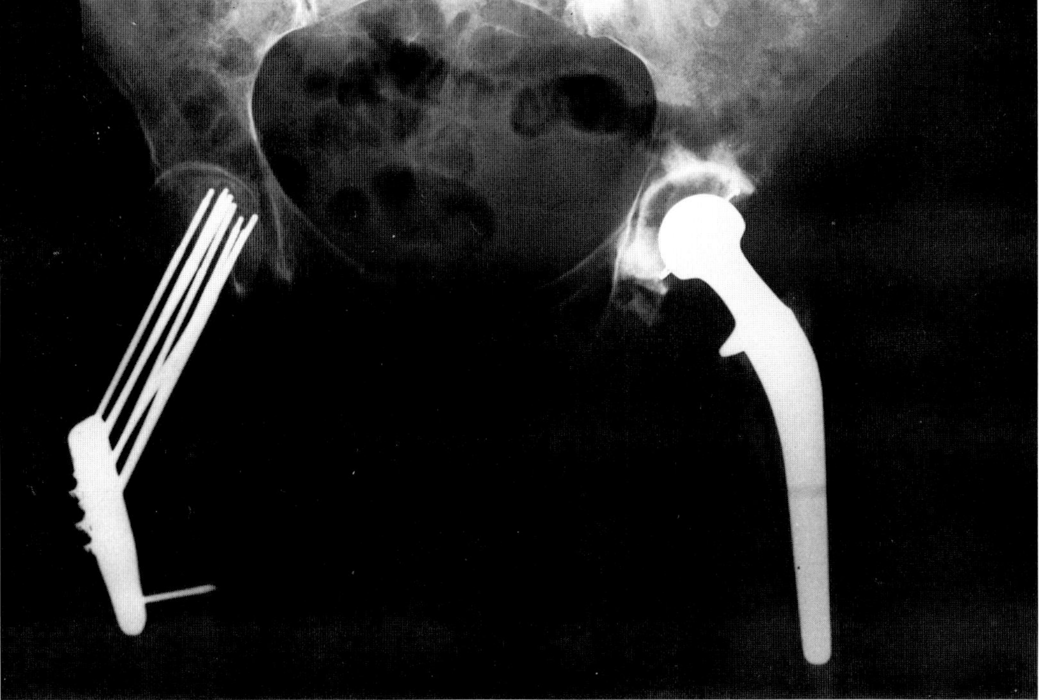

Fig. 13-20 *(Continued)*. **(C)** Displaced left femoral neck fracture with stage II disease. Healed right femoral neck fracture. **(D)** Primary total hip arthroplasty of the left hip for a femoral neck fracture in stage II disease.

dence.[6] Firm fixation was also desired to allow some weight-bearing and to relieve the stress of crutches on her arms.

When she fell again 8 years later and sustained a displaced left femoral neck fracture, the right hip was functioning well and was relatively pain-free. The left hip was painful prior to injury, consistent with stage II disease (Fig. 13-20C), and she subsequently underwent a total hip arthroplasty (Fig. 13-20D).

CASE REPORT 2

A 18-year-old woman with rheumatoid arthritis developed rapidly progressive, incapacitating right hip pain over a short period (Fig. 13-21A). Roentgenograms demonstrated severe articular cartilage loss in the right hip, whereas the left hip was thought to be uninvolved. Her medications included methotrexate and prednisone, and despite the latter medication her bone quality was excellent. Her young age and the quality of bone influenced the decision to employ a cementless (microfixation type) total hip replacement (Fig. 13-21B & C).

CASE REPORT 3

A 39-year-old woman with chronic rheumatoid arthritis underwent a "conservative" total hip replacement for severe involvement of the right hip (Fig. 13-22A & B). Four years subsequent to the arthroplasty, progressively severe pain with weight-bearing developed in the same hip. At the time of revision surgery, both components were loose. A cementless revision arthroplasty was done, utilizing a bipolar type acetabular component in the large recess remaining after removal of the primary acetabular component. The large bipolar component is necessary not only to fill the recess but to prevent further medial

migration of the acetabular component (Fig. 13-22C).

Today, a fixed cementless acetabular component would probably be used (Fig. 13-2B): Too many bipolar acetabula have failed, and the cementless, microfixation, fixed acetabula have a good record in both revisions and primary cases. Bone grafting is utilized as necessary for large defects.

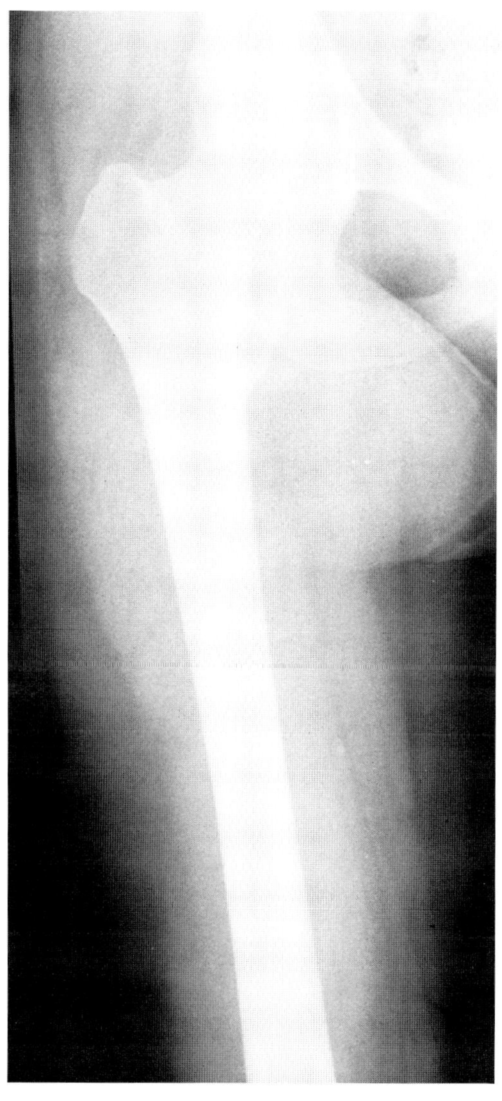

A

Fig. 13-21. **(A)** Right hip demonstrates severe articular cartilage loss (left hip was normal). (*Figure continues.*)

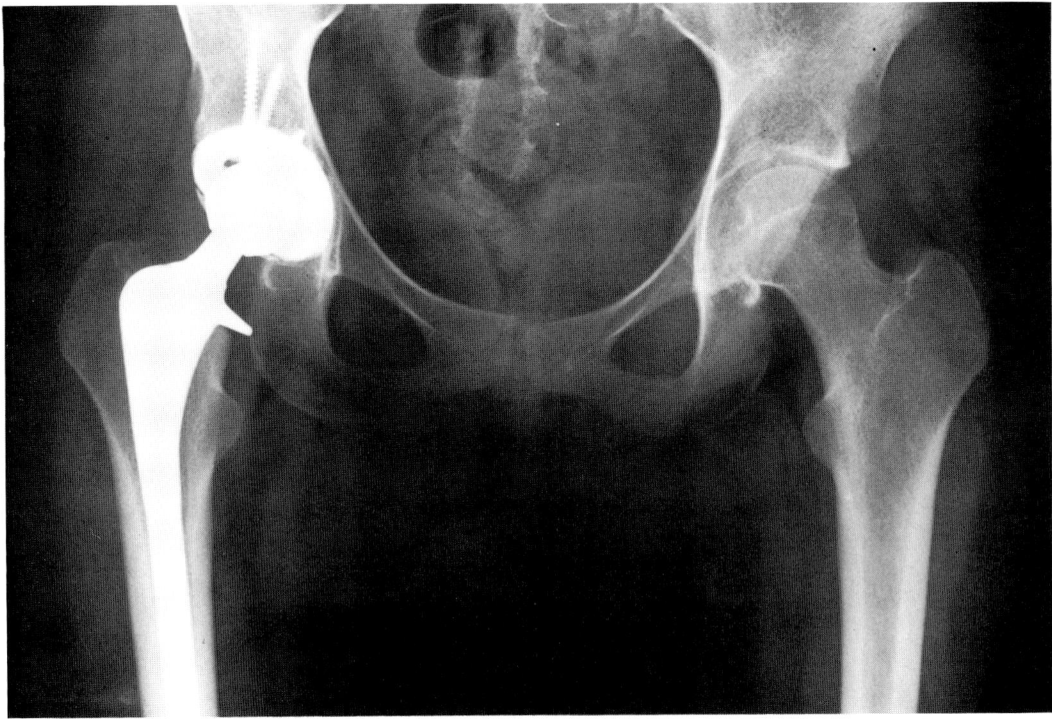

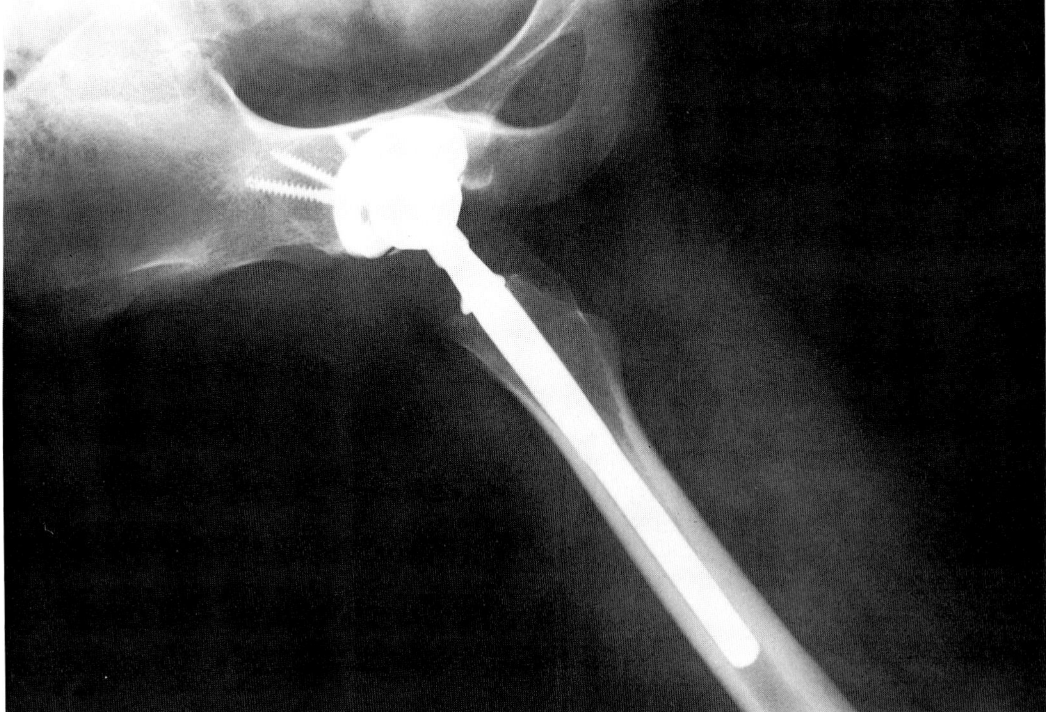

Fig. 13-21 (*Continued*). (**B & C**) Anteroposterior (**B**) and frog-leg lateral (**C**) views show cementless total hip arthroplasty. Care was taken to avoid screw placement in the pelvis of this young woman, who intends to bear children. Note the good bone stock, proper fit of all components, and equal leg lengths.

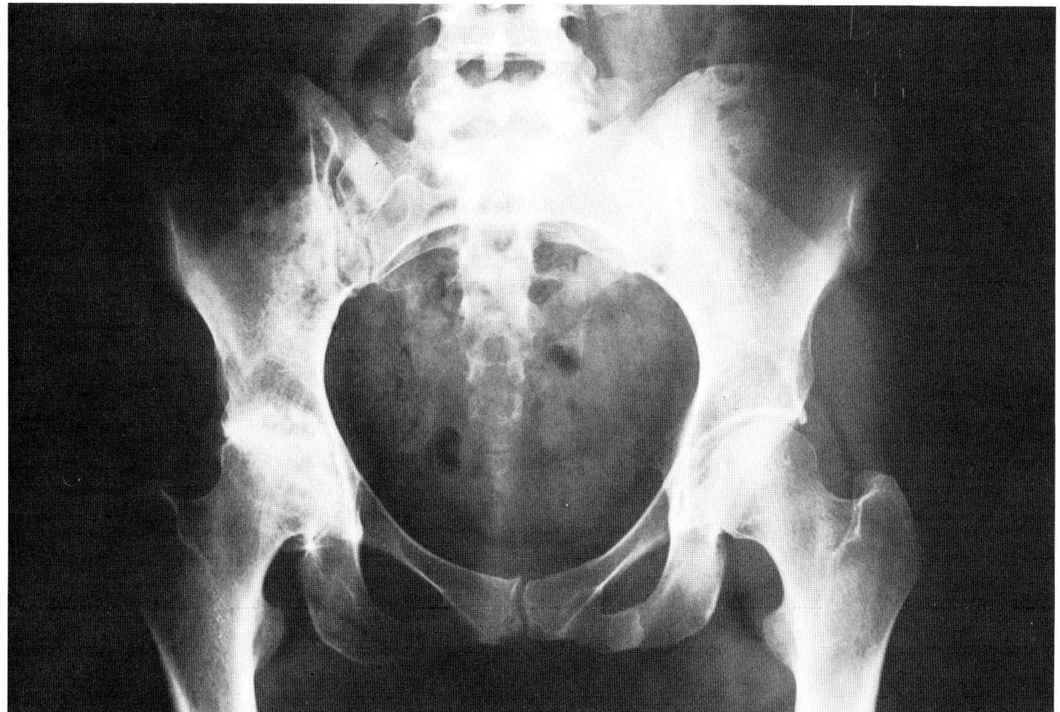

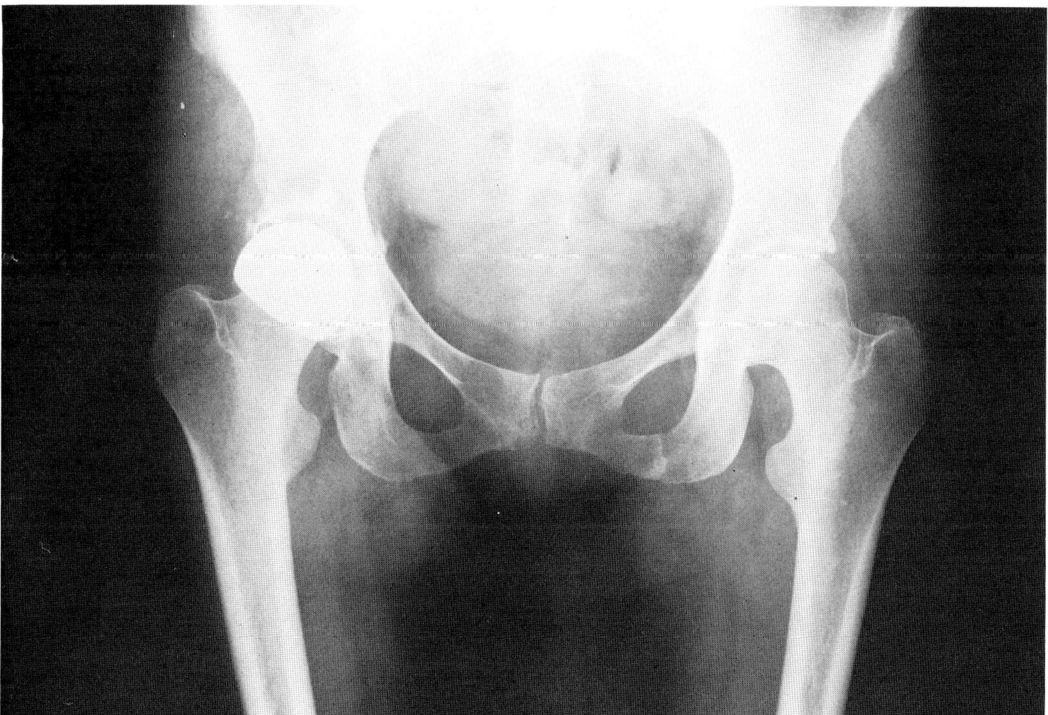

Fig. 13-22 **(A)** Preoperative roentgenogram demonstrates severe involvement of the right hip. **(B)** "Conservative" type total hip replacement prior to the onset of symptoms suggestive of failure. (*Figure continues.*)

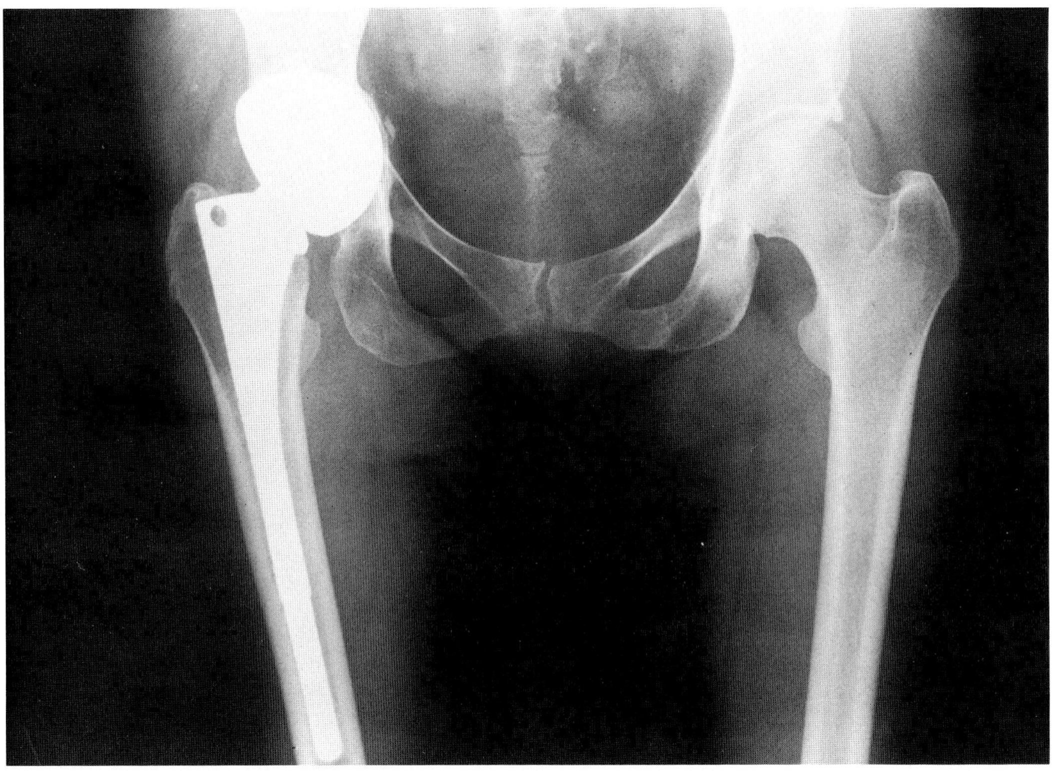

C

Fig. 13-22 (*Continued*). (**C**) Revision total hip arthroplasty. Note the large bipolar component and the thin, slightly protruded medial actabular wall.

REFERENCES

1. Aufranc OE: Constructive hip surgery with the vitallium mold: a report of 1,000 cases of arthroplasty of the hip over a 15-year period. J Bone Joint Surg [Am] 39:237, 1957
2. Bobyn JD, Engh CA: Human histology of the bone-porous metal implant interface. Orthopaedics 7:1410, 1984
3. Bombelli R, Santore R, Poss R: Mechanics of the normal and osteoarthritic hip. Clin Orthop 182:69, 1984
4. Charnley J: Arthroplasty of the hip; a new operation. Lancet 1:1129, 1961
5. Charnley J: Low friction arthroplasty. Clin Orthop 72:7, 1970
6. Clayton ML: Care of the rheumatoid hip. Clin Orthop 90:70, 1973
7. Clayton ML: Surgery of the lower extremity in rheumatoid arthritis. J Bone Joint Surg [Am] 45:1517, 1963
8. Clayton ML, Stringer T: Total hip arthroplasty with a new long-stem prosthesis. Clin Orthop 173:140, 1983
9. Clayton ML, Thirupathi RG: Dislocation following total hip arthroplasty: management by special brace in selected patients. Clin Orthop 177:154, 1983
10. Coventry MD, Beckenbaugh RD, Nolan DR, Ilstrup DM: 2012 Total hip arthroplasties: a study of postoperative course and early complications. J Bone Joint Surg [Am] 56:273, 1974
11. Cruess RL: Synovectomy of the hip in rheumatoid arthritis. p. 59. In Cruess RL, Mitchell NS (eds): Surgery of Rheumatoid Arthritis. 1971
12. Fackler CD, Poss R: Dislocation in total hip arthroplasties. Clin Orthop 182:109, 1984
13. Freeman PA: McKee-Farrar total replacement of the hip joint in rheumatoid arthritis and allied conditions. Clin Orthop 55:106, 1967
14. Galante J: Total joint arthroplasty without cement. Clin Orthop 176:2, 1983

15. Gschwend N: Surgical Treatment of Rheumatoid Arthritis. p. 174. George Thieme Verlag, Stuttgart, 1980

16. Harris WH: Traumatic arthritis of the hip after dislocation and acetabular fractures: treatment by mold arthroplasty. J Bone Joint Surg [Am] 51:737, 1969

17. Heywood AWB: Arthroplasty with a solid bone graft for protrusio acetabuli. J Bone Joint Surg [Br] 62:332, 1980

18. Jolley MN, Salvati E, Brown GC: Early results and complications of surface replacement of the hip. J Bone Joint Surg [Am] 64:366, 1982

19. Lord GA: Madreporique stemmed total hip replacement: five years' clinical experience. J R Soc Med 75:166, 1982

20. Mattingly DA, Hopson CN, Kahn A III, Giannestras NJ: Aseptic loosening in metal-backed acetabular components for total hip replacement: a minimum five-year follow-up. J Bone Joint Surg [Am] 67:387, 1985

21. McKee GK, Watson-Farrar J: Replacement of arthritic hips by the McKee-Farrar prosthesis. J Bone Joint Surg [Br] 48:245, 1966

22. Nelson JP: Musculoskeletal infection. Surg Clin North Am 60:213, 1980

23. Papenfus K, Clayton ML, Dennis DA et al: The Clayton total hip arthroplasty: a ten-year follow-up. Clin Orthop (in press)

24. Poss R, Maloney JP, Ewald FC et al: Six to 11-year results of total hip arthroplasty in rheumatoid arthritis. Clin Orthop 182:109, 1984

25. Poss R, Sledge CE: Surgery of the hip in rheumatoid arthritis. p. 2027. In Kelly WN, Harris ED, Ruddy S, Sledge CB (eds): Textbook of Rheumatology. 3rd Ed. WB Saunders, Philadelphia, 1989

26. Poss R, Thornhill TS, Ewald FC et al: Factors influencing the incidence and outcome of infection following total joint arthroplasty. Clin Orthop 182:120, 1984

27. Ring PA: Complete replacement arthroplasty of the hip by the Ring prosthesis. J Bone Joint Surg [Br] 50:720, 1968

28. Stauffer RN: 10-Year follow-up study of total hip replacement, with particular reference to roentgenographic loosening of the components. J Bone Joint Surg [Am] 64:983, 1982

29. Sutherland CJ, Wilde AH, Borden LS, Marks KE: A 10-year follow-up of 100 consecutive Muller curved-stem total hip-replacement arthroplasties. J Bone Joint Surg [Am] 64:970, 1982

30. Vainio K, Pulkki T: Rheumatoid arthritis of the hip. Presented to the Congress of the International League Against Rheumatism, Rome, 1961

31. Welch RB, Charnley S: Low friction arthroplasty of the hip in rheumatoid arthritis and ankylosing spondylitis. Clin Orthop 72:22, 1970

14

Management of the Rheumatoid Knee

Mack L. Clayton

The knee is one of the most common joints initially involved by rheumatoid arthritis, seen in approximately 20 percent of cases.[24] The involvement may remain monarticular for weeks or even years, but usually the disease process progresses to involve the opposite knee and continues to involve multiple other joints, becoming a generalized polyarticular disease. However, the knee is the most common joint involved in monarticular atypical rheumatoid arthritis.

The knee is a key joint for lower extremity function for activities for daily living. Most people, and particularly rheumatoid arthritics, sit more than they stand or walk; the most important function of the lower extremity has always been emphasized as stability, but in this modern age mobility is just as important and one should always strive to maintain or obtain mobility.

ANATOMY

The anatomy of the knee is different from that of other joints in that it is the largest joint in the body with the largest synovial cavity (Fig. 14-1). The knee joint should be thought of as a tricompartmental joint: medial femorotibial joint, lateral femorotibial joint, and patellofemoral joint. The large synovial cavity extends around the entire joint and up into the suprapatellar pouch as a single large synovium-lined cavity. It is designed to allow the relatively large range of motion from 0 to 145 degrees of flexion. The important ligaments around this joint are the medial collateral complex and the lateral collateral supporting structures, which provide stability against angular stresses. The anterior and posterior cruciate ligaments in the center of the joint are important for normal function. All of these ligaments are necessary for use of the knee when running, but most rheumatoid arthritic patients do not run. The anterior cruciate ligament is not necessary for walking. The posterior cruciate ligament is the strongest ligament in the body and important to normal gait and stair climbing or getting up from a chair.

Other important structures within the knee joint are the menisci or semilunar cartilages, which are wedge-shaped and essentially go around the tibial articulation medially and laterally, acting as shock absorbers. They increase the weight-bearing area of the flat or slightly convex tibia into a contoured surface to match the rounded femur. There is a fat pad at the inferior patella behind the patellar ligament, which is also synovium-lined. The synovium covers the cruciate ligaments as well.

The quadriceps muscle is the only extensor of the knee, with its insertion into the patella and the patellar ligament connecting the patella to the tibial tubercle. It is important to maintain this key function. Although it is the most significant muscle controlling knee motion, all of the muscu-

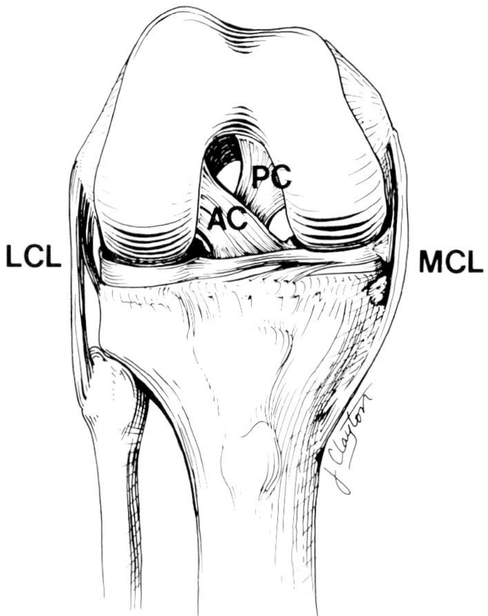

Fig. 14-1. Positions of the medial and lateral collateral ligaments (*MCL, LCL*) and the anterior and posterior cruciate ligaments (*AC, PC*).

lature is important. In general, the medial and lateral hamstrings are the flexors of the knee and control the important rotary element in the knee. The gastrocnemius musculature originates just above the posterior articular surface of the knee on the femur and helps provide posterior stability.

The knee is not a pure hinge joint. There is some rotation in the arc of motion as well as change in the axis of motion in that there is a gliding motion of the tibia on the femur as the knee is flexed and a partial hinging motion. The superb normal ligamentous complex around the knee provides stability in all ranges of flexion and extension.

There is considerable variation in the overall alignment of the knee regarding varus and valgus. Varus and valgus are commonly referred to as a measurement of the femorotibial angle (anatomic axis). This angle may be and frequently is determined by examining a small roentgenogram of the knee. Although this method is the usual way to measure these deformities, it is not a reliable one.

Of real interest is the mechanical axis (Fig. 14-2A), a line drawn through the center of the hip joint, center of the knee joint, and center of the ankle. Any deviation from this line is the true functional varus or valgus (Fig. 14-2B-C). The average or normal femur-tibia angle (anatomic axis) in a woman is about 8 or 9 degrees; in a man it is about 6 degrees. The ideal alignment for a knee is one that, when walking, causes no abnormal thrust in the mediolateral, anterior, or posterior direction. Of course, many people have a variation from the alignment mentioned, and the normal alignment in most men would be mildly toward a varus of the mechanical axis, which still represents a valgus of the anatomic axis. The mechanical axis is not the weight-bearing axis of the knee, as the normal center of gravity when walking is located to the side of S2. In a normal gait with a normal knee, weight-bearing is concentrated slightly to the medial tibial plateau area,

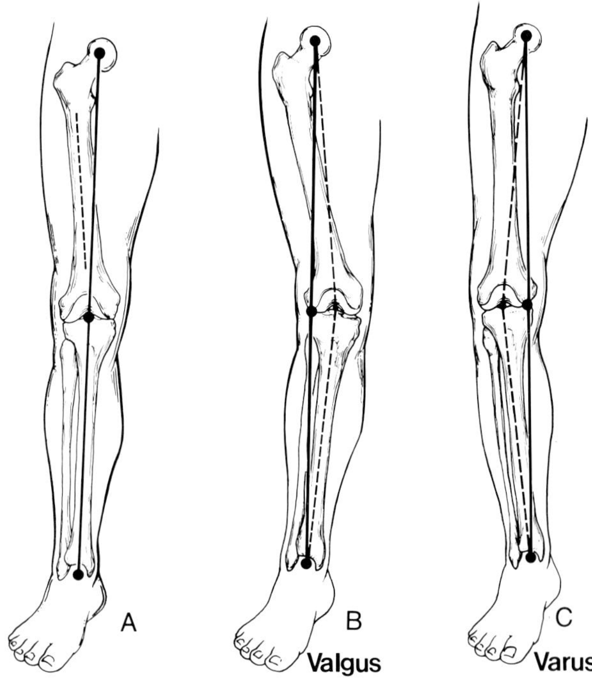

Fig. 14-2. (**A**) Normal mechanical axis. (**B & C**) Valgus alignment of the knee shifts weight laterally (dotted lines indicate mechanical axes for measurement). Varus alignment of the knee shifts weight medially.

which has a considerable larger weight-bearing area than the lateral tibial plateau.

DEFORMITIES

In patients with rheumatoid arthritis, the deformities that develop in the knee are often predisposed by the preexisting alignment of that joint in the individual patient. The common deformity that develops is valgus with flexion and external rotation because three-fourths of rheumatoid arthritic patients are women, and women tend to be in a more valgus position of the knees than men.

When the knee does become involved in rheumatoid arthritis patients, conservative treatment has the aim of controlling synovitis, thereby relieving pain, preserving function, and preventing deformities. Relative rest combined with range of motion exercises and isometric exercises to maintain full extension are important. The deformity that is most disabling in the leg is a flexion deformity of the knee. Part-time splinting and use of a cane or crutches may be prophylactic. Judicious intra-articular steroid injection can help control synovitis while the overall treatment plan is being instituted. Repeated injections (more than three or four per year) are not recommended and may be harmful. The aim is to prevent a flexion contracture of more than 10 degrees from developing. If the flexion contracture progresses, the disease in the knee is accelerated, and a flexion contracture often develops in the opposite knee, as it is difficult to walk with one knee in full extension and the other in fixed flexion. It is also necessary to control any hip flexion contracture and to ascertain that it is not the cause of a functional knee flexion deformity. Conversely, knee flexion contracture can also contribute to a hip flexion contracture.

As with other joints, there is a stiff type of rheumatoid arthritis,[2] and in these patients flexion contracture is more common without extensive synovial involvement.[3] The antithesis is the loose type of rheumatoid arthritic joint in which there is a progressive proliferative synovitis with

destruction of knee cartilage. In such joints motion is maintained and instability occurs. Flexion contracture is unusual, but the result is a knee that is unstable as well as painful and destroyed. With bony absorption and collapse, it can cause severe deformity.

Four factors contribute to the production of deformities in the rheumatoid knee: hip flexion deformity, synovial proliferation, contracture of the posterior capsular structures and ligaments, and abnormal bony configuration. The following sections present analyses of these knee flexion deformities and their treatment.

Knee Deformity Secondary to Hip Flexion (Type I)

Knee flexion deformity in the past commonly caused a patient to be confined to a wheelchair; and, conversely, any patient who has been wheelchair-bound for 6 months will have a knee flexion contracture. Sometimes a remission has been obtained in general arthritis patients, but the contracture is fixed and the patient unable to walk.

Flexion contracture in the 0- to 10-degree range is not a problem, but one of more than 20 degrees is a serious disability from a clinical standpoint. Therefore, 15 degrees is the approximate critical amount.[3] This clinical impression has been sustained by biomechanical analyses of pressure at the knee in various positions of flexion. The subpatellar pressure is minimal at 0 degrees, slightly increased at 15 degrees, and rises rapidly thereafter as flexion increases.[21]

When the standing flexion deformity of the knee is due to hip flexion contracture (Fig. 14-3), the hip must be corrected by conservative or operative means. If the knee flexion is a functional position, it can be fully extended in a semisitting position and no further knee treatment is necessary except exercises to maintain extension. The knee flexion deformity may also be due to other causes (see following sections). If hip and knee both have flexion deformity significant enough to require surgery, the hip should generally be corrected first.

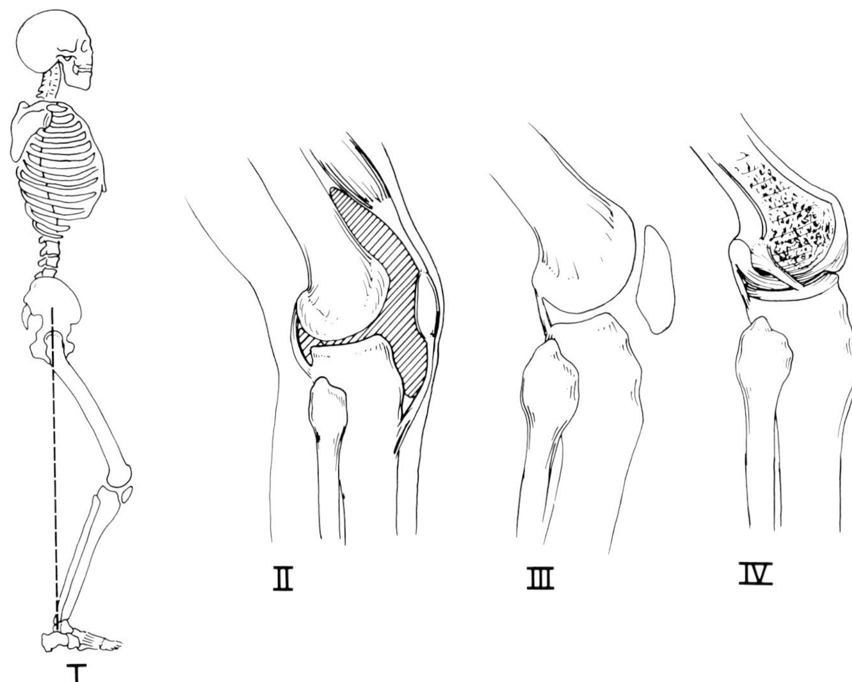

Fig. 14-3. Type I: functional flexion deformity of the knee due to hip flexion contracture. Type II: flexion deformity of the knee due to marked synovial proliferation. Type III: flexion deformity due to contraction of posterior structures; note posterior subluxation. Type IV: flexion deformity due to bony incongruity. Note incongruity with blocking of extension.

Knee Deformity Due to Synovial Proliferation (Type II)

Seventy-five percent of patients are female, and most of them tend to have a valgus alignment before their disease. The deformities developing, of course, depend a great deal on the type of joint before the arthritis develops. As a flexion contracture develops, the patient walks with flexion, valgus, and external rotation of the tibia. This gait is caused by distension of capsular structures by the synovitis and the forces acting on the joint. Although it has been described as a flexion-valgus-external rotation deformity, one should think of it in a global concept. It is a deforming force, with the foot fixed to the ground in the slightly externally rotated position and the body weight giving an increased thrust in the direction of flexion and valgus (Fig. 14-4). As the deformity progresses, the lateral knee flexors develop increased leverage for flexion and external

rotation, and the deformity perpetuates itself. The only specific way to control the progress is to control the synovitis and maintain full extension of the knee. Some patients learn to contract the muscles around the knee during the stance phase of gait with full extension of the knee, thus eliminating both the secondary deforming forces and painful friction. Some patients can be taught to walk this way, and it is an acceptable, barely discernible gait.

To help decrease the synovitis and maintain full extension, a resting cast or splint may be adjusted at intervals to help correct a mild flexion deformity. Rest alone helps diminish the synovitis, and a simple laced elastic knee support with side steels often alleviates pain. It is important to continue the active exercises.

Flexion contracture of up to 15 to 20 degrees can be due to synovial proliferation (Fig. 14-3). In such cases where there is preservation of articular cartilage, a synovectomy alone allows full

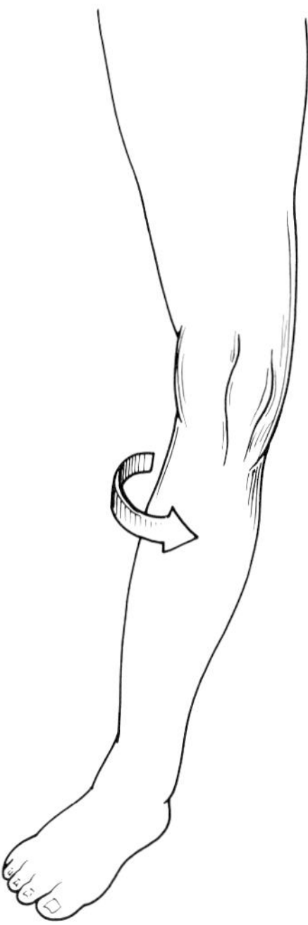

Fig. 14-4. Pathodynamic force leading to flexion, valgus, and external rotation deformity of the knee.

extension.[19] (Synovectomy is discussed in later pages.)

Deformity Resulting from Contracture of Posterior Capsule (Type III)

If posterior structures are contracted and joint cartilage is preserved, posterior release is indicated. Surgery for posterior release of the knee for flexion contracture was described by Wilson[28] in 1929 and Clayton[3] in 1963.

Surgical technique involves medial and lateral posterior incisions about 5 inches in length. The biceps tendon is lengthened in a Z fashion, and the peroneal nerve is protected. Gastrocnemius heads are released, and the posterior capsule is exposed completely from side to side. Posterior neurovascular structures are retracted gently with gauze. The capsule is incised about 2 cm above the tibia, with the incision continuing

slightly into the posterior portion of the collateral ligaments. If posterior subluxation persists (Fig. 14-3), the anterior cruciate ligament is released through the medial incision: With the knee flexed 90 degrees, a scissors is inserted into the lateral portion of the femoral condylar notch and the attachment released while an assistant performs an anterior drawer sign. It is rarely necessary to lengthen the medial hamstrings. In most cases the tensor fascia femoris (fascia lata) is divided transversely about 7.5 cm proximal to the knee joint (this step helps the correction of the external rotation and valgus deformity).

If the flexion contracture is mild and easily corrected, a long leg cast is applied. The cast is then bivalved or converted into a deep posterior shell within about 48 hours, and mobilization is begun with supervised physical therapy. The cast is used as a resting shell only (Fig. 14-5).

However, if a great deal of pressure is required, the deformity is more than 30 degrees, or full extension cannot be easily obtained, posterior subluxation is corrected through an upward pull on the proximal tibia using skeletal traction and a distal pin, both arranged to allow early motion.[3] Extensive pressure in a constant casted position leads to further cartilage damage and may also lead to peroneal palsy. Traction and early motion should encourage full extension within 10 to 14 days.

At the present time indications for posterior release alone are rare. A total knee arthroplasty is usually indicated in such cases, and a release can be an important part of the procedure; flexion contractures must be corrected during the operative procedure in a total knee arthroplasty. In unusual cases of more than 50 degrees flexion contracture, a posterior release may be necessary as a preliminary step of a total knee arthroplasty; complete extension is not necessary at the preliminary procedure. Such complex cases depend on the surgeon's experience as to how much can be safely corrected.

However, posterior release is still indicated in juvenile rheumatoid arthritis patients, especially before growth is complete. In these cases it is always important to release the iliotibial band to prevent progressive valgus with growth (Jakobowski, personal communication, 1972).[13]

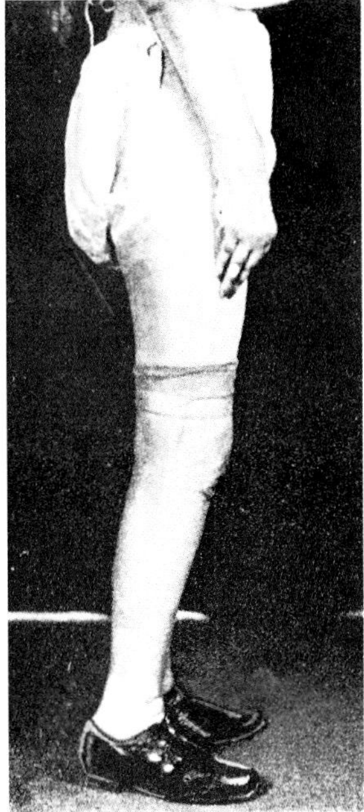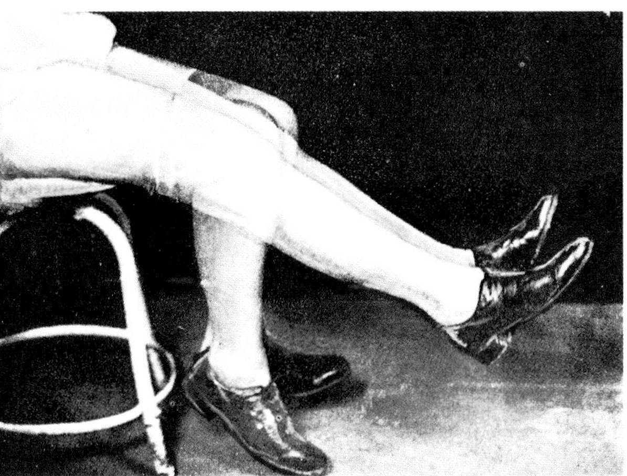

Fig. 14-5. A 55-year-old woman had been confined to a wheelchair for 6 months owing to rheumatoid arthritis flare-up in both knees. Preoperatively she had 55 degrees fixed flexion contractures bilaterally but some preservation of joint cartilage. Under anesthesia she extended easily to 30 degrees. Simple bilateral capsulotomy with release of anterior cruciate ligaments was performed at one operative procedure. This figure illustrates the condition 1 year postoperatively (retouched photograph). (Modified from Clayton et al.,[5] with permission.)

Knee Flexion Deformity Caused by Bone Changes (Type IV)

Flexion contracture due to bony configuration and cartilage destruction (Fig. 14-3) requires correction by either osteotomy or knee arthroplasty.[3] Today, total knee replacement is the usual procedure.

Extra-articular Synovial Cysts

Synovial involvement around the knee includes the bursae and the intra-articular synovitis. The bursae around the knee can be involved with rheumatoid synovitis, and the pathology of the synovium is the same whether it is in the bursa or the joint. The most commonly involved bursa is in the popliteal space, giving rise to a popliteal cyst.[15,16] With an active intra-articular synovitis, a popliteal cyst develops by way of an opening posteromedially just below the gastrocnemius origin (Fig. 14-6). Twelve percent of normal knees have communication from the joint into the popliteal area through this pathway. Also, with the development of rheumatoid synovitis and pressure, the synovitis may proceed through a preexisting opening or may develop a "rupture" of the synovium through this area. Fluid accumulates through this opening as the synovium proliferates, essentially as a one-way valve in that the fluid can go out but cannot come back. This cyst may become painful because of tension or may compress the deep veins and mimic thrombophlebitis (Fig. 14-7A). It is important to make the proper diagnosis; a venogram may be helpful (Fig. 14-7B). At times the cyst presents deep in the calf and is not palpable clinically, although it still gives rise to venous compression with distal edema.

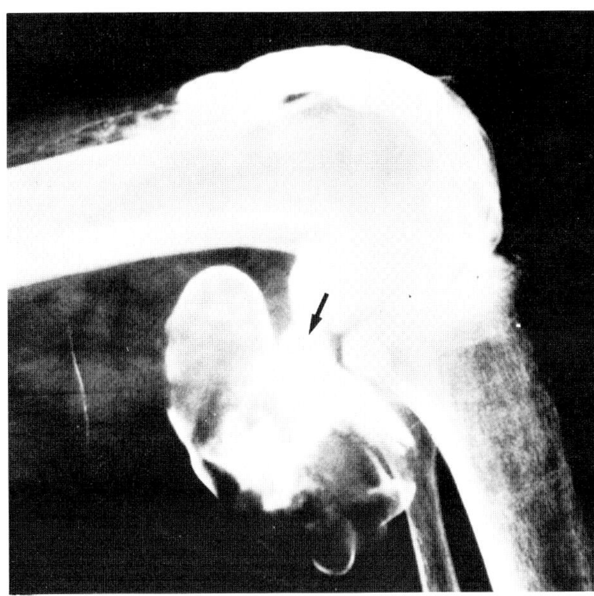

Fig. 14-6. Arthrogram of a rheumatoid knee. Note the passage of the dye through a "one-way" valve posteriorly (*arrow*) into the gastrocnemius-semimembranosis bursa, which has enlarged into the popliteal space and distally.

It is important to make the diagnosis, as several cases have been seen that were improperly treated with anticoagulants and had a hemorrhage into the cyst as a complication. Ultrasonography may help outline the cyst. A definitive diagnosis of thrombophlebitis should be obtained before anticoagulation treatment is started.

A steroid injection into the knee often provides temporary relief of both the intra-articular and cyst synovitis; local aspiration of the cyst provides a diagnosis, and a steroid injection temporarily calms the synovitis. In some cases the cyst is so small that it cannot be palpated, or it can be so large that it extends from above the knee to the level of the ankle (Fig. 14-7C & D). This popliteal cyst area is between the gastrocnemius and semimembranous, filling that bursa. As it extends, it usually dissects distally along the fascial planes, although it can dissect proximally as well.

Treatment of the symptomatic popliteal cyst in rheumatoid patients is by cyst excision and intra-articular treatment as indicated. In early stages with good articular cartilage, articular synovec-

tomy is the treatment of choice. When total knee arthroplasty is indicated, the cyst can be emptied and partially excised through the area of bone resection. These cysts do not recur.

OPERATIONS ACCORDING TO STAGE OF DISEASE

When conservative measures have failed to alter progression of the inflammatory process and control pain, and when deformities are increasing, treatment by surgical means should be considered. Procedures available for other rheumatoid joints are also used for surgical management of the knee. The most commonly employed include synovectomy, osteotomy, and arthroplasty.

Synovectomy

The knee has been the primary target of synovectomy through the years. It has the largest synovial cavity in the body and is superficial enough for easy evaluation of the synovial proliferation.

Indications for synovectomy of the knee are pain with marked synovial proliferation and an early stage of the disease where articular cartilage is preserved. There should also be a reasonable range of motion and stability of the joint, and the target joint should be involved out of proportion to other joints. The synovitis should have persisted despite good conservative treatment for 6 months or longer. The patient must be well educated and realize that the long-term result is unpredictable in any individual case. If a severe "malignant" type of disease is present, involving active synovitis of many joints, synovectomy is not indicated.

Technique
All synovium should be removed. Incisions are variable. We prefer medial and lateral short incisions (2.5 to 3.0 inches) with capsular incisions and additional medial capsular incisions posterior to the medial collateral ligament.[12,19] Today one must plan so the incisions allow for total

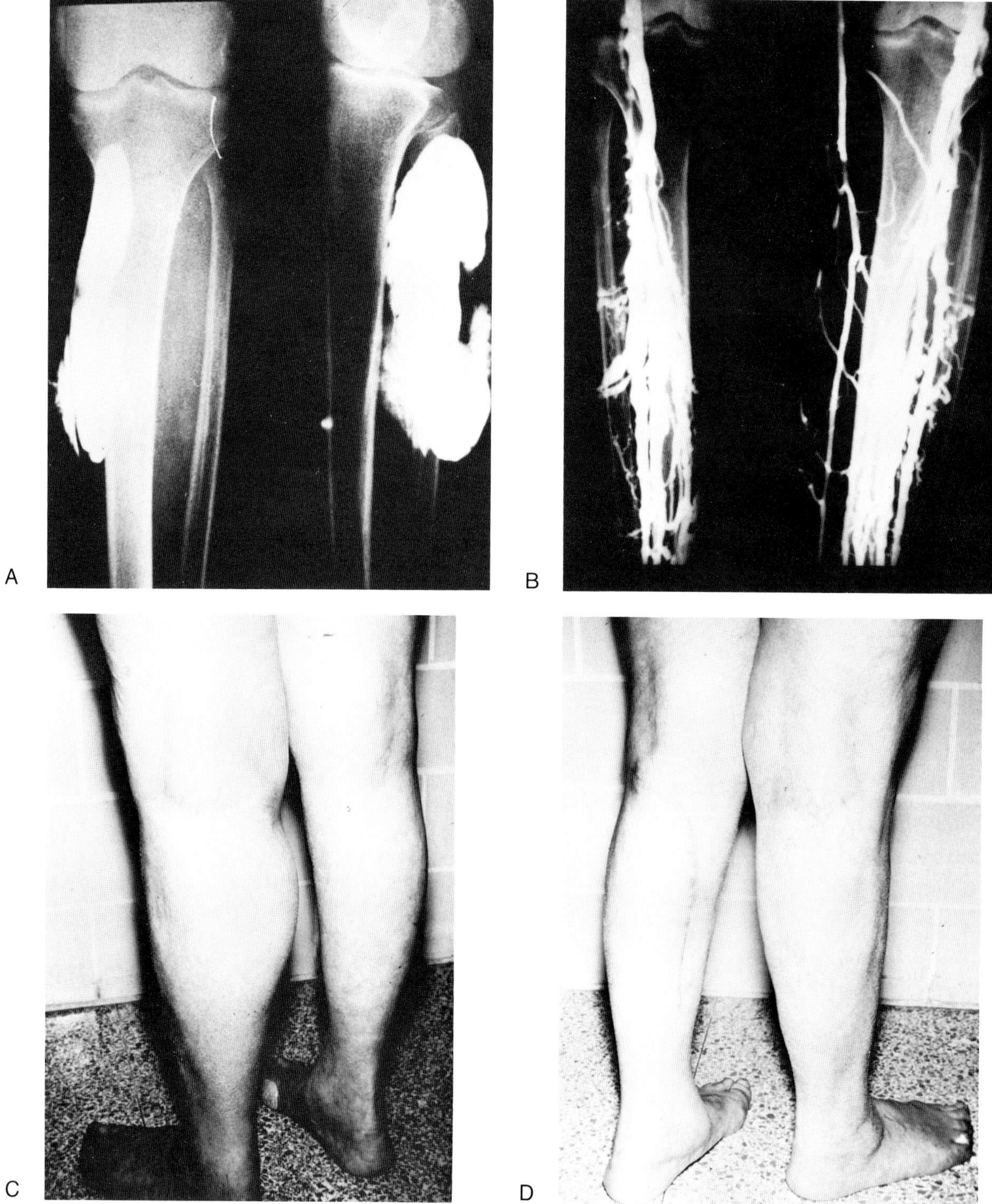

Fig. 14-7. **(A)** Large rheumatoid popliteal cyst with dissection far down the calf. This cyst was injected directly posteriorly to outline it, so it does not show the connection to the knee. **(B)** Venogram later revealed no evidence of active thrombophlebitis. **(C)** Preoperative photograph of the swollen calf. **(D)** Postoperative condition. Note the normal appearance of the calf after excision. (Today we would recommend intra-articular synovectomy at the same procedure.)

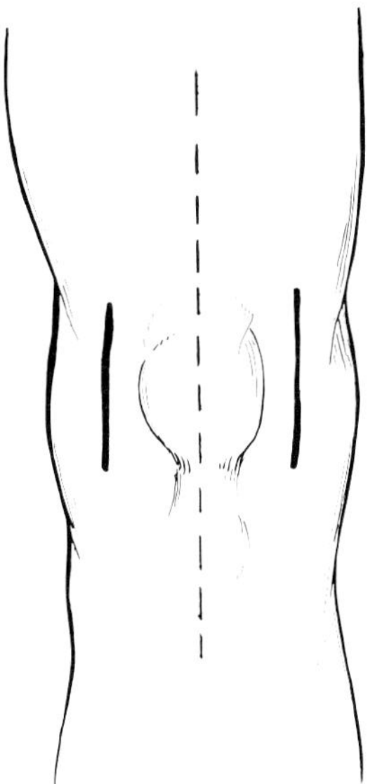

Fig. 14-8. Incision for synovectomy. Note the short medial and lateral skin incisions. Dotted line indicates the single long medial skin incision that may be utilized later if total knee arthroplasty is necessary.

knee arthroplasty in the future; a single long anterior incision may also be used (Fig. 14-8). The short medial and lateral incisions are far enough from the patella to allow a straight midline incision later if necessary. Surgeons should use the incision with which they are most comfortable. Synovium is removed one section at a time, and the synovium is separated in part just under the retinaculum before entering the joint proper.

The thickened synovium is easily peeled away, including the suprapatellar pouch, by dissecting upward through relatively small capsular incisions. It is important to preserve the yellow fat over the distal femur to provide a gliding surface. (Fat is the paratenon of large joints—and "fat is your friend.") If the menisci show marked involvement, they should be excised. Ronguers are useful for removing synovium from cruciate ligaments, which are usually found to be intact. The anterior cruciate ligament is destroyed in a few cases, but the posterior one is almost always intact, as it is almost extracapsular. Ronguers are also utilized to clean the posterior medial compartment through the posteromedial capsular incision. The posterior lateral compartment can be

exposed and cleared through the anterior lateral incision by placing the heel on the opposite mid-tibia ("figure four" position); a pituitary rongeur is helpful. It is important to clear synovium and pannus from the articular margins and the popliteus tendon (Fig. 14-8).

In later cases osteophytes should be débrided and rough surfaces smoothed. Patellectomy was often performed in the past but is rare today because convalescence is slower and results are poorer if total knee arthroplasty is necessary later.

Postoperative Care

Suction drainage is used for 24 to 48 hours, and the capsule is closed with nonabsorbable sutures. Early motion is important. Continuous passive motion (CPM) is an excellent adjunct, as motion can be gained rapidly with it. If CPM is not used, the patient is immobilize for 2 days and then active supervised physical therapy is begun. If motion is inadequate (<70 degrees) at 1 week, the knee is manipulated under anesthesia and injected locally with steroid: 1 ml prednisolone tebutate (Hydeltra-TBA). Prior to the mid-1970s 90 degrees flexion was considered adequate, but not today. Early and continued active mobilization prevents loss of motion.

Mobilization on crutches with partial (40 to 60 pounds) weight-bearing is utilized. Full weight-bearing is deferred for 3 to 6 weeks to allow muscle rehabilitation and the nutrition of the articular cartilage to return to normal.

Synovectomy with Popliteal Cyst

If there is a popliteal cyst present, it should be removed at the time of articular synovectomy (either open or arthroscopic). A small cyst may regress after synovectomy including the posteromedial compartment. A large cyst is less predictable regarding regression and should at least have its gross lining removed and the capsule decompressed into the fat and muscle; recurrence is rare. The small thin-walled cyst is similar to the usual nonrheumatoid popliteal cyst, which subsides with correction of the intra-articular pathology. However, chronic rheumatoid synovitis can develop into a thick-walled large synovial cavity that may be self-perpetuating and should be excised. At the very least, the proximal area near the knee joint should be excised and the cyst decompressed. Rheumatoid synovitis recurs to some degree in one-half of the patients within 2 years, if untouched the cyst may recur as well.[11]

The arthroscope is useful for synovectomy. For example, a 57-year-old man had had active rheumatoid arthritis for 10 years. He had had a painful left knee for 1 year with 2+ effusion, 3+ synovitis, 10 to 130 degrees motion, good stability, a small popliteal cyst, and roentgenographic stage II disease (minimal joint narrowing). Arthroscopy revealed proliferative synovitis into all compartments and the "corner" of the joint, meniscal involvement, and good articular cartilage with minimal changes (stage II). Arthroscopic synovectomy would not allow as complete an operation as indicated in this case, so open operation was performed. Medial and lateral incisions were made, including a posteromedial capsular incision. A complete synovectomy was also done, including the posterior compartment and partial removal of the popliteal cyst. Both menisci were involved and removed. CPM was utilized, and the patient obtained 90 degrees flexion within 3 days and was discharged on crutches. He regained full motion (0 to 135 degrees) and was pain-free at 2 years.

Arthroscopic synovectomy is being utilized in many centers today and is presented as a simple procedure that is associated with minimal morbidity, rapid regaining of motion, and relief from pain and swelling. A comparative study from Japan[17] showed slightly better results from arthroscopic synovectomy than from open synovectomy after several years. Synovectomy is not as complete as with the described open procedure, but if the surgeon is "arthroscopically oriented" it is a useful procedure.

As many as six arthroscopic portals may be indicated: superior medial and lateral, midmedial and lateral, and anteromedial and lateral (Fig. 14-9). Posteromedial and posterolateral portals also may be helpful. A high-speed, reversible, 4.5 mm synovial power resector is an essential tool. The resector should be a wide-opening side cutter (Fig. 14-9, inset). A high flow technique makes this procedure easier.

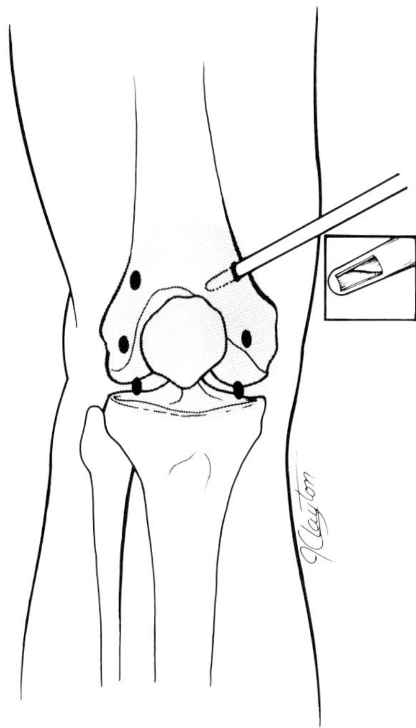

Fig. 14-9. Location of the six portals useful for arthroscopic synovectomy. **(Inset)** Synovial resector—an essential power tool for arthroscopic synovectomy. (From Mack and Clayton,[16] with permission.)

The arthroscopic synovectomy is best done systematically with wide, sweeping, semicircular movements pivoting around each portal. Synovial resection should be started in the suprapatellar pouch (medial and lateral) using the midanterior parapatellar portals (medial and lateral). The synovium is resected anteriorly to the joint line, including the fat pad as necessary. Using the anteromedial and lateral portals, the synovium can be resected from the medial and lateral gutters, the medial and lateral capsule, and under the medial and lateral meniscus (small end cutter, 2.8 mm). The arthroscope may be pushed through the notch into the posterior compartments; then with posteromedial and lateral portals the synovial resector can be introduced and posterior synovectomy performed.

Because of the extensive surface area involved, considerable bleeding may be encountered postoperatively. A large Hemovac drain and compression dressing may help prevent a postoperative hematoma. Early range of motion is facilitated by CPM, usually started on the first postoperative day. Ambulation with crutches or walker is started on day 2 with partial weight-bearing. Active range of motion and quadriceps isometric exercises are also begun on day 2. After arthroscopic synovectomy the patient generally regains preoperative motion rapidly, and manipulation is seldom required. Full weight-bearing is delayed until the patient demonstrates satisfactory range of motion and good quadriceps strength.

At the present time the popularity of synovectomy is at a low ebb in the United States, but we believe it will increase in the future.[25] (See Chapter 8.)

Osteotomy

Osteotomy above or below the knee is indicated to realign an angular deformity in a rare case of "burned out" inactive rheumatoid arthritis that essentially represents an osteoarthritis. The osteotomy functions to realign the weight-bearing, distribute pressures, and relieve pain. There should be some good articular cartilage remaining that can benefit from the weight redistribution.

The usual rheumatoid deformity is valgus with flexion and external rotation, which can be corrected by a supracondylar osteotomy.[3] Rigid internal fixation allows early motion. A good range of motion (70+ degrees) should be present, as osteotomy does not increase the range of motion but transfers it to a more functional range. Proximal tibial osteotomy is indicated for varus deformity; only a mild (10 degrees) flexion deformity should be corrected at the same time.

Many of the osteotomies were followed by a decrease in synovial activity for a period of time. It was due to relative rest after the procedure and to less stress on the knee after realignment. The procedure is rare today because the usual rheumatoid arthritic with angular deformity requires realignment and resurfacing, which can best be obtained with a total knee arthroplasty. In a personal series, good results were obtained early; but with active disease, most of them gradually deteriorated.[5]

Supracondylar Osteotomy of the Femur

Supracondylar osteotomy demands early motion to prevent stiffness due to binding of the gliding structures of the knee in the suprapatellar area.[3] A lateral skin incision with forward reflection of the vastus lateralis exposes the entire lateral shaft; the lateral side of the joint is opened, and synovectomy and débridement are performed as necessary. The osteotomy site about 2.5 inches above the joint level is outlined with multiple drill holes using one main lateral drill hole and changing the angle to produce many medial holes. (This type of osteotomy is almost performed with a drill.) Additional holes are drilled laterally.

The blade plate is inserted halfway into the femur. The position of the plate is determined by holding the leg in the deformed position of the valgus and flexion and then inserting the plate parallel to the lower leg (Fig. 14-10). The drill holes for osteotomy are next connected with an osteotome, and the proximal end of the femur is shaped with a rongeur as necessary for contact and impaction. After the osteotomy is completed, the leg is straightened. The nail is driven until the plate is flush. A few degrees of rotation can be accomplished as necessary and the plate clamped. Compression must be utilized with care because the bone can be "shattered." With screws added, the fixation is stable. A few degrees overcorrection is obtained by this simple alignment mechanism. Surgeons should use any system with which they are comfortable and can obtain proper alignment with rigid internal fixation to allow early motion.[3] The A-O system is excellent.[20] Overcorrection should be slight: 0 to 4 degrees beyond the mechanical axis. Often a long leg brace (cast brace) is utilized at 2 weeks; weight-bearing is limited until union occurs, about 4 months. The brace is continued with free motion for a number of months, after which the patients keep the brace ready and use it for intermittent flare-ups in the knee (Fig. 14-11).

The proximal tibial osteotomy for varus is performed by removing a lateral wedge of proper height to correct and overcorrect the mechanical axis 2 to 4 degrees. Osteotomy is just above the tibial tubercle, and the proximal one-half of the

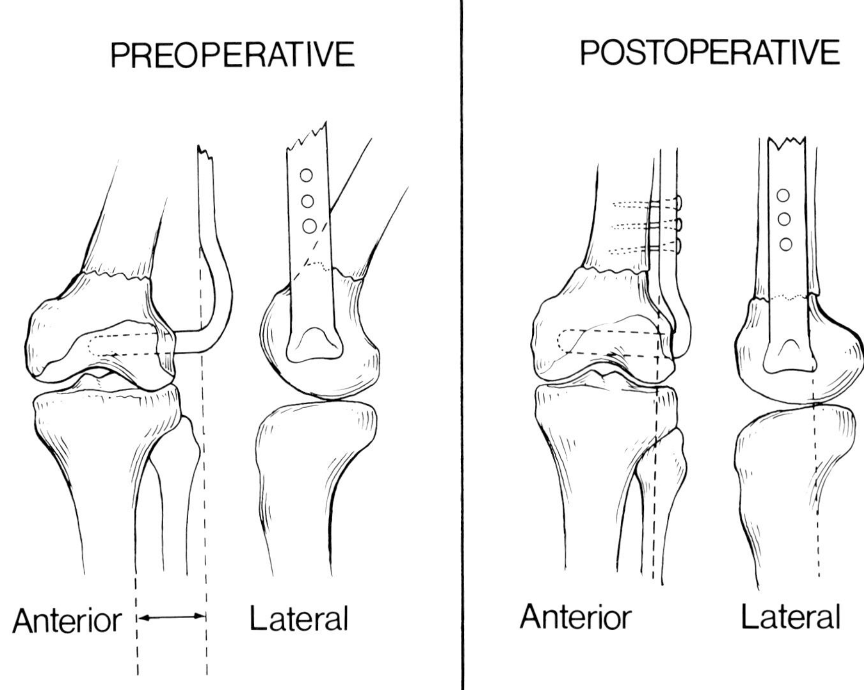

Fig. 14-10. Note placement of the blade plate before completing the osteotomy to correct both valgus and flexion. (From Clayton et al.,[3] with permission.)

fibular head is removed. The osteotomy is closed, staples are used for fixation, and a long knee splint is applied. A long leg cylinder cast is applied at about 1 week and is left in place until 6 weeks after operation. Supervised therapy helps mobilization; a cast-brace may allow early motion if good fixation is obtained.

These same operative techniques are used much more often today for osteoarthritis than rheumatoid arthritis. "The surgery for rheumatoid arthritis is not different; it is the rheumatoid arthritic patient who is different" (MLC).

Osteotomy of the knee for realignment of angular deformity in rheumatoid arthritis provides good results for a certain period of time depending on disease activity.[5] The only long-lasting results have been in relatively inactive, "burned out" cases. Today, patients with angular deformity are treated by total knee arthroplasty, at which time local synovectomy, realignment, and resurfacing are accomplished.

Arthroplasty

The most common surgical procedure for rheumatoid arthritis of the knee is total knee arthroplasty. In fact, it is probably the most common procedure for rheumatoid arthritis. The indications are pain with loss of weight-bearing articular cartilage (stage III or IV) and a lack of response to a general treatment regimen. Instability and angular deformity accentuate the pain by increasing the pressure of weight-bearing. Hip deformity may also emphasize the problem. Failed synovectomy, osteotomy, or hemiarthroplasty are also indications.

Historical Evolution
Arthroplasty of the knee began with resection and interposition with soft material such as fascia, cutis (skin), or nylon. Partial arthroplasty was performed with metallic replacement of the patella, femur, or tibial articular surface; these op-

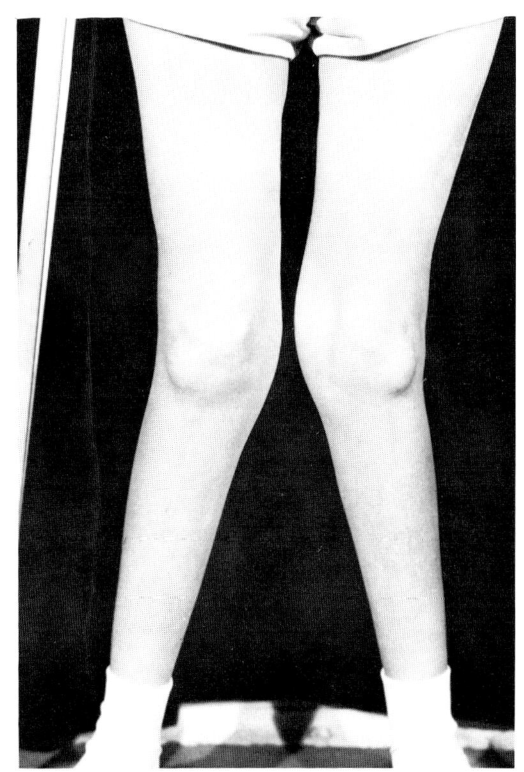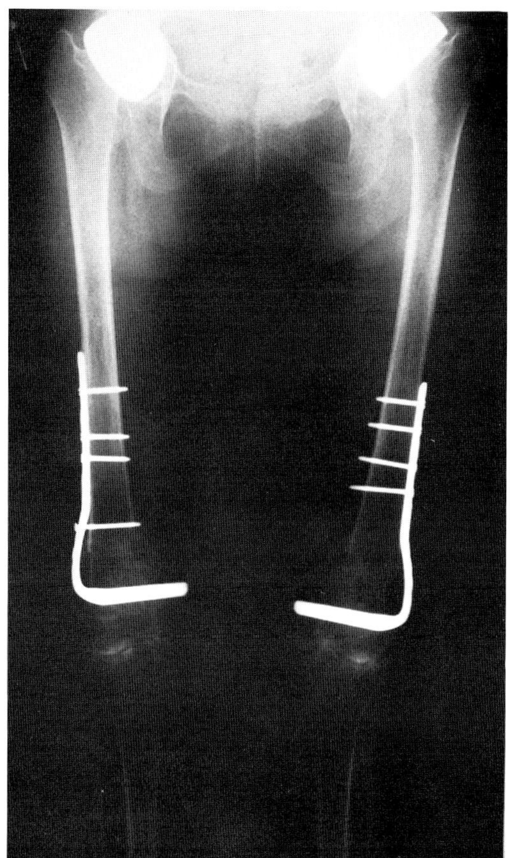

A   B

Fig. 14-11. **(A)** Preoperative stage IIIB knees and hips. Note the marked valgus with flexion deformity. **(B)** Roentgenogram shows bilateral cup arthroplasties followed by bilateral supracondylar osteotomies (operations done one at a time). Note overall alignment of the legs, which functioned for more than 10 years, at which time the left knee required further surgery.

erations are of historical interest, as they are not in use today. Even if reasonably good results were reported, the procedures continued to be modified.

Our personal experience with knee arthroplasty began in 1963 with a rigid hinge prosthesis of the Young type,[29] which was custom-made and required a patellectomy (Fig. 14-12). Later this prosthesis was modified to contain a patellar flange. Rigid Walldius hinges were also later utilized with and without cement. All had loosening problems, and most have been revised.

In 1966 hemiarthroplasties of the MacIntosh type were utilized with "satisfactory" early results (Fig. 14-13). In 1972 the Geomedic total knee using cement (Fig. 14-14) was employed with good or excellent results (18 of 20 rheumatoid arthritic knees were excellent after 2 years).[4] It did not allow patellar replacement and was too constrained, however. The early total knee replacements bore little resemblance to a normal knee.[12] They have largely been replaced, and the current trend is toward use of an "anatomic" knee. Of note is that most of the femoral components now in use are similar to Aufranc's Massachusetts General Hospital femoral prosthesis developed more than 30 years ago.[13,14]

In 1976 the total condylar knee was used with

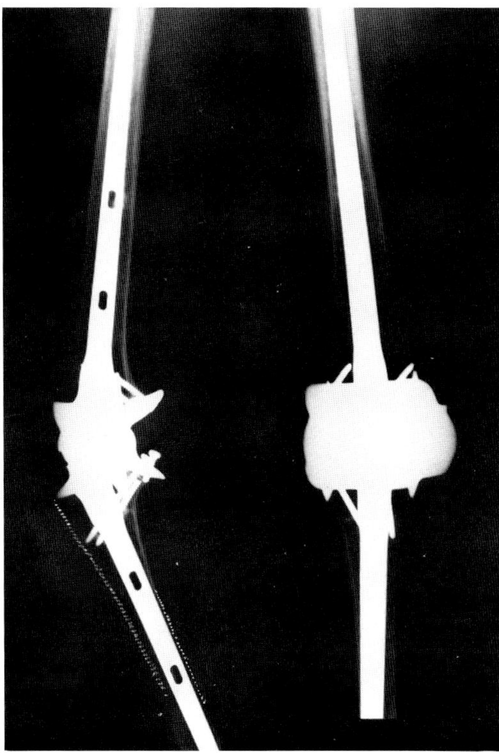

Fig. 14-12. Young hinge roentgenogram 26 years after insertion. Patient had 70 degrees of motion; but with the broken screw, patient has slight pain and loosening. Revision may be needed.

our modification to allow preservation of the posterior cruciate ligament[10] (Fig. 14-15). The Miller multiradius knee (a condylar type) was utilized in 1980 with low viscosity cement. The metal-backed tibial component enhanced cement fixation with a sintered surface. Low viscosity cement (LVC) is injected into the cancellous bone for micro interlock. Five years of experience with this artificial knee has revealed no progressive radiolucent lines at the bone–cement interface. This knee also is posterior cruciate sparing; it is semiconstrained with cupping of the tibia and must be inserted with a 10 degree posterior tilt. The average range of motion obtained was 108 degrees.

Other models have been introduced since 1984 that are designed for cement use or ingrowth, are posterior cruciate sparing, are less constrained, and have more sizes available (Fig. 15-13). Many sizes are available to obtain complete coverage of the tibia and proper fit of the femur. Some are modular and can be used as nonconstrained, partially constrained, or posteriorly stabilized devices.

The systems are probably no better than the surgeon's ability to insert them in individual patients. Results depend on the alignment of the leg and the prosthesis at the time of insertion, proper technique for bone and soft tissue, and the patient's ability to cooperate. There are a number of similar fine total knee systems available today. They are all condylar types and basically look the same. At the present time, we do not generally recommend ingrowth prostheses for rheumatoid arthritis because of the reproducible success of cement. (See Chapter 13, p. 12.) Osteoporosis is also part of the pathology in most cases. (The young patient with good bone stock is an exception.) In our experience, the average range of motion attained is 113 degrees with these newer modular protheses. There has been only a minimal difference in results beginning with the total condylar prosthesis in 1976. More than 90 percent have good or excellent results.

The prostheses mentioned are those that have been employed for the usual primary case. Salvage type cases with severe bone or ligament loss and revision procedures require a more constrained prosthesis. Rigid hinges are not now recommended.

There are revision prostheses that are partially constrained and provide reasonable stability. The Insall-Berstein posterior stabilized cemented revision prosthesis requires removal of little bone and is an excellent revision prosthesis; the porous-coated anatomic (PCA) revision can be used but has less stability. The old circle still exists: the more constraint, the more stability, which probably leads to more loosening. However, surgeons should use a model with which they are most familiar. Revision arthroplasty requires considerable experience. Hopefully, fewer revisions will be necessary as better original operations are performed (Fig. 14-15).

Because of better results since 1976, we have routinely performed patellar replacement, and it has been noted that a few patients with rheumatoid arthritis have had a recurrence of rheuma-

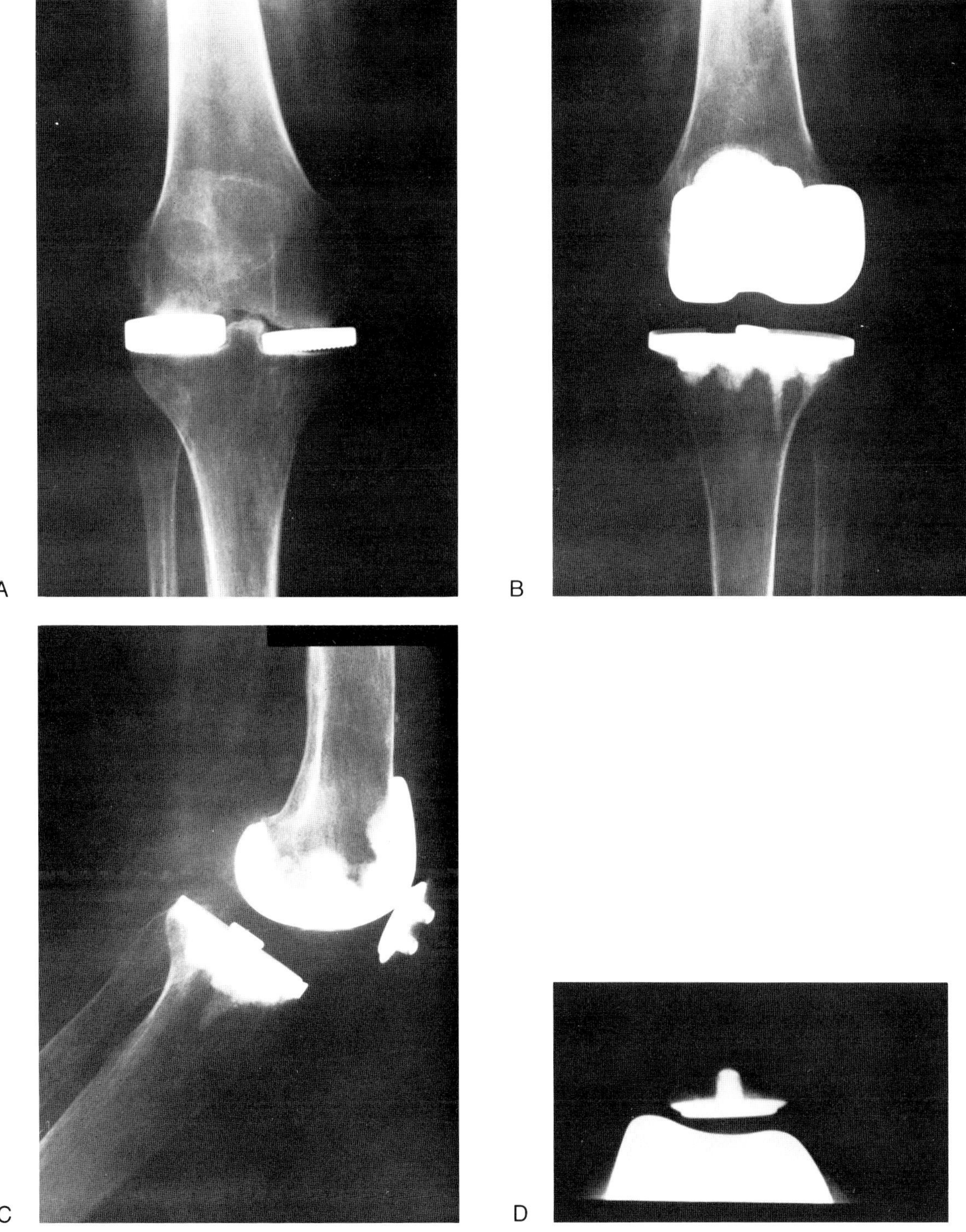

Fig. 14-13. (**A**) McIntosh tibial plateau replacements. Patient had good function for 14 years, but severe pain returned. (**B–D**) Revision to Miller Galante knee. Note the injected cement with irregular interlock to the cancellous bone. There was excellent function 6 years later. She has a contralateral ankylosed knee.

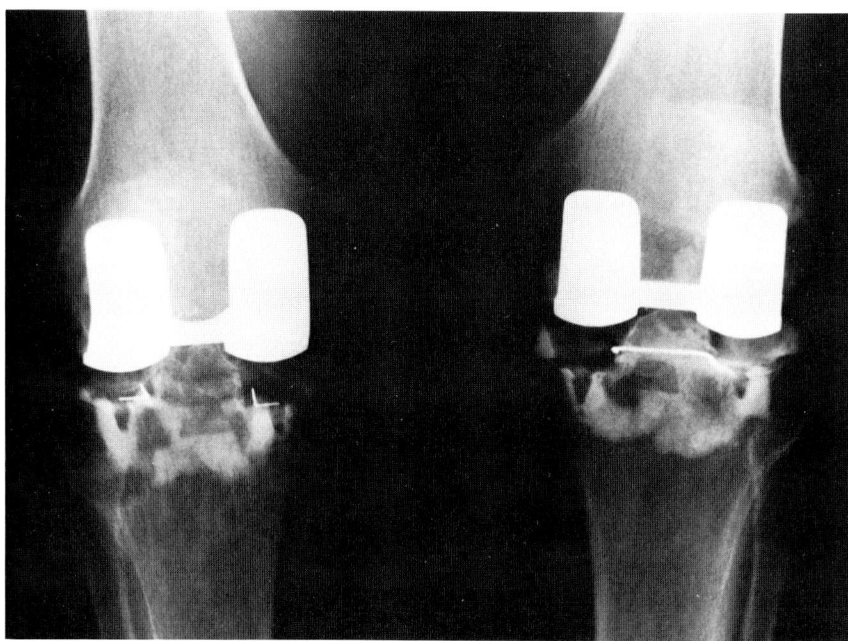

Fig. 14-14. Geomedic knees functioning well after 15 years.

toid synovitis if the patella had not been replaced. It appears that the rheumatoid synovial process requires articular cartilage to trigger the process. With the usual cemented knee, a plastic-only (non-metal-backed) patella is preferred.

The ancillary items used include intermittent compression air boots to prevent thromboembolism and continuous passive motion machines to gain motion more rapidly after surgery.

Evaluation and General Technique for Total Knee Arthroplasty

The indication for total knee arthroplasty is *pain*, loss of function despite good medical treatment, and loss of joint cartilage (stage IIIb or IV). Surgery is indicated when these factors interfere with the patient's way of life.

The general principles we have found to produce the best results are discussed here.[8] Many types of instrumentation are available. Every major total knee replacement system has an instrumentation recommended, and many are excellent. The surgeon should become familiar with the instrumentation but not be totally dependent on it.

Total knee arthroplasty for rheumatoid arthritis gives relief of pain for walking and enough mo-

tion for comfortable sitting. Ninety degrees flexion was an originally stated aim but is not enough for an excellent result. Approximately 200 degrees of combined hip and knee motion are necessary to get out of a chair easily. For a person of average 5 feet 6 inches height, the motion must be fairly evenly distributed.

The posterior cruciate ligament is the strongest ligament in the body. It is advised that it be preserved to prevent posterior subluxation yet allow knee flexion well beyond 90 degrees, thereby allowing better extension strength and stair-climbing ability. If necessary, the total knee replacement can then be slightly looser in flexion than extension and still be stable if the posterior cruciate is preserved. In full extension for weight-bearing, the knee is stable, and laxity in flexion encourages easier increased flexion without posterior subluxation. The tibial articular surface should be tipped slightly (up to 10 degrees) posteriorly, as is the normal knee. If the posterior cruciate is damaged, insufficient, or unsalvageable, a posterior stabilized type of knee is recommended, and collateral ligaments are balanced in flexion and extension.

The true key to success in a total knee arthroplasty is absolute alignment. Failure to obtain

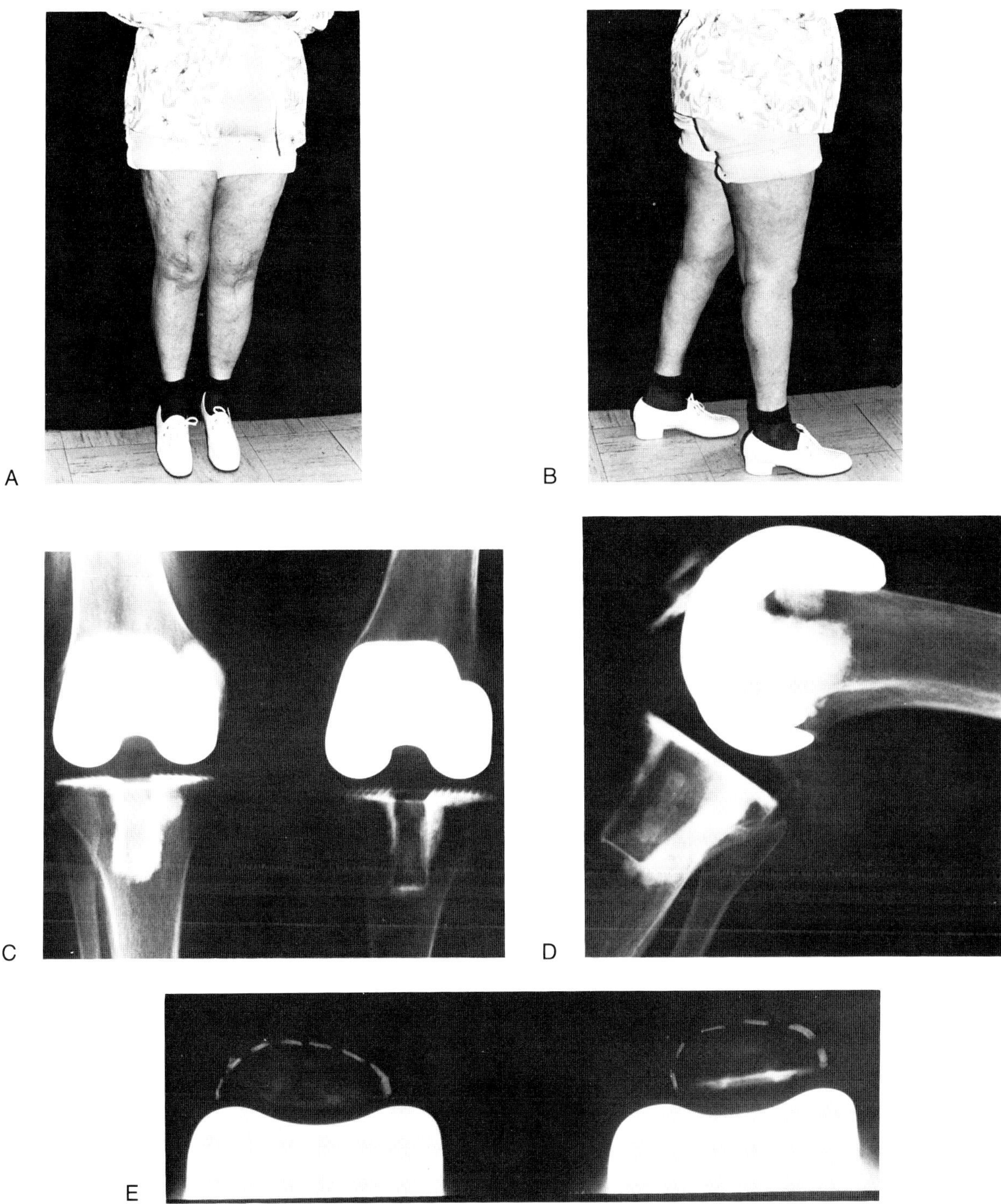

Fig. 14-15. Fourteen years after bilateral total condylar knee replacement (postcruciate saving). There are no signs of loosening; patella is well centered; and alignment is along the mechanical axis. She has 105 degrees of motion with no pain and no limp.

perfect alignment often means potential trouble. The mechanical axis (Fig. 14-2A) is the aim, with the center of the ankle, knee, and hip in a straight line. This alignment is empiric and does not portray the weight-bearing line. Total knee replacements have even-sized medial and lateral compartments, whereas the normal knee has a larger medial compartment weight-bearing area. Weight-bearing should be in full extension, which with the anteroposterior alignment allows weight-bearing with no abnormal movement either mediolaterally or anteroposteriorly. Alignment of the individual prosthetic components on the bony surfaces is also important and is illustrated in each manufacturer's technique brochure.

ROENTGENOGRAMS

Patients considered for surgery have the following films taken: 34 inches standing long-leg anteroposterior (Fig. 14-16A), lateral (Fig. 14-16B), tunnel (Fig. 14-16C), axial (Merchant) films (Fig. 14-16D), and varus (Fig. 14-16E) and valgus (Fig. 14-16F) stress films of the affected knee. A separate anteroposterior view of the pelvis is obtained to check for hip disease and proximal femur deformity (Fig. 14-16G). If the hips are well documented on the long film, a separate pelvic film can be omitted.

The standing long-leg film is taken with the patient placing weight on the affected side, as when walking (both feet touch the floor) (Fig. 14-16A). The stress films (Figs. 14-16E & F) record the amount of passive correctability of varus or valgus deformities. They also show the true thickness of the remaining cartilage joint spaces and indicate the maximum amount of collateral laxity present. They help to show, in conjunction with the tunnel view, the amount of bone loss present.

We plan for a specific type and size of prosthesis before surgery using these evaluation methods. The level of bone resection and estimated degree of soft-tissue release needed for realignment are planned before surgery, and the need for a special or custom-made prosthesis is recognized in advance. The series of films mentioned above were helpful in the preoperative planning for patients who were osteotomy candidates. This type of thorough preoperative evaluation aids in choosing between an osteotomy and a total joint arthroplasty in some cases.

Soft-tissue releases aid in exposure and in obtaining proper alignment for total knee arthroplasty utilizing any of the instrumentation systems.[8]

SURGICAL TECHNIQUE

Each total knee system and each surgeon has his or her "own" instrumentation and should use that with which he or she is most satisfied. Our preferred method is described in detail.

An electrocardiogram terminal marker is placed over the center of the femoral head using roentgenographic control. Unless circulation is poor, a tourniquet is used. An intraoperatively intermittent compression pumping system is utilized on the opposite leg during surgery and both legs postoperatively. Minimal impervious drap-

---

Fig. 14-16. **(A)** Long-leg weight-bearing film. Note the varus, marked narrowing medially, and some depression of the medial tibial plateau. **(B)** Lateral view. **(C)** Tunnel view. Note that the medial joint narrowing and bone loss are well emphasized on this view. **(D)** Axial view of the patella. Patellofemoral joint shows good alignment and a mild osteophyte laterally on the femur. **(E)** Varus stress films shows medial narrowing with slight "rocking" but good lateral ligament stability. **(F)** Valgus stress film shows the extent to which the varus can be passively corrected, the medial ligament stability, the joint spacing remaining laterally, and the medial bone loss and "rocking" on tibial spines. **(G)** Anteroposterior view of the pelvis shows mild varus conformation but essentially normal hip joints. (Hips are not visualized on the long film in this case.) (From Clayton et al.,[8] with permission.)

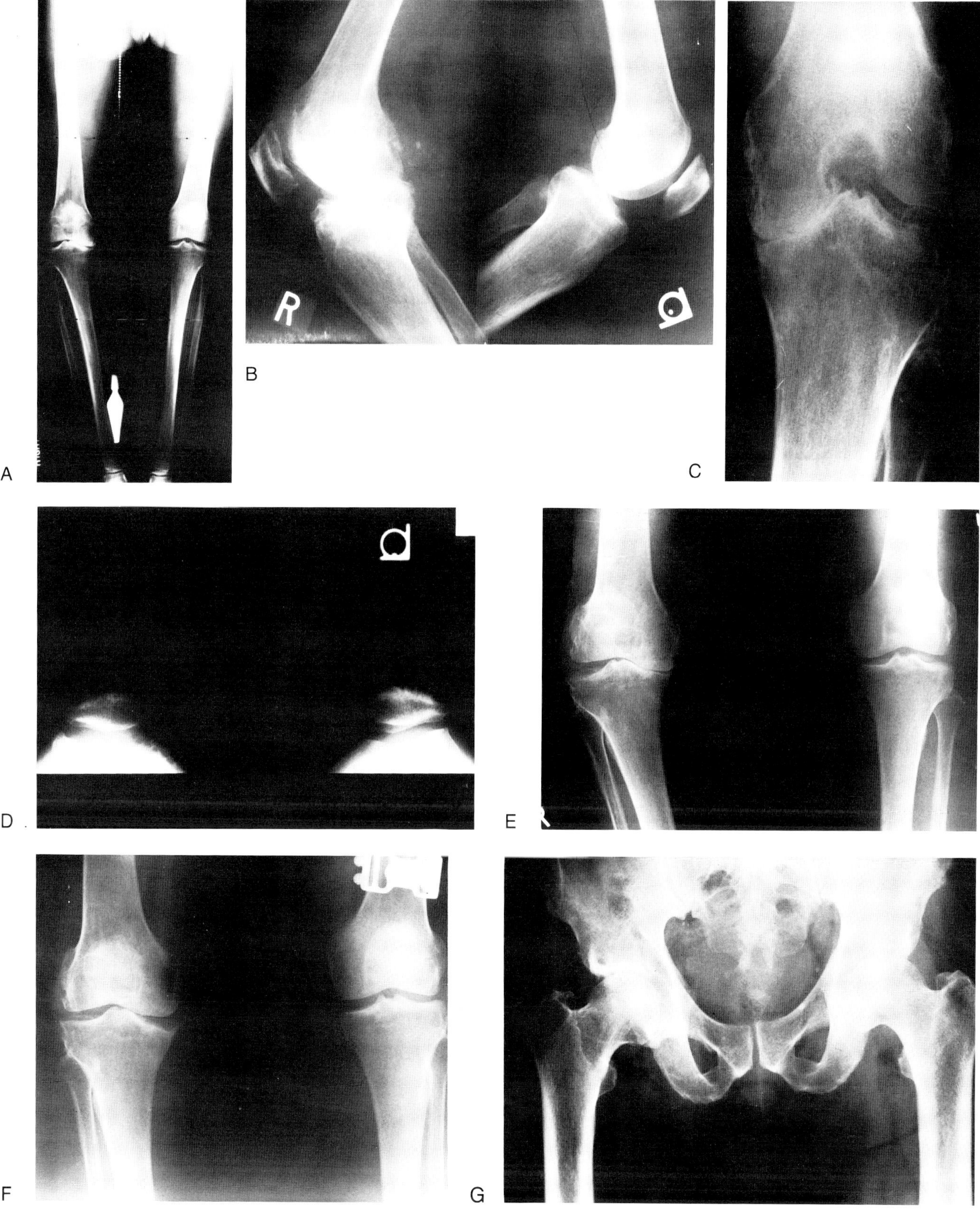

ing over the leg is used to allow easy palpation of the ankle for alignment. Steri-drape is utilized. In a "virgin" case, a long, straight, anterior (20 to 25 cm) skin incision (Fig. 14-17A) is made in the midline of the patella and down 2 to 4 cm below the tibial tubercle. The prepatellar bursa is incised and reflected medially. The joint is entered by a median parapatellar incision carried proximally for 5 cm, leaving 3 mm of vastus medialis tendon, and then carried 5 to 10 cm proximally separating medialis from rectus tendon (Fig. 14-17B). This step aids in exposure and allows later shifting of the vastus medialis as necessary for patellar alignment without buckling and weakening the rectus.

When exposure is difficult, the rectus tendon can be divided 5 to 7 cm above the patella in an oblique direction for about 3 cm, thus separating the vastus lateralis from the rectus proximally (Fig. 14-17C). This step allows eversion of the patella and knee flexion without avulsing the patellar tendon, and it is particularly helpful in the patient with a previous high tibial osteotomy. We are reluctant to elevate the tibial tubercle because of problems in the past.

The proximal tibia is exposed; the anterior cruciate ligament is excised; the fat pad is preserved to protect the patellar blood supply[6]; and the tibia is resected in a plane at a right angle to the vertical line bisecting the ankle. Inclination is desired at 5 to 8 degrees posteriorly, but it varies as some systems have it "built in" to the tibial component and individual instrumentation. Minimal tibial bone should be removed. If more than 1.5 to 2.0 cm needs to be resected on one plateau, a bone graft or custom-made prosthesis should be considered (preoperative planning). Care is taken to preserve the posterior cruciate ligament.

The femur is cut at the desired angle. At the present time the intramedullary system is utilized, but surgeons should use their favored system to achieve the mechanical axis. The level of the joint line should be maintained as close as possible.

If necessary, alignment by stage or graduated releases are performed at this time.[8] If the knee had a significant angular deformity, varus or valgus, staged soft-tissue releases are performed after osteophytes are débrided. Conservative soft tissue releases are often made prior to tibial resection to aid exposure for the saw cut. Releases are performed to allow the components to be inserted and maintain the mechanical axis of a straight line through the center of the ankle, knee, and hip. This line is to be obtained while maintaining equally taut collateral ligaments. Tightening of ligaments is not compatible with early motion, and subligamentous releases main-

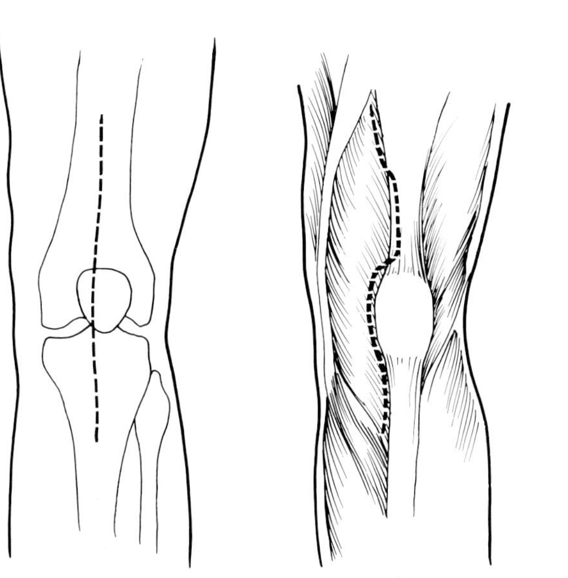
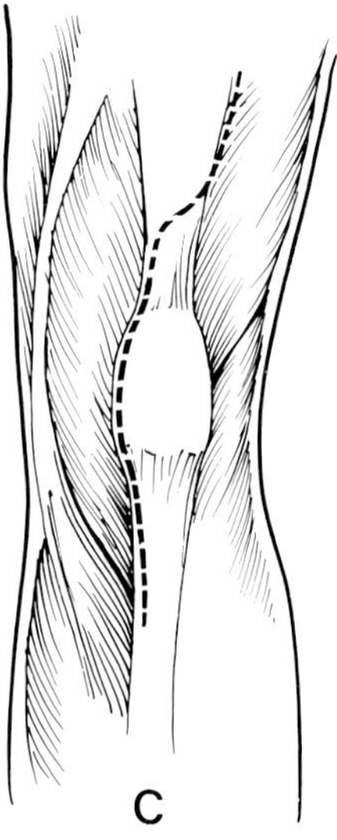

Fig. 14-17. (A) Midline skin incision. It may be varied slightly if there have been previous incisions. (B) Usual deep medial incision; note release of the vastus medialis from the rectus tendon proximally. (C) Deep medial incision where eversion of the patella is difficult (e.g., previous high tibial osteotomy). Note oblique incision across the rectus and release of the lateralis.

tain a periosteal sleeve and allow elongation with maintenance of stability. This plan of staged (graduated) releases prevents overcorrection and instability. Alignment along the mechanical axis is checked using any instrumentation. A Bovie card stretched from the center of the ankle to the electrocardiographic marker over the femoral head is a simple method.

Medial Release for Varus Deformity

Medial release for a varus deformity (Fig. 14-18) is performed as follows.

Stage I. Subperiosteally, expose the proximal 1 cm of medial tibia around to insertion of the semimembranosus. This maneuver releases the capsule and deep medial collateral ligament.

Stage II. Subperiosteally, release the superficial collateral ligament underneath the pes 5 to 6 cm distal to the joint line, and then release the medial capsule and semimembranous attachment from the tibia.

Stage III. Subperiosteally, release the anterior insertion of the pes and the anteroposterior capsule over to the posterior cruciate ligament. This step is facilitated by flexion and extension rotation of the tibia. Preserve enough of the pes attachment for closure as necessary later (Fig. 14-19).

Stage IV. Subperiosteally, release the medial collateral ligament on the femur, maintaining its continuity with the adductor tendon (Aufranc, personal communication). This stage does not provide a gradual release; a suture or staple can be utilized to restore a fixed point of rotation on the femur at the end of the operation. This stage was not employed in knee arthroplasty and would be used in an unusual case. It was used for tibial plateau arthroplasty until 1972. Additional bone resection or changing to a different knee prosthesis is indicated when correction is not obtained.

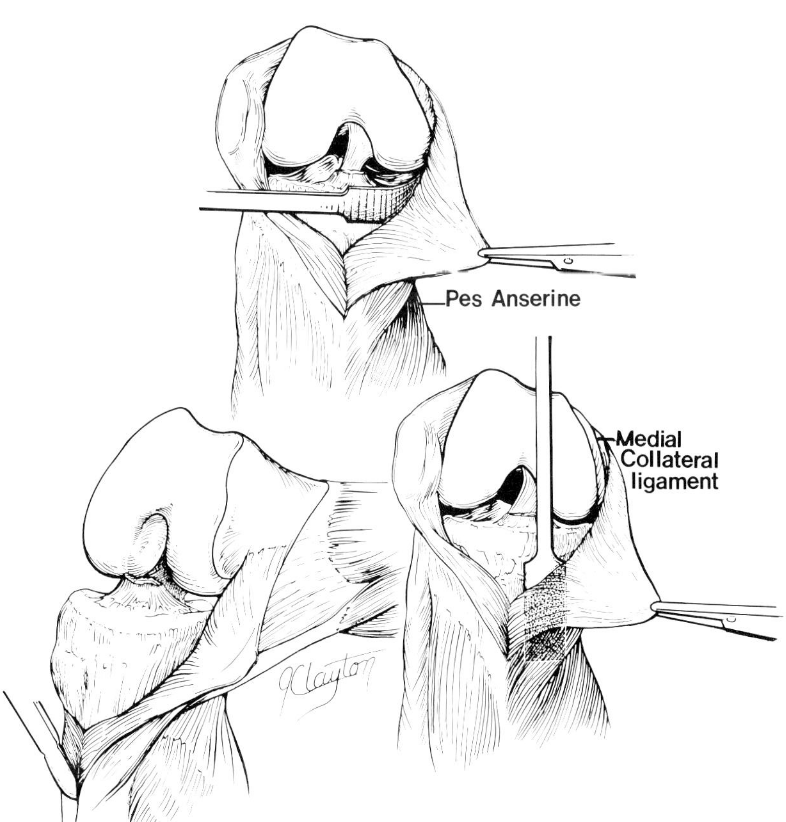

Fig. 14-18. Medial release of stages I, II, and III. All releasing is performed distally on the tibia. (From Clayton et al.,[8] with permission.)

Lateral Release for Valgus Deformity

Lateral release for a valgus deformity is performed as follows (Fig. 14-20).

Stage I. Subperiosteally, release the lateral collateral ligament and popliteus insertion from the lateral femoral condyle. Then, subperiosteally, release the lateral capsule from the proximal 1 cm of the tibia. Do not release the distal iliotibial band insertion.

Stage II. Subperiosteally, release the posterolateral capsule and lateral gastrocnemius origin. Subperiosteally, release the lateral intermuscular septum longitudinally off the femur for 7 to 8 cm, dividing the popliteus tendon.

Stage III. Make a transverse incision through the iliotibial band 10 cm above the joint line; expose subcutaneously.

Stage IV. Lengthen the biceps tendon in Z-plasty fashion while protecting the peroneal nerve. A separate incision may be necessary for biceps lengthening. A more laterally based skin incision is helpful when extensive lateral release is anticipated to eliminate the second (biceps) incision.

Flexion Contractures

Releases to correct varus or valgus are performed first, as this maneuver may correct the flexion.

Stage I. Subperiosteally, release the posterior capsule and gastrocnemius origin from the femur.

Stage II. Subperiosteally, release the attachment of the posterior cruciate ligament from the tibia for a short distance.

Stage III. Subperiosteally, release both medial and lateral collateral ligaments partially from both tibia and femur.

Stage IV. Perform biceps lengthening as for valgus release. If full extension is not obtained, further tibia may need to be resected, the posterior cruciate ligament sacrificed, and a more constrained prosthesis (posterior stabilized) utilized.

Recurvatum Correction

There are no releases for recurvatum problem, but it must be avoided. Proper fitting of components or use of a more constrained prosthesis usually corrects it. Mild hyperextension can be corrected by preventing full extension during postoperative care.

Realignment of Patella

Both facets are resected to give approximate normal thickness to the patella. Overly thin bone or too large anchoring holes predispose to fracture.[6] The patella should be restored as close to normal thickness as possible by intraoperative caliper measurements.

Additional Operative Features

After all components are cemented, the tourniquet is released to normalize tension of the musculature. The vastus medialis is anchored with a few key sutures while maintaining a taut patella tendon. The knee is flexed to 90 degrees while checking the patella tracking without support ("no thumb"). If subluxation or dislocation is noted, lateral release is performed during the interval between the vastus lateralis and the fascia lata or intermuscular septum. Avoid the lateral geniculate artery. Lateral release can usually be performed from within the joint, and the superior lateral geniculate vessels are easier to identify. One must be sure the release is extensive enough for proper patellar tracking. Lateral release performed adjacent to the patella has resulted in patellar complications, e.g., fractures.[6]

Selective distal and medial advancement of the vastus medialis tendon aids in patellar alignment. In some cases, slight medial placement of the prosthesis on available bone helps. It is important to obtain complete coverage of the tibia to get the strongest support for the tibial component. Right and left femoral components help somewhat in patella alignment. In rheumatoid

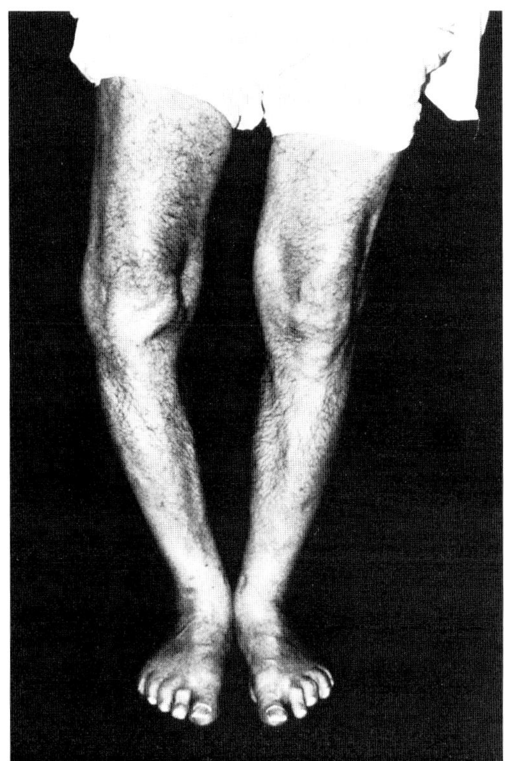

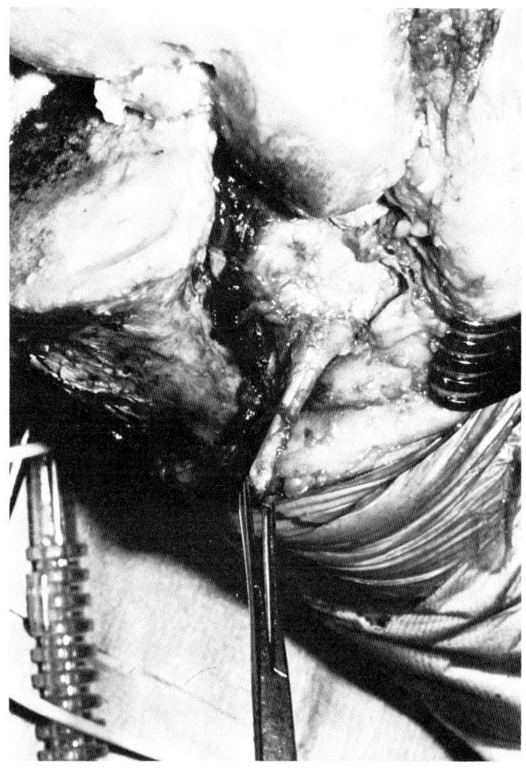

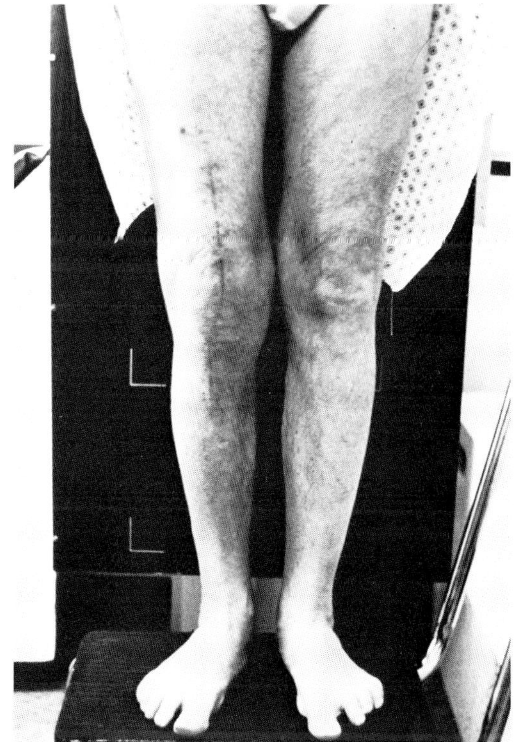

Fig. 14-19. (**A**) Preoperative view. (**B**) Intraoperative view (stage III varus release). Photograph was taken in flexion and external rotation. Note complete stripping of the proximal tibia around to the posterior cruciate ligament. The tenaculum inferiorly is around the pes anserinus, which has been released anteriorly. Arrow points to the depressed area of the tibial condyle. (**C**) After operation. (From Clayton et al.,[8] with permission.)

arthritis patients the valgus deformity predominates and is the most common release. About 25 degrees of valgus or varus can be corrected by release, as can about the same amount of flexion deformity. The necessary releases and alignment checking are important with any instrumentation system; too much reliance must not be placed on the instrumentation.

Alignment of the individual prosthetic components on the bone is also important and is illustrated in the manufacturer's directions for each total knee. The newer instrument systems are good, particularly the intramedullary femoral guides for resection. Lateral alignment of the femoral components is important; it should be at a right angle to the femoral shaft and avoid notching of the anterior femur.

One final factor regarding bone resection is that after posterior femoral condyle resection is performed one must check that posterior osteophytes have been removed and there is no bony obstacle to free flexion beyond the edge of the prosthetic femoral condyle (Fig. 14-21). This

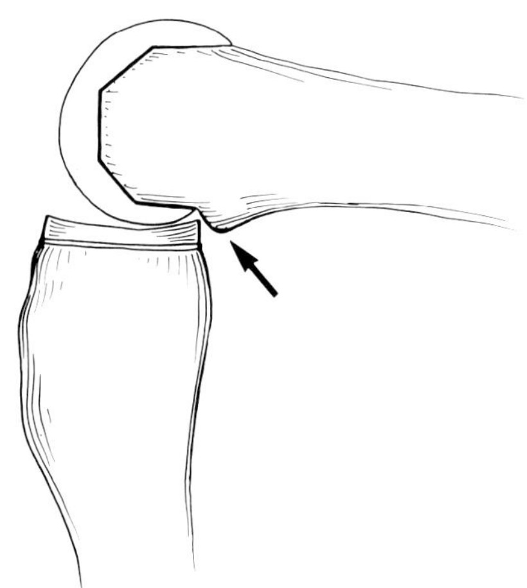

Fig. 14-21. Note the posterior osteophyte (*arrow*) blocking flexion.

point is important, as 110+ degrees flexion is desirable in the rheumatoid patient to aid arising from a chair or taking steps. It is generally preferable in rheumatoid arthritis patients to anchor the components with polymethylmethacrylate (PMMA). The cement is injected into the prepared cancellous bone of tibia, femur, and patella to a depth of about 3 to 4 mm in a low viscosity state.[18] To date there has been one loosening at 6 years in an osteoarthritic patient. During a period of more than 10 years, there have been no clinical loosenings with the use of hand-packed regular cement with total condylar knees, although some radiolucent lines have appeared.[9] Based on these positive experiences and only limited experience with the use of ingrowth prostheses, their use in the rheumatoid arthritic knee at this time is not established. The cementless prosthesis may be useful in the young patient if the bone stock is not porotic.

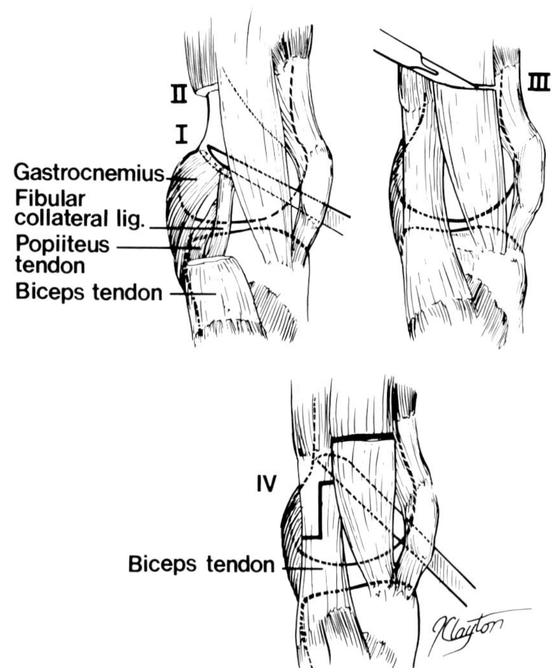

Fig. 14-20. Lateral releases for stages I, II, III, and IV. All releasing is performed proximally on the femur. (From Clayton et al.,[8] with permission.)

POSTOPERATIVE CARE

After checking and aligning the patella, two ³⁄₁₆ inch suction drains are inserted into the knee joint; musculotendinous layers are closed with No. 0 Dacron or No. 1 Vicryl; and the closure is tested to see that at least 90 degrees of flexion can be obtained.[4] Subcutaneous tissues are closed with absorbable suture and the skin closure with staples. A conforming dressing is applied. An intermittent pneumatic compression device is used on the opposite leg during surgery and is now also applied to the operated leg.[7] The leg is then placed in a CPM machine set for motion at 0 to 20 degrees of motion. (CPM may be delayed a day or two if desired.) If there has been correction of valgus flexion and the peroneal nerve is taut behind the fibular head, the knee is placed in 60 degrees and maintained in flexion for 24 hours. The CPM tends to maintain flexion, so the therapist daily assists extension gains to within the range of 0 to 5 degrees. Quadriceps exercises are taught preoperatively and continued postoperatively.

Intravenous cefazolin is used interoperatively and for 48 hours thereafter. Exacting, careful, aseptic technique is important. A rare case has been returned to the operating room during the early postoperative period because of a large or draining hematoma. Thorough evacuation (irrigation) was performed with closure of the wound and proceeding with the usual postoperative treatment. It is important to follow this regimen to prevent infection in such cases. Wound healing problems have rarely been encountered because of proper placement of the incision, careful handling of tissues, aseptic technique, proper closure, suction drainage for 48 hours, and meticulous attention to all aspects including the postoperative dressing. Rheumatoid skin must be handled with care, and skin sutures or staples should remain at least 2 weeks. A laminar airflow room is helpful but not as important as the overall care outlined above.

Hemovac tubes are removed in 2 days; a lighter dressing is applied at 2 to 4 days; and ambulation is started in a removable knee splint with protected weight-bearing of about 40 to 50 pounds. The pulsatile stockings are discontinued when ambulating regularly, usually at 4 to 7 days.

The CPM is advanced as rapidly as tolerated, striving for 90 degrees in 7 to 10 days. The patient is out of the machine at least 4 hours a day after the first day; it can be omitted at night also. Motion is gained faster, but it has little if any effect on the final range of motion.

Patients are discharged from the hospital at 7 to 10 days. This decision depends on the patient's general condition and the status of the operated knee.

Post-Hospital Care

Physical therapy is continued on an individual basis. Range of motion and partial weight-bearing (40 to 50 pounds) are the major aims for the first 6 weeks. Increased weight-bearing and strengthening exercises are then emphasized for the next 6 weeks. One crutch or a cane is used during this period, with the goal of full, unsupported weight-bearing at 3 months at the earliest. "Don't throw away the cane" (W. Blount). A cane or crutch should be used as long as the patient or the doctor believes it is necessary. Proper gait training and walking are the most important of all exercises. In the rheumatoid patient, other joints may dictate the continued use of crutches. In general, crutches are preferred to a walker because a more natural gait can be utilized; however, a walker may be necessary for patients who have other problems interfering with balance. Everything must be done to help prevent the patient from falling, as a fracture around a total joint replacement is a serious problem. Prevention is the best treatment. (See Chapter 13, p. 22.)

Special Considerations

If bilateral knee replacement is indicated, it can be performed at the same operative session, 7 to 10 days later, or 6 weeks later. The ultimate function is essentially the same. If there is a considerable bilateral flexion contracture (>25 degrees), operation at the same time accelerates ambulation. We prefer to do them simultaneously with two teams; otherwise it is preferable to do the worst knee first, send the patient home, and do the second knee 6 weeks later. In general, surgeons should handle these decisions so they are comfortable and their patients' needs are best served. Variations from the general regimen are individualized.

At times full extension can be obtained only by gentle pressure. If the rest of the criteria are met, a plaster splint or cast in full extension is used for 2 to 4 days, after which mobilization is begun.

Hyperextension is to be avoided at surgery. A slight amount of hyperextension can usually be overcome by keeping the knee in slight flexion at all times during the immediate postoperative period.

Stage IV cases with complete joint disorganization often have considerable loss of bone stock or marked ligamentous instability; a failed total knee arthroplasty often falls into this category. Such cases require a more constrained total prosthesis.

Marked loss of bone stock should be replaced by bone grafts or wedges where feasible rather than just cement. As much bone stock as possible must be preserved, as the long-term prognosis of total knee arthroplasty is unknown. Alignment again is the key, and the postoperative treatment is essentially the same.

COMPLICATIONS

Thromboembolism

Thromboembolism in the past has been a major complication of joint replacement in knees and hips. In 1980 a regimen of activity, air boots, and aspirin was initiated.[7] Each patient walked and practiced rehabilitation exercises the day before and the morning of surgery. The contralateral calf was intermittently pumped during surgery followed by bilateral pulsatile calf compression postoperatively until independently ambulatory (about 5 days). Aspirin was administered in the recovery room and was continued 600 mg twice a day until discharge. Early activity and ambulation postoperatively were expected.

In a prospective study of 100 total knee arthroplasties on this regimen, there were no clinical postoperative venous thromboses.[8] There was one "probable" pulmonary embolus based on a 1 week postoperative lung scan, and the patient was uneventfully treated with heparin.

There have been no deaths due to pulmonary embolus after total knee (or hip) replacement over a 10-year period with the outlined regimen. Surgeons should use the method of prophylaxis against thromboembolism with which they are most comfortable.

Hematogenous Infection

Late hematogenous infection has been encountered in a few cases. Rheumatoid arthritis patients have a higher incidence of deep joint infections than the general population, and the total joint arthroplasty is more susceptible to hematogenous joint infection than the original joint. The large foreign implant is the problem, with or without bone cement—the cement is not to blame. Prevention is attained by controlling infection in any part of the body. All of our patients have been given a card and a letter with the recommendations for prophylactic antibiotics (see Appendix at end of the book). It is similar to the prophylaxis recommended by the American Heart Association for heart valve problems.

If early or late infection does develop in a rheumatoid postoperative knee, the treatment is the same as for a nonrheumatoid patient, although the problem is magnified because of the usual immunosuppression in the rheumatoid. Any deep infection in a total joint is a serious problem,[27] and the infectious disease experts should be brought onto the team. Specific treatment is beyond the scope of this book.

A total of 42 total knee arthroplasties of the posterior cruciate-saving condylar design performed by us from 1975 to 1978 were reviewed with a follow-up of more than 10 years (Table 14-1). Fifteen patients had rheumatoid arthritic knees, six with bilateral involvement (21 knees). Twenty patients had osteoarthritic knees, one with bilateral involvement (21 knees). One patient had juvenile rheumatoid arthritis. The total, then, was 21 rheumatoid arthritic knees and 21 osteoarthritic knees. Polyethylene tibial components without metal backing were used in all knees; all components were cemented by the digital packing technique. There were no infections.

Table 14-1. Average Total Knee Arthroplasty
Results, by Diagnosis

Parameter	Rheumatoid Arthritis	Osteoarthritis
No. of arthroplasties	21	21
Age	54.6 years	71.1 years
Follow-up	11 years	11 years
Flexion		
Preop.	103.8°	108.6°
Postop.	104.5°	103.5°
Extension		
Preop.	−13.1°	−5.0°
Postop.	−1.9°	−1.3°
Postop. alignment	5.5° valgus	6.0°
Postop. HSS score[a]	84.7 points	84.6 points

[a]HSS = Hospital for Special Surgery.

All patients were evaluated postoperatively using the 100 point Hospital for Special Surgery Knee Rating Sheet, which categorizes knees as excellent (85 to 100 points), good (70 to 84), fair (60 to 69), or poor (<60).

There was *no difference in the results between the rheumatoid and the osteoarthritic patients.* Excellent or good results were achieved in 92.9 percent at 11 years with no femoral or tibial loosening (average range of motion 104 degrees). All knees were well aligned (3 to 9 degrees of femur-tibia valgus).

Late complications were mainly patellar, with two dislocations, two fractures, and one loosening; one posteriorly unstable knee with patellar tendon dislocation and one supracondylar fracture (late) were also seen. Proper alignment with weight-bearing was the single most important factor in determining the excellent results: "no abnormal moment medial or lateral, or anterior or posterior."

With these encouraging long-term results, we are reluctant to give up posterior cruciate ligament[22] and the use of cement, which remains the "gold standard." Similar results were obtained at the Brigham Hospital in Boston.[23] The only change in the results with "newer models" is that range of motion now averages 115 degrees, with many patients over 125 degrees.

Patellar Problems

Patellar problems are the main complications of total knee arthroplasty today.[6] Patellectomy has been necessary in one case with severe changes in the patella after a spherocentric type knee replacement that did not have a patellar flange. In another case the patella was fractured and was treated by patellectomy.

Subluxation or dislocation of the patella is a problem, but it is rare if proper alignment is obtained at surgery. Patellectomy is occasionally necessary, but useful function can still be maintained.

Wound Healing

Wound healing problems have rarely been encountered owing to proper placement of the incision, atraumatic technique, proper closure, and suction drainage. Meticulous attention to detail is important.

Revision surgery, always a difficult problem, may be compounded by the patient's general rheumatoid condition. Each case is different, and a detailed discussion of the subject is beyond the scope of this book.

CONCLUSIONS

Total knee arthroplasty is the most common operation in rheumatoid arthritis patients today. We prefer the nonconstrained condylar type replacement that preserves the posterior cruciate ligament. *Alignment* is the most important factor in the surgical procedure (alignment of the leg and of the individual prosthetic components). The operation is technically demanding with small tolerance for error. Installation is more important than the model, and results are excellent (>90 percent success rate). Cementing of components is preferred in usual cases of rheumatoid arthritis; loosening has occurred rarely in properly aligned cases. (See Chapter 20-7 Case Report.)

REFERENCES

1. Boegard T, Brattstrom H, Lidgren L: Seventy-four Attenborough knee replacements for rheumatoid arthritis; a clinical and radiographic study. Acta Orthop Scand 55:166, 1984
2. Clayton ML: Surgery of the thumb in rheumatoid arthritis. J Bone Joint Surg [Am] 44:1376, 1962
3. Clayton ML: Surgery of the lower extremity in rheumatoid arthritis. J Bone Joint Surg [Am] 45:1517, 1963
4. Clayton ML, Kagan A II: The rheumatoid knee. Curr Pract Orthop Surg 7:179, 1977
5. Clayton ML, Leidholt JD, Gamble WE: Realignment osteotomy at the knee for chronic arthritis (degenerative and rheumatoid). J Bone Joint Surg [Am] 47:1284, 1965
6. Clayton ML, Thirupathi R: Patellar complications after total condylar arthroplasty. Clin Orthop 170:152, 1982
7. Clayton ML, Thompson TR: Activity, air boots and aspirin as thromboembolism prophylaxis in knee arthroplasty; a multiple regimen approach. Orthopedics 10:1525, 1987
8. Clayton ML, Thompson TR, Mack RP: Correction of alignment deformities during total knee arthroplasties; staged soft tissue release. Clin Orthop 202:117, 1986
9. Dennis DA, Clayton ML, O'Donnell S, Stringer EA: Posterior cruciate condylar knee arthroplasty; average 11-year follow-up. Submitted for publication
10. Ewald FC, Jacobs MA, Miegel RE et al: Kinematic total knee replacement. J Bone Joint Surg [Am] 66:1032, 1984
11. Geens S, Clayton ML, Leidholt JD et al: Synovectomy and débridement of the knee in rheumatoid arthritis. I. Historical review. II. Clinical and roentgenographic study of thirty-one cases. J Bone Joint Surg [Am] 51:617, 1969
12. Gunston FH: Polycentric knee arthroplasty; prosthetic simulation of normal knee movement. J Bone Joint Surg [Br] 53:272, 1971
13. Jones WN: Mold replacement in the rheumatoid knee. p. 35. In Cruess RL, Mitchell NS (eds): Surgery of Rheumatoid Arthritis. Lippincott, Philadelphia, 1971
14. Jones WN, Aufranc OE, Kermond WL: Mold arthroplasty of the knee. J Bone Joint Surg [Am] 49:1022, 1967
15. Harvey JP, Corcos J: Large cyst in lower leg originating in the knee occurring in patients with rheumatoid arthritis. Arthritis Rheum 3:218–28, 1960
16. Mack RP, Clayton ML: Synovial and bursal lesions about the knee. p. 3539. In Evarts CM (ed): Surgery of the Musculoskeletal System. 2nd Ed. Churchill Livingstone, New York, 1990
17. Matsui N, Taneda Y, Ohtas H et al: Arthroscopic versus open synovectomy in the rheumatoid knee. Int Orthop 13:17, 1989
18. Miller J, Clayton ML, Dunn H: Composite structure fixation in total knee arthroplasty; a preliminary report of a multicenter clinical trial. J Bone Joint Surg [Br] 66:300, 1984
19. Mori M, Ogawa R: Anterior capsulectomy in the treatment of rheumatoid arthritis of the knee joint. Arthritis Rheum 6:130, 1963
20. Muller ME, Allogower M, Schneider R, Willenegger H: Manual of Internal Fixation. Techniques Recommended by the AO-Group. 2nd Ed. Springer-Verlag, New York, 1979
21. Perry J, Antonelli MS, Ford W: Analysis of knee joint forces during flexed knee stance. J Bone Joint Surg [Am] 57:961, 1975
22. Ritter MA, Gioe TJ, Stringer EA, Littrell D: The posterior cruciate condylar total knee prosthesis; a five-year follow-up study. Clin Orthop 184:264, 1984
23. Scott RD, Sledge CB: Total knee arthroplasty in rheumatoid arthritis. Ann Chir Gynaecol 74:70, 1985
24. Short CL, Bauer W, Reynolds E: Rheumatoid Arthritis. Harvard University Press, Cambridge, 1957
25. Sledge CB, Archer RE, Shortkroff S et al: Intra-articular radiation synovectomy. Clin Orthop 182:37, 1984
26. Sledge CB, Walker PS: Total knee arthroplasty in rheumatoid arthritis. Clin Orthop 182:127, 1984
27. Wiedel JD: Arthrodesis for the failed total knee replacement. Complications Surg 1:7–11, 1986
28. Wilson PD: Posterior capsuloplasty in certain flexion contractures of the knee. J Bone Joint Surg 11:40, 1929
29. Young HH: Use of a vitallium prosthesis for arthroplasty of the knee. J Bone Joint Surg [Am] 53:1658, 1971

15

Management of the Rheumatoid Ankle

Mack L. Clayton

The ankle is initially involved in only 4 percent of the cases,[9] but about twice this many are later involved.[11] "Ankle pain" is a frequent complaint because the patient does not distinguish ankle (tibiotalar) from hindfoot problems. In a survey of 300 rheumatoid arthritis patients with 10 years' duration of disease, Gschwend and Steiger found ankle and subtalar joint involvement in 52 percent.[4]

In general, ankle involvement of significant disabling degree is infrequent compared to foot involvement.[2] The ankle joint mortise with the attached ligaments allows plantar flexion and dorsiflexion but essentially no inversion or eversion and only a jog of rotation. Synovial involvement can be palpated anterior to each malleolus. The normal range of motion is about 10 degrees dorsiflexion and 50 degrees plantar flexion, but an active rheumatoid synovitis decreases the range. With involvement, and as the joint cartilage is destroyed, the ligaments are occasionally destroyed. Careful physical examination is necessary to determine the exact joints that are the source of pain in the area of the ankle and the hindfoot. Standard weight-bearing anteroposterior and lateral roentgenograms of the foot and ankle are helpful. If surgery is to be considered, inversion and eversion stress films may also be helpful.

Tenosynovitis exactly as seen at the wrist may also involve any of the tendons within the sheaths around the ankle, and even tendon ruptures may be noted; the ruptures are analogous to those at the wrist and are caused by tenosynovitis in the closed tendon sheaths. The etiology of the rheumatoid arthritic tendon ruptures are (1) direct invasion of tendon by rheumatoid synovial nodules; (2) friction against the tunnel with synovitis; (3) aseptic necrosis of tendon due to constricting tenosynovitis cutting off the blood supply; and (4) attrition by erosion over a bony irregularity.

Posterior tibial tendon rupture is the most common tendon injury in the foot and leads to a severe valgus deformity; one must be suspicious of it in a patient with a severe planovalgus deformity with rapid progression. The treatment has been by triple arthrodesis. (For a passively correctable hindfoot, talonavicular arthrodesis can be utilized—see Chapter 16.) Tendon transfer is generally not indicated in the rheumatoid patient. In early cases with clinical tenosynovitis of the posterior tibial tendon, tenosynovectomy is indicated to prevent tendon rupture (Fig. 15-1). Tenosynovectomy should relieve pain and prevent rupture.

A tarsal tunnel syndrome can develop from compression of the tibial nerve at the ankle in the compartment for the toe flexors in a manner similar to carpal tunnel syndrome due to rheumatoid tenosynovitis.[7] Symptoms are pain and paresthesias on the sole of the foot. Hypalgesia may be present; electromyography and nerve conduction measurements are usually necessary to confirm the diagnosis. In definite cases treatment is by tenosynovectomy and decompression of the tib-

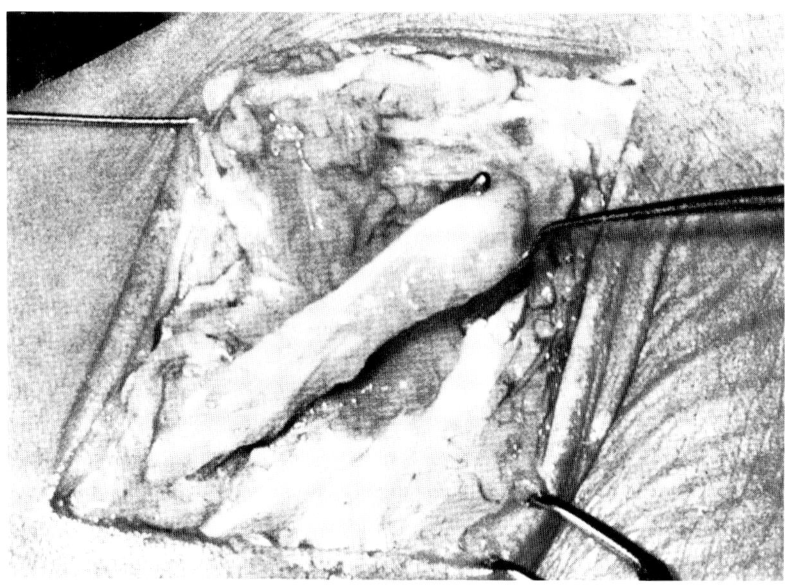

Fig. 15-1. Tenosynovitis of the posterior tibial tendon. Note the formation of irregular nodules, a precursor to tendon rupture.

ial nerve down and into its branches. The tarsal tunnel syndrome is rare in comparison to the carpal tunnel syndrome.

The Achilles tendon has also been noted to rupture in several cases. One patient had pain, slight swelling, and tenderness over the distal Achilles tendon at the level of the os calcis; 80 percent rupture was found at surgery due to attrition over the bony irregularity at the posterior corner of the os calcis. The irregular corner of the bone was widely excised, the tendon repaired, and the foot immobilized in slight equinus for 6 weeks in a short leg walking cast. Identical involvement and findings were noted on the other side 1 year later, and an identical procedure was performed. She has had no recurrent problems in these areas for 6 years and has good strength.

No rupture was noted in the anterior compartment tendons, but it could occur. Tenosynovectomy is indicated for pain and swelling and the technique is similar to that used for the wrist. One important difference of the treatment is that a pulley of the retinaculum must be retained over the extensors at the ankle (or over peroneal tendons posterior to the fibula). Bowstringing or subluxation of these tendons is a serious problem at the ankle, whereas it is not at the wrist (Fig. 15-2).

Stress fractures of the fibula just above the ankle may occur along with a marked valgus foot.

One must be suspicious when the pain is not at the joint level. These injuries can be easily missed, as the rheumatoid patient usually has many pains (see Fig. 17-1A). Stress fracture of the tibia occurs less frequently.

With symptomatic involvement of the ankle joint, proper shoeing in the early cases may be helpful. This treatment includes the usual type of shoe supports, addition of a high shoe or a boot, or addition of a strut hidden in the boot to increase support similar to a short leg brace. Such treatment may be helpful even in later, more involved cases.

Synovectomy may be beneficial for cases of nonresponding synovitis and persistent pain when good cartilage (stage II or IIIa) is present. Short (3 to 4 cm) incisions over the anterior medial and lateral malleolar joints expose the capsule, which is entered laterally above the fibulotalar ligament and in a similar manner medially. The synovium and capsule are excised until the entire ankle joint is cleared; small rongeurs are helpful. In an unusual case with enough posterior synovitis, the posterior medial incision can be utilized just posterior to the medial malleolus and following subligamentously to the joint, which can be cleaned with a pituitary rongeur. A similar posterolateral incision is utilized occasionally. Associated tenosynovectomy may be performed when indicated by enlarging the inci-

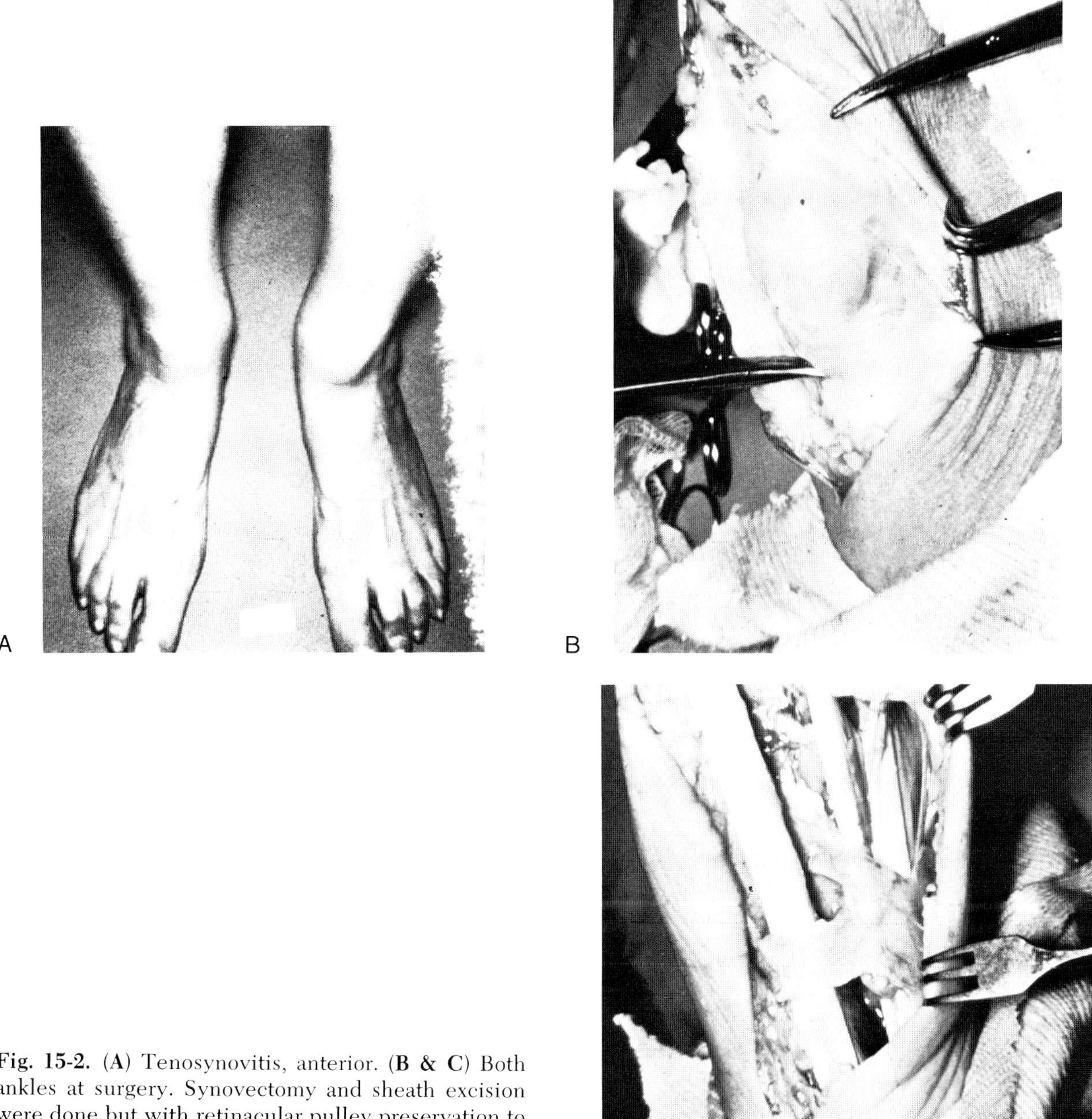

Fig. 15-2. (**A**) Tenosynovitis, anterior. (**B** & **C**) Both ankles at surgery. Synovectomy and sheath excision were done but with retinacular pulley preservation to prevent bowstringing.

sions as necessary. A compression dressing and a simple posterior splint is utilized for a few days, after which active motion and protected weight-bearing are started. Protection is utilized for 2 to 3 weeks or for as long as 6 weeks as indicated.

Pahle and Teigland[8] reported that 73 percent of 63 patients were free of pain 5.7 years after ankle synovectomy using the anterior and posterior approach in two stages; seven of their cases later failed and the patients underwent fusion or arthroplasty. Mori (personal communication) found about 70 percent good results. We have had too few cases to evaluate; most have been done in conjunction with a triple arthrodesis.

In a few cases of foot ankle deformity with moderate rigidity, Heywood[5] utilized a supramalleolar osteotomy to place the foot in plantigrade position. Pain relief was obtained, with some motion maintained to avoid the marked stiffness of a pantalar arthrodesis.

If the patient has severe pain and the ankle joint is markedly involved (stage IIIb or IV), ankle fusion or total ankle replacement is indicated. In a few cases bracing such as was mentioned earlier relieves the pain, and after a number of months the boot or brace may be taken off or worn intermittently. If the foot is in a good neutral position, considerable wear of the ankle joint may be tolerated for a long time. If the foot is in a deformed position, underneath the ankle joint, the pain is often severe.

Until the mid-1970s, the only procedure available was arthrodesis, which was associated with several months' immobilization and a significant number of pseudoarthroses.[10] At the time of the fusion, if the hindfoot joints are mobile, the foot should be placed at 90 degrees neutral position in relation to the tibia in the lateral aspect, the heel should be in slight valgus (neutral), and the forefoot should rest plantigrade. Holding the forefoot up to 90 degrees at the time of fusion later allows 10 degrees plantar flexion through the subtalar and midtarsal joints. In time it will increase to about 20 degrees motion, which allows wearing of about 1.25 inch heels for dress occasions as well as a basic low heel oxford shoe.

If the hindfoot joints are also painful and involved, a pantalar arthrodesis may be necessary, and in this case the foot should be in neutral or about 5 degrees equinus and forefoot plantigrade; little variation in heel height is allowed. At times a shoe with a rocker sole and a well padded inner sole and heel is helpful.

Ankle fusion with good motion in the hindfoot joint gives an excellent result. In some cases, ankle fusion leads to painful hindfoot involvement of a progressive nature, which must be converted to a pantalar arthrodesis. However, triple arthrodesis or talonavicular fusion rarely leads to increased ankle involvement. In fact, ankle pain may diminish after proper realignment of the hindfoot. General disease activity is also an important factor. Pantalar arthrodesis gives a satisfactory result in the severe salvage type case.

There are many techniques of ankle fusion, and surgeons should use the technique with which they are most comfortable. Anterior or lateral or medial approaches have been used with special indications. The important common denominator is proper position of the arthrodesis and good bony contact with immobilization by internal or external fixation aided by bone grafts as necessary. There is no worry about leaving anatomy suitable for later conversion to a total ankle arthroplasty, as no success has been reported.

TECHNIQUE OF ANKLE FUSION

Gschwend, Wagner, and coworkers[3,4,12] recommended the use of internal fixation by compression screws. After an anterolateral incision is made (Fig. 15-3A) the fibula is exposed, transected approximately 3 inches from the distal tip, and reflected posteriorly, thus hinging on the posterior tissues and leaving intact the blood supply and peroneal tendons in their sheaths. The anterior aspect of the ankle is also completely exposed subligamentously and subperiosteally. The joint surfaces are prepared with either flat surfaces or simple removal of the articular cartilage according to the bony changes present; congruity and bony contact are the important factors. Two large compression screws are inserted with the foot at a right angle and the heel in neutral position (slight valgus). The first screw is inserted from the sinus tarsi obliquely upward and posteriorly to end near the posterior medial tibial cortex or vice versa. The other screw is inserted from the lateral tibia obliquely into the medial and anterior portion of the talus, and a slot is cut to fit a washer proximally. The screws are finally tightened alternately after an intraoperative roentgenogram is obtained to check the screws and positon of the foot. If fixation is not perfect, supplementary staples can be added using one anterior and one posterior from the lateral side. The fibular and an adjacent bed are prepared. The fibula is placed across the ar-

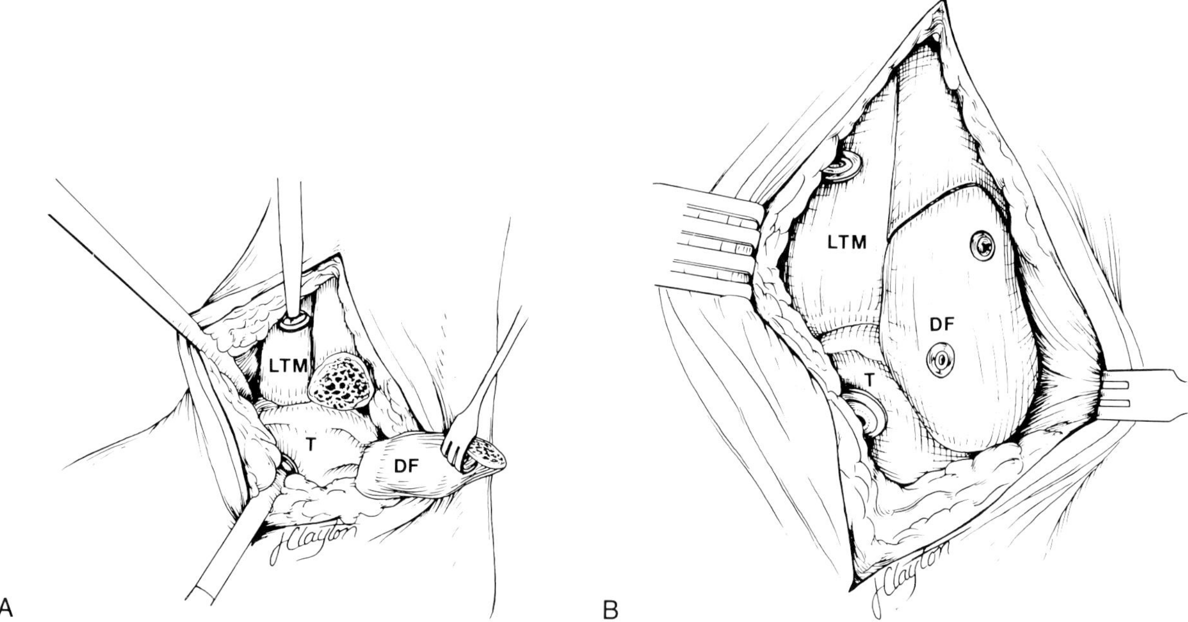

Fig. 15-3. (**A**) Completion of a 6.5 mm cancellous screw insertion obliquely across the ankle arthrodesis sit. The proximally directed screw (32 mm thread) is inserted through the talus (*T*) at the sinus tarsi to engage the medial cortex of the distal tibia. The distally directed screw (16 mm thread) is placed from the lateral tibial metaphysis (*LTM*) to engage the medial aspect of the body of the talus. Screws are alternatively tightened to apply compression across the arthrodesis. The distal fibula (*DF*) is reflected posteriorly to provide adequate exposure. (**B**) Completed ankle arthrodesis. The sagitally split distal fibula has been secured to the lateral aspect of the ankle as a bridge graft with two additional 4 mm cancellous screws (From Dennis and Clayton et al.,[3] with permission.)

throdeses area and is anchored with small screws or a staple; it then acts as a living bone graft. This step keeps the peroneal tendons in a proper location and gives a more normal configuration to the ankle (Fig. 15-3B). A posterior splint or a cast can be utilized.

If fixation is completely stable, gentle exercises may be started early. A posterior splint and soft dressing are used for 2 weeks, a non-weight-bearing short leg cast for 6 weeks after surgery, and then weight-bearing until union. For a virgin tibiotalar fusion, union occurs at 8 to 12 weeks (average 9.5)[3] (Fig. 15-4).

If the osteoporosis is so severe that compression screws do not grip, alternative technique should be used, e.g., external fixation. Pantalar arthrodesis can be performed in one or two stages. We had a patient with nonunion of the ankle due to infection after single-stage pantalar

procedure. Union was obtained with revision and external fixation, but only after prolonged drainage from a pin site. In many cases it is advisable to do the triple arthrodesis first and the ankle later.

The Denver Orthopedic Clinic has reported 16 primary ankle screw fixation fusions using internal fixation as described with 15 unions; three were rheumatoid ankles, and all united.[3] In one case faulty technique left threads across the fusion line, and nonunion developed; union was achieved after a secondary operation using proper technique. Intraoperative roentgenograms should be obtained, as image intensifier is not reliable.

Uuspaa and Raunio,[10] reporting on 148 ankle fusions in rheumatoid arthritis patients (the world's most extensive reported study), had 22 percent nonunions. However, 80 percent of the

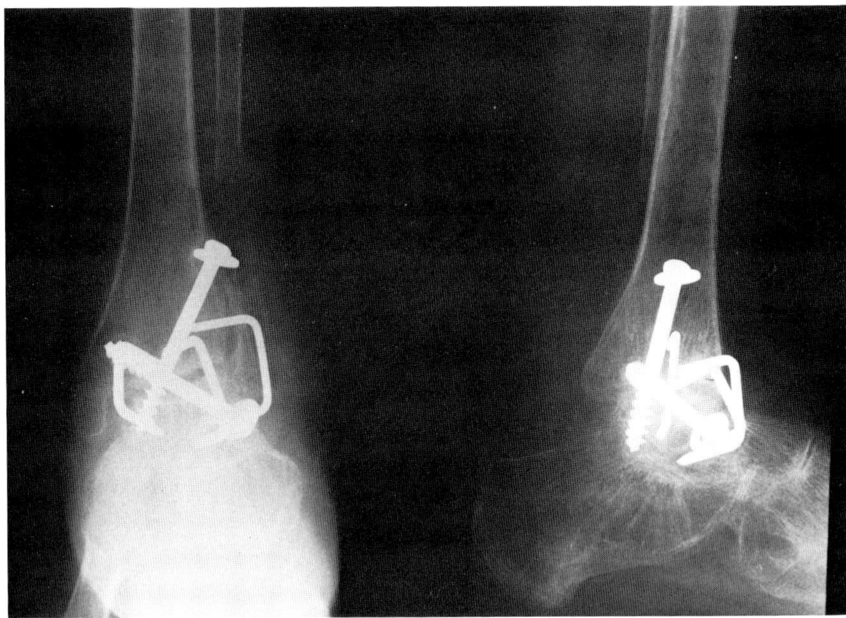

Fig. 15-4. Ankle fusion in a 38-year-old woman. It is a pantalar fusion, as the hindfoot joint was ankylosed; the foot is about 5 degrees equinus. Compression screws from the lateral talus to the medial tibia would be better at more of an angle, but the sinus tarsi was obliterated by bone. She has no pain 3 years later and can walk or stand for several hours. (From Dennis et al.,[3] with permission.)

patients with union had no pain, and 50 percent could wear normal shoes and walk at least 1 km. The triangular external fixation clamp of Calandruccio (Richards Manufacturing Co., Memphis, TN) gives excellent immobilization, although the device with which the surgeon is most comfortable should be used. This clamp may be used for arthrodesis to salvage a failed total ankle arthroplasty when there has been too much bone destruction to use compression screws (Fig. 15-5).

TOTAL ANKLE ARTHROPLASTY

Total ankle arthroplasty is a desirable type of procedure in rheumatoid arthritis patients because there is usually involvement of the hindfoot also. If the hindfoot is involved (as well as the ankle joint) to the point that surgery is necessary and a triple arthrodesis is indicated, it should be per-

formed first. The ankle replacement is performed 6 weeks or longer after union. If the hindfoot has the indications for arthrodesis and is passively correctable, a talonavicular fusion can be combined with the ankle arthroplasty. In general, total ankles are metal to plastic and have been anchored with methylmethacrylate. There are round-topped ankles that are less constrained; however, they may shift into progressive valgus or varus, and they have not proved helpful. Each of these techniques is well described in the brochure from the manufacturer.

In general, an anterior incision is utilized with the necessary bone excision.[6] In some of these devices there is a metal-backed tibial component, and pressurization of cement enhances fixation. They are inserted with an anterior incision; if necessary, a posteromedial short incision is helpful for clearing posterior cement, which is almost always present. The dorsal retinaculum over the extensor tendons must be repaired to prevent bowstringing.

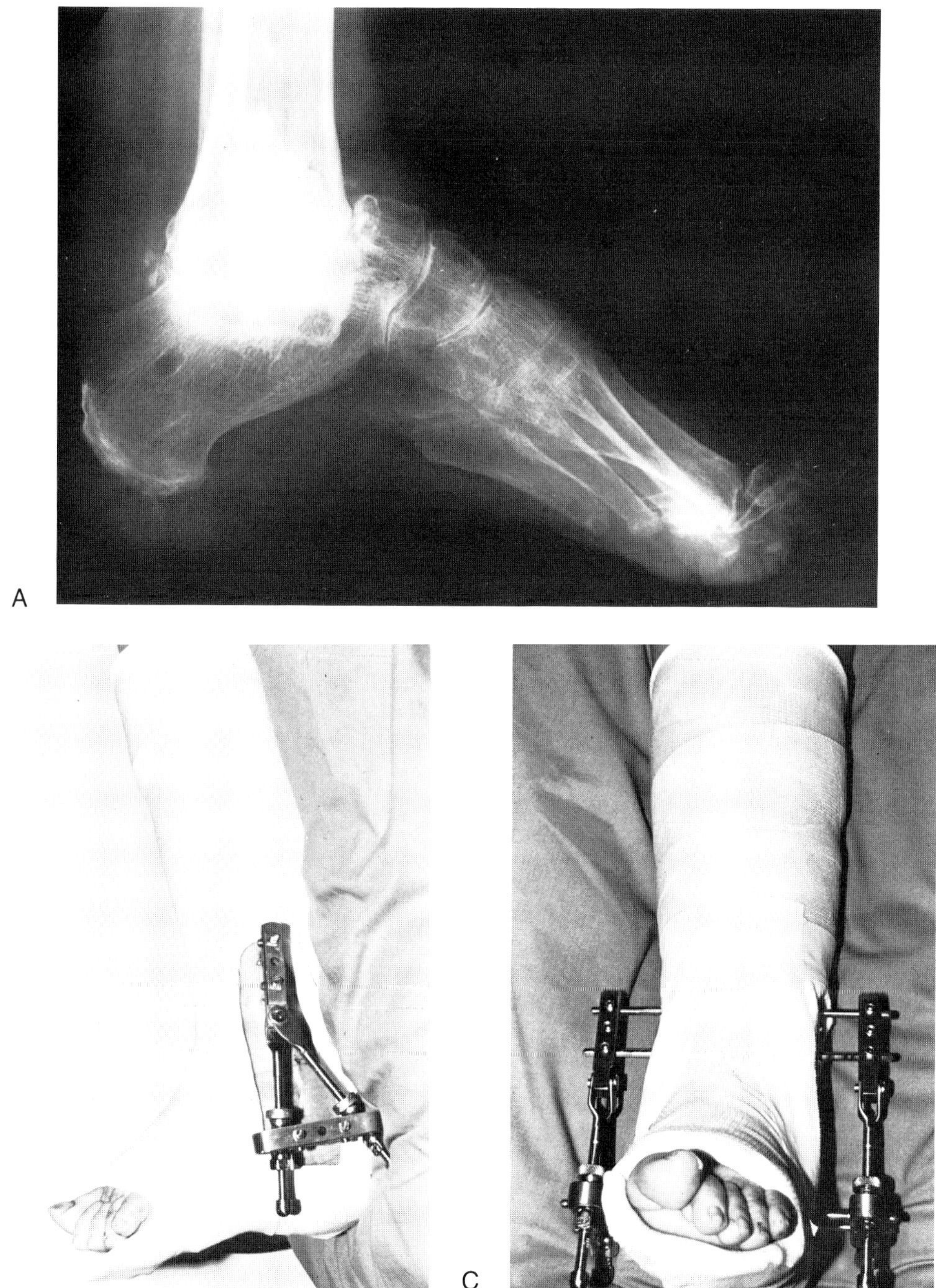

Fig. 15-5. (**A**) Roentgenogram 5 years after fusion for a failed total ankle arthroplasty. The talus had been essentially destroyed. Bone grafts (autogenous iliac and femoral head allograft) fill the large tibial defect and bridge into the os calcis. (**B & C**) Triangular external pin fixation was used for 3.5 months and a walking cast for another 3 months. These cases are difficult, requiring much longer to fuse than a primary procedure, and the result is not as good. This technique is a "limb salvage" type procedure.

If ligament reconstruction or a talonavicular fusion has been performed, cast immobilization is continued for 6 to 10 weeks. Only 20 to 25 degrees of ankle motion is expected, and the immobilization time does not seem to change this figure. In uncomplicated cases the immobilization is used for only 2 to 3 weeks.

Total ankle arthroplasty is recommended in **unusual** cases of rheumatoid arthritis only. In 13 years 32 cemented prostheses have been implanted, and no ankles have had malleolar replacement. Reasonable overall early pain relief has been obtained, although a number of patients still complain of pain, some of which is probably from the hindfoot or due to early loosening. Four patients have had severe pain with clinical and roentgenographic evidence of loosening, resulting in removal of the components and fusion. Il-

iac grafts, fibular grafts, and banked bone allografts have been used at times to help fill the space and maintain length, and the triangular external fixation clamp of Calandruccio has been utilized. As mentioned, these ankles have been immobilized in the clamp for 4 to 5 months, with the patient then spending a number of months in a short leg walking cast; three of these ankles have united (Fig. 15-5). One patient developed a separate deep severe infection in the forefoot, and nonunion resulted; amputation was performed.

A number of the ankles that are still functioning have ominous radiolucent lines around the tibial component or have tipped into a valgus or varus deformity. Patients are mostly satisfied with their results (70 percent), however; and there are several patients with excellent results

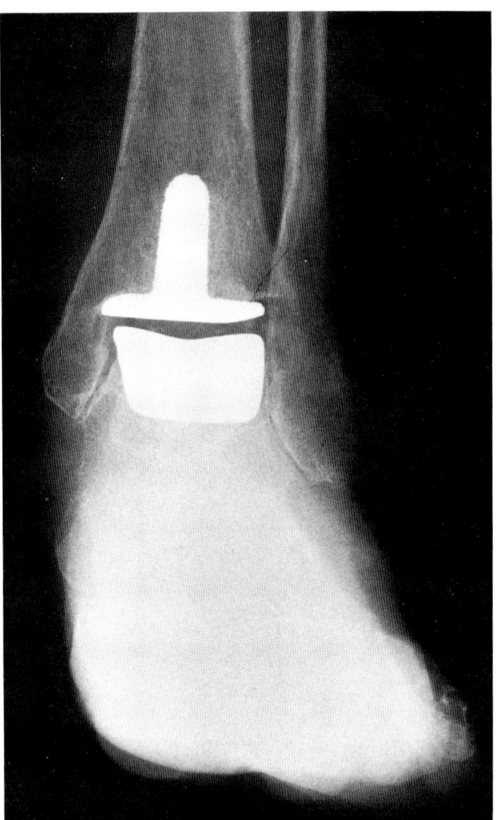

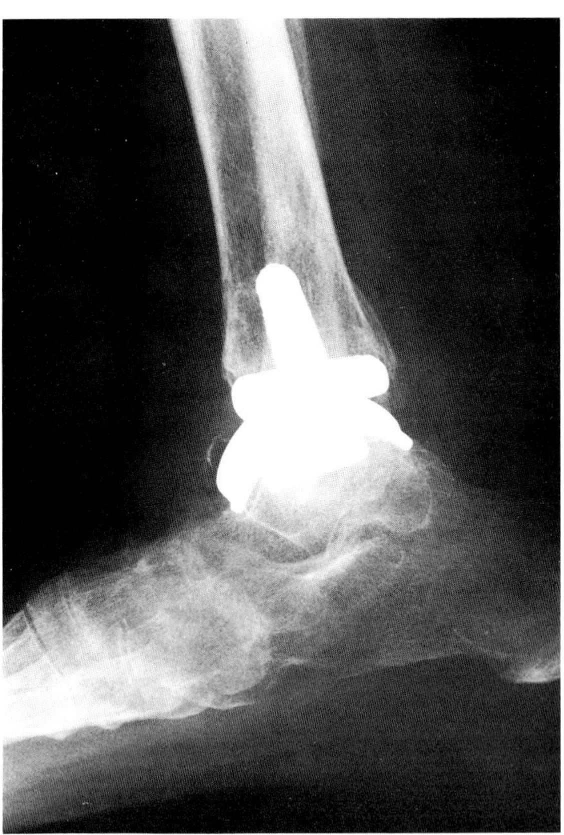

Fig. 15-6. **(A)** New Jersey total ankle (cementless) replacement with an interposed polyethylene bearing at 6 months. **(B)** Ankle showed no signs of loosening, no pain, and 25 degrees of motion at 3 years. She is having pain and swelling at 4 years and may need re-operation.

who walk with a good gait and have had no pain over 10 years.

There are few enthusiastic reports of total ankle replacement.[6] Pahle and Teigland[8] reported that of 66 total ankle (cemented) arthroplasties followed for 5 years, there were more than 80 percent good results and an average range of motion of 30 degrees. They recommended the procedure only for rheumatoid arthritis.

Raunio reported on the experience of total ankle arthroplasty at the Rheumatism Hospital in Heinola, Finland at the ERASS meeting in 1985

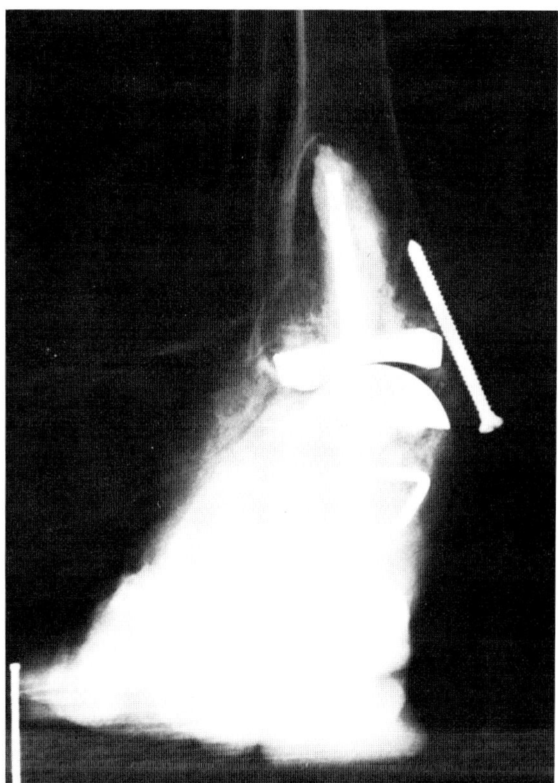

A

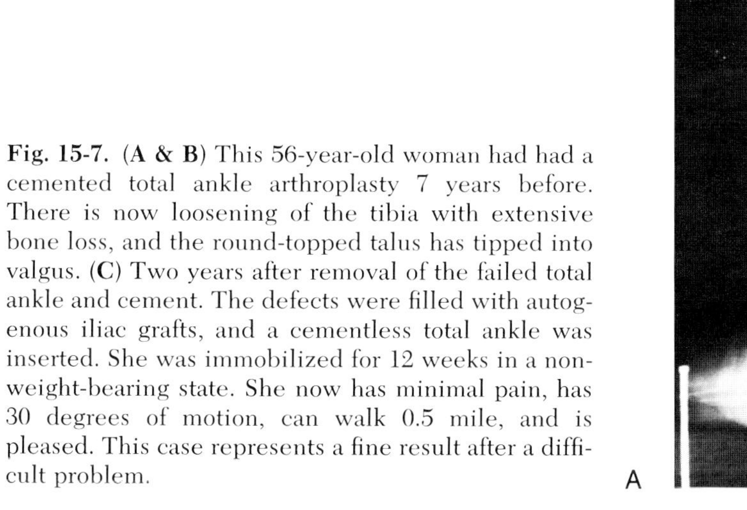

Fig. 15-7. (**A & B**) This 56-year-old woman had had a cemented total ankle arthroplasty 7 years before. There is now loosening of the tibia with extensive bone loss, and the round-topped talus has tipped into valgus. (**C**) Two years after removal of the failed total ankle and cement. The defects were filled with autogenous iliac grafts, and a cementless total ankle was inserted. She was immobilized for 12 weeks in a non-weight-bearing state. She now has minimal pain, has 30 degrees of motion, can walk 0.5 mile, and is pleased. This case represents a fine result after a difficult problem.

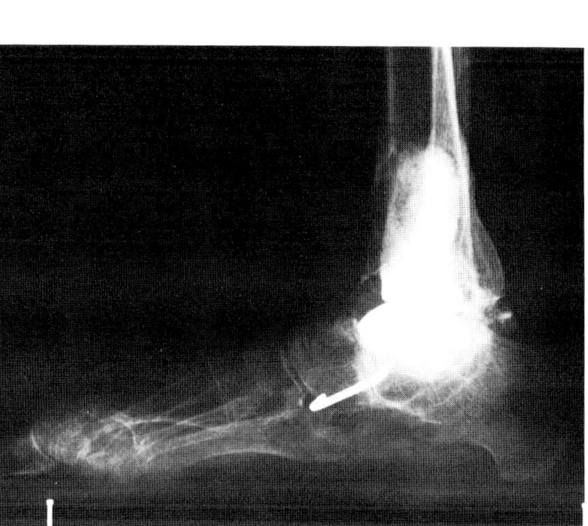

B

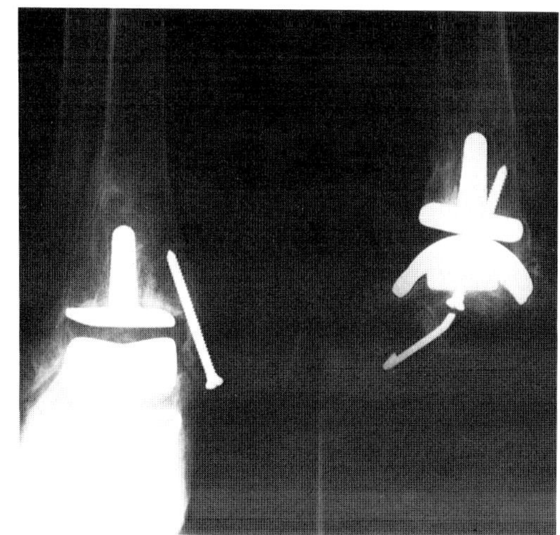

C

(personal communication). He reported on 41 cemented ankles in 34 patients with rheumatoid arthritis (average follow-up 5 years). There were many complications: Delayed healing was present in six, one had a deep infection, and 24 percent were loose at follow-up. Three failed ankles were fused but required a long healing time. Two-thirds of the roentgenograms showed talar subsidence. Results were much worse than those with total hip or total knee replacement, and Raunio ceased performing total ankle arthroplasties in 1981.

We have been investigating a porous-coated ankle prosthesis with an interposed mobile bearing ankle[1] (DePuy, Warsaw, Indiana) (Figs. 15-6 and 15-7). Early results were promising, but the ankle is no longer generally available. If it should fail, bone loss would be minimal.

At the present time, total ankle arthroplasty cannot be recommended except in the unusual rheumatoid arthritic when motion of the ankle would make a great difference. There are some successful total ankles (Fig. 15-8), but the failures are terrible and are too frequent. Arthrodesis remains the standard recommendation today.

SUMMARY

Ankle involvement is relatively uncommon in rheumatoid arthritis compared to the foot. In some cases it is difficult to distinguish ankle pain from hindfoot pain, and in fact they may coexist. For pain relief shoe supports, a boot, or a short leg brace may give symptomatic relief in early or some later cases. Synovectomy has been helpful in a few cases in the early stages and does not "burn any bridges" in terms of further treatment. For pain relief in severely involved later cases, ankle fusion is the recommended procedure at this time (synovectomy). Total ankle arthroplasty has not yet become a reliable, reproducible procedure using the cemented type components. A better prosthesis will surely be available in the future.

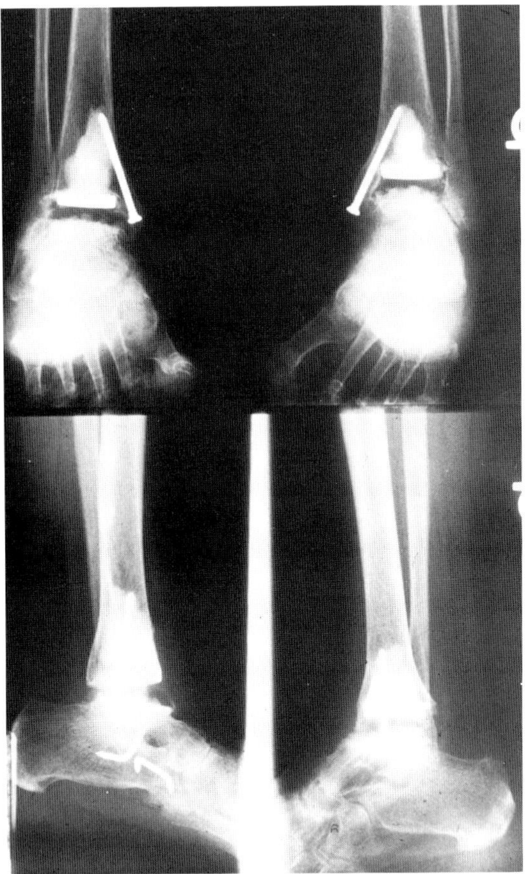

Fig. 15-8. At 14 years after bilateral total ankle arthroplasty the patient had no pain and 20 degrees of motion. At 16 years the left ankle has loosened and requires surgery.

REFERENCES

1. Buechel F, Pappas MV: New Jersey low contact stress total ankle replacement, biomechanical rationale and review of 23 cementless cases. Foot Ankle 8:279, 1988
2. Clayton ML: Surgical treatment of the rheumatoid foot. p. 444. In Giamestras NS (ed): Foot Disorders. Lea & Febiger, Philadelphia, 1973
3. Dennis DA, Clayton ML, Wong DA et al: Internal fixation compression arthrodesis of the ankle. Clin Orthop 253:212, 1990
4. Gschwend N, Steiger U: Stable fixation in hindfoot arthrodesis; a valuable procedure in the complex RA foot. Rheumatology 11:114, 1987
5. Heywood AW: Supramalleolar osteotomy in the

management of the rheumatoid hindfoot. Clin Orthop 177:76, 1983
6. Johnson K: Ankle replacement arthroplasty. p. 1173. In Morrey B (ed): Joint Replacement Arthroplasty. Churchill Livingstone, New York, 1991
7. Keck C: The tarsal tunnel syndrome. J Bone Joint Surg [Am] 44:180, 1962
8. Pahle JA, Teigland JC: The complex foot. I. Synovectomy of the ankle and subtalar joints. II. Total replacement arthroplasty of the ankle joint. Rheumatology 11:179, 1987
9. Short CL, Bauer W, Reynolds E: Rheumatoid Arthritis. Harvard University Press, Cambridge, 1957
10. Uuspaa V, Raunio P: Ankle arthrodesis; a material of 148 ankle fusions on 130 ankle joints of 118 patients. Rheumatology 11:104, 1987
11. Vainio K: The role of surgery on the rehabilitation of rheumatoid arthritis patients. In Proceedings IV European Rheumatology Congress. Istanbul Press, Istanbul, 1959
12. Wagner H, Puck HG: Die Verschraubungsarthrodese der Sprunggelenke. Unfallheilkunde 85:280, 1982

16

Management of the Rheumatoid Foot

Mack L. Clayton

In 16 percent of rheumatoid arthritic patients the disease originates in the feet, and in 4 percent the ankle is the initially affected joint.[9,35] About the same percentage experience the condition initially in the hands as in the feet. This observation tends to disprove the theory that in most patients rheumatoid arthritis is first apparent in the hands or in the feet and hands. Although 30 percent of the patients have unilateral involvement initially, 9 percent of the involvement eventually becomes bilateral. One large series of patients showed that the metatarsophalangeal (MTP) joints were involved in 46 percent of the cases, tarsals in 46 percent, toes in 23 percent, ankles in 68 percent, knees in 78 percent, and metacarpophalangeal (MCP) joints in 71 percent.[21]

The authors, working in conjunction at the Arthritis Clinic at the University of Colorado far more than 20 years, believe that there are two definite clinical subtypes of chronic rheumatoid arthritis. The first is the group of patients in whom the joints tend to stiffen with gradual loss of motion and even progress to ankylosis. Here the predominant aspect is progressive loss of joint function and is considered the "stiff" type. The second type is the group in whom soft-tissue and bursal involvement predominate and cause secondary joint deformity. In this group, joint destruction is slow and does not always lead to ankylosis. In fact, there may be gradual destruction of the joint with developing instability ("loose" type). This type predominates in patients with hand and foot involvement. Whether steroid treatment plays a causative role in the development of this feature is still open to question. However, it is not certain if a definite subclassification can be established along these lines, as the microscopic pathologic changes are the same in both groups, and many cases overlap. Definite cases are nevertheless seen representing each extreme. These two subtypes may account for the marked difference in the results obtained with reconstructive surgical procedures in rheumatoid arthritis patients. In the first, or stiff, type, ankylosis is prone to occur, arthrodeses are easy to obtain, but mobility may be difficult to regain after arthroplasty. In the second, or loose, type, arthrodesis may be more difficult to obtain than in an ordinary case.

DEVELOPMENT OF FOOT DEFORMITIES

During the early active stages of rheumatoid arthritis, the disease usually manifests in the forefoot as puffiness and tenderness. There may be mild heat and redness, and increased perspiration is common. Manual lateral compression of the metatarsal heads is a useful test. Pain between the metatarsal heads indicates involvement of periarticular non-weight-bearing structures, which are involved in rheumatoid arthritis but are not usually involved in a mechanical type of MTP joint abnormality. The exception to this rule is a plantar neuroma with its characteristic findings. As a result of synovitis, the toes tend to assume a cock-up position with active and passive limitation of flexion at the MTP joints. In the early stages, roentgenograms reveal only osteoporosis with soft-tissue swelling, but they soon show surface erosions of the metatarsal heads in most cases (Fig. 16-1).

In the early stages, proper shoeing and supports with a graduated exercise regimen are helpful; some deformities may even be prevented (Fig. 16-2). Considerable rest may be indicated during early acute exacerbations. Despite conservative measures, many cases progress to severely painful, disabling deformities in the forefoot. Deformity of the knees often accentuates the foot deformity. The most common combination of deformities is hallux valgus, bunions with forefoot spread, depressed metatarsal heads, and varying degrees of cock-up of the toes. Some toes remain slightly flexible, whereas others are rigid

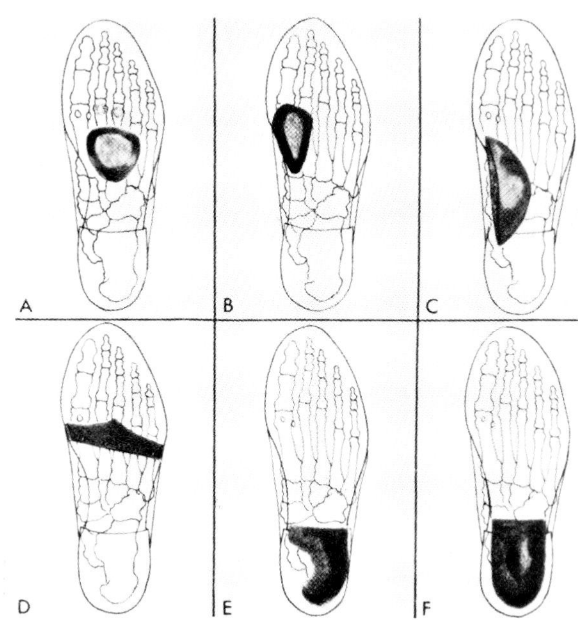

Fig. 16-2. Shoe supports should be rubber and leather and must be adjustable. They are designed to relieve pressure areas and give mechanical support to the foot. (From Clayton,[10] with permission.)

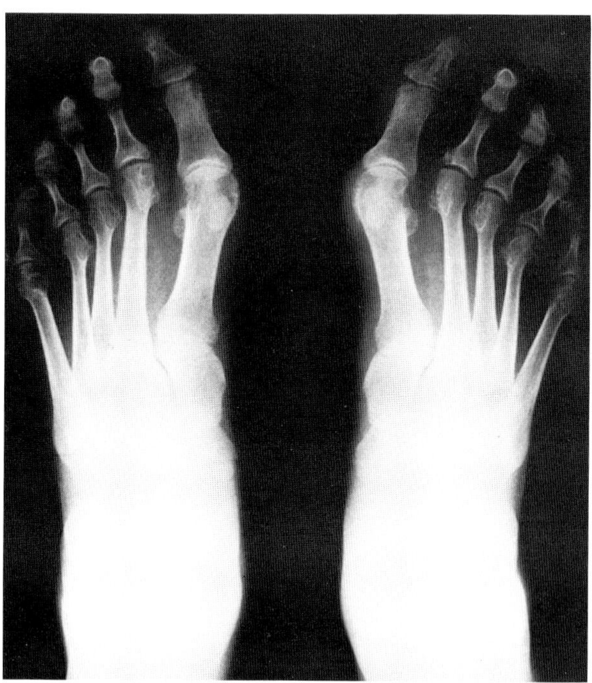

Fig. 16-1. Erosions of bone at MTP joints (stage IIIA), particularly of the metatarsal heads and IP joints of the great toes. Joint space is well preserved (stage II) in the lesser toes. (From Clayton,[10] with permission.)

with dorsal subluxation or complete dislocation of the proximal phalanges on the metatarsal heads. This problem increases the height of the forefoot and makes shoeing difficult. Painful corns develop over the dorsum of the middle joints, and calluses develop underneath the depressed prominent metatarsal heads on the sole of the foot (Fig. 16-3).

With walking, pain arises from abnormal pressure underneath the metatarsal heads on the sole or against the shoe on the dorsum of the toes. Attempts to support the metatarsal areas often produce increased pressure on the dorsum of the toes owing to the inflexibility. There is contracture of the soft tissues, including muscles, tendons, fascia, and skin, which often leads to fibrous ankylosis. However, spontaneous bony ankylosis of the MTP joints (stage IV) is rare (about 1 percent). When active synovitis continues, the intrinsic muscles are overpulled by the long extensors and flexors, and the cock-up deformity of the toes becomes similar to that often seen with paralysis of the intrinsic muscles of

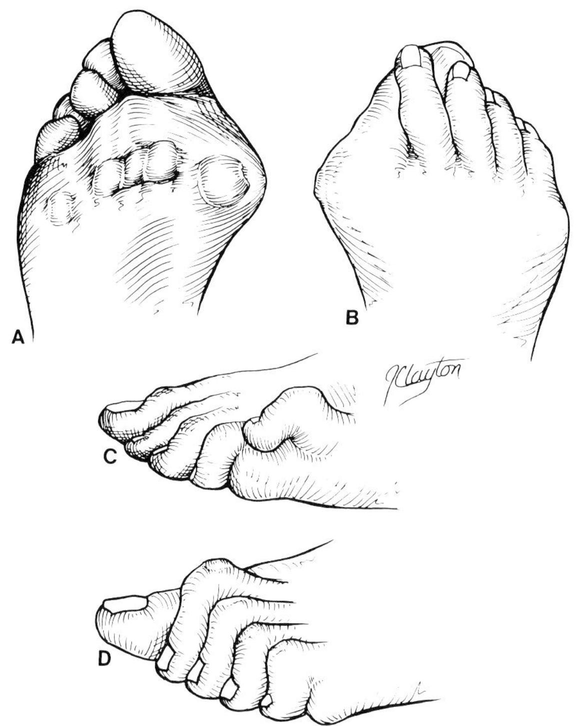

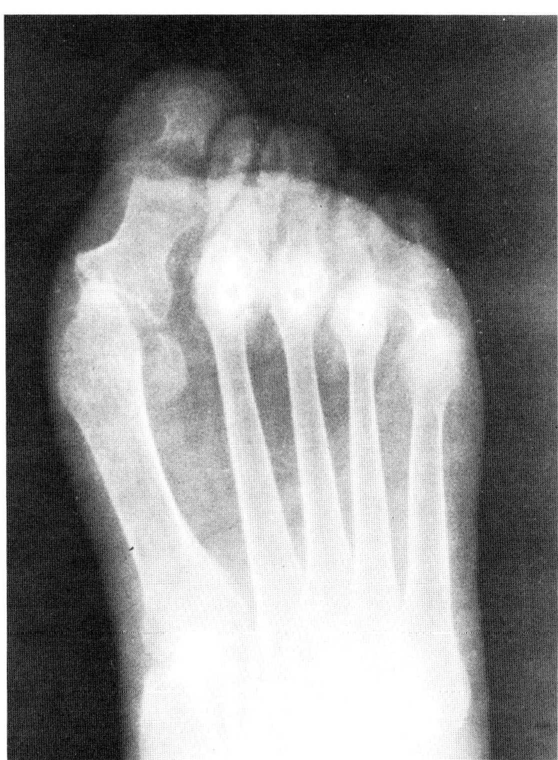

Fig. 16-3. **(A & B)** The most frequent deformity is hallux valgus, bunions, depressed metatarsal heads, and cock-up toes. **(C & D)** Various deformities may occur. (From Clayton,[10] with permission.)

Fig. 16-4. Late rheumatoid arthritis with a 90-degree dislocation at MTP joints two, three, and four (stage IV). The proximal phalanges appear "gun barrel." (From Clayton,[10] with permission.)

the foot. The flexor tendons subluxate to the side and migrate dorsally until they no longer exert flexor action on the proximal phalanx and actually increase the cock-up deformity. This defect does not resemble the so-called intrinsic-plus deformity commonly seen with rheumatoid arthritis of the hand.

Of course, there are many variations of pathology in the involved tissues that would give rise to other deformities, but most have the basic pattern of hallux valgus, bunions, and cock-up toes with depressed metatarsal heads. Roentgenograms help to reveal the abnormalities. Erosions of the metatarsal heads or bases of the phalanges are usually greater than is suspected on clinical evaluation. Joint spaces are narrowed; subluxation or dislocation of the MTP joints may be noted and can be seen on anteroposterior roentgenograms as overlap of the proximal phalanx over the metatarsal head. In instances when

there is marked dorsal dislocation of the phalanges to the extent approximating 90 degrees with the metatarsal (Fig. 16-4), a "gun barrel" sign can be noted, which is simply an axial view of the proximal phalanx in which the bony cortex is outlined as if it were a gun barrel. Varying degrees of osteoporosis are present in cases of this type.

Several patients in this group had complete spontaneous dislocation at the first MTP joints (Fig. 16-5), and we have seen this problem only with rheumatoid arthritis. The deformity represents spontaneous rupture of the dorsal portion of the capsule and the abductor halluces tendon, caused by rheumatoid synovial involvement and aided by friction against the underlying irregular first metatarsal head. The pull of the unopposed muscles dislocates the proximal phalanx in a fibular direction; this problem is illustrated by the

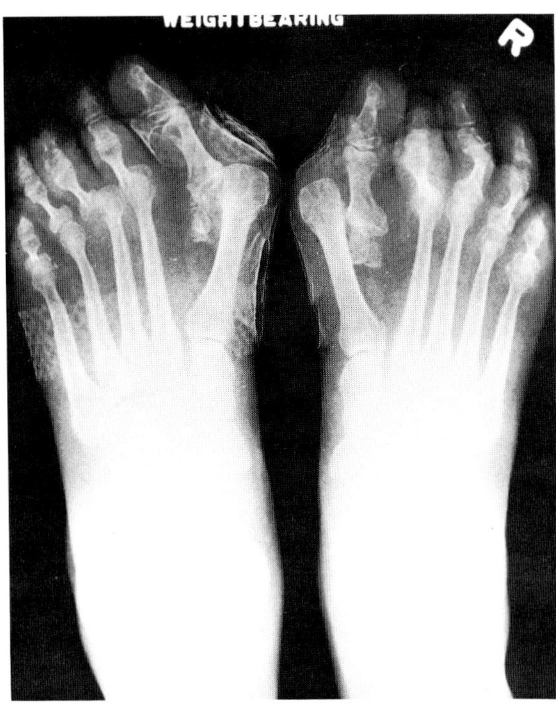

Fig. 16-5. First MTP joint dislocations (stage IV) seen only in rheumatoid arthritis and due to complete rupture of the abductor tendon and tibial capsular structures from synovitis. Sesamoids follow the base of the proximal phalanges, and typical changes are noted in the lesser toes. (From Clayton,[10] with permission.)

sesamoids following the base of the phalanx on the roentgenogram. This dislocation greatly increases the metatarsus primus varus with pressure on the bunion of the first metatarsal head and gives rise to large, painful bursae that on occasion become infected and drain intermittently.

Also noted were three feet with spontaneous hallux varus, an unusual deformity in untreated feet (Fig. 16-6). The varus deformity was due to a rupture of the adductor halluces by rheumatoid synovitis, which was identified at surgery.[41,42] Similar tendon ruptures as a cause of certain hand deformities are well known.

Deformity of the hindpart of the foot is usually a progressive valgus (loose type), with changes first in the talonavicular or subtalar joint and later through the midtarsals. In other cases the deformity is minimal, but there is limited motion with pain in the hindpart of the foot due to arthritic joint changes (stiff type). Cavovarus deformity is also seen; it is more common with juvenile rheumatoid arthritis but often is not symptomatic until adult years.

Bursitis (or tenosynovitis) may develop around the tendocalcaneus, and several cases of rupture of the Achilles tendon have been noted. Tenosynovitis may occur near the plantar fascia insertion. Tenosynovitis may develop around any of

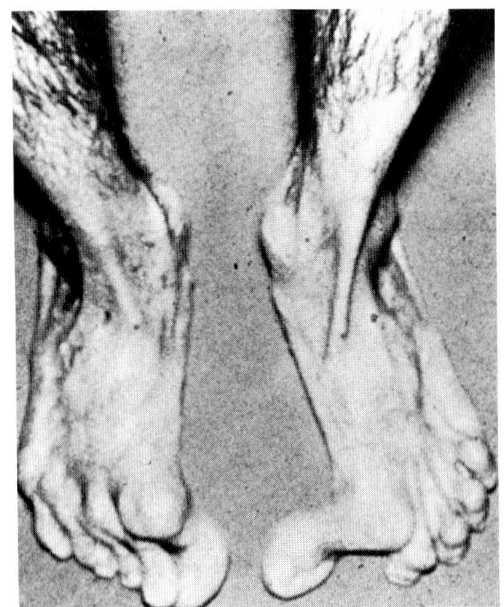

A

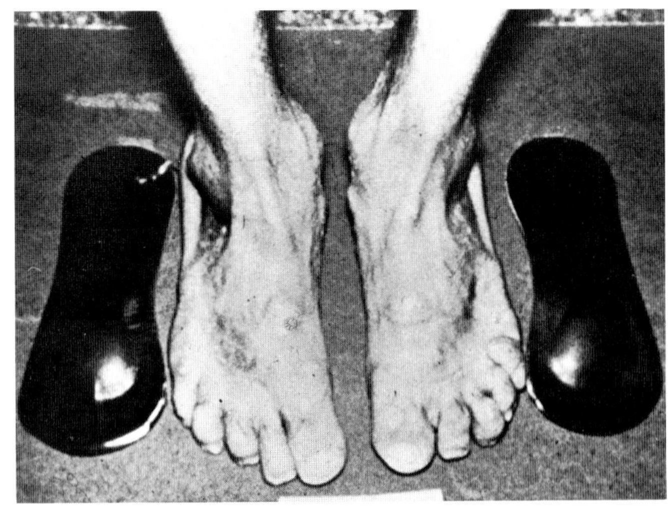

B

Fig. 16-6. (A) Hallux varus in a 24-year old man caused by rupture of the adductor tendon due to rheumatoid synovitis. **(B)** Two years after bilateral reconstruction (MTP resection arthroplasty as illustrated in Figure 16-11). The feet functioned well for 18 years (patient is now deceased). (A from Clayton and Reis,[12] with permission.)

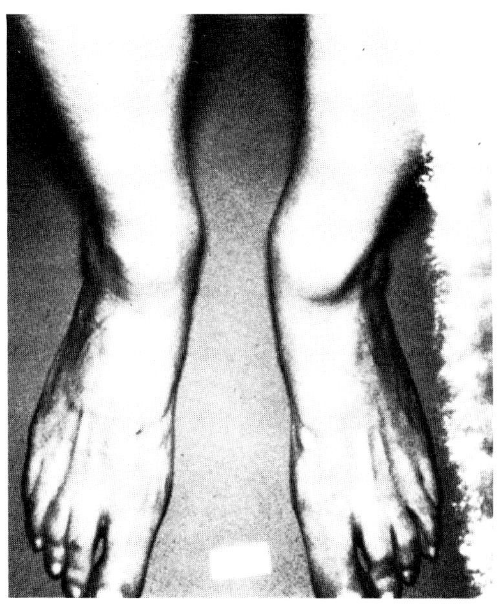

Fig. 16-7. Bilateral swelling just proximal to the dorsal retinaculum of the ankle due to a tenosynovitis of the anterior tibia and the common toe extensors.

the tendon sheaths at the ankle level, as is seen in the hand and wrist, occasionally causing tendon rupture (Fig. 16-7). Rupture of the posterior tibial tendon may cause rapid, severe valgus of the hindfoot. Nodules often develop on the weight-bearing aspect of the os calcis and may erode the bone (Fig. 16-8).

CONSERVATIVE TREATMENT

The conservative measure of proper shoeing with simple orthopaedic supports should be used in early stages with a proper exercise regimen to keep the toes flexible. Basic oxford shoes with a low to medium heel and closed toes and heels are recommended (Fig. 16-9). Metatarsal pads, long arch pads, or heel wedges are added when indicated (Fig. 16-2). Arch supports are usually of firm rubber and are leather-covered. Steel or firm plastic alone is usually too rigid for the rheuma-

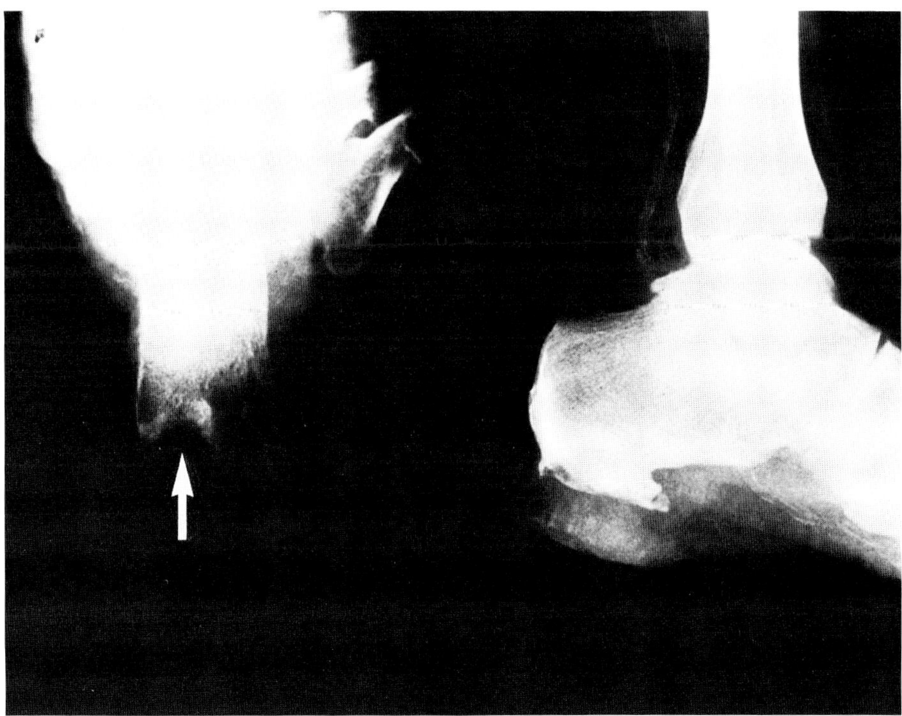

Fig. 16-8. Erosion of the weight-bearing aspect of the os calcis due to a painful rheumatoid nodule (*arrow*).

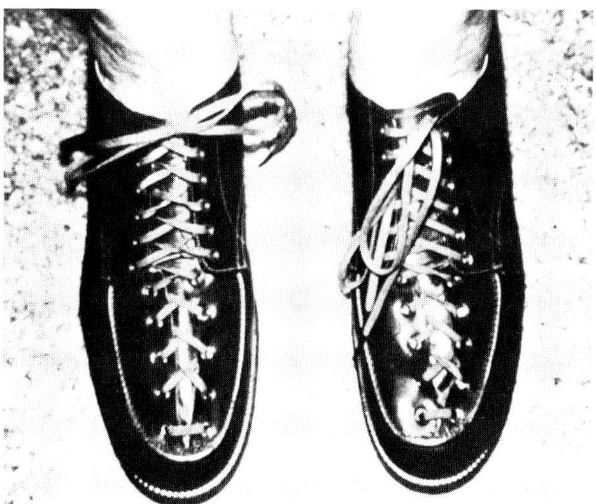

Fig. 16-9. Simple basic oxford shoes with extra depth that may be split and laces added to use as convalescent shoes after surgery.

toid foot. The supports must be custom-made for each patient and frequently require secondary alterations for pressure relief;[31] at times plaster impressions of the feet are helpful for seeing that the arch supports fit precisely. Extra-depth shoes are also commercially available, and special inserts of plastizoate with the extra-depth shoes have been helpful. Running shoes are also useful, especially as a postoperative shoe, and are

stylish and popular today (Fig. 16-10). Berg et al.,[3] utilizing the successful pressure distributing footwear Paul Brand developed for insensitive neurotrophic feet, has treated many rheumatoid feet without surgery. The milder cases utilize an extra-depth shoe with plastizoate liner. More severe feet utilize a sandal with special plastizoate inserts. Severe deformities require a specially made shoe with inserts. The principle is always relief of abnormal areas of pressure. The pain due to long-standing deformity is primarily pressure, as the active stage of inflammatory synovitis is passed. It takes constant supervision of the shoe correction and close cooperation with a knowledgeable pedorthist (shoe expert). Despite proper shoeing for a period of time, a number of patients may want surgery so they can wear a reasonable shoe, a natural desire in today's society. The rheumatoid patient has many problems, and one is to remain within the realm of social acceptance.

The same care must be used for postoperative supports, which are necessary in practically all cases. Usually these supports are simple metatarsal additions, with or without longitudinal pads; but with progression of the disease, more pressure relief may be indicated and necessary. These devices are simply the same basic orthopaedic supports used for mechanical foot deformities due to any other cause (Fig. 16-2).

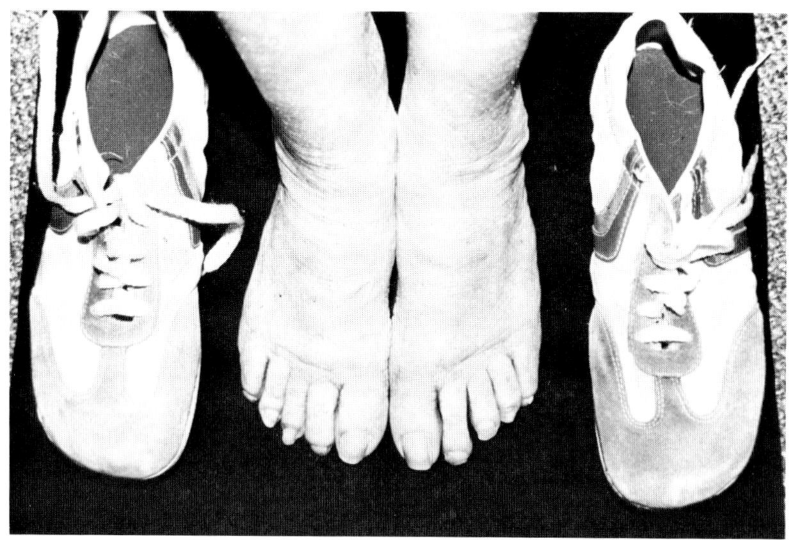

Fig. 16-10. Running shoes may be utilized as pre- or postoperative shoes. Note good alignment of the toes after bilateral forefoot reconstruction and how well the "square" toe of the shoe fits the foot shape. These feet had been reconstructed 6 months earlier. (From Clayton,[10] with permission.)

A brace is occasionally necessary for the valgus deformity of the hindpart of the foot. However, it usually provides only temporary relief; and if the arch supports do not suffice, surgical stabilization may be necessary. A simple outside iron, short-leg brace with an inner T strap has been used when the ankle joint is not particularly painful. If the ankle is painful, a double upright brace with limited ankle motion may be used. Some patients obtain pain relief within a few months even if the deformity remains, and they can then wear the brace part-time.

HISTORICAL REVIEW OF SURGICAL MANAGEMENT

At the meeting of the American Orthopaedic Association in 1911, Hoffmann[23] presented an excellent treatise with many valid principles, and it came to represent the first important report in the literature on surgery of the rheumatoid forefoot.

Several of Hoffmann's patients had "infectious arthritis" (rheumatoid arthritis), and his description of a suitable case was as follows: "The toes are strongly dorsiflexed at the metatarsophalangeal joints and plantar-flexed at their interphalangeal ones and are retained in this position by shortening through adaptation of tendons, ligaments and other soft structures, and by bone changes due to long-continued new relationship of articular surfaces." His operation consisted in excision of the heads and, if necessary, parts of the neck of the metatarsal bones of all affected toes through a transverse curved plantar incision just behind the web of the toes. In the closing discussion Hoffmann stated that "the operation is simply to get rid of the metatarsal heads because they make the patient's life miserable. Every step he takes hurts him so he is afraid to get up from his chair. Mild grades of contracted toes should not be operated upon in this way."

In Hoffmann's first cases, "timidity, due to uncertainty of the outcome, prompted him to remove barely enough bone to allow the articular surface of the phalanx to come in contact with the cut end of the metatarsal bone. Experience taught that it is better to remove the entire metatarsal head and enough of the neck to permit the phalanx to drop into line with the resulting metatarsal stump without crowding against it. This always resulted in freely moveable and serviceable joints, and in feet that were painless and, functionally, surprisingly good." Most of the cases in this original report were cavus feet, which is probably why he removed only metatarsal heads and considerable bone well back into the neck. His technique allowed toes to straighten and relieved the cavus.

In 1937 Thompson[38] outlined surgical procedures useful for correcting deformities of the arthritic foot, including (1) the Keller procedure (exostectomy and proximal hemiphalangectomy of the great toe to correct hallux valgus or hallux rigidus); (2) dorsal dislocation of the toe at the MTP joint corrected by excising the metatarsal head; (3) hammer toe with painful corn corrected by excising the corn and fusing the interphalangeal (IP) joint; (4) painful hammer toe with pressure on the toenail corrected by terminal Symes amputation to remove the toenail and the distal phalanx; and (5) claw toe projecting dorsally corrected by excising the proximal phalanx.

Aufranc and Larson[1] reported a series of patients with chronic rheumatoid arthritic feet seen at the Boston Orthopaedic Club in 1949. Surgery had been performed with varying degrees of MTP joint resections through multiple dorsal incisions. Key[25] in 1950 mentioned a number of surgical procedures with a certain amount of excellent philosophy regarding the care of the arthritic foot. He stated, "I find it possible to benefit a greater number of patients to a greater degree by a few relatively simple operations on the feet than by any of the elaborate procedures on the larger joints which occupy so much of the time and thought of the modern orthopaedic surgeon." He recommended a Keller operation to correct bunions and hallux valgus and occasionally used a proximal osteotomy of the first metatarsal to narrow the metatarsus primus varus. Hammer toe was corrected by dorsal capsulotomy of the MTP joint, excision of the corn transversely, and excision of the distal half of the proximal phalanx. For marked depression of the metatarsal heads, either the base of the phalanx, the metatarsal head, or both were excised. He wrote, "Surgery tends to be destructive or at least ablative and should be moderately radical. Deformities are corrected by extensive removal of bone, and movement is restored to joints by wide excision rather than by meticulous arthroplasties . . . . Many patients with deformed and painful arthritic feet can be greatly benefitted by multiple relatively minor surgical procedures."

In 1959 Fowler[18] discussed how metatarsal heads and bases of phalanges were removed through a dorsal incision that divided skin, veins, and extensor tendons. He also excised a wedge of skin on the plantar aspect of the foot to help pull the toes down and bring the fat pad back under the metatarsal ends. Twelve patients had rheumatoid arthritis, and in these instances he reported satisfactory results. That same year, the first of a series of articles were published that appeared over the next two decades involving resection of the MTP joints.[6–13,36] This type of procedure (see below) has been widely adopted in many parts of the United States and throughout the world.

The following year, Flint and Sweetman[17] reported a procedure for amputation of all toes through the MTP joints. For 12 patients with rheumatoid arthritis they reported six excellent, four good, and two fair results. This procedure is not recommended today because the metatarsal heads remain prominent in the sole of the foot and the result is often unsatisfactory.

Potter[30] in 1961 noted that a forefoot spread due to involvement of the intermetatarsal ligaments was seen in 40 percent of the patients and hallux valgus in 28 percent. Also illustrated were examples of bursitis, tenosynovitis, rheumatoid nodules, and a Morton's neuroma due to rheumatoid involvement.

In 1964 Schwartzmann[34] presented an average 6-year follow-up study of patients with forefoot metatarsal head resections using a single dorsal transverse or multiple longitudinal incisions. Results were generally good, although 8 percent required a second operation.

Kates et al.[24] modified a procedure described by Hoffmann[23] and Fowler[18] and presented their results in 1965. They described an appropriately placed curved plantar incision, convex proximally, with a generous excision of all the metatarsal heads performed to produce a flat anterior arch. Furthermore, they recommended that the great toe be held in line with the first metatarsal using a Kirschner wire (K-wire) and that realignment of the toes and fat pad be accomplished by excising an ellipse of skin with the center part about 1 inch in breadth.

Funk,[19,20] using the same technique as Clayton, obtained good results in 50 feet during 1969 and 1971. He observed that wound healing following the transverse dorsal incision was rapid and recommended that complicated forefoot reconstructive procedures be avoided and immobilization of any lower extremity rheumatoid joint be kept to a minimum. He has now used K-wire fixation of the toes in many cases.

Brattstrom and Brattstrom[4,5] presented their experience with 300 forefoot procedures in rheumatoid patients (average 30 months' follow-up). The best results occurred when the four lateral MTP joints were resected as described by Clayton.[7] However, a transverse plantar incision was preferred, and surgery of the great toe was done only if the toe was symptomatic. Among those patients whose great toe was not primarily operated on, 16 percent later developed hallux valgus.

Lipscomb et al.[26] reported 20 of 22 patients with an average 3-year follow-up who improved after a procedure these surgeons developed for the typical rheumatoid forefoot deformity. Three dorsal longitudinal incisions were recommended. The standard procedure for severe deformity included tenotomy of the extensor tendons, smooth resection of all or part of all the metatarsal condyles flush with the metatarsal shafts, and excision of part or all of the proximal phalanges together with MTP joint synovectomy. A Keller or fusion procedure was performed on the great toe. K-wire fixation of the "floppy" toes was kept in place for 3 weeks. It was thought that preservation of metatarsal length improved stance and balance, and that fusion produced a more stable great toe.

Barton[2] compared the results of various techniques of rheumatoid forefoot resection and found that the operative technique probably makes little difference to the end result, provided the metatarsals are trimmed to approximately equal length. The metatarsal stumps should form a smooth arc toward the fifth metatarsal. Although the subjective results were good, objectively they were less satisfactory. The lateral four toes were usually functionless, and the gait was never normal.

In another large series of patients with rheumatoid arthritis, Marmor[28] presented the results of 272 Clayton-type forefoot resections. There were 85 percent good or excellent results and only 2 percent failures in 128 patients (average 4.7 year follow-up). Most patients could wear regular shoes and walk long distances. If recurrent deformity developed, it was usually because of a long metatarsal shaft.

Gschwend[21] has a long experience with forefoot reconstructions and now generally utilizes a plantar incision with some wedge skin excision for the second through the fifth metatarsal heads, with a separate incision for the great toe. Previously he had 85 percent good results using the MTP resection procedure with the dorsal approach.

OTHER FOREFOOT PROCEDURES

Helal[22] described oblique osteotomy of the distal metatarsal shafts to correct a single deformity; or, in more deformed feet, all five were used. Tillmann[39] preferred to operate through a plantar approach similar to that used by Gschwend.[21] There is a great deal of material of a review nature in his book. It should be noted that excisional type surgery, i.e., forefoot resection, is a basic procedure, but many variations are described. Forefoot reconstruction better describes the procedures today.

Raunio and Laine[32] reviewed MTP joint synovectomies in a small series of 33 procedures on 28 patients whose disease activity was judged mild. By using comparative roentgenograms and Calkin's criteria for disease activity, an attempt was made for objectivity. With an average follow-up period of 25 months, good results were found clinically and roentgenographically in up to two-thirds of the cases. Overall disease activity did affect the results, which were unpredictable; and synovectomy was rarely utilized.

HINDFOOT PROCEDURES

Vahvanen,[40] in a 1967 review of triple arthrodeses, published a controlled series on rheumatoid hindfoot surgery (average 3.7 years follow-up). When the subtalar joints become inflamed, swelling and pain on weight-bearing and the development of planovalgus are early signs; deformity usually develops within 3 years of the occurrence of the first signs in the foot. The most severe radiologic changes occur in the talonavicular joint with the exception of osteoporosis, which is most severe in the area of the calcaneocuboid joint. The symptoms of subtalar inflammation almost completely resolve with triple arthrodesis, and correction of deformity is often achieved. Slight to moderate valgus (10 to 25 degrees) frequently remains but does not cause discomfort with walking. Union usually occurs with the procedure. When nonunion occurs it is most often in the talonavicular joint (3 percent). Autogenous bone grafting is recommended in the most severe cases. The use of bone graft and staples helps with hindfoot reconstruction, but in severe cases it does not prevent the calcaneus from slipping into valgus if weight-bearing is permitted sooner than 6 to 8 weeks. Triple arthrodesis does not adversely affect the stability of the ankle joint, nor does it increase progression of disease in that joint. Vahvanen recommended the operation be done before a hindfoot deformity becomes fixed—usually within 3 years of the development of progressive symptoms in the hindfoot.

Potter[30] and Elbaor et al.[15] reported that the talonavicular joint was the earliest hindfoot joint to demonstrate involvement with rheumatoid arthritis. The initial occurrence was often peroneal muscle spasms, creating eversion of the hindfoot. For the patient unresponsive to conservative measures but in whom the hindfoot is still flexible, talonavicular fusion alone can relieve pain and correct the deformity. Progression of the deformity does not occur, and the hindfoot is stabilized in neutral position (slight valgus) by the single fusion. Their patients did not require later triple arthrodesis. As noted in the review of the hindfoot procedure, the basic procedure is stabilization by arthrodesis.

INDICATIONS FOR SURGERY

Surgical intervention is indicated when there is increasing deformity of the foot or continued pain upon weight-bearing despite conservative measures. In such advanced cases, relief of the abnormal weight-bearing pressure in the forefoot can be obtained by surgery. Such joints are extensively damaged: The feet are already weak, and the toes have lost their usual function. Not only do these patients lack the "takeoff" to their gait, they avoid pressure on the forepart of the foot. Surgery on the forepart of the foot does not further weaken the damaged arthritic foot or impair the patient's gait. In fact, the gait is improved, and with improved gait there may be a decrease in pain in the involved knees and hips.

ANESTHESIA

Surgery to correct arthritic defects in the feet is normally performed under general anesthesia, although regional anesthesia has been used with success and is desirable. Most patients have been on steroid medication at the time of surgery or have recently received steroids. They should receive supplementary steroid medication. No difficulty in healing of the soft tissues has been attributed to the steroids either during the immediate operative phase or postoperatively. Although final wound healing has not been affected, the rate of healing is slower. The tissues of the foot tend to be fragile and must be handled atraumatically. Magnification is used at surgery in the same manner as it would be for hand surgery. Modern motorized power equipment is also utilized. Foot surgery must not be relegated to a minor category. Perioperative intravenous antibiotics are used for the day of operation, usually cephalosporin.

SURGERY OF THE FOREPART OF THE FOOT

The marked contracture of soft tissues accompanying these deformities demands adequate bony resection for correction and pain relief. As previously indicated, the basic procedure has been MTP joint resections of varying degree with excision of an adequate amount of bone to correct the deformity. In the more markedly involved cases the tendency has been to resect all the metatarsal heads and a portion of the necks. The proximal portion ($<$50 percent) of each of the proximal phalanges is also removed as indicated. The distal joints of the toes have been manipulated straight to correct the cock-up deformities, but formal fusion of the distal joints of the small toes has not been performed.

Ten toes are corrected at one operative exercise in most patients. Occasionally, despite the lack of underlying skin changes such as a callus, a metatarsal head must be resected because it would otherwise remain too prominent after removal of the offending adjacent head. The surgical procedure is tailored to fit the individual patient's deformity. It is often preferable to operate through a transverse dorsal incision at the base of the toes, and this incision was utilized in nearly all cases from 1957 to 1972[6–9,11] (Fig. 16-11). With the transverse dorsal approach, there is less disturbance of the major blood and nerve supply to the toes, which enters through the plantar aspect. Exposure is also easier than through multiple dorsal incisions.

Technique

Two surgical teams working simultaneously can help to shorten the anesthesia and operating time and thereby diminish the stress placed on the patient. An Esmarch bandage is used as a tourniquet around the ankle applied over a good layer of padding to prevent skin pressure, or a midthigh tourniquet can be applied.

A transverse dorsal incision is made at the base of the toes in a slightly proximal curve over the first and fifth metatarsal heads (Fig. 16-11). In the

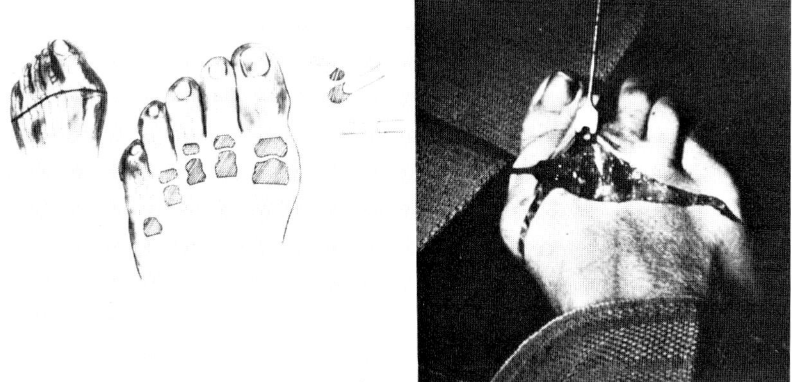

Fig. 16-11. Single dorsal transverse incision with MTP joint reconstructions. Relative amount of bone was resected as well as the remaining fifth phalanx. Note the excellent exposure. (From Clayton,[10] with permission.)

usual case, which is without marked rigid deformity, the extensor tendons are severed except for the great toe, and the base of each proximal phalanx is exposed. The bases of the proximal phalanges are excised except for the fifth toe, and subsequently the metatarsal heads are easily delivered and adequately resected. The plantar aspect of each of the lateral four metatarsals is beveled to give a smooth weight-bearing surface.

The second toe is operated on first and then, moving laterally, the third, fourth, and fifth, thus leaving the great toe until last. The fifth toe is rarely dislocated, and in most cases only the fifth metatarsal head is excised. This method also helps to prevent later fibular drift of the toes. The PIP joints of the lesser toes are gently manipulated straight, waiting until the bone resected has relieved tension on the neurovascular structures. The toes should not be hyperextended in order to prevent damage to vascular structure. After the lesser toes have been corrected, the entire incision can be drawn slightly medially, and exposure of the first metatarsal head and proximal phalanx is simplified. The proximal one-third to one-half of the proximal phalanx of the great toe is resected. The dorsal and tibial surface of the first metatarsal should be beveled to prevent later pressure. The first and second metatarsal stumps should be approximately the same length with gradual tapering evenly across the third, fourth, and fifth. The sesamoids are usually not excised; if they are fused to the metatarsal head or unduly prominent, they are excised. Through the single incision, the exact contour of the distal ends of the metatarsal can be determined and adjusted as desired. Small power saws, double-action bone-cutting forceps, and rongeurs simplify the procedure. The excess capsule of the great toe is often interposed and the capsule closed with a few absorbable sutures. At this stage all of the toes can be placed in the desired position; it is well to shift them slightly medially. Intramedullary K-wires help give stability; they are currently used in most cases, and plantar plate arthroplasty is also performed.

Prior to closure of the soft tissues, the tourniquet should be released. Pressure over the forepart of the foot is applied for several minutes, and major bleeders are subsequently cauterized. Penrose or suction drains are often used. The skin incisions should be carefully closed with fine interrupted sutures or small skin staples. The less trauma to which one subjects these tissues, the better and more rapid is the healing. When closing the incision it is not necessary to suture the tendons, as loss of extension does not occur.

Postoperative Care

The postoperative dressing (Fig. 16-12) is a large conforming dressing applied to hold the toes exactly in the desired position without trying to abduct the great toe. Wet Dacron batting applied over nonadherent dressing with gauze over the incision is held in place by a bias-cut stockinette. A wooden shoe or a cardboard or plaster of Paris

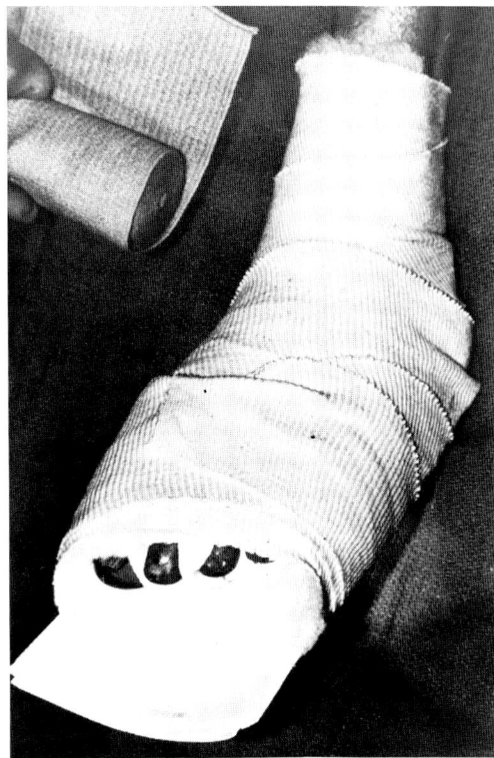

Fig. 16-12. Typical postoperative dressing including wet Dacron batting and a bias-cut stockinette. A wooden shoe is commonly used today to protect the toes and can be used for ambulation later.

splint is used, extending slightly beyond the tips of the digits and incorporated into the dressing. This device protects the foot from the bedclothes and provides some anteroposterior support rather than round-and-round support, which tends to compress the forefoot from side to side.

Elastic bandage may be utilized to wrap from the hindfoot up with slight compression, similar to an elastic stocking. The same gentle care is necessary as when applying a postoperative hand dressing. The drains are usually removed on the second day; dressings are changed at 2 to 3 days and the toes wrapped in the desired position.

If there has been no evidence of circulatory difficulty in the toes, patients are permitted to take a few steps on approximately the third to sixth postoperative day. Sutures remain in place for 2 to 3 weeks. The dressings are changed as

necessary. Ambulation is started with a wooden-soled, laced-top convalescent-type shoe.

Patients have usually been discharged from the hospital after 5 to 7 days in bilateral cases and sooner if unilateral. Only rarely has there been persistent swelling of the forefoot 2 months after surgery. K-wires remain 3 to 4 weeks, depending on the individual. A convalescent-type split shoe is fitted as indicated at 3 to 4 weeks, and the patient is gradually moved into a simple medium-heel oxford shoe.

Patients who do not require crutches for any other disability do not require crutches after forefoot surgery. A metatarsal pad, approximately 3/16 inch to 1/4 inch in height, is generally recommended for patients postoperatively because of the altered configuration of the distal metatarsal. In some patients, a 3/16 inch metatarsal bar may be added. As a rule, no attempt is made to resect corns, calluses, or thickened bursae between the metatarsal heads at the time of surgery. With relief of abnormal pressure of these corns, the calluses and bursae gradually disappear (Fig. 16-13).

Alternate Surgical Approaches

A dorsal transverse incision of the lesser MTP joints may be combined with a dorsal longitudinal incision for the great toe and is the most common approach today. The separate incision for the great toe is particularly useful when a silicone implant is to be utilized (Fig. 16-14A).

A plantar approach (Fig. 16-14B) to the lesser metatarsals, excising a swathe of skin including the callus, is useful for feet with marked depression of the metatarsal heads. The skin closure (dermodesis) helps to pull the toes down; the separate longitudinal dorsal incision for the great toe is again utilized. The plantar incisions are not painful, but the operation is more difficult. Any skin healing complication on the sole is a major problem compared to one on the dorsum of the foot. The cosmetic result is good.

We used three longitudinal skin incisions (Fig. 16-14C) in our first cases, and they are still utilized in feet that have previous longitudinal incisions or those with borderline circulation, as the

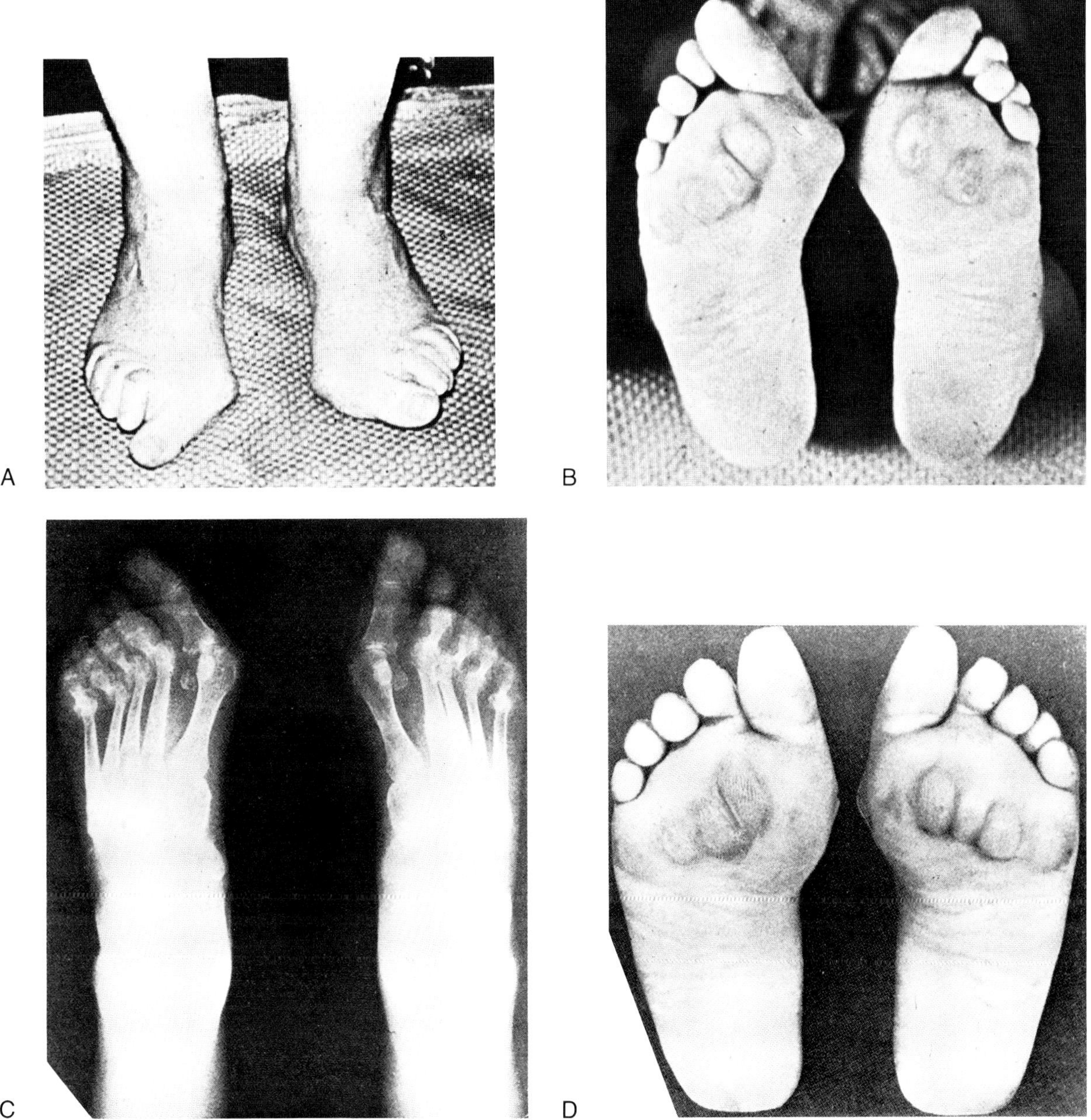

Fig. 16-13. (**A & B**) Typical forefoot deformity. (**C**) Preoperative roentgenogram. (**D**) At 12 days after operation. (*Figure continues.*)

arterial and venous supply is undisturbed to at least one side of each toe (a tourniquet is unnecessary). In general, surgeons may use the incisions with which they are most comfortable.

Recent Developments

Overrefinement of a successful operation in a progressive disease such as rheumatoid arthritis

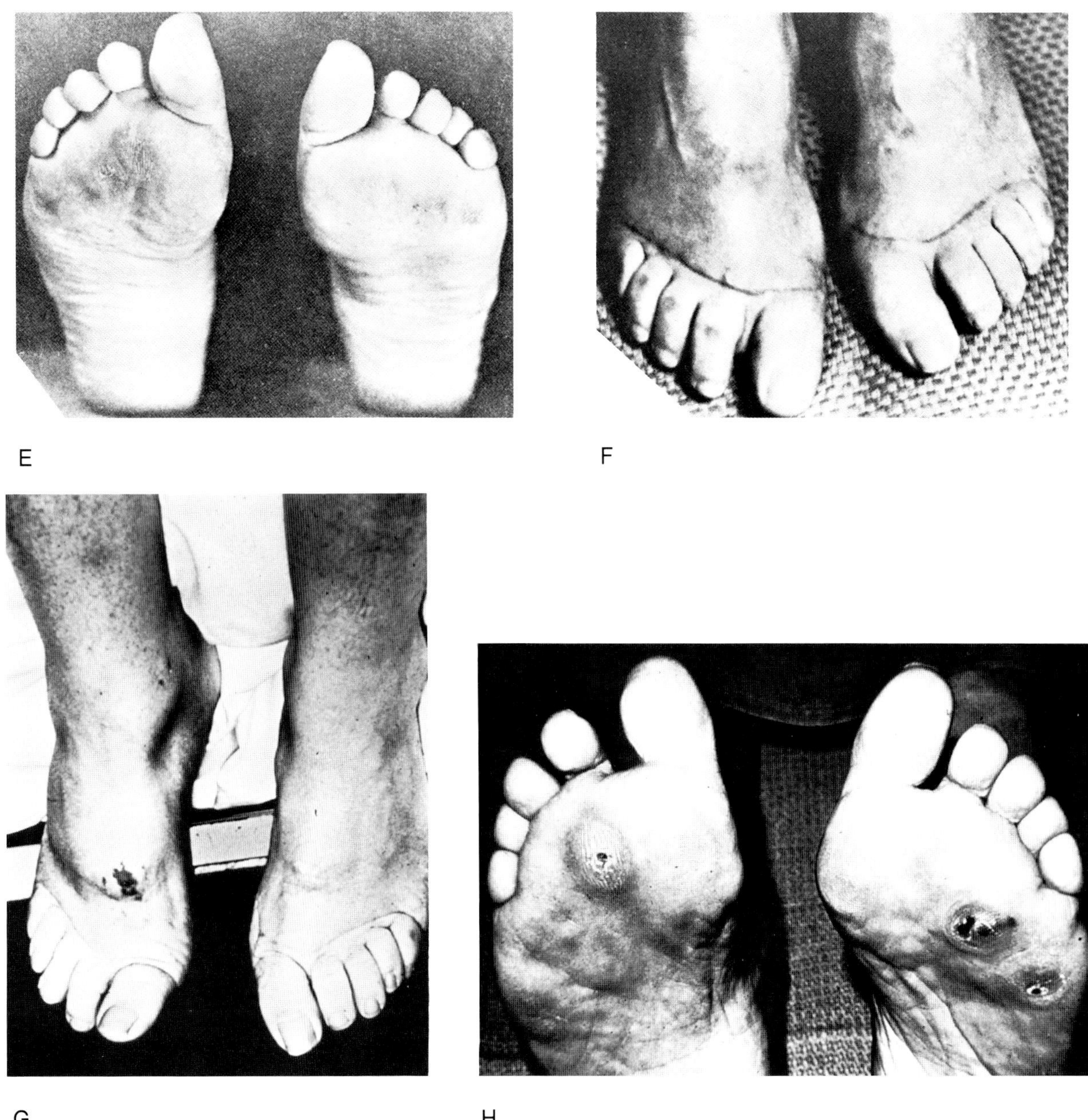

Fig. 16-13 (*Continued.*) (**E & F**) At 3 months after operation. (**G & H**) At 13 years after operation. Recurrent pressure problems were partially relieved by supports. The major pain was in the right foot; osteotomy of the second metatarsal on the right was performed during other surgery, and the pain was relieved. (Figs. A–H from Clayton,[10] with permission.)

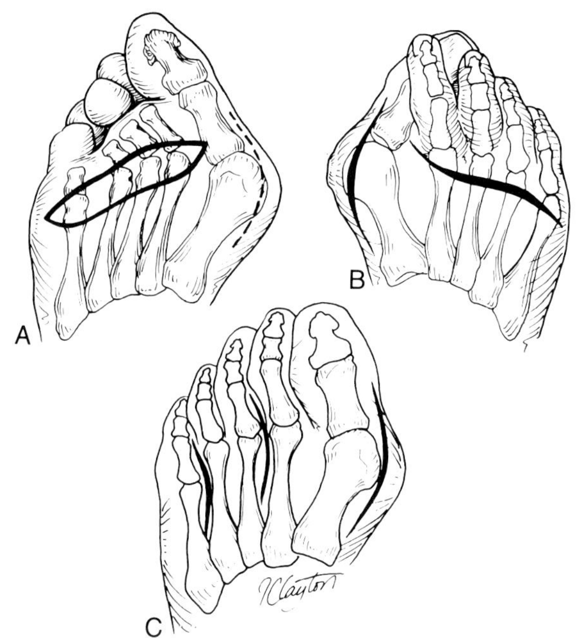

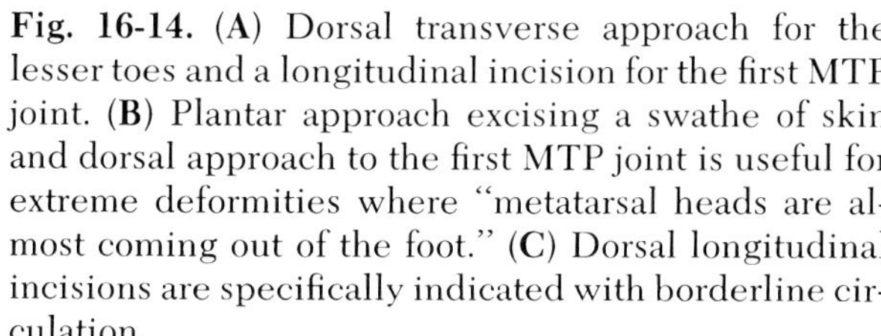

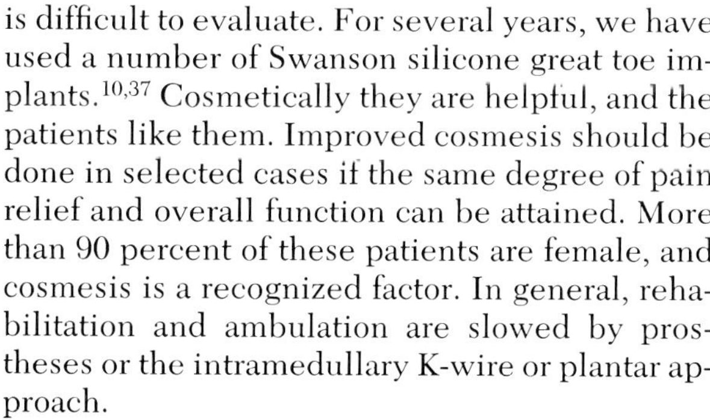

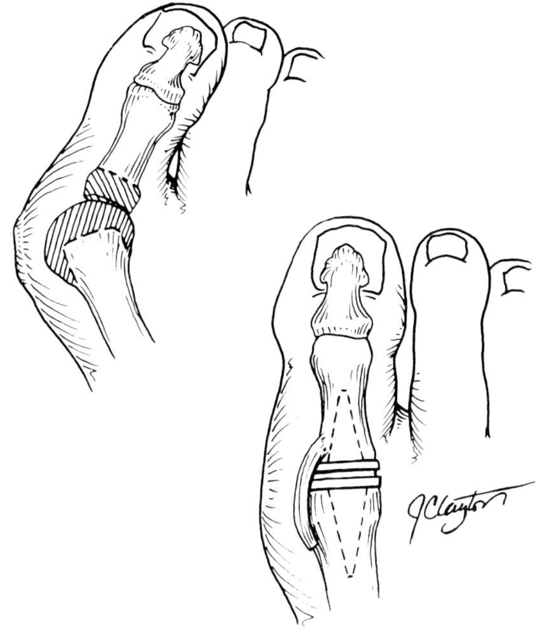

Fig. 16-14. (**A**) Dorsal transverse approach for the lesser toes and a longitudinal incision for the first MTP joint. (**B**) Plantar approach excising a swathe of skin and dorsal approach to the first MTP joint is useful for extreme deformities where "metatarsal heads are almost coming out of the foot." (**C**) Dorsal longitudinal incisions are specifically indicated with borderline circulation.

Fig. 16-15. Silicone (Swanson) double-hinge implant for the great toe. Its use requires the same precise rebalancing of the soft tissues around the implant as it does in the hand. Key reconstruction of the tibial collateral ligament and capsule is necessary, and the toe should remain in the fully corrected position at the end of the procedure. (From Clayton,[10] with permission.)

is difficult to evaluate. For several years, we have used a number of Swanson silicone great toe implants.[10,37] Cosmetically they are helpful, and the patients like them. Improved cosmesis should be done in selected cases if the same degree of pain relief and overall function can be attained. More than 90 percent of these patients are female, and cosmesis is a recognized factor. In general, rehabilitation and ambulation are slowed by prostheses or the intramedullary K-wire or plantar approach.

In the prosthesis for the great toe, the double-hinged type is now preferred, and the procedure is an exacting one[37] (Fig. 16-15). The single-stem silicone implant has too often led to "silicone" synovitis, including disturbing cysts.[16] This complication has been rare with the double-stem implant. An independent longitudinal dorsal incision is utilized. The soft tissue rebalancing is all-important to maintain the realignment of the

great toe. A distally based capsular flap is utilized to expose the MTP joint and the bunion in the usual manner. The metatarsal head is resected in a conservative manner, and the base of the phalanx must be resected to give a flattened surface. Overall shortening of approximately $1/8$ to $1/4$ inch through the metatarsal head is desirable for decompression; an excessive amount of the metatarsal head should not be removed. If the short flexor has become detached from the base of the proximal phalanx, it should be resutured. Closure of the distally based capsular flap with absorbable sutures should have the toe exactly in the desired position at the end of the procedure.

Because the prosthesis contributes to the length of the great toe, less bone is removed from the lesser MTP joints; often only the metatarsal heads are removed and, if necessary, a small amount of the base of the phalanx. K-wires are used across the lesser MTP joints.

Convalescence is slow (3 to 4 weeks), and postoperative therapy and supervision are necessary. An outrigger with elastic tension along with active and passive exercises may be used to guide the formation of encapsulation around the implant. The toes can be simply taped in position but must allow exercises, both active and passive, for the great toe. Toes must be trained exactly in the desired position and adequate dorsiflexion obtained for a good gait. Wooden shoes are used for ambulation for 3 to 4 weeks until K-wires are removed. Convalescent-type shoes are then utilized, and toes are strapped into position for more time if necessary. A night splint for the great toe may be used for a few weeks. Metatarsal pads and other supports as indicated are utilized.

Another important development has been the plantar plate arthroplasty[10,29,36] of the lesser MTP joints (Fig. 16-16). After the usual MTP joint resection from a dorsal approach, the plantar plate is released from the flexor tendons for about 1 cm distally by simply incising the sheath. The plate is drawn upward over the end of the resected metatarsal exactly centering the flexor tendons underneath the end of the metatarsal and transfixing with an intramedullary K-wire, which is left in place for 3 to 4 weeks. The extensor tendon is not sutured, providing an interposition arthroplasty and tending to prevent recurrence of deformity as it centers the flexor tendons underneath the end of the metatarsal. It adds minimal time to the procedure. If K-wire fixation is not desired, the plantar plate can be sutured to the dorsum of the resected metatarsal through a small drill hole. A medial capsular arthroplasty can be performed in the great toe in a similar manner if a prosthesis is not indicated or desired (Fig. 16-17). The medial capsular arthroplasty

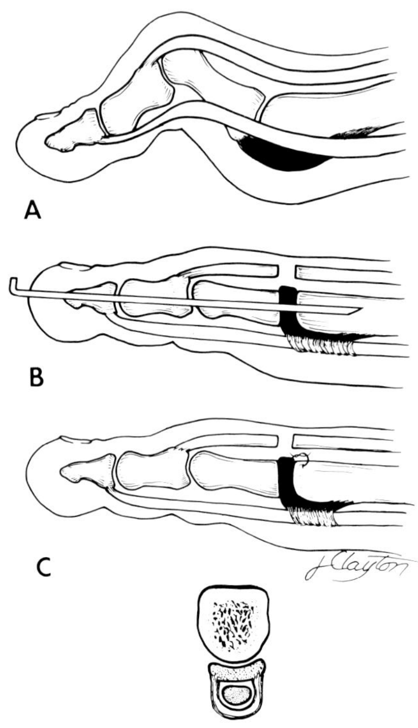

Fig. 16-16. (A) Plantar plate interpositional arthroplasty. Flexor tendon deformity and rotation of the plantar plate off to the side of the metatarsal head are present, causing the flexor to become a deforming force. **(B & C)** Postoperative diagram after MTP joint resection shows K-wire fixation of the plate with proper flexor tendon orientation seen on cross section. The long extensor tendon is not sutured. Wires are usually left in for 3 to 4 weeks. (From Clayton,[10] with permission.)

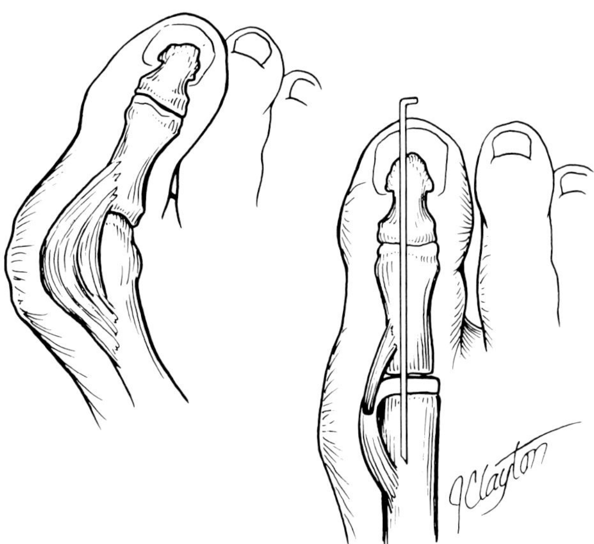

Fig. 16-17. Medial capsular arthroplasty after MTP joint resection. The excess medial capsule is released on the volar aspect almost to the sesamoid, preserving a small slip, which is to be resutured as a collateral ligament. The medial capsular flap is interposed and speared with the K-wire, which holds the great toe in proper alignment. Tension adjustment on the medial flap at the time of interposition controls the position of the sesamoids.

provides a slightly better result than simple resection, as one can control the position of the sesamoids underneath the first metatarsal head. After MTP joint resection, excess medial capsule is interposed and fixed with the K-wire. It is important to save a small portion with which to reconstruct the tibial collateral ligament, as illustrated.

Occasionally, the first MTP joint fusion is useful to correct pain and deformity. Mann and Thompson[27] reported this operation to be their procedure of choice, combined with MTP resections of lesser toes. They had 14 excellent and 2 good results and 2 failures in 18 feet, which approximates the percentages reported for forefoot resection reconstruction (Table 16-1). Raunio et al.[33] compared 35 resection arthroplasties with 30 arthrodeses of the first MTP joint. They reported that "functional and anatomical assessment of the results performed by the doctor as well as by the patient did not reveal superiority of either series. Failures of the arthrodeses almost constantly resulted from incorrect position of the fusion." We have little personal experience with arthrodeses in rheumatoid arthritis, as arthroplasty has given good results, the recovery period is simpler, and there is no subsequent abnormal stress on the IP joint.

In one case (Fig. 16-18), arthrodesis was performed by removing articular cartilage, usually leaving the rounded contours. Fixation was obtained by crossed K-wires and interosseous wiring. This step provides excellent compression for contact and rigid fixation, which allows early weight-bearing in a wooden shoe. Pins do not violate the IP joint, which is important as it will be under increased strain later; also the fixation materials are buried and usually do not require removal. The desired position of fusion is at 15 to 20 degrees valgus and 10 to 20 degrees dorsiflexion in the plane of the foot. It usually is at 25 to 30 degrees in the plane of the first MTP angle, but this angle varies according to the angle of the first metatarsal and the floor. At the time of surgery a sterile piece of Plexiglas underneath the foot is helpful for estimating the proper angle and the pressures across the foot.

When lesser metatarsal heads alone are resected, K-wire fixation is sometimes used to keep the base of the phalanges properly centered over the end of the metatarsal, and it places the plantar plate directly underneath the metatarsal head and helps keep the flexor tendon centrally located.

Recurrent cock-up deformity is due not only to contraction of the extensors but mainly to the flexor tendons sliding off to one side. The flexor tendons actually becoming extensors of the MTP joint and flexors of the proximal IP joint, which causes recurrent deformity.

Special Considerations

For the forefoot with less severe deformity, several isolated procedures utilized the same basic principles of adequate bony resections: (1) the Keller procedure with or without medial capsular arthroplasty or silicone implant (Fig. 16-19) for hallux valgus and bunion; (2) partial proximal phalangectomy or middle-joint resection, with or without arthrodesis, for individual hammer toe (Fig. 16-20); (3) bony fusion is usually not desired, and if a pin is used it should be removed in about 3 to 4 weeks; (4) oblique resection of the fifth metatarsal head for a bunionette or intractable callus underneath it. Again, the basic principle is adequate bony resection.

If three metatarsal heads require surgery, it is preferable to perform the entire forefoot reconstruction so that a new weight-bearing alignment may be achieved across the entire MTP portion of the foot. Such alignment is determined by the relative alignment of the metatarsal ends. Further decompression is obtained by resecting the base of the phalanges as necessary for proper re-

Table 16-1.   Results of Forefoot Reconstruction

Result	No. of Patients at 1 to 5 Years of Follow-up			
	1	*2*	*3*	*5*
Good	58	50	30	16
Fair	5	4	1	1
Failure	3 (0)[a]	3 (1)[a]	2 (1)[a]	—
Total no.	66	57	33	17

[a] Number of patients who had a better result after supplementary surgery.
(Data from Clayton.[9])

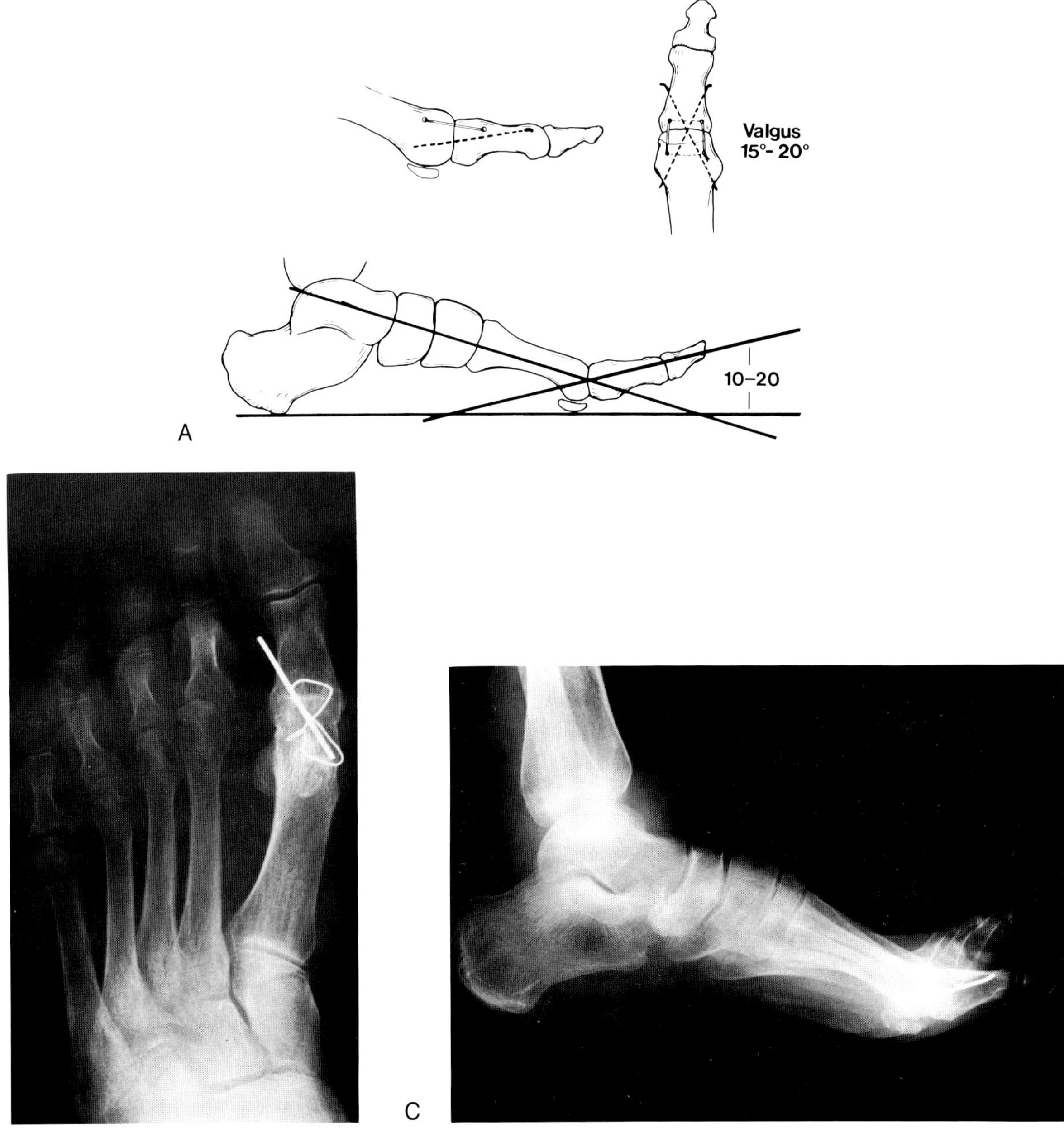

Fig. 16-18. **(A)** Position for first MTP joint fusion, crossed K-wires, and the interosseous wire loop. **(B & C)** Roentgenograms of a 60-year-old woman who had had rheumatoid arthritis for 20 years and developed painful hallux valgus and metatarsalgia. Arthrodesis relieved the great toe pain and most of the metatarsalgia.

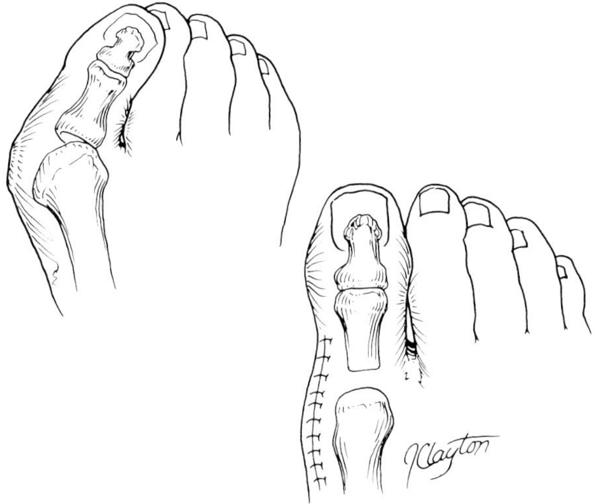

Fig. 16-19. Simple Keller procedure with proximal phalanx resection, where early ambulation is desired. Medial capsular arthroplasty or double-hinge silicone arthroplasty may be used if desired. (From Clayton,[10] with permission.)

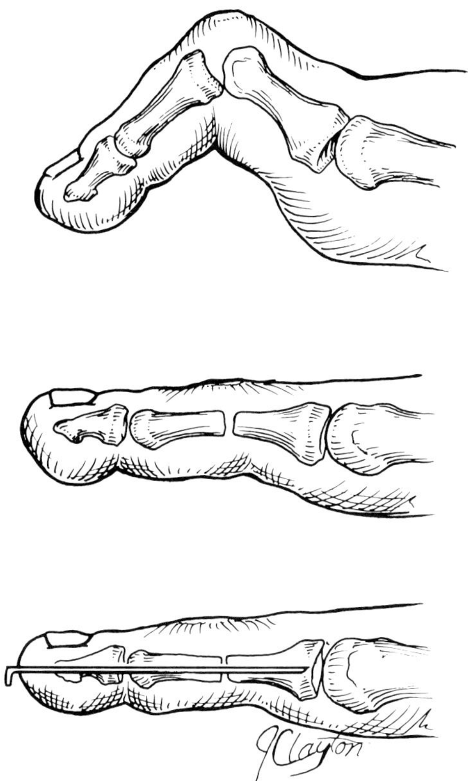

Fig. 16-20. Middle joint resection for hammer toe (ankylosis of toes is neither necessary or desirable). If a pin is used, it should not cross the MTP joint unless necessary to maintain correction; it is left in place for 3 to 4 weeks for soft tissue healing. (From Clayton,[10] with permission.)

alignment without unnecessary shortening the metatarsals. If the patient has a short first metatarsal head, its resection may not be necessary (Fig. 16-21). Only the bunion exostoses should be removed. It is the final relative length that is important. There is a little more leeway in the exact length of the first metatarsal, as the sesamoids are not usually removed; however, if they are adherent or immobile, both should be excised. They usually retract slightly and give a fairly wide area to transmit weight to the first metatarsal head. In some cases with painful prominence of only one or two lesser metatarsal heads, simple osteotomy through the distal shaft is performed; if shortening is desired as well, it can be done obliquely. The latter can be performed as an individual correction under local anesthesia or, in case of a recurrent deformity, with an operation to relieve pressure callus and pain.

Other forefoot procedures recommended in unusual cases include arthrodesis of the IP joint of the great toe for hyperextension deformity with painful callus underneath the distal condyles of the proximal phalanx but with a well-aligned, serviceable MTP joint. We have referred

to this deformity as functional hallux rigidus[12] and believe it is due to involuntary spasm of the intrinsic muscle of the great toe in an attempt to unload the lateral metatarsal heads. It prevents normal dorsiflexion at the first MTP joint and causes hyperextension of the IP joint with a painful callus such as is seen with hallux rigidus (Fig. 16-22). Another operation is the terminal Symes procedure, which is excellent to correct marked nail deformity or terminal joint deformity (Fig. 16-23). Subcutaneous tenotomy is also a useful operation. For an early case of flexion deformity of an IP joint or extension deformity of an MTP joint, simple subcutaneous tenotomy of the flexor or extensor tendon, respectively, with manipulation of the toe (in com-

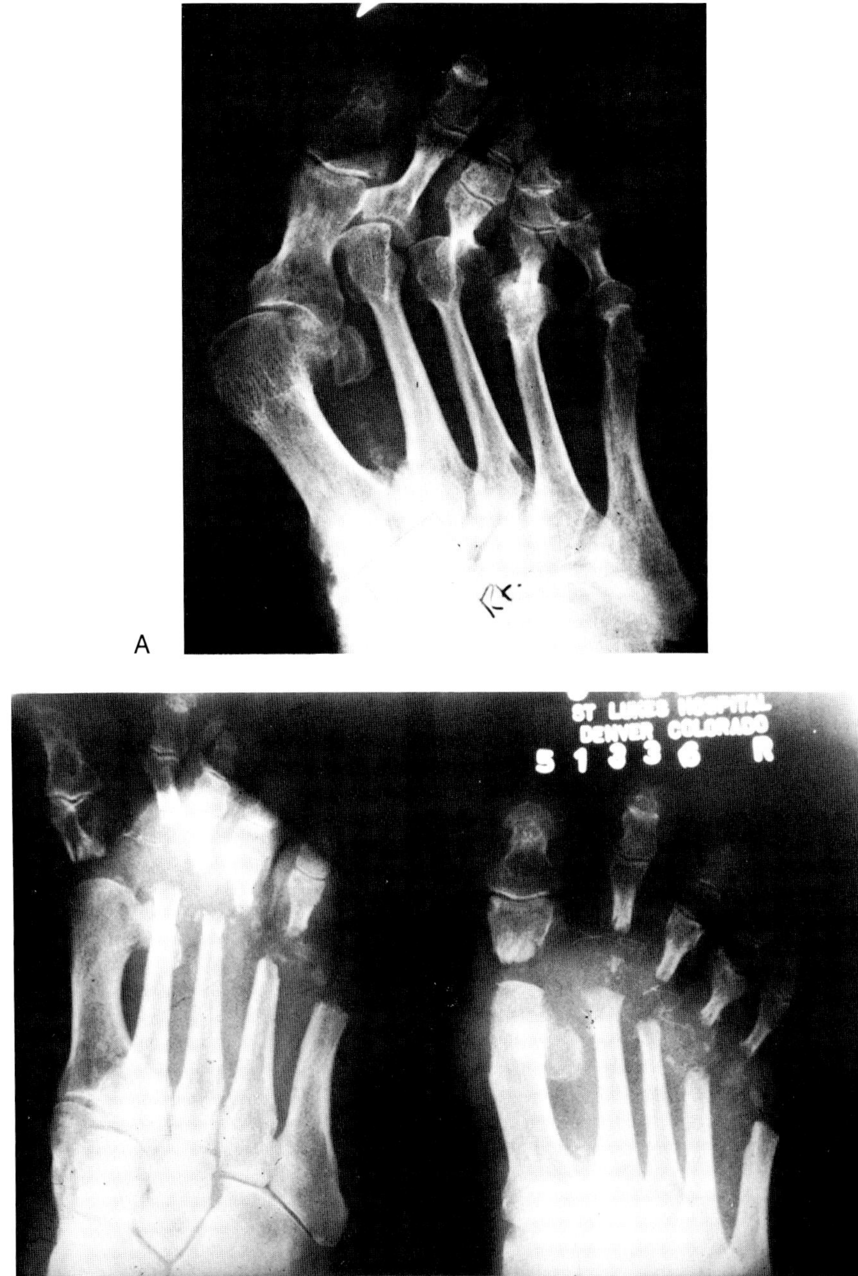

Fig. 16-21. **(A)** Classic forefoot deformities: hallux valgus, bunions, dislocated MTP joints, erosions of the fifth metatarsal head, and a short first metatarsal. **(B)** After reconstruction. First metatarsal head remains, but the relative length of the metatarsals is now correct.

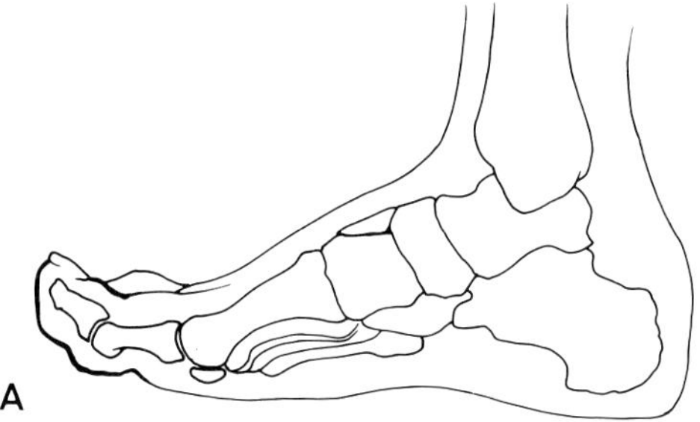
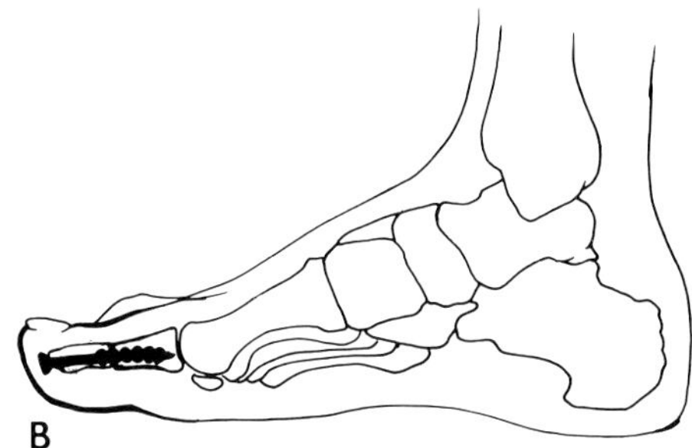

Fig. 16-22. (**A**) Functional hallux rigidus. The great toe has a good MTP joint but an IP hyperextension deformity. The MTP joint is held in flexion with weight-bearing owing to spasm of the intrinsic musculature from painful lesser MTP joints. (**B**) If the MTP joint is in good condition, arthrodesis of the IP joint with screw fixation is indicated (the screw is purposely overemphasized here). Lag screw threads should not cross the arthrodesis line. (From Clayton and Reis,[12] with permission.)

bination with proper support) may produce adequate correction of the subjective and objective symptoms.

Morton's neuroma or interdigital neuroma may require excision along with the rheumatoid synovium in the bursa. In a case of forefoot reconstruction, resection of the metatarsal heads relieves the pressure on a neuroma and obviates dissection of the nerves. However, in an isolated case without other forefoot deformities, excision of the neuroma is indicated the same as for a nonrheumatoid case.

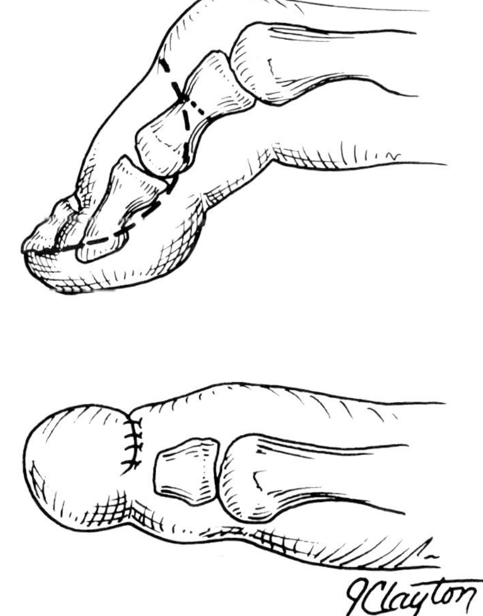
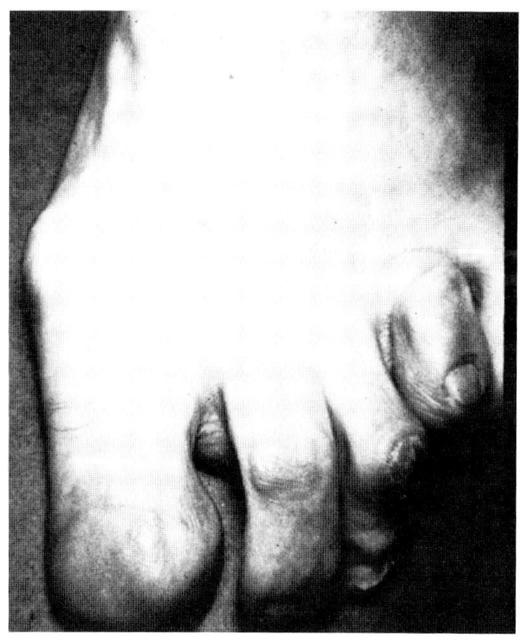

Fig. 16-23. (**A**) Terminal Symes procedure of a lesser toe, which would be through either the distal IP joint or the middle phalanx. It is a more common procedure for severe deformity of the nail bed of the great toe. It is important to remove all of the nail bed. If desired, the patient can "paint" a toenail on the dorsum later. (**B**) Five years after operation.

Results of Forefoot Resection

Results of complete forefoot reconstruction without K-wires have essentially good results (Table 16-1). About 10 percent of the patients have required further surgery because of disease progression or alterations with abnormal pressure. A single recurrent pressure point underneath a metatarsal end is best treated by a metatarsal osteotomy under local anesthesia with minimal incision (or trimming the metatarsal end) and continued walking in a stiff shoe. At certain times a single cock-up toe requires a procedure to correct the hammer toe deformity or a tenotomy. The toes are usually "loose" and function as shoe fillers after the resection. Deformed arthritic toes have already lost their function before the surgery (Fig. 16-13). The important factor determining the result is not the incision but the proper realignment of the metatarsals for weight-bearing. Variations of the incisions have been utilized for many years in selected cases (Fig. 16-14).

The cosmetic results obtained from prostheses and plantar plate arthroplasty have been good, and functional results seem the same or better than standard resections over a 2-year personal follow-up. There have been no cases of severe displacement or cock-up at the MTP joints, although there have been a few reports of abnormal pressure areas underneath metatarsal heads. It should be noted that procedures that remove less bone have had more recurrent problems with time.

The overall level of function usually depends on the general rheumatoid disease activity; for example, a few patients are able to play tennis or ski, whereas others require walking aids because of other involved joints. In general, refined cosmetic procedures are reserved for younger patients. In an older patient for whom early resumption of activity is important, simple excisional forefoot resection arthroplasty without additional fixation provides early mobilization and good results.

SURGERY OF THE HINDFOOT

Progressive valgus deformity of the hind part of the foot often resembles a paralytic valgus deformity with its insidious progression. Surgical stabilization is indicated when conservative measures fail to give relief of pain or to control the deformity.

The talonavicular joint is the keystone of the arch of the foot. If the valgus can be passively corrected, fusion of the talonavicular joint stabilizes the hindfoot and blocks 90 percent or more of the motion of the subtalar joint. Subtalar fusion alone is not as satisfactory and has allowed breakdown in the talonavicular and calcaneocuboid joints with progressive rheumatoid arthritis.

Arthrodesis

Arthrodesis is the surgery of choice for the hindfoot involved by rheumatoid arthritis and is indicated if progressive pain and deformity not responding to shoe supports are present. The most common deformity is progressive valgus deformity; in time, it is often as severe as a paralytic valgus. Posterior tibial tendon rupture due to rheumatoid tenosynovitis has been seen as a cause of rapid severe valgus. Tendons can rupture around the foot exactly as around the hand. However, cavovarus is also seen, particularly in patients with juvenile rheumatoid arthritis.

If the deformity is not passively correctable, triple arthrodesis with joint excision to correct the deformity is utilized (Fig. 16-24). A generous longitudinal incision just anterior to the lateral malleolus and distally over the calcaneocuboid joint protecting the sural nerve is recommended; a second medial incision is utilized over the talonavicular joint. The usual small incision laterally is not recommended in rheumatoids because of skin healing problems probably due to too forceful retraction; rheumatoid tissues, especially the skin, are fragile. Also, triple arthrodesis is an uncommon operation today. The markedly deformed rheumatoid foot requires extensive release around the talus to obtain correction. However, just as for the forefoot, the incision is not the determining factor, and surgeons should choose the incision with which they are most comfortable. In the severe valgus foot after releasing around the talus, the os calcis must be translocated underneath the talus with minimal bone excision. Simple wedge excision does not

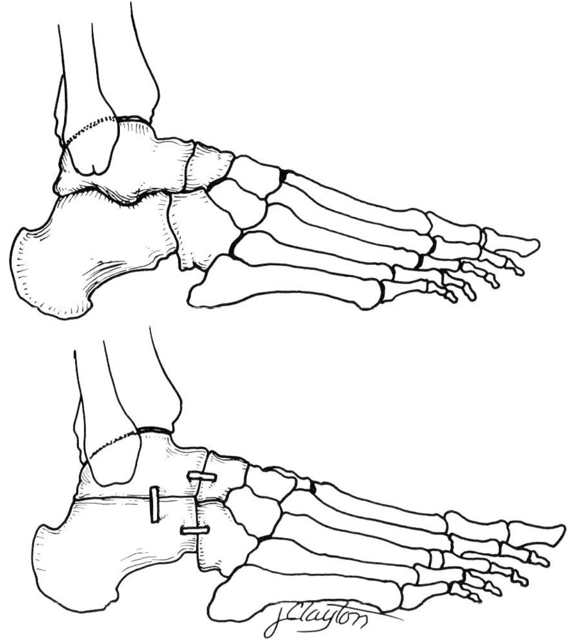

Fig. 16-24. Triple arthrodesis (talocalcaneal, talonavicular, and calcaneocuboid). Additional bone graft may not be necessary. Staples are used for internal fixation.

correct the deformity. The talocalcaneal joint must be stapled in the physiologic slight valgus ("Thou shall not varus"); the forefoot is then derotated and stapled first at the talonavicular and then at the calcaneocuboid to give a plantigrade forefoot (Fig. 16-25). Bone grafting may be necessary as well. Cracchiolo, an experienced foot surgeon and past President of the American Orthopedic Foot and Ankle Society, and his group[14] reported excellent results using a dowel bone grafting technique. They emphasized correction of the deformity before grafting and used staples when internal fixation was necessary.

Staple fixation is usually utilized and in some cases allows earlier weight-bearing in a short leg cast. In unstable cases however, immobilization is necessary in a short leg non-weight-bearing cast for 6 to 8 weeks and then a walking cast for another month. Screw fixation also can be utilized instead of staples. The principle is to obtain internal fixation.

When multiple hindfoot involvement can be passively corrected, triple arthrodesis utilizing

plug grafting is recommended. Local, tibial, or iliac bone can be utilized with additional staples as necessary. If stable, this technique allows early weight-bearing in a cast. In the illustrated case (Fig. 16-26), proper alignment has been maintained, but progressive loss of cartilage produced a painful foot; such a case is ideal for "plug" bone grafting.

In some cases the talonavicular joint is the first joint affected and is involved out of proportion to the others (Fig. 16-27A). This situation is an indication for talonavicular arthrodesis alone, as reported by Elbaor et al.[15] (Fig. 16-27B). The prominence of the navicular is excised; a bone graft is then inlaid ("plugged") across the joint and fixed with a staple or two. An iliac graft may be used.

The talonavicular fusion also immobilizes and stabilizes the subtalar joint; more than 90 percent of the motion is prevented. The talonavicular joint is the keystone of the arch of the foot, and none of these cases has had to be converted to triple arthrodesis. It is the operation of choice for early cases. We often plug-graft other triple joints along with the talonavicular joint if they show marked changes, even when it is not absolutely necessary.

The arthrodesis of the hindfoot should be positioned in slight valgus (neutral) as for any other condition; varus is a disaster. **The foot must be aligned with the ankle**, not the knee. Most rheumatoid patients have an external rotation deformity through the knee, so alignment of the foot with the knee would lead to varus. Triple arthrodesis often requires up to 3 months of immobilization in a cast and another 3 months for maximum rehabilitation. Underestimation of time to recovery creates an unhappy patient; conversely, if the time in a cast turns out to be shorter, the patient is pleased. Talonavicular arthrodesis alone requires at least 8 weeks of immobilization and about 4 months for maximum rehabilitation.

If an ipsilateral angular deformity at the knee and an arthroplasty is indicated, the knee should be treated before the triple arthrodesis. Hence the foot can be positioned plantigrade during the final alignment of the leg.

One unusual complication after triple arthrodesis has been noted with rupture of the deltoid ligament and severe valgus deformity through the ankle joint. Treatment of two such cases has

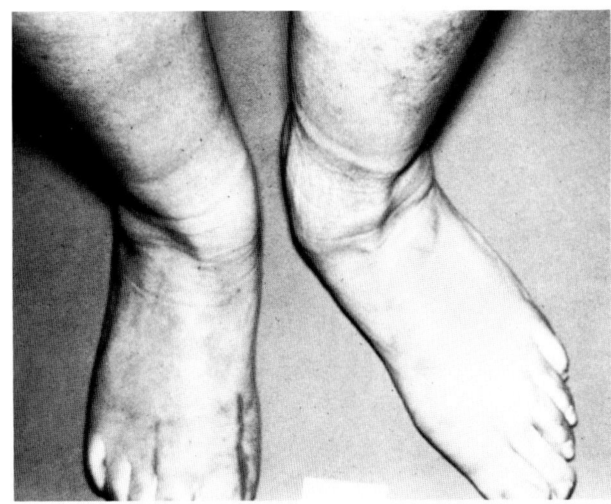

A

Fig. 16-25. **(A)** Preoperative photograph. Note valgus deformity of the left foot; this severe unilateral deformity is often associated with posterior tibial rupture or dysfunction. **(B & C)** Lateral weight-bearing roentgenograms of both feet. Note the valgus and depression of the long arch on the left and the talonavicular changes (arrow). (*Figure continues.*)

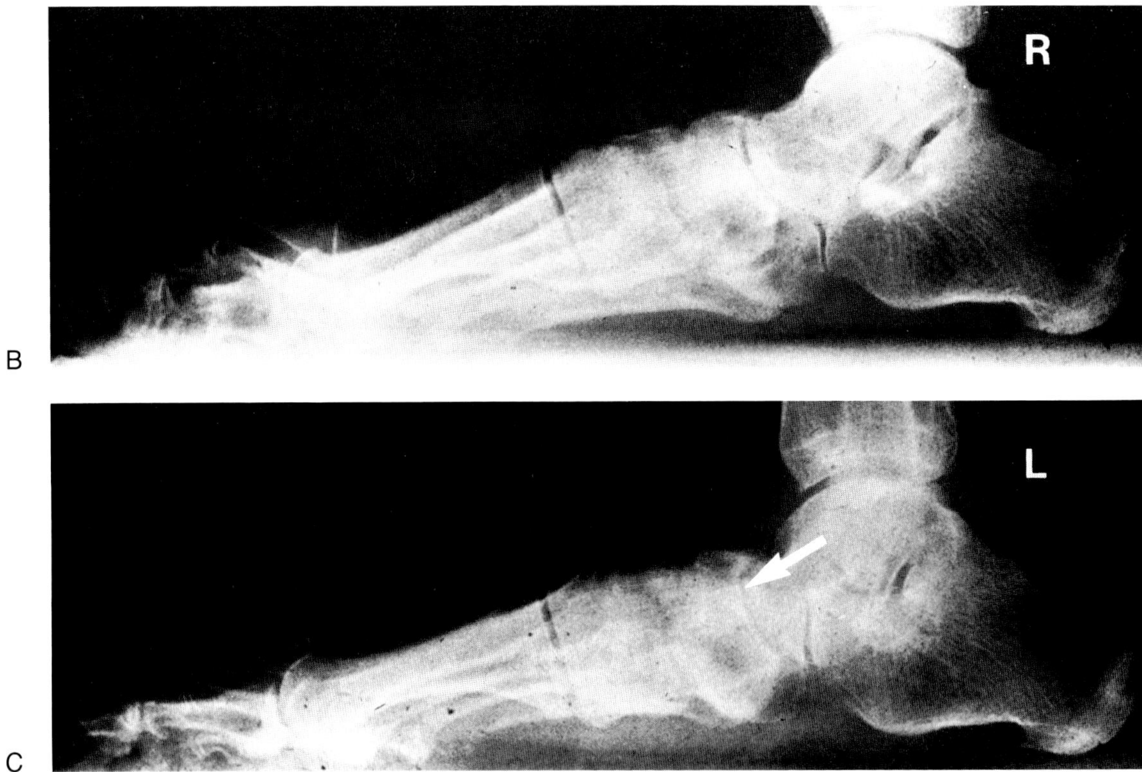

B

C

been ankle fusion through a medial approach with a longitudinal osteotomy of the medial malleolus that is hinged posteriorly and replaced as a living bone graft.

Hindfoot arthrodesis provides the usual good result with relief of pain at the expense of mo-tion. Triple arthrodesis is not a common operation today, and proper stabilization of the severely deformed rheumatoid foot is not a simple procedure: It is exacting and often time-consuming. Rheumatoid nodules over pressure areas such as the os calcis may require excision; recur-

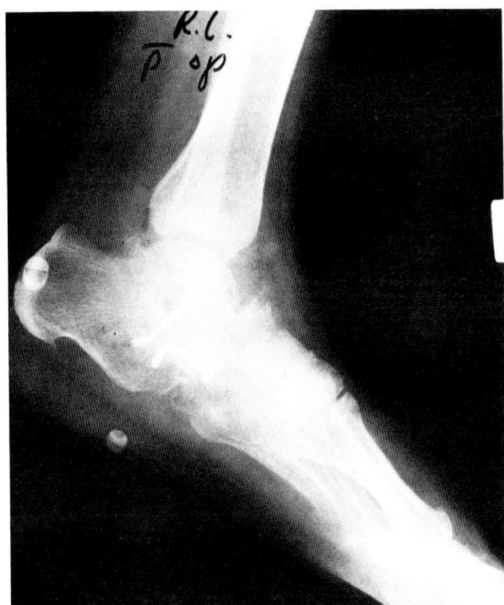
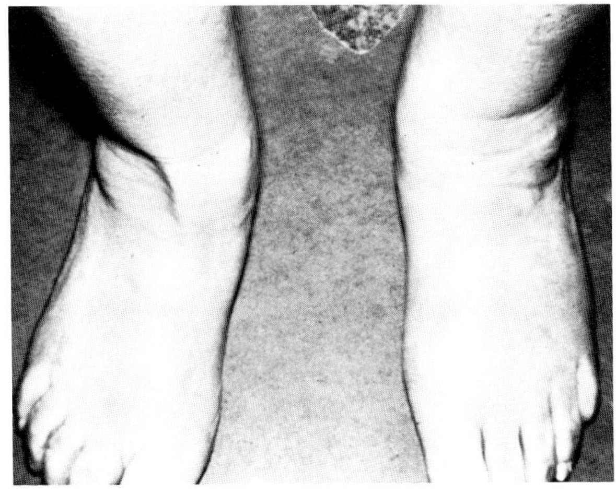

Fig. 16-25 *(Continued).* **(D & E)** Postoperative roentgenograms of triple arthrodesis. Staples were used in the subtalar and calcaneocuboid joints. Deformity of the left foot is corrected.

rence is common unless shoeing alterations are used to prevent recurrent pressure (Fig. 16-8).

Tenosynovitis occurs around the foot and ankle exactly as in the hand and wrist, but it is much less common. Dorsal tenosynovectomy is similar to that in the wrist except that a narrow portion (1.5 to 2.0 cm) of the dorsal retinaculum must be maintained as a pulley at the ankle to prevent bowstringing (Fig. 16-7). Tenosynovectomy of the posterior tibial tendon (see Fig. 15-1) should be performed if it is involved with release of the tarsal tunnel. This procedure can relieve pain and help prevent rupture. Several cases of rupture of posterior tibial tendons have led to severe planovalgus feet that have had to be treated with triple arthrodesis.

While the patient is in the hospital and in bed recovering from the foot surgery, other involved joints are treated using selected apparatus and regimens. Medical treatment as indicated is resumed so no time is wasted. Often improvement can be obtained in other joints by conservative measures utilizing the necessary period of rest after surgery. Many upper extremity procedures can be carried out at the same time as forefoot surgery by using teams.

Results

For forefoot surgery, the object is to relieve the pain from abnormal weight-bearing pressure and to obtain a weight-tolerant foot. No attempt is made to retain strong toe function. When evaluating the forefoot procedures, the partial loss of active toe motion is considered an acceptable loss. Functional and cosmetic results have generally been gratifying to both patient and surgeon. In the experience of orthopaedists who have worked with arthritic patients and who have been able to follow them carefully, the consensus is that these patients have been satisfied with the results; rarely has one regretted having undergone the operation.[21] Usually such patients have been grateful for the relief of pain. Results of surgery for this chronic progressive generalized disease cannot be compared with those obtained for any other type of static condition, as the goal here is to attain a limited gain in function.

When evaluating the procedure in 1967,[9] a decision was made about rating the end results of these cases, and it seemed advisable not to include a category of "excellent" in this type of excisional surgery. This decision has remained

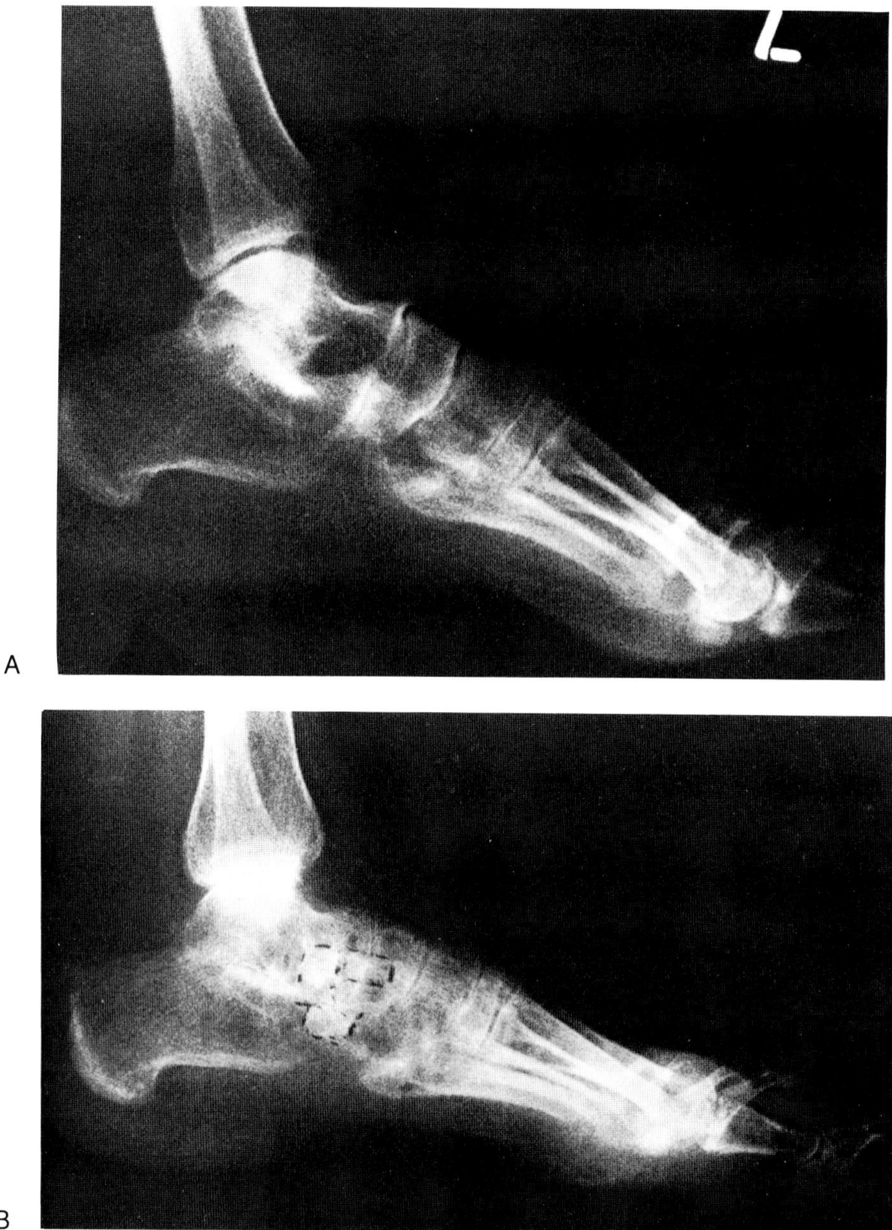

Fig. 16-26. **(A)** There is overall good alignment of the foot but marked narrowing and irregularity of the triple joints. **(B)** After inlay plug grafting with iliac bone of the triple joints, fusion has occurred after 2.5 months in a walking cast. The dotted lines outline the plug grafts; grafts were inserted with small medial and lateral incisions, and the joints were not otherwise resected.

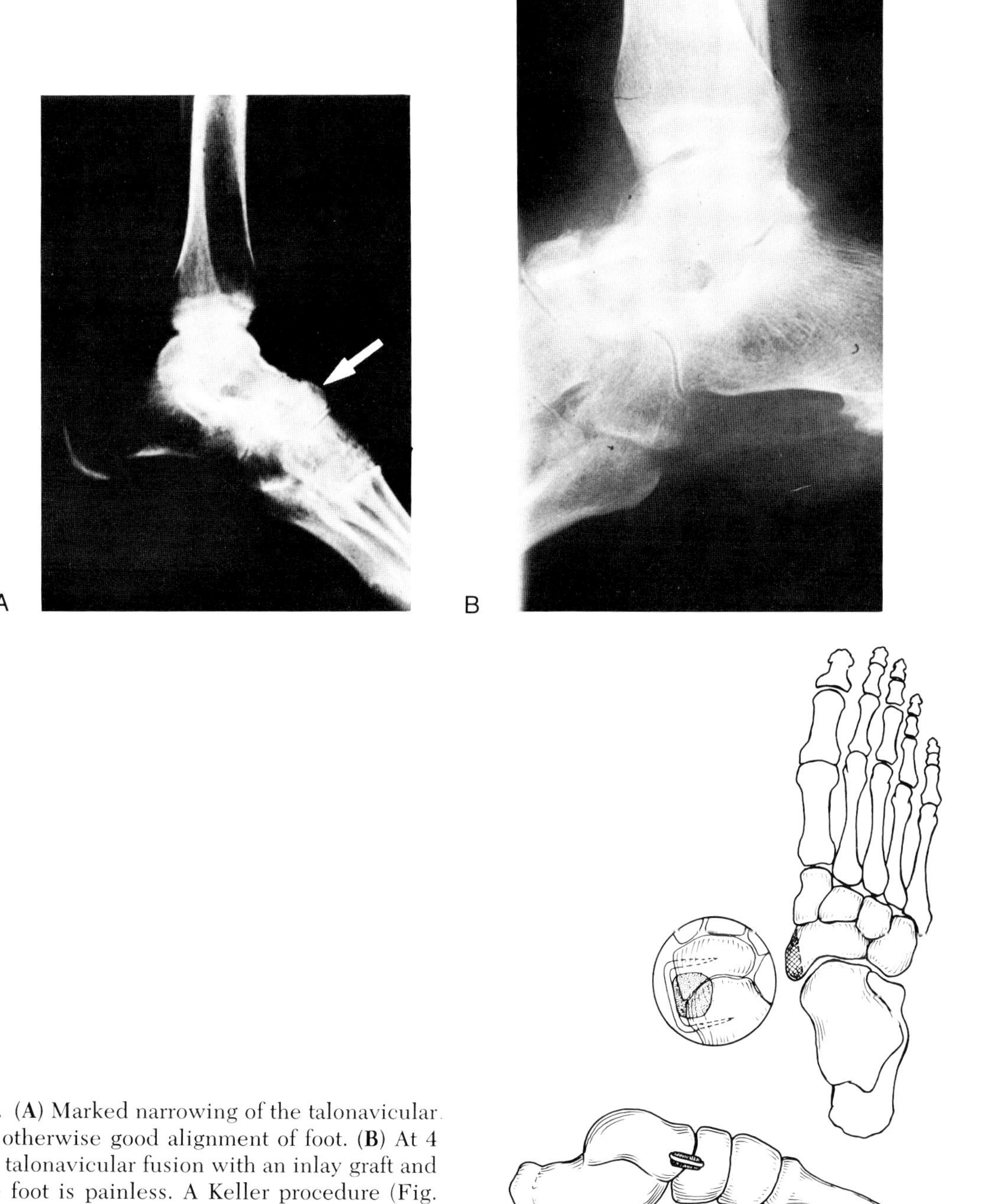

Fig. 16-27. (**A**) Marked narrowing of the talonavicular joint with otherwise good alignment of foot. (**B**) At 4 years after talonavicular fusion with an inlay graft and staple, the foot is painless. A Keller procedure (Fig. 16-19) was performed at the same time. (**C**) Talonavicular fusion technique.

the consensus (Table 16-1). Many times the difference between excellent and good results depends on the patient's overall condition. The criteria for a good result include absence of pain or only minimal pain with no more than mild calluses, ability to wear regular shoes with simple supports, and forefoot pain of such a mild degree that it does not interfere with gait. Results are considered fair in those patients who have moderate pain or moderate calluses in the forepart of the foot. Such a patient may require special shoes. Only mild improvement has been obtained with surgery. For any condition other than rheumatoid arthritis, this result would be considered poor. Today "failure" is a result regarded as worse than the condition prior to surgery.

Revision Arthroplasty

Supplementary surgery is necessary in approximately 10 percent of patients with rheumatoid arthritis. It is usually for minimal "tailoring" of the length of one of the metatarsals that was either too long initially or in which a spike of bone has regrown. A metatarsal osteotomy may be used to relieve the pressure under the metatarsal end. Rheumatoid arthritic patients are abnormally sensitive to pressure, and there are some recurrences with time, no matter what type of surgery has been employed.

Among the patients with extensive surgery, such as those requiring silicone hinge prostheses or medial capsular arthroplasty in the great toe and plantar plate arthroplasty, 2-year postoperative results have been 90 percent good or excellent. The feet have better cosmetic appearance and "look like feet." A number of patients paint their toenails and some wear open-toed shoes. Procedures that commonly removed less bone in the past have led to more recurrences; these patients need to be followed longer.

Arthrodesis of the hindfoot has given generally good results with relief of pain, but of course it is accompanied by the loss of motion. It does not appear to increase ankle joint disease.

CONCLUSIONS

Surgery of the rheumatoid arthritic foot can produce satisfactory results despite the fact that it is a progressive, crippling disease. Adequate bony excision at the MTP joint level (forefoot resection and reconstruction) is the basic principle for correcting a severe forefoot deformity to obtain a weight-tolerant foot. Some innovations that give better cosmetic results and the same early functional results have been described. Eighty percent of the patients are female and appreciate the cosmetics. One of the great problems with rheumatoid arthritis is keeping the patient in the realm of social acceptance. Resection of the forepart of the foot has been a good procedure for rehabilitation of the lower extremity.

These good results (85 percent) have been repeatedly confirmed by many investigators,[18–20,27] and the newer, more complicated techniques have not yet been proved to give better functional results. After 2 years' follow-up of rheumatoid arthritis patients, we believe the result cannot be attributed to the surgery but to the mercy of the course of the disease. Forefoot reconstruction, in use for more than 35 years, has been a very successful procedure in the rheumatoid lower extremity—longer than any other procedure in wide use today.

The surgical procedures employed to correct foot deformities in rheumatoid arthritis patients do not differ from the basic orthopaedic procedures performed for a similar deformity due to other conditions. It is exemplified in surgery of the hindpart of the foot in which the basic procedure is stabilization with a talonavicular or triple arthrodesis when either is necessary.

CASE REPORT 1

In 1972 a patient had a plantar "neuroma" excised from her right foot, cleft three–four. After doing well for 2 years she developed pain again and had swelling with increased separations of toes three and four and hypalgesia of the clef. Roentgenograms showed spreading of toes three

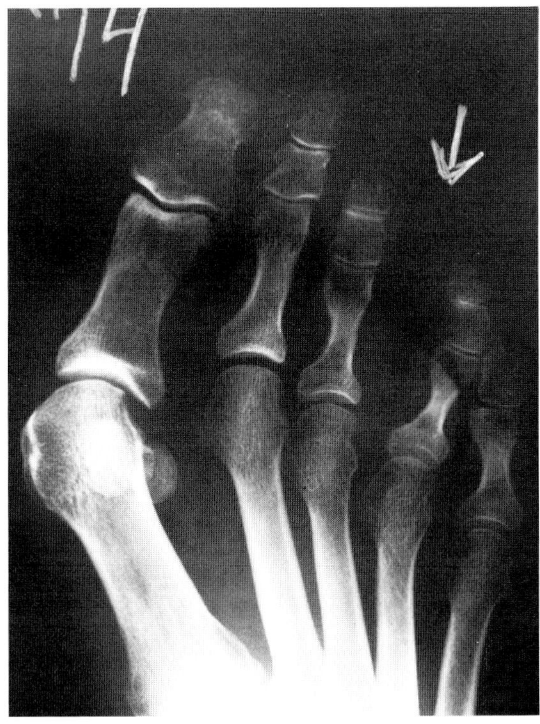

Fig. 16-28. Preoperative roentgenograms show hallux valgus, bunions, and spreading of toes three and four.

and four with soft tissue swelling, hallux valgus, but no joint changes (Fig. 16-28).

Surgery was performed, and a grayish yellow nodule was found adherent to the scar and extending down to the capsule of the third MTP joint. The nodule was excised and the nerve resected. The capsule of the third MTP joint was opened and a large amount of thickened synovium removed; a small amount was also removed from the fourth MTP joint. The diagnosis was rheumatoid arthritis of the MTP joint and neuroma. She has had no further pain in that area.

In 1977 she had pain and swelling over the bunions on both feet, more marked on the right (Fig. 16-29). Surgery was performed on the right foot with synovectomy, bunionectomy, Keller procedure with silicone single stem implant (Swanson), and transfer of adductor tendon to metatarsal head through a drill hole. The repair held the toe in good neutral position with a flexor and extensors recentralized.

In 1981 she had increasing pain in the left bunion area, although the right foot was not painful (Fig. 16-30). The overall alignment of the bunion

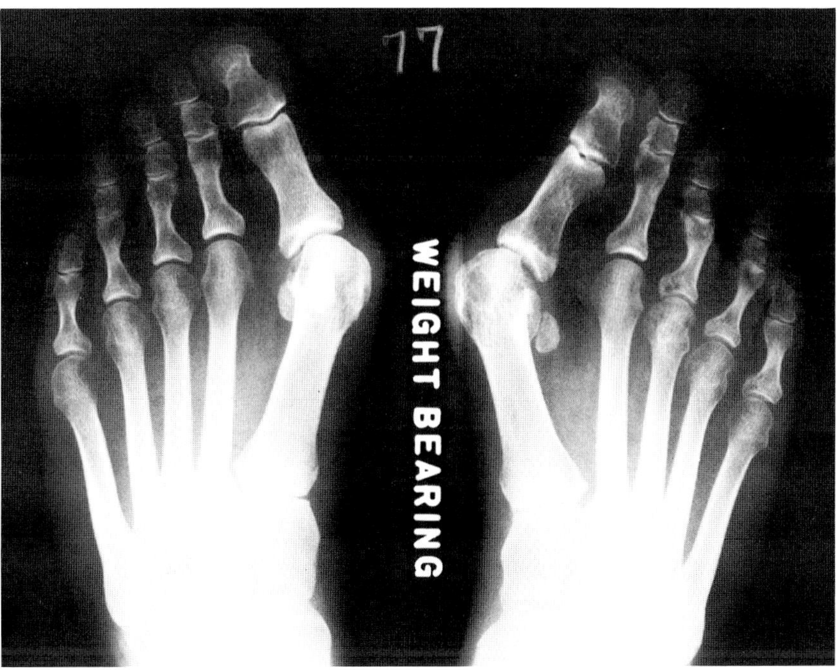

Fig. 16-29. Joint narrowing and erosions at the third MTP joint and an increase in hallux valgus and bunions.

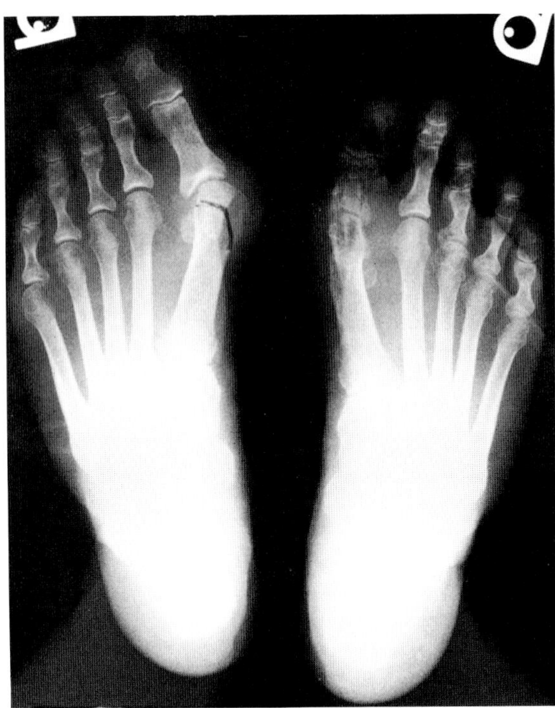

Fig. 16-30. Reaction around the single stem silicone implant of the right great toe and planned Stone bunionectomy on the left.

area on the right foot was good, but there was evidence of some wear of the silicone prosthesis and some bone absorption in the canal of the proximal phalanx.

Because of the findings around the opposite silicone implant, a left Stone bunionectomy was performed with an oblique biplane removal of the first metatarsal head, leaving a longer portion on the distal fibular plantar aspect to rest on the sesamoids. All bone removal was from the metatarsal to help narrow her foot and to diminish a slight cavus.

In 1983 she had no pain in the left foot but had developed pain and swelling of the right first MTP joint. Roentgenograms showed good position of the left Stone bunionectomy (Fig. 16-31). The right great toe showed soft tissue swelling, marked bone absorption around the stem of the silicone prosthesis, and a large cystic area involv-

ing two-thirds of the metatarsal head. Because of pain and the local reaction, surgery was performed with synovectomy, removal of the prosthesis, and medial capsular interposition arthroplasty (Fig. 16-32A). Pathologic examination revealed that multiple sections contained synovial elements with abundant acute and chronic inflammation, palisading granulomas, foci of fibrinoid degeneration, and focal areas of multinucleate giant cells containing birefringent foreign material, but no evidence of malignancy.[16]

She had had no further pain for 6 years in the great toe. She did, however, develop dislocations and subluxations of the lesser toes (Fig. 16-32B), due in part to the proximal retraction of the sesamoids. The mild pain was relieved by metatarsal supports.

Comment: Rheumatoid arthritis can start in an extra-articular area and produce plantar neuroma symptoms and signs. A number of cases of known rheumatoid arthritis have been seen with spreading of a pair of toes (either two–three or three–four) with pain; and at surgery a mass of rheumatoid synovial or nodular tissue has been found that may or may not communicate with an MTP joint.

The single stem silicone prosthesis used in the Keller procedure has produced silicone synovitis in a number of cases. The small wear particles cause the phenomenon. Almost any substance in small particles can cause a reaction. Wear has also been a problem with breakage or bone absorption around the stem. Several patients with broken prostheses, however, have no symptoms.

We do not recommend the single-stem prosthesis. The double hinge has been used in some patients with rheumatoid arthritis and is associated with a low incidence of problems. It is not recommended for heavy usage, as in people who what to run. Patients with silicone implants should be followed at least annually for 5 years. The prosthesis is removed if reaction and bone loss are noted. The toes still function as a resection arthroplasty, which is the original alternative. Patients should be informed that "anything implanted in the body may have to be removed one day."

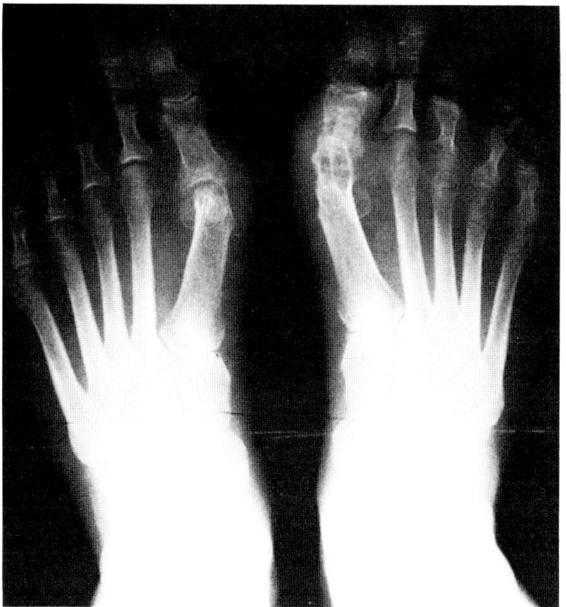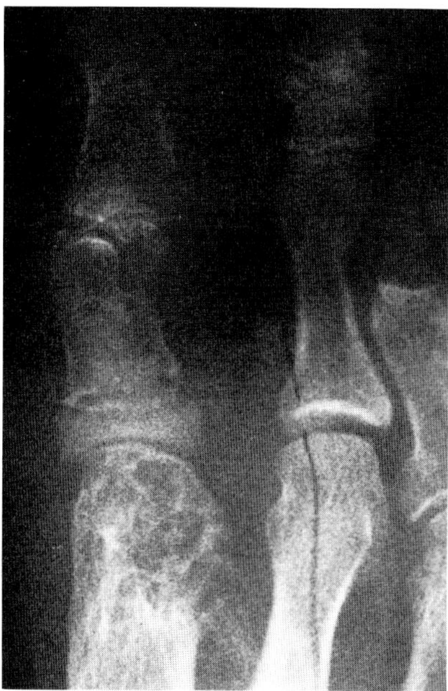

Fig. 16-31. (A) Good position of the Stone bunionectomy and sesamoids directly underneath the first metatarsal head. The right great toe was painful; note the cystic area in the first metatarsal head and the reaction around the single stemmed implant in the great toe. (B) Marked cystic changes in the metatarsal head.

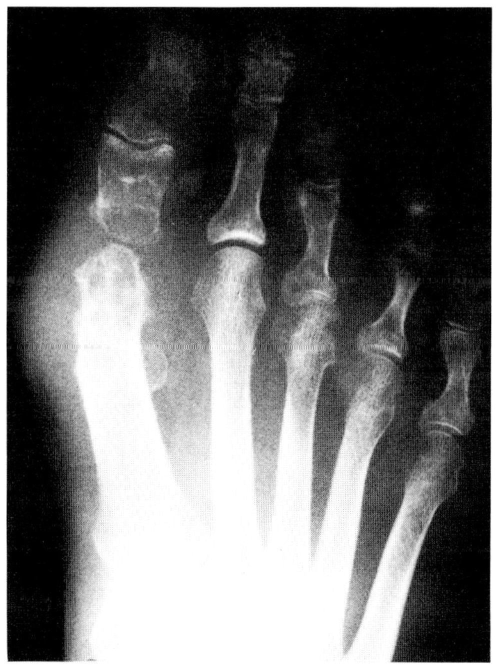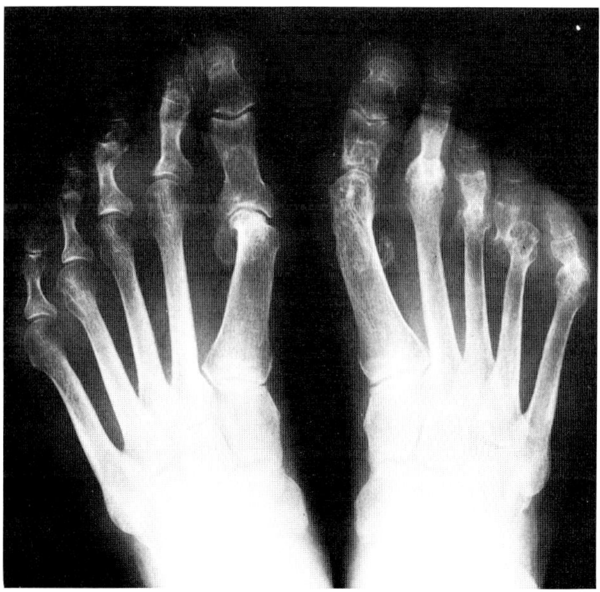

Fig. 16-32. (A) Prosthesis has been removed, and synovectomy and medial capsular interposition have been performed. There is overall good alignment but shortening of the great toe and retraction of the sesamoids. Patient now has a resection-type arthroplasty and no pain in the great toe. (B) Six years later there is good alignment of the great toe with no further bone lysis; the sesamoids are retracted. Note the dislocations of the MTP joints that have occurred but with minimal pain.

CASE REPORT 2

A 17-year-old young woman with juvenile rheumatoid arthritis and painful feet was seen. She had worn custom-made shoes for 2 years but wanted to wear shoes like those of her peers (Figs. 16-33 and 16-34). There was marked forefoot spread with hallux valgus, bunions, metatarsus primus varus, cock-up hammer toes with corns, and depressed metatarsal heads with calluses and cavus feet. The hindfoot was at neutral.

Surgery was planned with a plantar incision, excising a swathe of skin, including the calluses (Fig. 16-14b) underneath metatarsal heads two to five (Fig. 16-35). Note the flexor tendons, which are dislocated between the heads and have become a major deforming force. The metatarsal heads were resected well back into the necks,

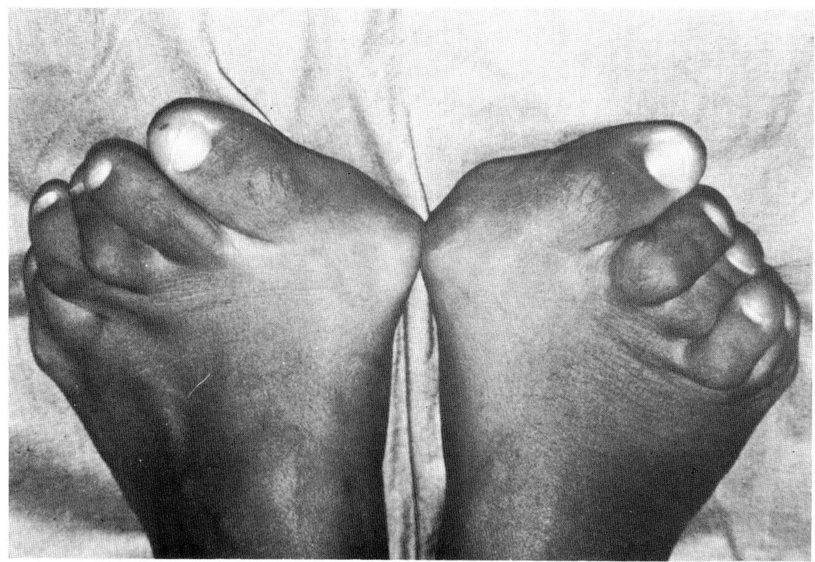

A

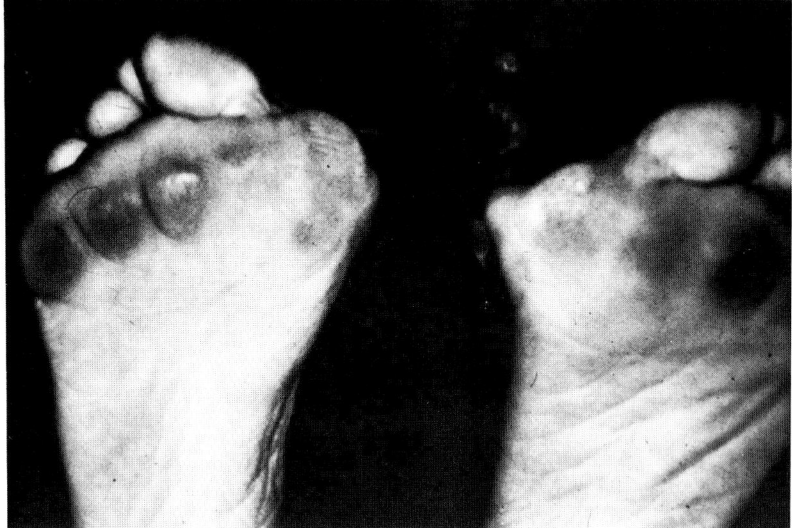

B

Fig. 16-33. Severe deformity due to hallux valgus, bunions, depressed metatarsal heads, splay foot, and cock-up toes.

which helped correct the cavus, and no bone was removed from the proximal phalanges.

The first MTP joint was exposed through a dorsotibial incision (Fig. 16-14b) and a silicone double hinge prosthesis inserted (Fig. 16-15). Because of the primus varus, a closing wedge osteotomy at the base of the first metatarsal was performed and stabilized with a K-wire. Each of the lesser toes were stabilized by intramedullary K-wires after gently manipulating the PIP joints into a straight position.

Closure of the plantar incision helped hold the toes down. K-wires were removed from the toes at 4 weeks. Postoperative roentgenograms at 2 months (Fig. 16-36) and 1 year (Fig. 16-37) revealed union of the osteotomy at the base of the first metatarsal. She had no pain, and the plantar incisions were not tender. She could wear dress shoes with low or medium heels.

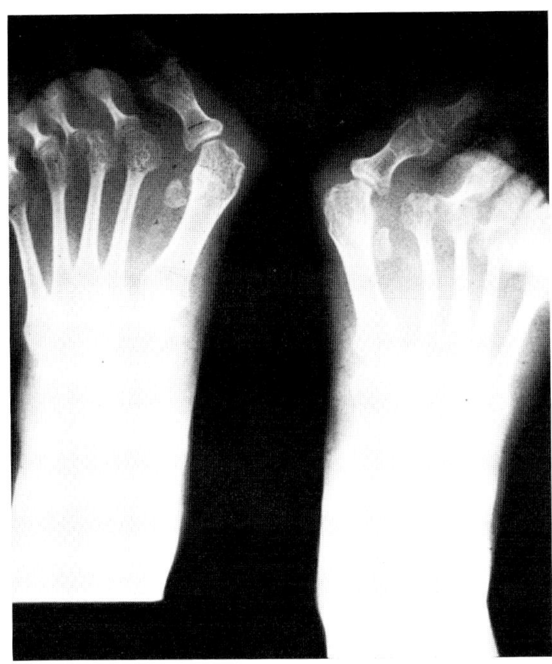

Fig. 16-34. Same deformities on roentgenograms: hallux valgus and bunions with involvement of all MTP joints. Note the metatarsus primus varus.

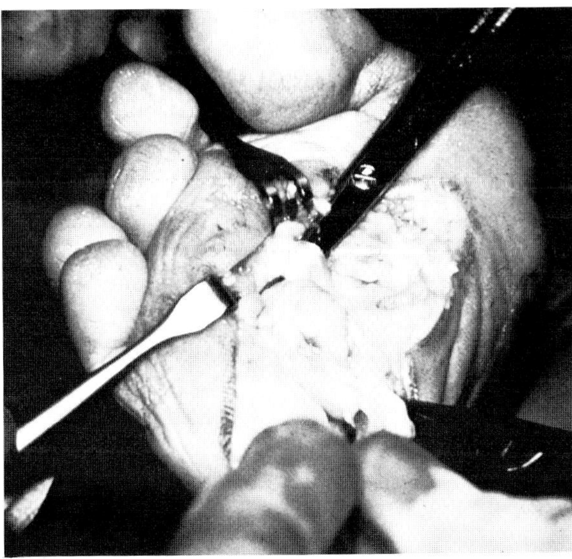

Fig. 16-35. Plantar incision for heads two to five, excising calluses and a swathe of skin. Flexor tendon (under scissors) is dislocated between the metatarsal heads.

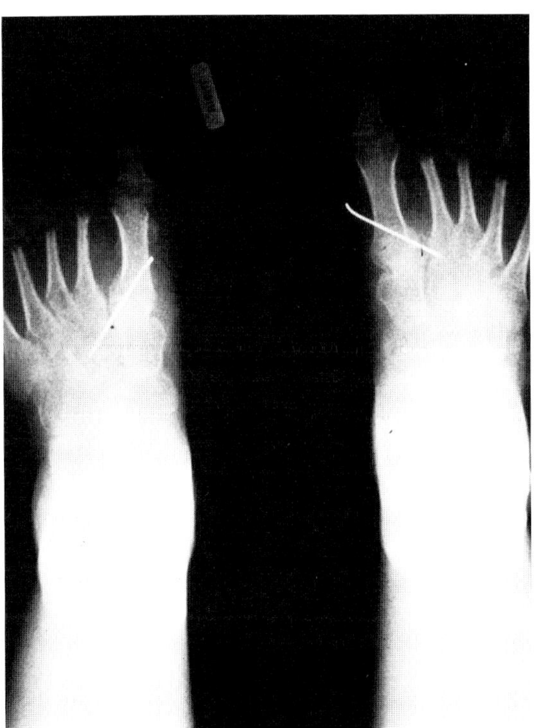

Fig. 16-36. Roentgenogram at 2 months reveal union of the osteotomy of the first metatarsal; toes and a silicone-hinge prosthesis are in excellent position.

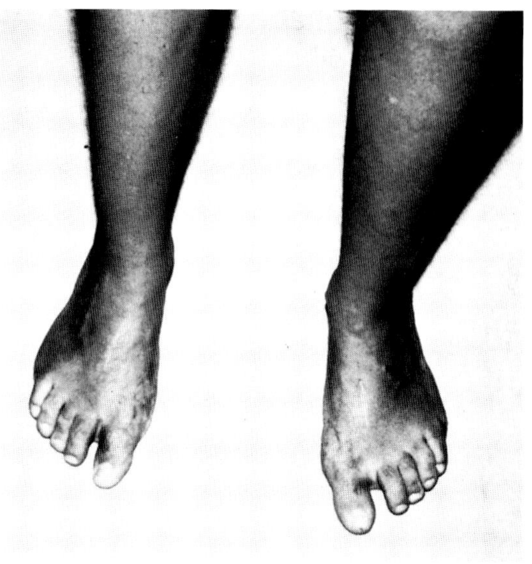
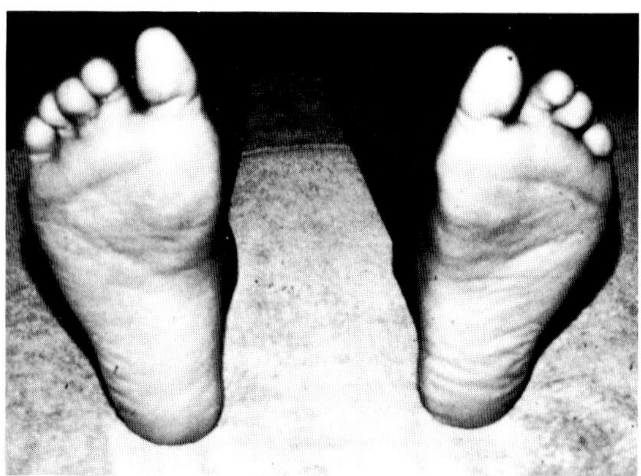

Fig. 16-37. Excellent appearance of the feet at 1 year. All incisions are healed, and the patient has no pain.

However, 7 years after surgery she returned with pain and swelling in each great toe. The left foot had a painful callus underneath the fourth metatarsal; the right foot had hammer toes with crossing of toes three and four. Roentgenograms showed bone absorption around the stems of the silicone (Fig. 16-38).

Supplementary surgery was performed and the silicone implants were removed. One was cracked at the hinge but not completely fractured. The bone was eroded, but synovitis was minimal. The great toes were realigned, preserving the capsule. On the right foot, hammer toes three and four were corrected by resecting the PIP joints and syndactyly. The IP joints of the great toes were arthrodesed to correct the cock-up deformities. Pain was relieved and the deformity corrected. Two years later she was still pleased with the surgical procedures.

Comment: This patient illustrates many facets of surgery of the rheumatoid forefoot. Pain unrelieved by acceptable conservative measures is the indication for surgery. The plantar approach was utilized excising a swathe of skin, as the metatarsal heads were depressed and prominent, "coming through the sole of the foot." All bone resection was from the heads to help diminish

the cavus and preserve more normal appearance of the toes.

The silicone double-hinge implants were utilized to correct the hallux valgus and gave a normal appearance to the great toes; implants alone could not give an adequate correction without correcting the primus varus by a basal osteotomy. In this case elevation of the first metatarsal also helped correct the cavus and gave more valgus to the heel. The operation was tailored to the deformity and to the patient as a young, attractive woman. The feet were operated on at two sessions, each requiring about 3 hours (two teams are often utilized).

After 2 years, the results of rheumatoid surgery without replacement depend on the course of the disease. The silicone implant has a synovium lined capsule and can suffer from recurrent synovitis; silicone synovitis due to wear particles may develop, as may bone resorption, in a small percentage of cases. Historically, about 10 percent of all forefoot reconstructions have required supplementary surgery, and the newer procedures have not changed this need. The supplementary surgery is usually much simpler than the original operation. If a silicone implant has to be removed, there is still a resection arthroplasty

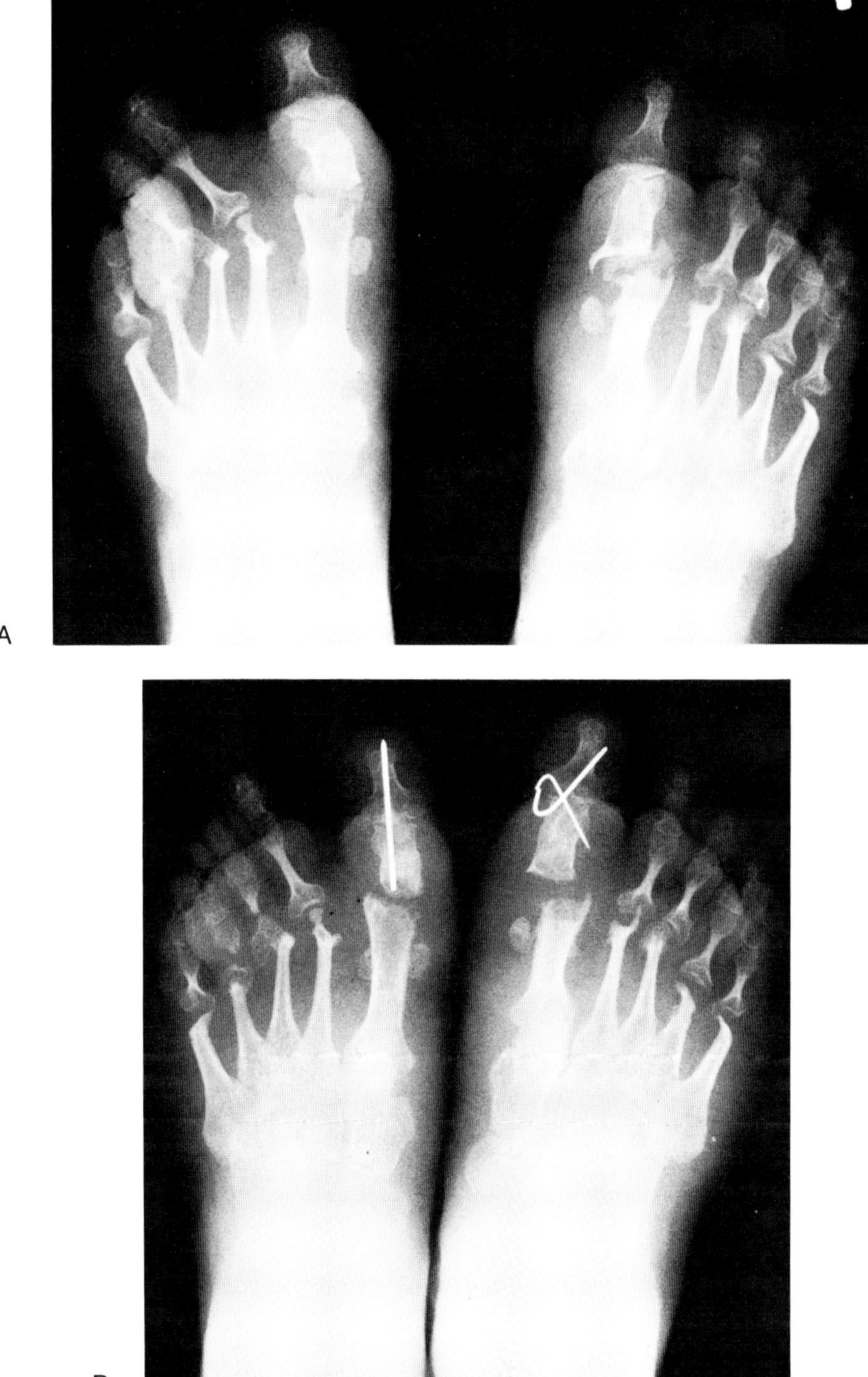

Fig. 16-38. (A) Roentgenogram 7 years postoperatively. There is deformity of the silicone prostheses in the great toes and bone erosion around the stem and proximal phalanges. The great toes were "cocked up," and toes three and four were crossed. Bone growth on the ends of several lesser metatarsals is irregular. (B) Postoperative roentgenogram. Silicone hinges have been removed, the IP joints of the great toes fused, and the hammer toe deformities of toes three and four corrected. The osteotomy of the fourth metatarsal is not well visualized.

due to the encapsulation that forms around the implant.

REFERENCES

1. AuFranc O, Larson CB: Surgery of the rheumatoid forefoot. Presented to the Boston Orthopaedic Foot Club, Boston, 1949
2. Barton NJ: Arthroplasty of the forefoot in rheumatoid arthritis. J Bone Joint Surg 558:126, 1973
3. Berg E, Bailey JP Jr, Mealing HG Jr, Childress F: Nonoperative care of the painful rheumatoid foot. AAOS Exhibit, 1978
4. Brattstrom H: Surgery in metatarsophalangeal joints II–V in rheumatoid arthritis. Acta Orthop Belg 48:107, 1972
5. Brattstrom H, Brattstrom M: Resection of the MP joints in rheumatoid arthritis. Acta Orthop Scand 41:213, 1970
6. Clayton ML: Surgery of the forefoot in rheumatoid arthritis. Arthritis Rheum 2:84, 1959
7. Clayton ML: Surgery of the forefoot in rheumatoid arthritis. Clin Orthop 16:136, 1960
8. Clayton ML: Surgery of the lower extremity in rheumatoid arthritis. J Bone Joint Surg [Am] 45:1517, 1963
9. Clayton ML: Results of surgery in rheumatoid feet. Excerpta Medica Int Congress Ser 165:October, 1967
10. Clayton ML: Correction of arthritic deformities of the foot and ankle. p. 889. In McCarty DJ (ed): Arthritis and Allied Conditions: A Textbook of Rheumatology. 11th Ed. Lea & Febiger, Philadelphia, 1989
11. Clayton ML, Leidholt JD, Smyth CJ: Surgery of the forefoot in rheumatoid arthritis. Motion picture available through AAOS, Park Ridge, IL, 1961
12. Clayton ML, Reis MD: Functional hallux rigidus in the rheumatoid foot. Clin Orthop 271:233, 1991
13. Clayton ML, Smyth CJ: Situation of the foot regarding early synovectomy in rheumatoid arthritis. p. 146. In Hijams W et al (eds): Early Synovectomy in Rheumatoid Arthritis. Excerpta Medica Foundation, Amsterdam, 1969
14. Cracchiolo A III, Pearson S, Kitaoka H, Grace D: Hindfoot arthrodesis in adults utilizing a dowel graft technique. Clin Orthop 257:193, 1990
15. Elbaor JE, Thomas WH, Weinfeld MS, Potter TA: Talonavicular arthrodesis for rheumatoid arthritis of the hindfoot. Orthop Clin North Am 7:821, 1976
16. Ferlic DC, Clayton ML, Holloway M: Complications of silicone implant surgery in the metacarpophalangeal joint. J Bone Joint Surg [Am] 57:991, 1975
17. Flint M, Sweetman R: Amputation of all toes: a review of forty-seven amputations. J Bone Joint Surg 428:90, 1960
18. Fowler AW: A method of forefoot reconstruction. J Bone Joint Surg [Br] 41:507, 1959
19. Funk FJ Jr: Surgery of the foot in rheumatoid arthritis. J Med Assoc Ga 58:8, 1969
20. Funk FJ Jr: Surgery of the foot in rheumatoid arthritis. Semin Arthritis Rheum 1:25, 1971
21. Gschwend N: Surgical Treatment of Rheumatoid Arthritis. George Thieme Verlag, Stuttgart, 1980
22. Helal B: Metatarsal osteotomy for metatarsalgia. J Bone Joint Surg [Br] 57:187, 1975
23. Hoffman P: An operation for severe grades of contracted or clawed toes. Am J Orthop Surg 9:441, 1911–12
24. Kates A, Kessel L, Kay A: Arthroplasty of the forefoot. J Bone Joint Surg [Br] 49:552, 1967
25. Key JA: Surgical revision of arthritic feet. Am J Surg 79:667, 1950
26. Lipscomb PR, Benson GM, Sones DA: Resection of proximal phalanges and metatarsal condyles for deformities of the forefoot due to rheumatoid arthritis. Clin Orthop 82:24, 1972
27. Mann RA, Thompson FM: Arthrodesis of first M.P. joint for hallux valgus in rheumatoid arthritis. J Bone Joint Surg [Am] 66:687, 1984
28. Marmor L: Resection of the forefoot in rheumatoid arthritis. Clin Orthop 108:223, 1975
29. Netter F, Clayton ML, Susman MH: Surgery of the rheumatoid foot. In Ciba Collection of Medical Illustrations. Vol 8. Musculoskeletal System, Part II. Excerpta Medica, Amsterdam, 1990
30. Potter TA: Rheumatoid arthritis of the foot. AMA Exhibit, Denver, 1961
31. Potter TA, Kuhns JG: Correction of arthritic deformities. p. 428. In Hollander JL (ed). Arthritis and Allied Conditions. 7th Ed. Lea & Febiger, Philadelphia, 1966
32. Raunio P, Laine H: Synovectomy of the metatarsophalangeal joints in rheumatoid arthritis. Acta Rheumatol Scand 16:12, 1970
33. Raunio P, Lehtimaki M, Erola M et al: Resection arthroplasty versus arthrodesis of the first metatarsophalangeal joint for hallux valgus in rheumatoid arthritis. Rheumatology 11:173, 1987
34. Schwartzmann JR: The surgical management of foot deformities in rheumatoid arthritis. Clin Orthop 36:86, 1964

35. Short CL, Bauer W, Reynolds WE: Rheumatoid Arthritis. Harvard University Press, Cambridge, 1957
36. Susman MH, Clayton ML: Surgery of the rheumatoid foot. Ann Acad Med Singapore 23(2):1, 1983
37. Swanson AB, Swanson GD, Mayhew DE, Khan AN: Flexible hinge results in implant arthroplasty of the great toe. Rheumatology 11:136, 1987
38. Thompson TC: The management of the painful foot in arthritis, Med Clin North Am 21:1785, 1937
39. Tillmann K: The Rheumatoid Foot. Georg Thieme, Stuttgart; Thieme Medical Publ., New York, 1979
40. Vahvanen VA: Rheumatoid arthritis in the pantalar joints. A follow-up study of triple arthrodesis on 292 adult feet. Acta Orthop Scand, Suppl 107:3, 1967
41. Vainio K: The rheumatoid foot; a clinical study with pathological and roentgenological comments. Ann Chir Gynaecol Fenn, suppl. 1, 45, 1956
42. Vainio K: Hallux varus rheumaticus. Z Orthop 89:271, 1957

17

Management of the Rheumatoid Complex Foot and Ankle

Mack L. Clayton

A surgical rheumatoid arthritis foot problem becomes complex when multiple areas are involved, including ankles, knees, or hips. If the patient's major complaint is the forefoot, and the hindfoot is mobile, forefoot reconstruction is the best initial procedure. Severely deformed forefeet often have pressure areas with infection or are prone to break down and become infected. In such a case the forefoot should always be corrected first (Figs. 17-1 and 17-2). As noted by Souter,[4] "Begin with a winner."

If the proximal joints are so involved that walking is not practical, a total hip or total knee arthroplasty is indicated. In general, total hips are done before knees (Fig. 17-2). (See Chapter 13, p. 8.)

When both the hindfoot and forefoot are so involved that the hindfoot does not have enough mobility to compensate, any angular deformity of the knee should be corrected by total knee arthroplasty before a hindfoot arthrodesis is contemplated. The foot can thus be made plantigrade through hindfoot arthrodesis. In such a case, forefoot reconstruction would be the last procedure, as final tailoring of the metatarsophalangeal (MTP) resection could compensate for mild residual deformity and yield a weight-tolerant forefoot. For example, a cavus foot bone would be removed only from metatarsals, as described by Hoffmann.[3] It would lower the high arch as well as relieve increased metatarsal head pressure. More bone would be removed from the metatarsal than in the usual case with metatarsal head and proximal phalangeal resection. With a

mild *varus*, slightly more bone is resected on the fourth and fifth metatarsals, and the base of the fifth may be partially excised.

With ankle and hindfoot involvement, triple arthrodesis for the hindfoot should be done first, followed by ankle fusion or total ankle arthroplasty. When involvement is severe, pantalar arthrodesis (ankle and triple arthrodesis) can be performed at the same time. Realignment of the foot under the ankle by triple arthrodesis often diminishes ankle pain for a long period. Fusion or a total ankle replacement can be performed later. (We are still looking for a good total ankle prosthesis; total ankle arthroplasty is utilized only in unusual cases.) If talonavicular fusion alone is necessary, it can be performed at the same time as the ankle replacement.

Complex rheumatoid foot and ankle problems consist in interconnected parts that are intricately involved by rheumatoid arthritis. In general, the ankle and hindfoot are treated by fusion and the forefoot by resection arthroplasty with reconstruction. Each case requires careful analysis of the entire problem involving hips, knees, and the overall situation (Fig. 17-2).

When planning treatment in surgical stages, the first operation should be a winner, but it should also benefit the patient even if the next procedure is not performed. We are convinced that early hindfoot stabilization would give better results, but the process is usually bilateral, requiring crutches and several months of cast immobilization; and it is much more difficult for the

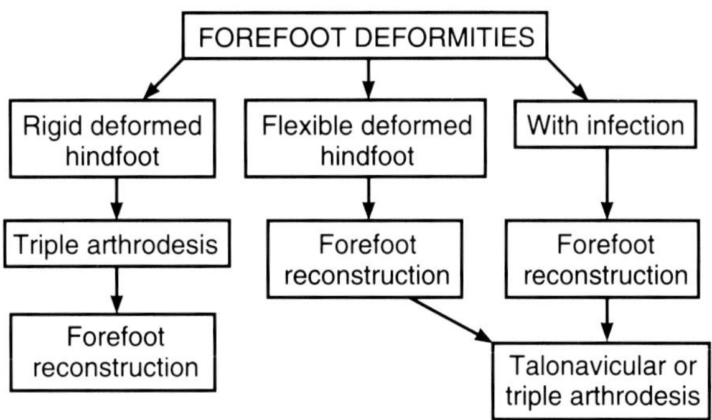

Fig. 17-1. Flow chart depicting complex foot deformities and sequential surgical management.

patient than forefoot surgery. At the present time, severe hindfoot and ankle abnormalities are some of the most difficult surgical problems in the lower extremity. The following case reports illustrate complex problems utilizing the team approach and the procedures described in preceding chapters.

CASE REPORT 1

A 54-year-old woman presented with long-standing chronic rheumatoid arthritis. In 1983 she had a triple arthrodesis of the left foot and was referred 2 years later because of increasing pain in the foot and ankle. On examination she had a

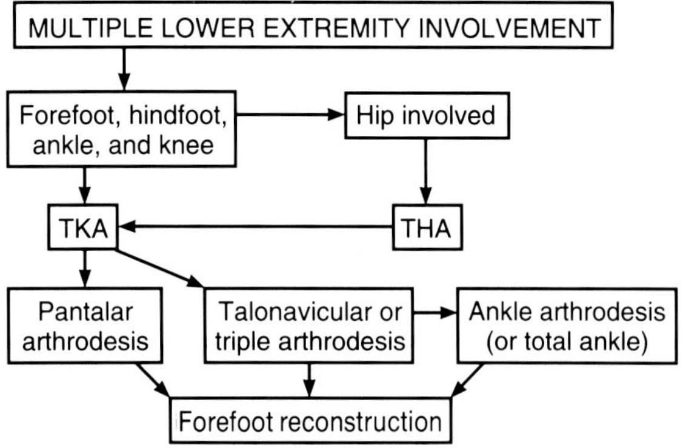

Fig. 17-2. Flow chart depicting complex multiple lower extremity involvement and sequence of indicated surgery.

marked limp on the left and a marked valgus through the hindfoot with abduction of the forefoot. With weight-bearing she was essentially walking on the medial border of her foot.

Three-way weight-bearing roentgenograms of the foot and ankle (Fig. 17-3A–C) showed evidence of considerable foot deformity below the ankle; hence she was not considered a candidate for total ankle arthroplasty. Ankle fusion was recommended, and surgery was performed utilizing a slightly anterior medial approach to expose the ankle joint. The medial malleolus was osteotomized in line with the joint and excised; there was no remaining cartilage. The joint surface was slightly cut to get a good, flat surface, and the talus was similarly positioned. An anterolateral incision was made, the distal fibula excised, and the talus transposed completely to the medial aspect of the tibia, thus correcting the lateral displacement and excess hindfoot valgus. With slight rotation, part of the abduction through the forefoot was also corrected to essentially line up the foot with the knee.

The ankle joint fusion was stabilized using one lone AO screw through the sole by way of a stab wound through the os calcis and into the tibia. Another screw placed obliquely through the lateral incision into the tibia and across into the talus gave good fixation. The abnormal position of the foot was corrected at the time of the ankle fusion and a plantigrade foot obtained with 5 to 10 degrees equinus of the foot (Fig. 17-3D & E). Immobilization in a short leg cast without weight-bearing was necessary for the first 6 weeks because of the marked osteoporosis of the bones, which could have collapsed with early weight-bearing. A weight-bearing cast was then worn for another 2 months.

Comment: Internal fixation of ankle fusions is a desirable method to utilize at this time, particularly in a rheumatoid arthritic.[2] Abnormal positions of the foot can sometimes be corrected through the ankle, leaving the foot in a plantigrade position; the foot can then be realigned with the knee. (When performing a triple arthrodesis alone, the foot must be realigned with the ankle, not the knee.) Pantalar type of arthrodesis in 0 to 10 degrees plantar flexion in a markedly involved rheumatoid arthritic gives a good result,

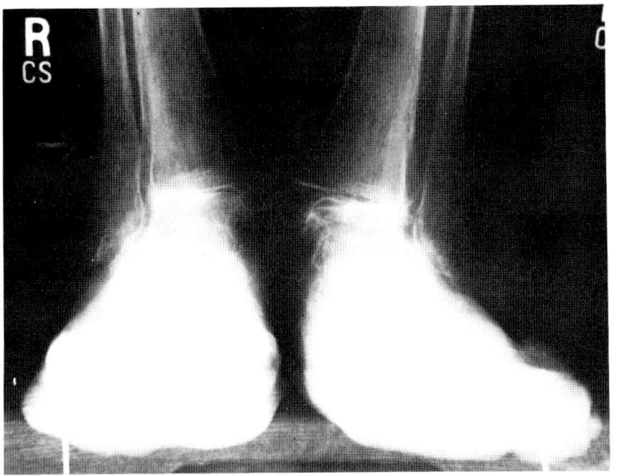

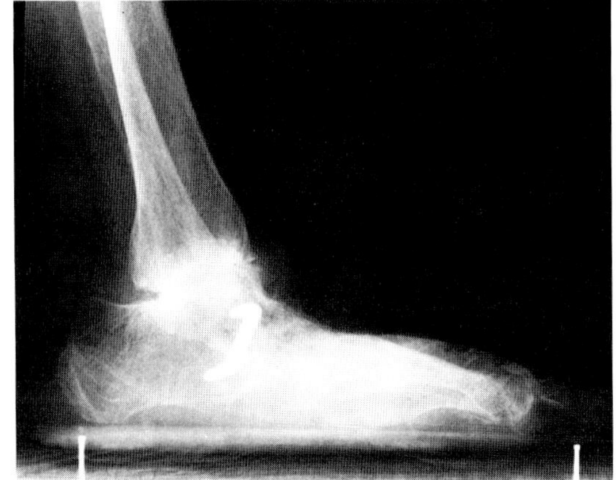

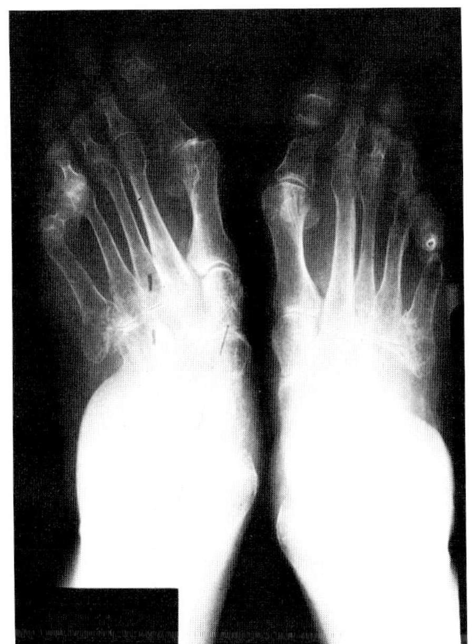

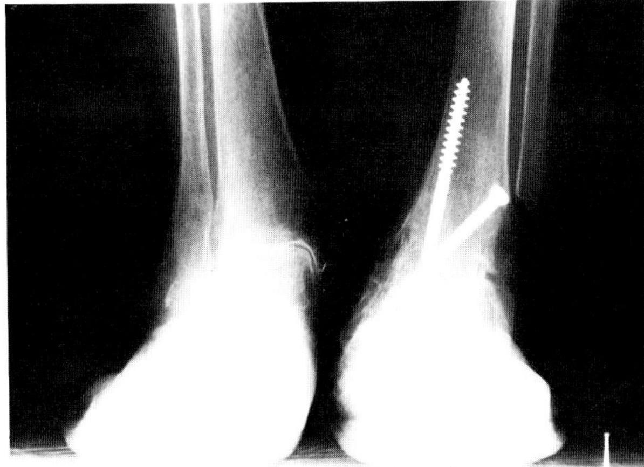

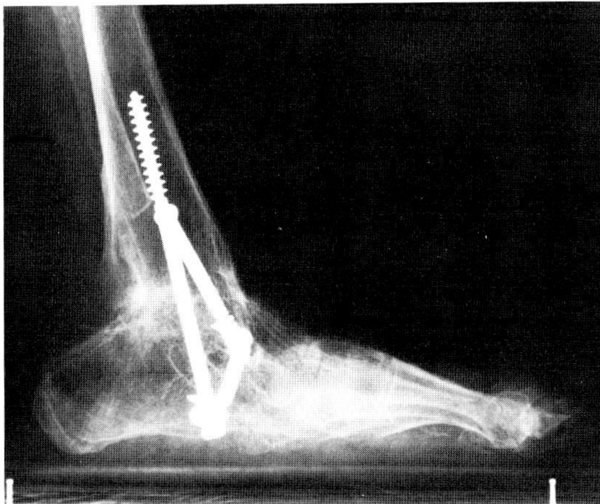

Fig. 17-3. (A) Marked narrowing of the left ankle with bone loss and valgus. The staple is present from the previous triple arthrodesis. White line across the medial malleolus denotes the planned level of removal for the arthrodesis. Stress fracture can be seen on the right distal fibula. (B) Complete narrowing of the joint and marked valgus with flattening of the longitudinal arch. (C) Anteroposterior weight-bearing of both feet with dotted lines denoting left. Staple and triple arthrodesis are on the left; note the marked valgus. Dotted lines illustrate the present axis of the talus, os calcis, and marked forefoot abduction. (D) Ankle fusion with excision of the medial malleolus and medial displacement of the talus to better position the foot under the ankle. The compression screws were utilized for arthrodesis. (E) On the lateral view, ankle fusion is in slight equinus and the plantigrade position with weight-bearing. The long lag screw has backed out a few millimeters away from the washer. This type of screw should have threads gripping just above the fusion line, or it could have been inserted on the medial tibia into the talus to get a better grip. The ankle has been fused varus to give a plantigrade foot.

as the patients are essentially free of pain. If necessary, they can walk with a rocker-bottom shoe to help the gait; usually a simple, well-padded ordinary oxford shoe or a running type shoe is sufficient.

CASE REPORT 2

A 51-year-old man had had a progressive, "malignant" type of rheumatoid arthritis for 8 years. During the last 2 years he had operations on both wrists and both hands. He was forced to discontinue work as an electrician because of his inability to grip and utilize the tools with his hands.

At this time he had painful feet with *severe* valgus deformities on both feet as well as marked forefoot deformities of hallux valgus, bunions, and depressed metatarsal heads with cock-up toes (Fig. 17-4). He had triple arthrodeses of both feet performed simultaneously with two teams; a longitudinal lateral approach and a medial approach were utilized with staple fixation. After 2 weeks he was mobilized in bilateral weight-bearing casts until 3 months after surgery, at which time there was union of the triple arthrodesis. However, he developed increasing valgus of the left ankle due to a rupture of the deltoid ligament (Fig. 17-5A).

Four months after the triple arthrodeses, he underwent an ankle arthrodesis of the left ankle using a medial approach. A longitudinal osteotomy of the medial malleolus was utilized, leaving the posterior soft tissue attachments to provide a blood supply and "living bone graft" (Fig. 17-5B). He was initially immobilized in a plaster cast and then in a short leg weight-bearing cast approximately 2 weeks later; he was out of plaster at 3 months. He had no further pain in the hindfoot on either side (Fig. 17-5C & D).

He had problems with his forefeet, and as he walked more they became increasingly painful. After he had been out of the casts a few months, a bilateral forefoot reconstruction was performed utilizing medial capsular arthroplasty of the great toes and plantar plate arthroplasty of the lesser toes with intramedullary wire fixation of all toes (Fig. 17-6). Six years later he was having minimal pain in his feet, and his left foot with the pantalar

arthrodesis had about 8 degrees total plantar-dorsiflexion through the midtarsal area. He was satisfied with each foot. He has had a total of 13 hospitalizations for surgeries on the upper and lower extremities, including a total hip replacement.

Comment: This patient illustrates a number of points. He had a malignant type of progressive rheumatoid arthritis that continued to progress despite basic medical treatment. The first surgeries were on his wrists and hands because they bothered him the most and were the reason he had stopped working. Although his wrists and hands improved, he was not able to work as an electrician. As he began to develop more problems, surgery was performed when indicated.

His feet illustrate the problems of a complex rheumatoid foot with involvement of both hindfoot and forefoot. Three-way views of foot and ankle weight-bearing roentgenograms (anteroposterior view of the foot, anteroposterior view of the ankle, and lateral views of the foot and ankle) are important when analyzing the problem and planning treatment.

This patient had a painful, fixed deformity of valgus in both hindfeet and probably had a rupture of the posterior tibial tendon on the left side. This diagnosis is sometimes difficult in a rheumatoid patient, but it is one of the causes of rapid progression to a severe valgus foot. The treatment of a rigid, severe valgus rheumatoid foot is a triple arthrodesis, and in this case it was performed bilaterally. He was allowed early weight-bearing because of marked involvement of the upper extremities. (At this time, we would not operate on both feet at the same time, nor do we recommend early weight-bearing for a foot this severely affected. Allowing 6 to 8 weeks of non-weight-bearing prevents loss of position.)

The triple arthrodeses united, but he developed an unstable valgus ankle on the left side due to rupture of the deltoid ligament. (We have seen this occurrence in another case, which developed several years after successful triple arthrodesis. We have found no previous reports of ruptured deltoid ligaments in rheumatoid arthritis.)

This approach is an unusual one for ankle fusion, but it was an excellent solution to this problem. We currently use AO fixation compression

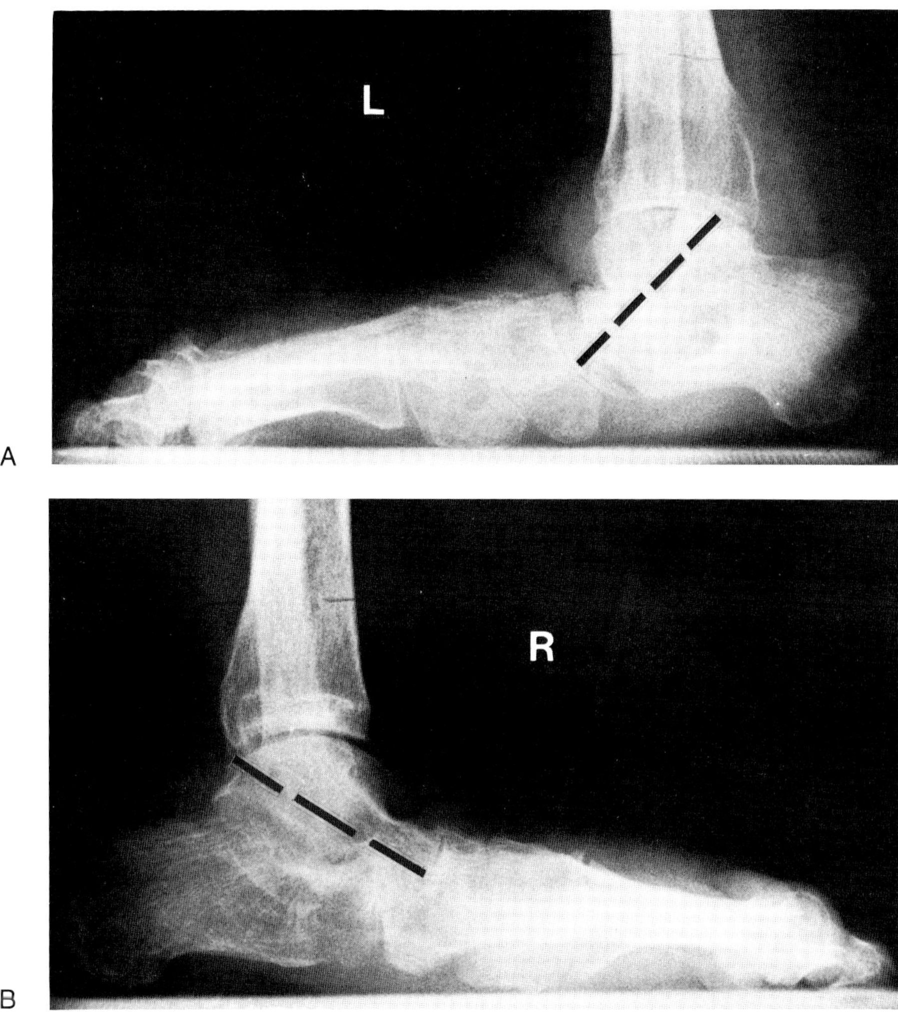

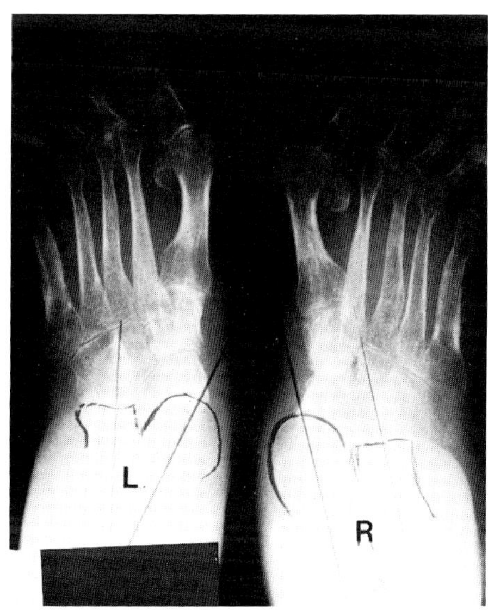

Fig. 17-4. (**A & B**) Weight-bearing films show marked valgus in both views with depression of the long arch. The left foot (**A**) has marked plantar-flexed talus. Note the bilateral forefoot deformity with hallux valgus and destructive changes in the MTP joints. (**C**) On the anteroposterior view, the line of the talus should point toward the first metatarsal ray, and the os calcis should point toward the fifth ray.

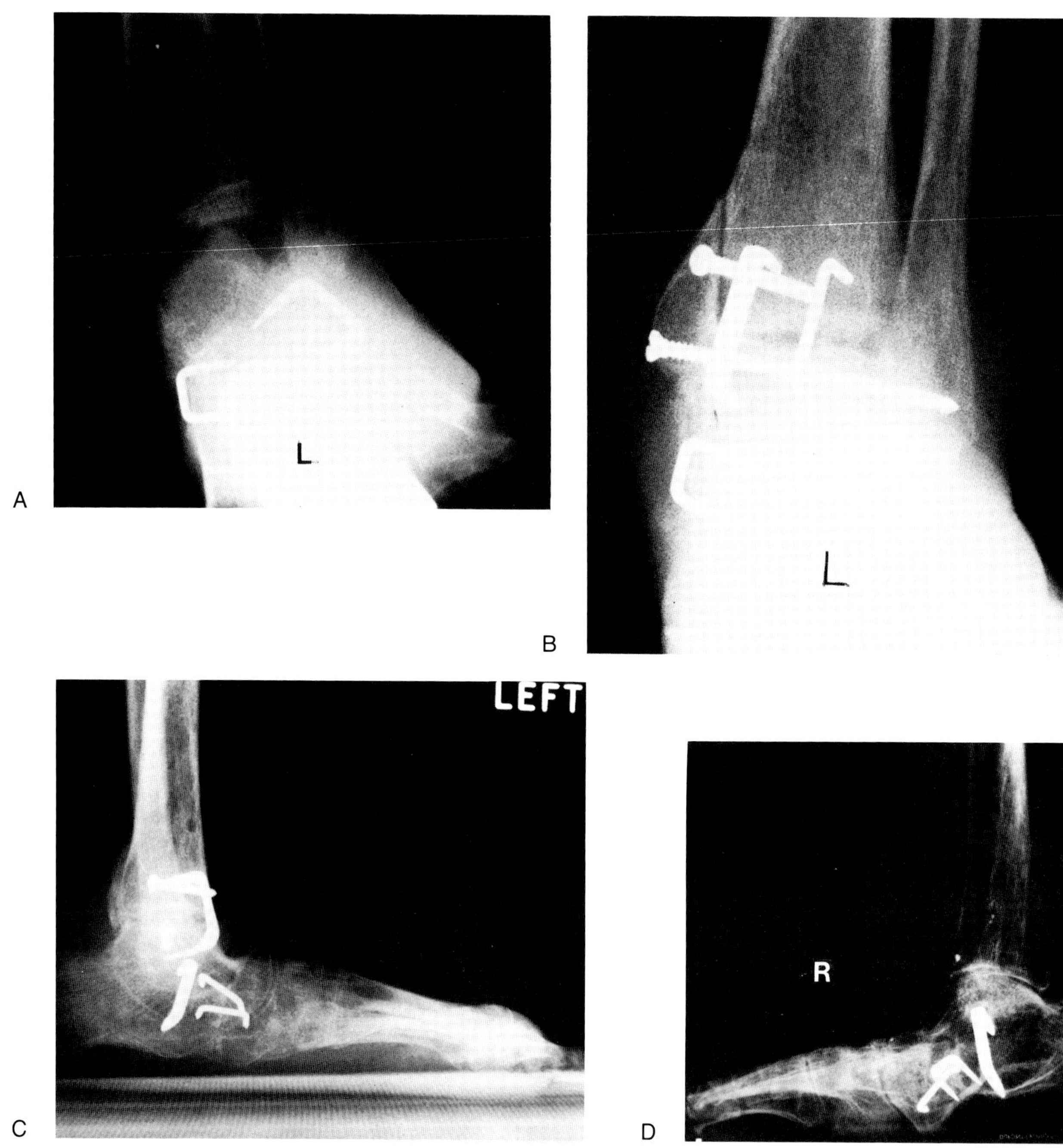

Fig. 17-5. (**A**) Three months after triple arthrodesis. Stress film reveals a marked valgus tilt of the ankle, indicating rupture of the deltoid ligament. Staples are from the triple arthrodesis. (**B**) Postoperative roentgenogram of the left ankle after arthrodesis. (**C**) Postoperative lateral roentgenogram of the left foot and ankle following triple arthrodesis and ankle arthrodesis (pantalar arthrodesis). The foot is at a right angle to the tibia. (**D**) Lateral weight-bearing of the right foot and ankle following triple arthrodesis and union. There is a slight loss of correction due to early weight-bearing.

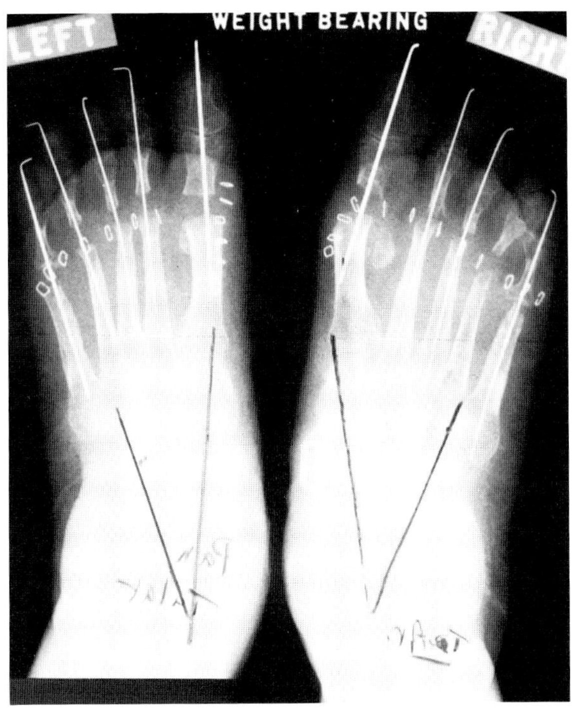

Fig. 17-6. Anteroposterior weight-bearing roentgenogram following pantalar arthrodesis on the left and triple arthrodesis on the right. Superimposed lines show the current positon of the os calcis and talus in relation to the forefoot. Forefoot reconstruction has been performed with medial capsular arthroplasty of the great toe and plantar plate arthroplasty of the lesser toes. Staples outline the skin incisions.

screws, but surgeons should use the type of fixation with which they are most comfortable.[2] With a pantalar arthrodesis, about 0 to 5 degrees of plantar flexion is an ideal position, and that was the amount obtained for this patient.

After the hindfoot and ankle healed, he underwent forefoot surgery,[1,5] as the forefoot resection could now be tailored to fit the position of the hindfoot. In this case, the hindfoot position was adequate (neutral) to do a standard type of a forefoot reconstruction as illustrated.

Six years later he had good results, with minimal pain in his feet, and he can wear regular shoes with small pads in the metatarsal area. His left foot with the pantalar arthrodesis has about 8 degrees dorsiflexion and plantar flexion through the midtarsal area, allowing him to walk quite well. This man would not be considered a "heavy user" of his lower extremities, and he is able to ambulate within the limits of his arthritis; he does not prefer one foot over the other. The patient has expressed the opinion that "without surgery, I would be in a wheelchair."

REFERENCES

1. Clayton ML: Correction of arthritic deformities of the foot and ankle. p. 889. In McCarty DJ (ed): Arthritis and Allied Conditions: A Textbook of Rheumatology. 11th Ed. Lea & Febiger, Philadelphia, 1989
2. Clayton ML: Surgical treatment of the rheumatoid foot. p. 444. In Giamestras NS (ed): Foot Disorders. Lea & Febiger, Philadelphia, 1973
3. Hoffmann P: An operation for severe grades of contracted or clawed toes. Am J Orthop Surg 9:441, 1911–12
4. Souter WA: Planning treatment of the rheumatoid hand. Hand 11:3, 1979
5. Susman MH, Clayton ML: Surgery of the rheumatoid foot. Ann Acad Med Singapore 23:225, 1983

18

Management of the Rheumatoid Spine

David A. Wong
Alan E. Heilman

CERVICAL SPINE
Alan E. Heilman
David A. Wong

Neck pain is a common complaint of many patients. Those patients who have morning stiffness combined with an insidious onset of neck pain should be further evaluated for the possibility of inflammatory arthritis. It is beyond the scope of this chapter to delve into the subtle differences among the various inflammatory diagnoses. We concentrate attention on rheumatoid arthritis as the model disease for involvement of the spine.

Classes of Cervical Spine Involvement

There are many classification systems currently in use for rheumatoid arthritis. The two most common are the American Rheumatism Association (ARA), or Steinbrocker, scale[99] and the Ranawat scale.[72] The ARA system is a general function scheme, and the Ranawat system is a functional neurologic grading scale (Table 18-1).

General Pathomechanics of Rheumatoid Arthritis

Rheumatoid arthritis is an inflammatory process that can result in ligamentous destruction or distension, with secondary rupture, synovitis, articular cartilage destruction, and pannus formation.[10,67] The effects of rheumatoid arthritis on bone are osteoporosis, cyst formation, and erosion. Postmortem dissections of the cervical spine have revealed synovial and granulomatous rheumatoid lesions in the joints of Luschka, although no radiographic evidence of cervical rheumatoid arthritis was evident.[86] Thus the pathomechanics of the overall disease process do not necessarily correlate with the roentgenographic findings.

Involvement of the cervical spine may be found in 25 to 90 percent of patients with rheumatoid arthritis.[10] In a prospective study of patients with rheumatoid arthritis, Pellicci et al. found that 70 percent of patients had radiologic evidence of cervical spine involvement and 36 percent had progressive neural abnormalities over a 5-year period.[72] Other authors have found that only 10 to 15 percent of patients develop

353

Table 18-1. Functional Classification Schemes for Rheumatoid Arthritis

Class	Criteria
Steinbrocker or American Rheumatology Association	
1	Complete ability to carry out all usual duties without handicaps
2	Adequate for normal activities despite handicap of discomfort or limited motion of one or more joints
3	Limited to few or no duties of usual occupation or self-care
4	Incapacitated largely *or* wholly bedridden *or* confined to wheelchair; little or no self-care
Ranawat	
I	No neurologic deficit (normal neurologic condition)
II	Subjective weakness with hyperreflexia and dysesthesia (paresthesia, subjective weakness, e.g., cannot do buttons or walk as well as before; tingling in limbs)
IIIa	Objective weakness and long-tract signs but able to walk (on examination, definite weakness and increased tone)
IIIb	Quadriparetic or nonambulatory (bed bound or wheelchair bound)

spinal cord involvement.[37,67,69,97] The lumbar spine is only involved in approximately 5 percent of cases. Similarly, the thoracic spine is rarely involved.[8]

Several techniques have been investigated to determine the extent of spinal cord involvement. These include plain and dynamic roentgenograms, myelography, computed tomography (CT), dynamic CT, plain magnetic resonance imaging (MRI), dynamic MRI, and bone scanning.[2–4,12–15,23,24,28,29,38,46,47,51,57,73,74,88,113–115] Other testing methods to monitor the patient during surgery, e.g., somatosensory evoked potentials, are currently under investigation.[53,101]

Care must be taken not to miss other diagnoses when a patient with rheumatoid arthritis presents with neurologic symptoms. These patients may have strokes, Brown-Sequard cord infarcts, and peripheral neuropathies as well. A careful physical examination is usually sufficient to sort out the diagnosis, but other tests, including laboratory studies and electromyography (EMG), may be necessary. The patient with rheumatoid arthritis is at a higher risk of infection and the wound takes longer to heal owing to al-

tered immune responses. Normal signs of fever and leukocytosis may not be present in the rheumatoid patient with an infection.[55,64]

Instability

The inability of a patient to lift the head off a pillow in the morning or the feeling that the head is about to fall off the shoulders are signals that spinal instability exists in the rheumatoid patient. Also, the patient may complain of a loss in function of the hands or legs with neck flexion or extension. This last complaint signifies involvement of the spinal cord secondary to the bony instability.

The cervical spine is commonly divided into two regions for analysis of instability problems. The upper cervical region includes the occiput C1 and C2 articulations. The subaxial (lower cervical region) encompasses the C3 to C7 levels.

Wiesel and Rothman have shown that the normal range of sagittal translation of the C1–C2 articulation in flexion and extension does not exceed 1 mm.[110] A finding of more than 4 mm of translation anterior to the dens is indicative of instability of the C1–C2 joint. The distance between the base of the occiput and the top of the dens is 4 to 5 mm. An increase of more than 1 mm in flexion and extension is indicative of instability.[107] Biomechanically, 50 percent of head rotation occurs in the C1–C2 complex. When a patient complains of pain with rotation of the head, the likely instability level is the upper cervical junction. Many instability symptoms can be lessened when a patient is supine with the head supported on a pillow. If the patient is asked to actively lift his or her head off the pillow, instability elicits either weakness or a feeling of impending doom (Fig. 18-1A). Subtle instabilities are magnified if resistance is added to lifting the head (Fig. 18-1B). If these symptoms are present, flexion and extension roentgenograms are obtained with careful observation. Motion should never be forced during dynamic roentgenograms, and the patient is instructed to stop if there is discomfort. Motion into neck flexion or extension should be stopped at the first sign of pain or any abnormal feeling.

Subaxial Instability.   Patients with subaxial, or C3–C7, instabilities usually present with severe posterior or occipital neck pain and headaches.

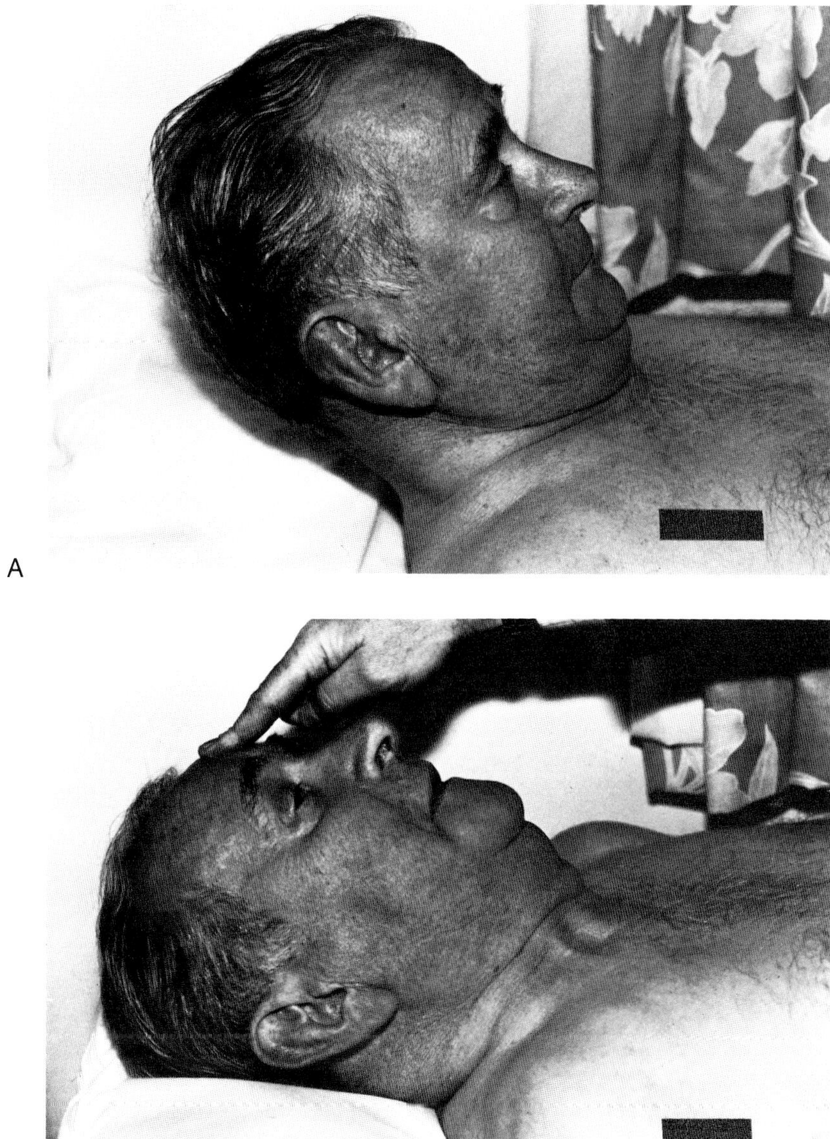

Fig. 18-1. Supine head elevation test for cervical spine instability. (**A**) Without resistance. (**B**) With resistance.

Some patients have neural involvement such that when leading forward the spinal cord becomes compressed and causes arm or leg symptoms. Typically, these patients avoid any flexion of the spine and tend to hold the head in extension to avoid any neurologic compromise.

Instability is assessed using carefully observed flexion and extension roentgenograms. If the translation is less than 3.5 mm, the patient is observed clinically and with serial roentgenograms, unless there are obvious neurologic complaints.[107] If the translation is more than 3.5 mm, the patient may be a candidate for posterior fusion over the involved segments.[19] Fusion includes adjacent hypermobile segments; i.e., if there is C4–C5 subluxation of more than 3.5 mm and C5–C6 translates 2 mm, C4–C6 is fused.

Iatrogenic or Postlaminectomy Instability. The presence of swan-neck deformity after cervical laminectomy is not a new concept. Sim et al.

have written extensively on the postlaminectomy swan-neck deformity.[90] Rheumatoid patients who have been treated with extensive posterior laminectomies without fusion should be carefully watched for development of secondary instabilities.

Neck Pain

It is not uncommon for the patient to present with severe posterior occipital neck pain and headaches.[83] He or she may also have intrascapular pain and pain into the ears and temples. If the problems are secondary to bony instability, these symptoms may be elicited with flexion or extension. The cutaneous and deep innervation of the posterior neck and head may be seen in Figure 18-2.[43]

The greater occipital nerve exits deep behind the vertebral artery. It then travels between the rectus capitis posterior and the semispinalis capitis and exists subcutaneously in the posterior occipital area. Any instability or irritation on the occipital or C1–C2 facet articulations may irritate this nerve. Also, the posterior ramus of the C1

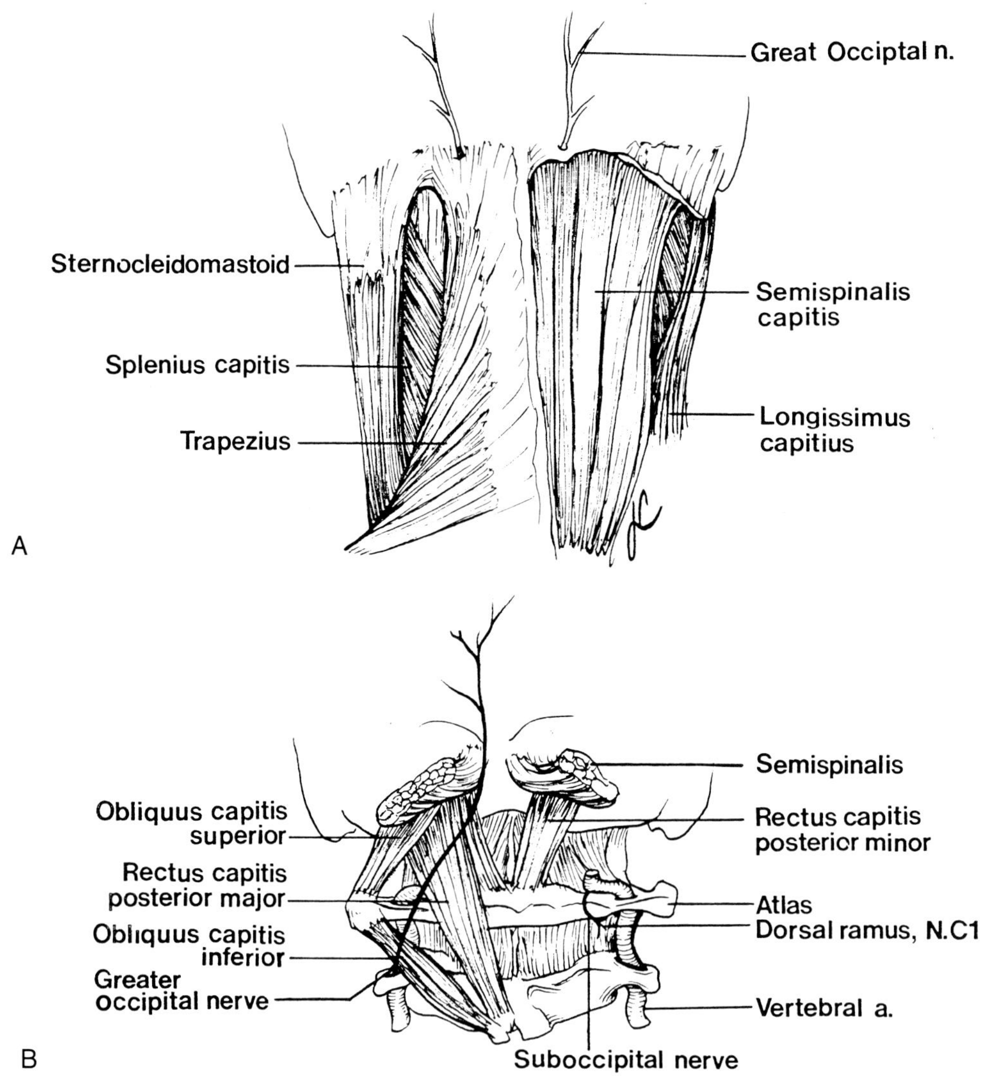

Fig. 18-2. Innervation of the posterior cervical spine. (**A**) Superficial dissection. (**B**) Deep dissection showing course of greater occipital and suboccipital nerves. (From Hollinshead,[43] with permission.)

root swings around the posterior ring of C1 and may refer pain via the suboccipital nerve.

Cranial Subluxation

The occipital condyles have oblique facets that are laterally related to the C1 facets. With degeneration of the joints secondary to inflammatory arthritis, the cervical spine may migrate proximally into the foramen magnum, causing the patient to have superior migration of the odontoid onto the brainstem. This condition is termed *basilar impression*. These patients may initially complain of little neck pain but may have dizziness or episodes of fainting. In any patient with these symptoms, a lateral roentgenogram of the cervical spine is advised.

Myelopathy

The symptoms of spinal cord compression are termed *myelopathy*. They include spasticity of the arms or legs and a loss in the fine control of the hands. The problem often manifests as a de-

crease in penmanship. For example, if a patient attempts his or her signature ten times, there is usually deterioration in writing quality across the repetitions (Fig. 18-3). Spasticity of the lower extremities is exhibited as gait alterations, such as tripping or an inability of the patient to walk rhythmically or control the legs.

Grading Systems of Myelopathic Involvement. The Japanese have developed a point scale to evaluate, through the use of chopsticks, the severity of myelopathy.[20,72] However, in the United States, it is difficult to apply this rating system because we are not chopstick users. Instead, the Ranawat grading is employed. A series of dexterity tests are given for the upper extremities, including mazes and Jebson hand function evaluation. To determine lower extremity involvement, the Nurick grading system is used, as well as timed gait analysis at 30 feet and timed stair climbing.

If the patient has cord involvement as well as instability, it is imperative to determine whether the cord symptoms are secondary to the instability or the result of a fixed cord compression independent of the associated instability. To help in this evaluation, flexion and extension roentgenograms are obtained in the office. If there is any evidence of neurologic compromise of the cord, flexion and extension CT myelography or flexion and extension MRI is indicated (Fig. 18-4). During flexion the odontoid has an anterior translation force applied to it. If there is insufficiency of the alar or transverse ligament, the odontoid is no longer held in approximation to the alar ring. The odontoid then translates posteriorly to cause spinal cord compression (Fig. 18-5).

Part of the inflammatory process secondary to inflammatory arthritis is bursal enlargement. There is a bursa posterior to the odontoid peg, and with inflammation a pannus of inflammatory tissue may develop. This tissue may itself cause direct spinal cord compression (Fig. 18-6). When the disease is in remission, the pannus may decrease in size. Some investigators believe it may resolve spontaneously with a solid posterior fusion.[116]

The atlas may also translate in a rotatory fashion (Fig. 18-7) if the inflammatory process selectively involves one side of the ligament/facet or ligament/odontoid mecha-

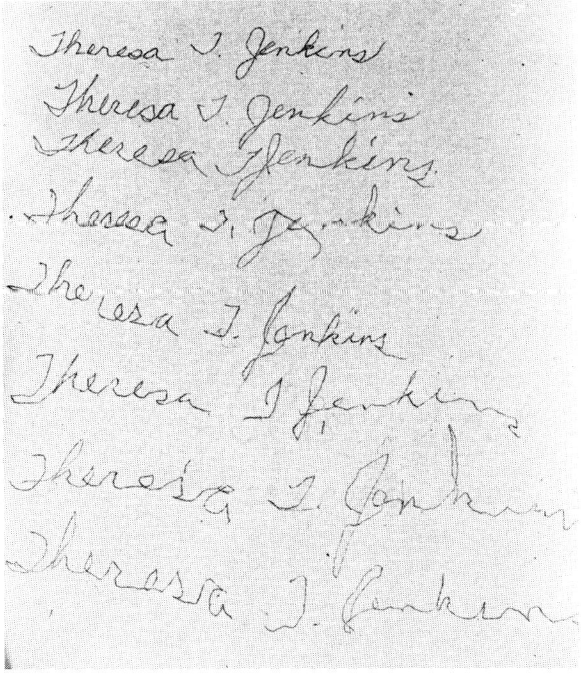

Fig. 18-3. Handwriting test of a patient with cervical myelopathy. Note the deterioration of writing quality with repetition of the signature.

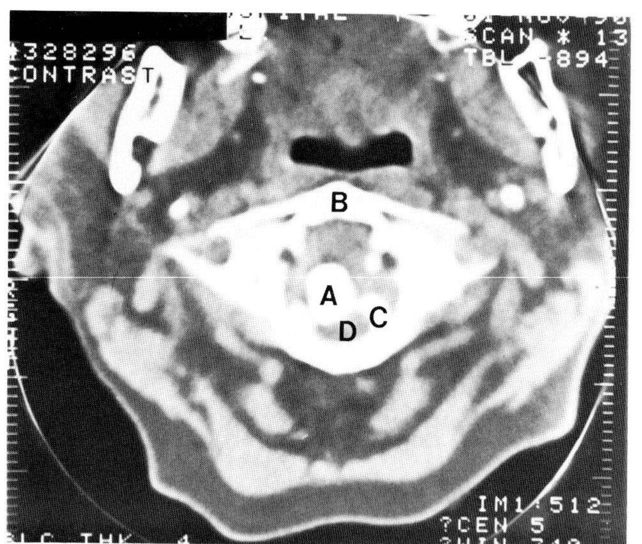

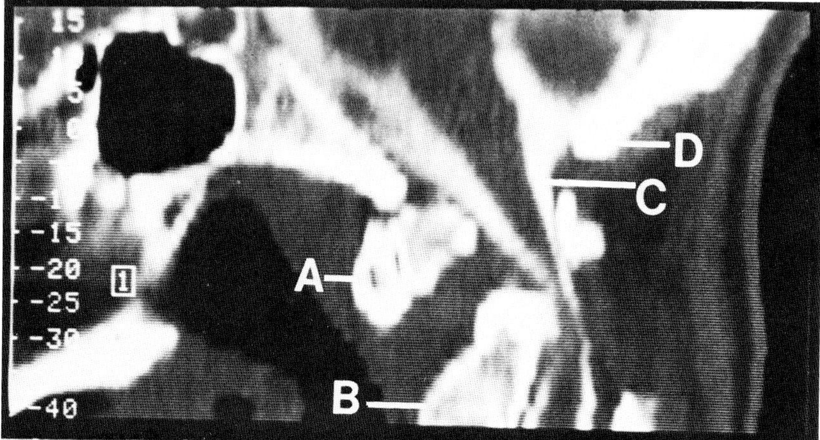

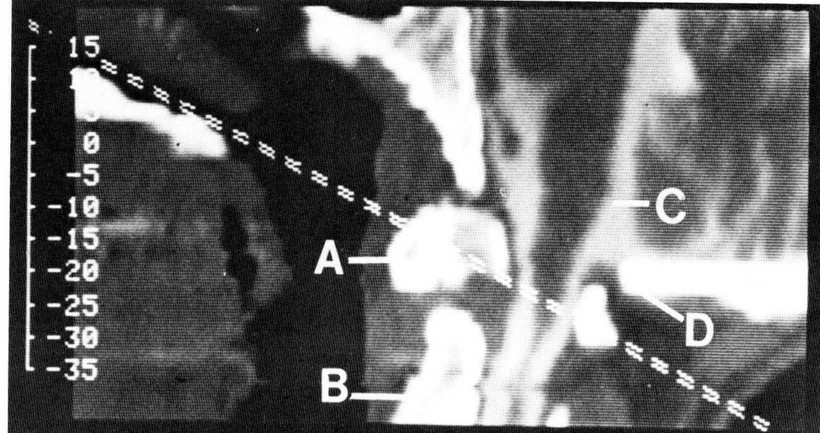

Fig. 18-4. (**A**) CT myelogram in flexion. The odontoid (A) is displaced from the anterior ring of C1 (B), which is impacting on the dural sac filled with contrast (C) and the spinal cord (D). (**B**) MR scan in flexion. This sagittal cut is through the occipitocervical region of the anterior ring of C1 (A), which is displaced anterior to the odontoid (B). Odontoid is impinging on the spinal cord (C). D = occiput. (**C**) MR scan in extension. Canal diameter is adequate for the spinal cord.

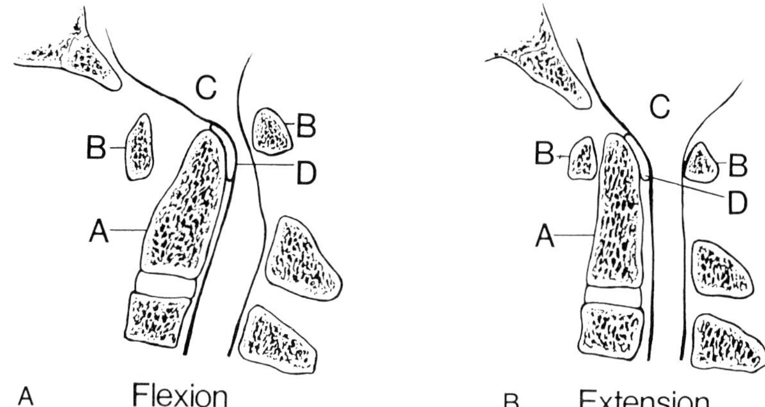

Fig. 18-5. Relation of the odontoid (A) to the C1 ring (B) and spinal cord (C). (**A**) In flexion, the odontoid compresses the spinal cord. (**B**) In extension, the canal diameter is adequate.

nism.[11,26,48–50,72,75,77,82,91,96,100,103,105] If this situation occurs, the odontoid may mover vertically or in an anterior or posterior direction. Special CT studies are required to identify rotatory subluxation, but vertical, lateral, or anteroposterior subluxation can often be seen on plain films. It is important to determine if these translations are fixed or mobile. If the deformity is fixed and not causing neural compression, a posterior fusion may be necessary to reduce the neck pain associated with these deformities. If the deformity is mobile or causes neural compression, a fusion and decompression of the spinal cord is indicated.

Treatment

There are many excellent review articles about the treatment options for rheumatoid arthritis.[5,20,27,29,32,56,58,59,62,66,67,85,106] The treatment of patients with rheumatoid involvement of the spine is divided into two types: that for patients with occipital C1–C2 involvement and that for those with subaxial instabilities. In many patients both of the deformities exist together.

Bracing

Many patients can be treated conservatively for their neck symptoms with a soft collar or Phila-

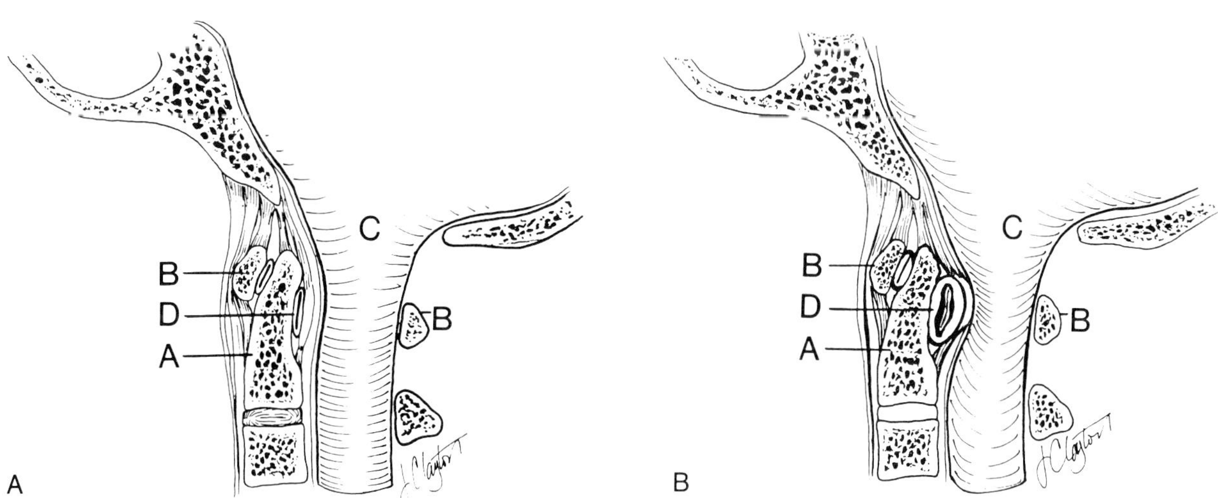

Fig. 18-6. (**A**) Normal odontoid (A), C1 ring (B), spinal cord (C), and bursal (D) relations. (**B**) Posterior odontoid bursal enlargement causes compression of the spinal cord.

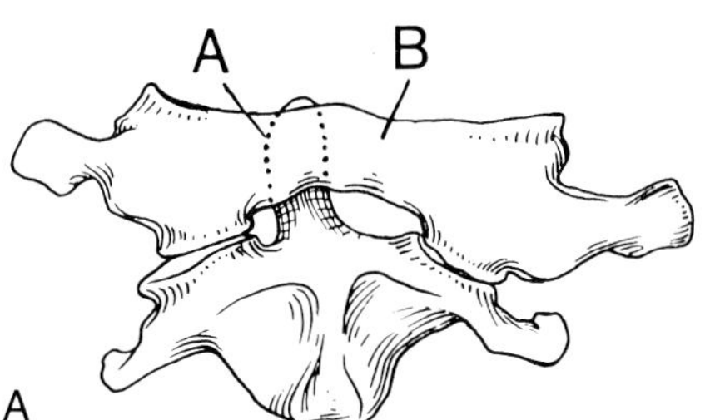
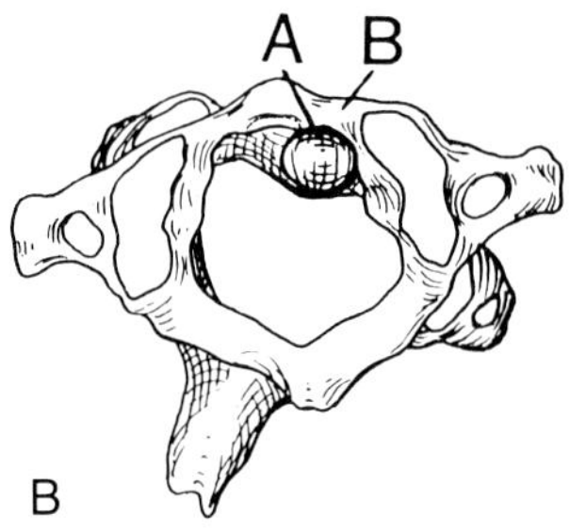

Fig. 18-7. Rotatory subluxation of the odontoid. (**A**) Anteroposterior view. Note the narrow space between the odontoid (A) and the C1 lateral mass (B). (**B**) Axial view showing the asymmetric position of the odontoid (A) relative to the anterior C1 ring (B).

delphia collar. Once there is evidence of significant neural compression, surgery is commonly recommended. Patients are mobilized as rapidly as possible, and a halo is applied if required. Whitehill et al. reported halo brace immobilization failure in rheumatoid patients.[108] However, close supervision of rheumatoid patients with a halo may reduce problems.[80] Patients are seen and the collar tightened on a regular basis. Usually the fusion consolidates in about 12 weeks, at which time the halo can be removed. A collar is employed until the patient has regained neck control and musculature.

Timing of Treatment

The longer the spinal cord is compressed, the less chance there is of recovery of neural function. In a study of patients with myelopathy following odontoid fractures, it was also observed that the cross-sectional area of the cord atrophies distal to the site of maximal compression.[40] It may be due to a block in the vascular supply to the cord, as at the upper cervical level the blood supply slows proximally to distally. With a bony block this high, there may be ischemic changes over a longer area of the cord than simply the area of direct bony compression. Thus early treatment of patients with neurologic symptoms should be considered.

Instability Without Myelopathy

The levels of translation are determined from the preoperative flexion and extension roentgenograms. These patients are usually treated with posterior wiring and fusion. If the deformity is more than two levels, we use a Bohlman triple wire technique. For fusion of the C1–C2 ring, we use the Gallie technique or Halifax clamps. For

fusion of the occiput to C2, we use either a Luque custom loop (Ransford), Cotrel-Dubousset occipital ring, or more commonly the iliac graft and wire technique of Bohlman.

Instability With Myelopathy

A previously noted, flexion and extension radiographs are obtained initially. Flexion and extension MRI or CT myelography is employed to determine if the cord compression is fixed or dynamic. These patients are highly unstable, and sudden death has been reported if the condition is not treated appropriately.[71] If the compression is fixed, anterior decompression of the cord with a subsequent posterior fusion of the involved levels is performed.

The anterior decompression relieves the source of compression of the cord. If the patient has posterior compression from ligamentum flavum hypertrophy, posterior laminectomy and fusion are also done. If acute deterioration of spinal cord function occurs, the patient is placed in Gardner-Wells traction until appropriate studies can be obtained. This treatment often produces improved neurologic status. Some investigators recommend treating these patients with prolonged traction, but we have not been able to reproduce their results.[72,75]

Transoral Surgery

There are many patients with fixed anterior compression of the cord who do not improve after posterior fusion alone. If a fixed deformity of the cord from bony impingement of the odontoid is present, a transoral odontoid resection followed by a posterior fusion may be elected. Transoral surgery is technically demanding. The surgeon must be familiar with the use of the microscope and pay particular attention to the handling of the posterior pharyngeal mucosa. The Codman/Crockard instrumentation is useful. It allows excellent visualization of the spine while preventing pharyngeal irritation.[21]

Other Surgical Techniques

McAfee et al. described the retropharyngeal approach to the upper cervical spine.[63] We have not been as impressed with the ability of this procedure to obtain decompression of the entire cord when compared to the transoral route. The advantage of this approach is a lower risk of infection. Also available are a variety of posterior stabilization techniques other than the standard wiring techniques of Bohlman and Gallie.[22,34,44,84]

Subaxial instabilities without myelopathy are treated with posterior fusion.[27] The fusion must not be ended on a hypermobile segment. For a single level fusion, a simple Roger's technique may be used, and for multiple levels the triple wire technique of Bohlman is commonly utilized.

Patients who have neural symptoms with isolated subaxial instability are evaluated with flexion and extension MRI or CT myelography. If the compression is posterior, a laminectomy with fusion is usually performed. If the patient has fixed compression anteriorly, a sequential vertebrectomy and strut grafting is used to decompress the cord, followed by a posterior fusion if needed. The patient is routinely placed in a halo if no posterior fusion is done.

Parenthetically, the anesthetic management of the myelopathic patient requires a skilled anesthesiologist trained in techniques of awake fiberoptic intubation and well versed in the use of spinal cord monitoring.[70]

Conclusions

Treatment of patients suffering from inflammatory arthritis of the cervical spine requires a careful, stepwise approach. The patients who are at greatest risk of developing spinal problems are the rheumatoid patients in whom the disease develops late in life and patients with severe peripheral involvement.[19,21,72,75] Patients with subtle translations should be followed with spinal

dynamic films, but only a small number require surgery. If a neurologic deficit develops, early surgery is favored.

DESTRUCTIVE SPINAL LESIONS IN INFLAMMATORY ARTHRITIS
David A. Wong

Bony erosions of the vertebral bodies have, for many years, been recognized in association with inflammatory arthritis, particularly ankylosing spondylitis (Marie-Strumpell disease, Bechterew's disease, rheumatoid spondylitis, pelvospondylitis ossificans).[35,111] Such lesions are generally acknowledged to be part of the pathogenesis of the disease, although the exact etiology of the destruction, the relation of the disease to clinical pain, and the optimum methods of treatment remain issues for debate.

History

Crawley et al.[18] credited the first descriptions of destructive spinal lesions in inflammatory spondylitis to Andersson and Edstrom. Recognition of these lesions was uncommon during the first half of the twentieth century. Andersson's report described localized bony destruction of the spine in two patients and Edstrom's in only one patient. Forestier et al.[30] reviewed 200 patients with ankylosing spondylitis and found two patients with bony erosions of the spine.

Early investigators were unclear as to the etiology of the destructive lesions observed roentgenographically. Bony erosion and occasional involvement of the disc space led to suspicion of septic discitis (pyrogenic, tuberculous brucellosis), multiple myeloma, crush fracture, fracture pseudarthrosis, and metastatic malignancy.[60,78]

More recent clinicopathologic studies have recognized two major classes of bony erosions in the spine.[31] Anterior spondylitis is a localized, destructive process located at the anterior rim of the vertebral body. Spondylodiscitis involves the discal surface of the vertebral body and may result in changes in the disc space.

Anterior Spondylitis (Romanus Lesions)

Anterior spondylitis was described by Romanus and Yden[81] as a short-lived erosion occurring at the point where the outer fibers of the annulus attach to the anterior and anterolateral corners of the vertebral body. These lesions occur early in the course of the disease. Pathology studies by Ball[7] suggested that these changes are manifestations of the inflammatory component of ankylosing spondylitis involving the vascular portion of the annulus. The vascular area has been identified by the injection studies of Rathburn and MacNab.[76] Healing of the Romanus lesion stimulates new bony formation leading to the appearance on radiographs of syndesmophytes (Fig. 18-8). These bony spurs eventually coalesce to form the continuous, bony bridges characteristic of the "bamboo spine" of ankylosing spondylitis (Fig. 18-9). Clinically, anterior spondylitis is thought to be related to the chronic, aching back pain seen with the early, inflammatory stages of the disease.

Spondylodiscitis

Spondylodiscitis, the second major group of erosive spinal lesions, involves the discal surface of the vertebral body. Cawley et al.[18] described five subtypes of spondylodiscitis (Fig. 18-10). Lesions are grouped according to the area of the discal surface involved and the degree of destruction. Subtypes A and B involved the area of the vertebral rim, and subtypes C and D involved the cartilaginous end-plate. Subtype E lesions show severe erosions of both the vertebral rim and cartilaginous end-plate. The classification (A to E) generally reflects the degree of clinical symptomatology, with subtype E lesions being recognized as the most painful. The lesions of spondylodiscitis have a chronologic as well as anatomic separation from anterior spondylitis. Anterior spondylitis is seen in the early stages, whereas spondylodiscitis occurs late in the course of the disease. Wholey et al.[109] and Rivelis and Freiberger[78] noted lesions of the spondylodiscitis only in patients known to have the disease for longer than 10 years. Little et al.[60] noted asymptomatic spondylodiscitis in six patients. Only one patient had ankylosing spondylitis for less than 10 years.

Although it is generally conceded that the degree of spinal involvement is greater in those patients with long-lasting disease, the reported incidence of spondylodiscitis varies widely in the literature from 1 percent to 28 percent.[18] The severe subtype E lesions are the rarest and are the only subtype that seems to have a predilection for a particular anatomic area of the spine. These lesions are most often found in the lower thoracic and lumbar areas.[18] The etiology of spondylodiscitis is not definitively known. Biopsy has not revealed bacteria in any reported case,[45] and cultures and smears for fungi have been negative.[61] Bagenstoss et al.[6] obtained autopsy material from one of the three patients in their series. The histology demonstrated granulomatous lesions similar to nodules found in the patient's other tissues, including the subcutaneous tissue and synovium.

Lorber et al.[61] biopsied one patient and found chronic inflammatory changes with fibrosis. Wholey et al.[109] obtained tissue for histology from two of their ten patients and found chronic inflammatory changes in both samples.

More recently, Rivelis and Freiberger[79] found histologic changes suggestive of fracture pseudarthrosis in their patients. Osteoclastic resorption of bone was observed with associated areas of new bone formation and invasion by vascular fibrous tissue. They also noted that the le-

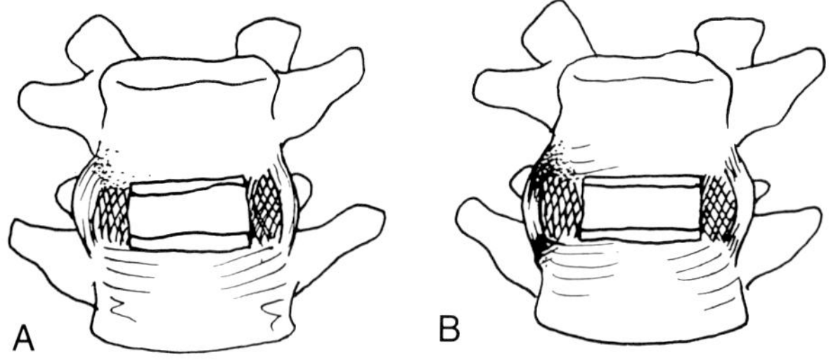

Fig. 18-8. Erosion and inflammation where outer fibers of the annulus attach to the body (**A**) and (**B**) lead to the formation of bony syndesmophytes, which eventually coalesce to form the typical "bamboo" spine.

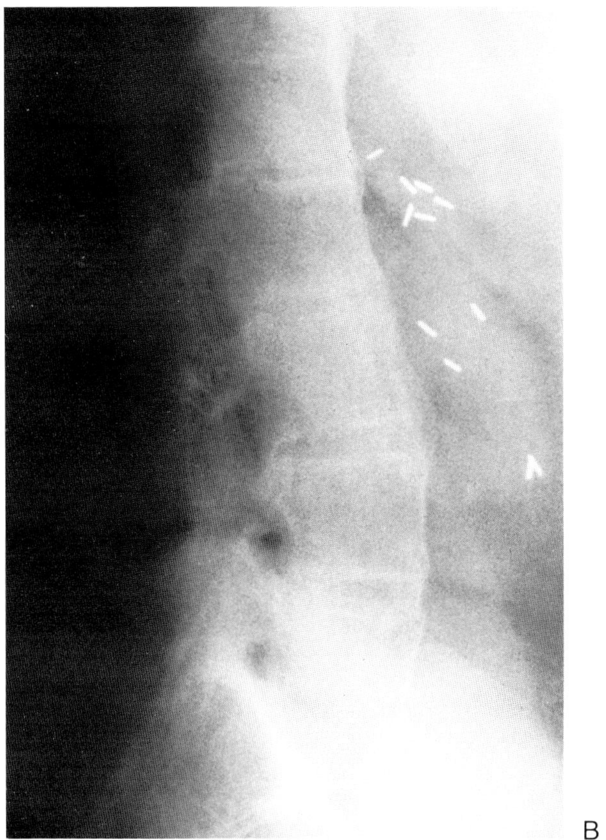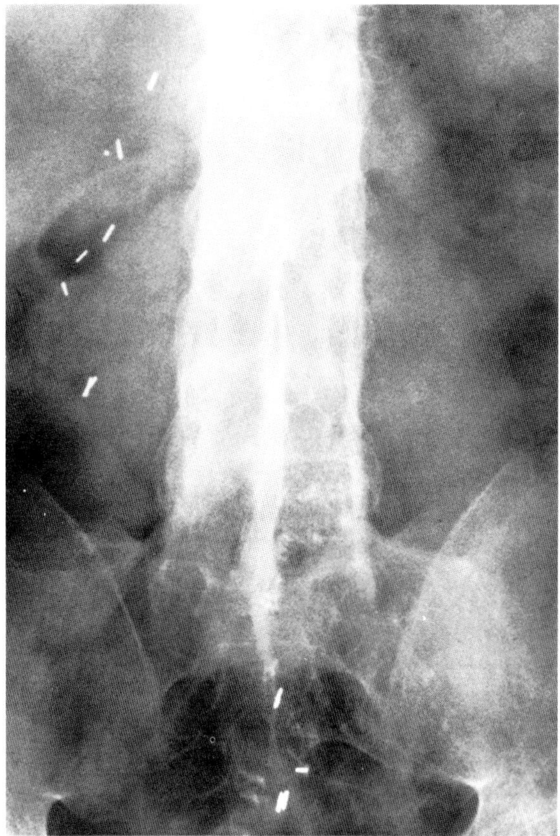

Fig. 18-9. (A) Lateral roentgenogram showing the typical "bamboo" spine of ankylosing spondylitis. **(B)** Anteroposterior view.

sions they identified occurred in areas with a segment of fused spine above and below the lesion, enhancing their conviction that the lesion represented a fracture pseudarthrosis. Cawley et al.[18] and Kanefield et al.[45] agreed that the severe destructive lesions may arise from repeated trauma to an unfused segment in chronic ankylosing spondylitis. In one of Kanefield's patients, a fracture through the posterior elements actually preceded the development of spondylodiscitis at that level. Calin and Robertson[17] described spondylodiscitis in association with enteropathic spondyloarthropathy treated by steroids.

Seaman and Wells[87] suggested that cortisone treatment may be an etiologic factor. Fifty percent of their patients had been on steroid therapy. Lorber et al.,[61] however, noted that none of their patients had been on steroids.

Clinical Presentation

Patients with spondylodiscitis generally presented with localized complaints of back pain. The pain is increased by mechanical movement. Symptoms generally appeared some years after abatement of the more diffuse pains encountered in the early stages of ankylosing spondylitis. All of the patients of Cawley et al.[18] were involved in manual work. The patients of Kanefield et al. gave a history of minor injury.[45] Cases of asymptomatic spondylodiscitis have been noted by Little et al.[60] and Seaman and Wells.[87]

Spondylodiscitis can be responsible for significant clinical deterioration.[36] Kanefield et al.[45] reported one case of paraplegia below the level of spondylodiscitis at T9–T10. Surgical intervention was undertaken, and the compression was

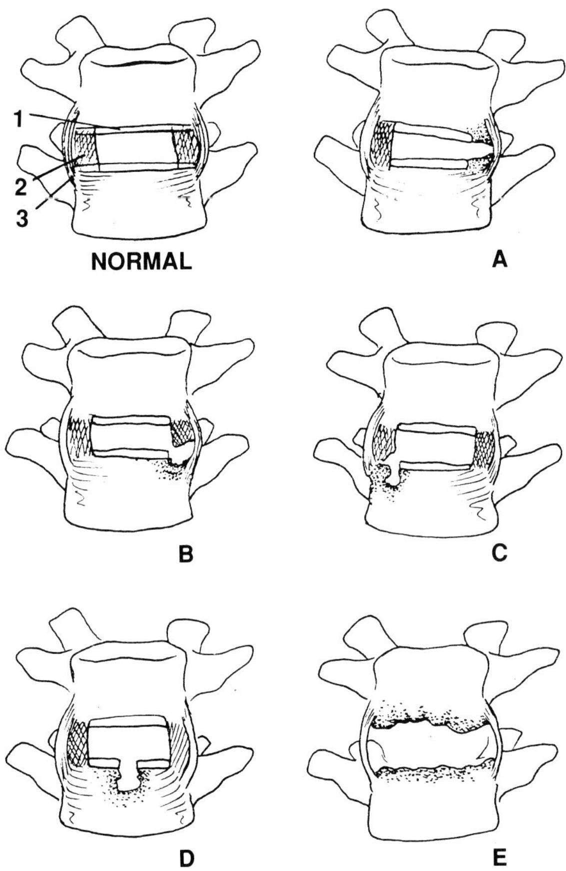

Fig. 18-10. Cawley's classification of spondylodiscitis. Normal spinal motion segment: epiphyseal plate (1); inner fibers of annulus (2); outer fibers of annulus (3). Inflammation (**A**) and erosion (**B**) of vertebral rim. Involvement of peripheral (**C**) and central (**D**) endplate. Severe erosions (**E**) involving vertebral rim and endplate.

found to be resulting from a mass of granulomatous fibrous tissue with no active signs of inflammation on histology. Lorber et al.[61] had also undertaken surgical decompression in a case with signs of neurologic compromise; epidural granulation tissue was found in their case also.

Treatment

Treatment of spondylodiscitis is essentially determined by the degree of symptomatology present. Little et al.[60] followed six patients with asymptomatic spondylodiscitis for an average of 14 years with no need for therapeutic intervention. The general rationale for treatment of symptomatic spinal lesions is rest, immobilization of the affected level, and control of the overall disease process. Rest and immobilization may simply involve an alteration in the patient's activity level, or it may involve bracing and even surgical fusion of the involved level.[9] Simmons (personal communication, 1985) has reported that spondylodiscitis has healed after osteotomy of the spine at a level removed from the area of spondylodiscitis. Osteotomy realigns the spine into a vertical orientation rather than the more horizontal position in the kyphotic position. The tension or shear force that often exists as a result of the kyphotic spinal deformity and the force of gravity is transformed by osteotomy[68] into a force of compression at the level of spondylodiscitis.

Discussion

Two distinct destructive lesions have been noted in inflammatory spondylitis. The lesions of anterior spondylitis (Romanus lesions), which involves the anterior rim of the vertebral body, are generally seen early in the course of the disease. Their etiology is thought to be related to the inflammatory process involving the vascular portion of the annulus.

Spondylodiscitis involves bony destruction of the discal surface of the vertebral body and may involve the disc space. It is usually seen late in the course of the disease and may be asymptomatic or the cause of severe pain and neurologic compromise. The etiology of spondylodiscitis is not clear. The most widely regarded explanation is that the lesions result from repeated trauma to an unfused segment of spine or represent a fracture pseudarthrosis.

Other destructive processes may mimic anterior spondylitis or spondylodiscitis. Serial roentgenograms and other imaging studies may be of benefit in identifying such pathologic processes.[95] Disc narrowing usually precedes bony destruction with pyogenic infection. With ankylosing spondylitis, bony erosions may be seen without disc narrowing or, in some cases, with disc widening. CT scans may identify paravertebral masses often found with pyogenic as well as tuberculous osteomyelitis. In cases where the presence of a metastatic neoplasm is questioned, a biopsy may be the only definitive investigation.

Treatment of anterior spondylitis and spondylodiscitis is generally symptomatic. Some cases require surgical intervention for fusion of the involved segment, decompression for neurologic compromise, or osteotomy for spinal realignment.

SPINAL OSTEOTOMY IN INFLAMMATORY ARTHRITIS
David A. Wong

Although diffuse spondyloarthropathy can occur with any inflammatory arthritis, including rheumatoid arthritis, it is most commonly seen in ankylosing spondylitis. Spinal involvement in ankylosing spondylitis is found in more than 80 percent of patients with a duration of symptoms longer than 5 years and in nearly 100 percent of patients with symptoms of more than 15 years duration.[111] Some patients develop a progressive flexion deformity of the spine, which occasionally reaches a degree where significant functional impairment is produced. Such patients may be candidates for correction of the deformity by spinal osteotomy.[9]

Prevention of spinal deformities should be a primary goal of treatment in spondyloarthropathy. Early diagnosis, appropriate medical treatment, and adjustment of daily activities and work environment are essential segments of treatment.[94] Bracing has been advocated as a preventive measure when early deformity is found.[65,89] Despite these measures, some patients continue to develop a progressive flexion deformity of the spine, a distortion of normal alignment that may lead to embarrassment of abdominal and thoracic structures. However, of more immediate and practical concern to the patient is the resulting restriction in field of vision, which leads to difficulties with interpersonal communication, mobility in the community, and work performance. Severe flexion deformity of the cervical spine leading to the "chin on chest" deformity can cause problems with basic activities of daily life. Food ingestion may be impaired because of restricted jaw opening and swallowing difficulties. Personal hygiene is difficult owing to an inability to shave or wash under the chin. Any severe deformity and its associated functional limitations has obvious adverse psychological effects.

Indications for Extension Osteotomy of the Spine

The primary indication for surgical correction is the presence of a flexion deformity of the spine causing restricted, nonfunctional field of vision. Secondary indications include difficulties with food ingestion, personal hygiene, and psychological considerations. The patient should be in good general medical health with adequate control of their disease. They should have a good range of motion of major joints and acceptable muscle strength. In general, involvement of musculoskeletal and other organ systems should be limited so a reasonable level of function can be anticipated following surgery. Most candidates for surgery are in their fourth or fifth decade of life.

Contraindications to surgery include significant medical problems, neurologic involvement, and fixed deformity of major joints, particularly the hips. Fixed flexion deformities of the hips are treated with total hip replacement, if feasible, prior to consideration for correction of spinal deformities.

Preoperative Evaluation of Spinal Deformity

The site and extent of flexion deformity must be carefully determined by clinical assessment and radiologic examination. As part of the overall clinical assessment, the patient's mobility and functional level are noted as he or she moves around the office and examining room, gives a history, and undresses for the physical examination.

Clinical evaluation of the spinal deformity is made by observing the patient from the front, back, and side. The side view is the most important. The site of major deformity (cervical, thoracic, or lumbar spine) can be determined and the extent of the deformity measured (Figs. 18-11 and 18-12). The frontomental line is used as the baseline for assessing the deformity. This line is normally vertical when erect and looking straight ahead. In a patient with a flexion deformity, the severity is measured by noting the angle of the frontomental line from the vertical. The patient is asked to place the neck in the most comfortable position. A large goniometer is used to estimate the angle between the frontomental line and the vertical. This measurement reflects the overall degree of spinal deformity and thus estimates the angle of required surgical correction. The aim of surgery is to correct the flexion deformity to the point where the patient is looking nearly straight ahead (frontomental line 0 to 15 degrees flexed

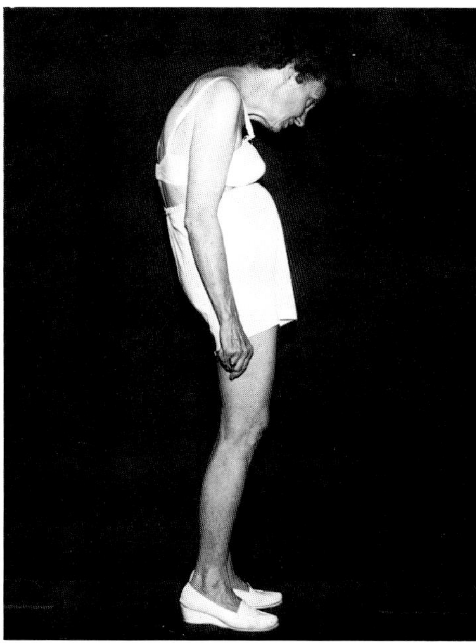

Fig. 18-11. Lateral view of a 58-year-old woman with ankylosing spondylitis. Note that the major flexion deformity is in the neck. Contrast this patient with the one in Figure 18-12, in whom the major deformity is in the lumbar spine. The frontomental line in both patients is approximately 45 degrees from the vertical. A corrective osteotomy of 45 degrees would thus allow the patients to look straight ahead.

forward from the vertical). In this position, the patient is able to see the horizon when in a standing or sitting position and is also able to use ocular movements to visualize his or her feet when standing.

Site of Osteotomy

The choice of osteotomy site is determined by the location of the major deformity, which is more commonly in the lumbar spine (Fig. 18-12). However, a number of patients have their major deformity in the cervical spine with its associated "chin on chest" phenomenon (Fig. 18-11). Patients whose major flexion deformity lies in the hip joints are treated with bilateral total hip replacement before consideration is given to spinal osteotomy.

Anatomic factors dictate that the osteotomy be performed in either the lumbar or lower cervical spine. The thoracic area is not favorable because of the small canal diameter relative to cord size, thereby increasing the chance of cord damage. The presence of ankylosed costovertebral joints also make angular correction difficult.

The lumbar spine, anatomically, is the best location for spinal osteotomy.[65] The spinal canal is wide, and the osteotomy can be performed below the level of the spinal cord. Thus any compression of the dural sac would result in a cauda equina lesion rather than spinal cord lesion. The L2–L3 or L3–L4 levels are usually designated as the sites of osteotomy or the apex for multiple level osteotomies.

In the cervical spine the osteotomy is located at the C7–T1 level.[102] The spinal canal is widest at this point in the cervical spine. The vertebral arteries usually pass anterior to the C7 transverse processes to enter the foramen transversarium of C6. An osteotomy at C7–T1 is therefore less likely to damage the vertebral arteries than a similar procedure at higher levels.

Technique of Extension Osteotomy

A number of variations in the technique of spinal osteotomy have been described. Techniques generally vary in one or more of four areas.

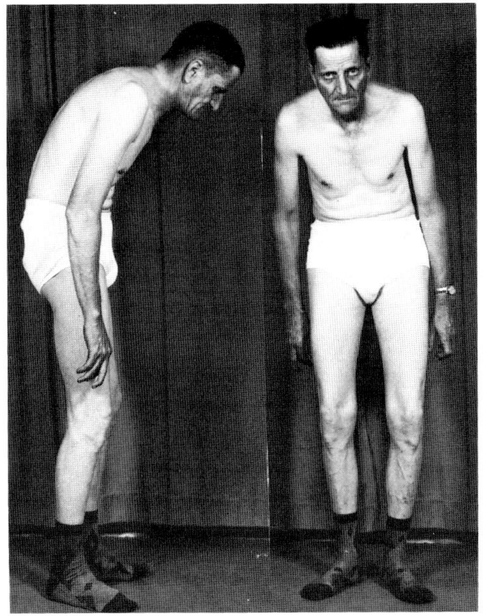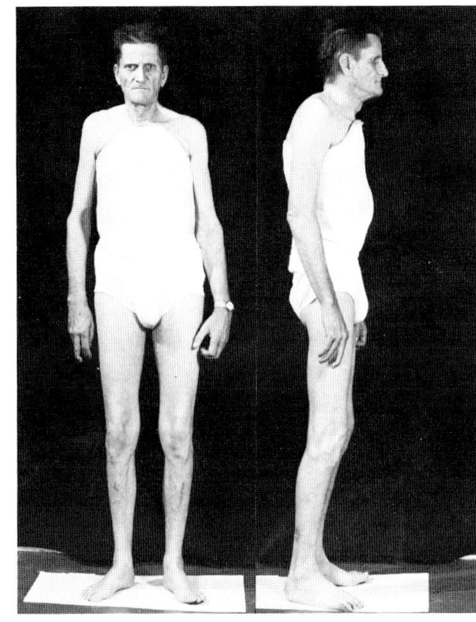

Fig. 18-12. (**A**) Preoperative photographs of a 47-year-old man prior to lumbar osteotomy. Frontomental line is approximately 45 degrees off vertical. Major deformity is in the lumbar spine. (**B**) Postoperative photographs following lumbar osteotomy showing frontomental line vertical. The patient is now able to look straight ahead.

1. Position of the patient (prone or lateral decubitus)
2. General or local anesthesia
3. One-stage posterior approach only or two-stage posterior and anterior approach
4. Number of levels being osteotomized

Surgical osteotomy in ankylosing spondylitis was first described in 1945 by Smith-Petersen and colleagues,[98] who reported six cases. The patients were positioned prone, general anesthesia was used, and one to three osteotomies were used for correction in a one-stage posterior approach. LaChapelle[52] used a two-stage approach. He first performed a posterior osteotomy, followed in 2 to 3 weeks by an anterior sectioning of the anterior longitudinal ligament. Adams[1] used the lateral position to perform a posterior osteotomy at one level only. Simmons has used local anesthesia,[92,112] which eliminates some of the anesthetic concerns, particularly the necessity for endotracheal intubation, and allows patients to monitor their own neurologic status; they can then inform the surgeon if any signs of cord or nerve root pressure occur. Hehne et al.[39] have advocated multilevel osteotomies and segmental pedicle screw instrumentation for correction of lumbar deformities.

Complications

Extension osteotomy of the spine is associated with some specific complications.

Intraoperative Complications

The obvious difficulties with airway management due to the fixed attitude of the cervical spine and jaw have been previously mentioned. The other major complication encountered intraoperatively is compression of the neural elements. Translation of the spine at the osteotomy level can result in neural compression at either the cervical or lumbar level. This complication can be avoided by careful construction of the osteotomy wedges and by the use of segmental instrumentation so there is locking of the bony elements with correction of the spine. Correction should be done slowly with precise control of the segments above and below the osteotomy.

Infolding of the posterior aspect of the dural sac may also be responsible for compression, particularly in the cervical spine where there is relatively little room for accommodation due to the presence of the cord itself and the bony architecture of the canal at this level. The central portion of the osteotomy in the cervical spine is made somewhat oval to accommodate this possible infolding of dura. Simmons (personal communication, 1985) described a case in which paraplegia was reversed by immediate splitting of the infolded dura posteriorly. The eighth nerve root in the neck is also relatively fixed and may be stretched with the correction of a cervical osteotomy. Although this problem may give rise to numbness and tingling along the ulnar border of the hand and weakness of the intrinsic hand muscles, it is still compatible with good function.[92]

Fracture of an ankylosed segment of spine remote from the site of osteotomy has occurred.[1] The danger of fracture in ankylosed cervical spine is particularly high when a lumbar osteotomy is performed in the prone position. This danger is alleviated to a great extent by using the lateral position.

Catastrophic aortic rupture has been reported in association with aortic calcification and a single level osteotomy.[104]

Postoperative Complications

Acute gastric dilatation is probably the most common and most dangerous of the early postoperative complications in lumbar osteotomies.[33] It is generally thought to result from stretching of the superior mesenteric artery across the third part of the duodenum when the spine is extended and the deformity is corrected.[1] A nasogastric tube is inserted intraoperatively and kept in place until bowel sounds have returned in order to try to avoid significant problems resulting from this condition. The dilatation and its associated paralytic ileus usually clear within a few days.

Early postoperative displacement of the osteotomy resulting in neurologic compromise has occurred,[65] and it has occasionally been fatal.[42]

Skin lesions may occur when contracted skin in the concavity of flexion deformity is stretched during the hyperextension maneuver. Skin can actually split with the degree of stretch applied. Lower abdominal and thigh pain can occur owing to stretching of the lateral femoral cutaneous nerve.[41] Pressure ulcers are also a significant problem in these patients, as the patients have often been on steroids and are immobilized in bed, a halo vest, or TLSO.[25]

Nonunion has rarely occurred in the cervical spine. Simmons has treated two nonunions by anterior fusion with good results.[93]

The last major long-term difficulty is a recurrence of the deformity.[16,54] Simmons believes that it occurs more often when an inadequate correction has been performed (E. Simmons, personal communication, 1985). His aim is to correct the deformity to the point where the weight-bearing line from C7 to T1 is redirected posteriorly and falls directly above the pelvis. The weight-bearing line is behind the apex of the osteotomy.

Summary

Extension osteotomy for correction of fixed flexion deformity of the spine has a definite place in the treatment of ankylosing spondylitis. Candidates for surgery must be carefully chosen. The surgical technique is precise and demanding. Significant risks are associated with the procedure. Nevertheless, gratifying results to both the patient and the surgeon are obtainable.

REFERENCES

1. Adams J: Technique, dangers and safeguards in osteotomy of the spine. J Bone Joint Surg [Br] 34:226, 1952
2. Aisen AM, Martel W, Ellis JH, McCune WJ: Cervical spine involvement in rheumatoid arthritis: MR imaging. Radiology 165:159, 1987
3. Althoff B, Goldie IF: Cervical collars in rheumatoid atlanto-axial subluxation: a radiographic comparison. Ann Rheum Dis 39:485, 1980
4. Anda S, Nilsen G, Roysland P: Periodontoid changes in rheumatoid arthritis. MRI observa-

tions: report of two cases. Scand J Rheumatol 17:59, 1988

5. Awerbach MS, Henderson DRF, Milazzo SC et al: Long term follow-up of posterior cervical fusion for atlanto-axial subluxation in rheumatoid arthritis. J Rheumatol 8:423, 1981

6. Baggenstoss A, Bickel W, Ward L: Rheumatoid granulomatous nodules as destructive lesions of vertebrae. J Bone Joint Surg [Am] 34:601, 1952

7. Ball J: Enthesopathy of rheumatoid and ankylosing spondylitis. Ann Rheum Dis 30:213, 1971

8. Benhamou CL, Roux C, Viala JF, Gervais T: Thoracic and lower cervical spine involvement in a case of rheumatoid arthritis. Rheumatol Int 9:39, 1989

9. Bennett GJ: Ankylosing spondylitis. Clin Neurosurg 37:622, 1991

10. Bland JH: Rheumatoid subluxation of the cervical spine. J Rheumatol 17:134, 1990

11. Bogduk N, Major GAC, Carger J: Lateral subluxation of the atlas in rheumatoid arthritis: a case report and post-mortem study. Ann Rheum Dis 43:341, 1984

12. Braunstein EM, Weissman BN, Seltzer SE et al: Computed tomography and conventional radiographs of the craniocervical region in rheumatoid arthritis: a comparison. Arthritis Rheum 27:26, 1984

13. Breedveld FC, Algra PR, Vielvoye CJ, Cats A: Magnetic resonance imaging in the evaluation of patients with rheumatoid arthritis and subluxations of the cervical spine. Arthritis Rheum 30:624, 1987

14. Bundschuh C, Modic MT, Kearney F et al: Rheumatoid arthritis of the cervical spine: surface-coil MR imaging. AJR 151:181, 1988

15. Bywaters EGL: Rheumatoid and other diseases of the cervical interspinous bursae, and changes in the spinous process. Ann Rheum Dis 41:360, 1982

16. Calabro JJ: An appraisal of the medical and surgical management of ankylosing spondylitis. Clin Orthop 60:125, 1958

17. Calin A, Robertson D: Spodylodiscitis and pseudarthrosis in a patient with enteropathic spondyloarthropathy. Ann Rheum Dis 50:117, 1991

18. Cawley MI, Chalmers TM, Ball J: Destructive lesions of vertebral bodies in ankylosing spondylitis. Ann Rheum Dis 30:539, 1971

19. Clark CR, Goetz DD, Menezes AH: Arthrodesis of the cervical spine in rheumatoid arthritis. J Bone Joint Surg [Am] 71:381, 1989

20. Conaty JP, Mongan ES: Cervical fusion in rheumatoid arthritis. J Bone Joint Surg [Am] 63:1218, 1981

21. Crockard HA: Anterior approaches to lesions of the upper cervical spine. Clin Neurosurg 34:389, 1988

22. De los Reyes RA, Malik GM, Wu KK, and Ausman JI: A new surgical approach to stabilizing C1–2 subluxation in rheumatoid arthritis. Henry Ford Hosp Med J 29:127, 1981

23. Einig M, Higer HP, Meairs S et al: Magnetic resonance imaging of the craniocervical junction in rheumatoid arthritis: value, limitations, indications. Skeletal Radiol 19:341, 1990

24. El-Khoury GY, Wener MH, Menezes AH et al: Cranial settling in rheumatoid arthritis. Radiology 137:637, 1980

25. Emneus H: Wedge osteotomy of spine in ankylosing spondylitis. Acta Orthop Scand 39:321, 1968

26. Fehring TK, Brooks AL: Upper cervical instability in rheumatoid arthritis. Clin Orthop 221:137, 1987

27. Ferlic DC, Clayton ML, Leidholt JD, Gamble WE: Surgical treatment of the symptomatic unstable cervical spine in rheumatoid arthritis. J Bone Joint Surg [Am] 57:349, 1975

28. Fezoulidis I, Neuhold A, Wicke L et al: Diagnostic imaging of the occipito-cervical junction in patients with rheumatoid arthritis: plain films, computed tomography, magnetic resonance imaging. Eur J Radiol 9:5, 1989

29. Floyd AS, Learmonth ID, Mody G, Meyers OL: Atlantoaxial instability and neurologic indicators in rheumatoid arthritis. Clin Orthop 241:177, 1989

30. Forestier J, Jacqueline F, Rotes-Querol J: Ankylosing spondylitis: Clinical Observations, Roentgenology, Pathological Anatomy and Treatment. p. 249. Charles C Thomas, Springfield, IL, 1956

31. Frank P, Gleeson J: Destructive vertebral lesions in ankylosing spondylitis. Br J Radiol 48:755, 1975

32. Glynn MK, Sheehan JM: Fusion of the cervical spine for instability. Clin Orthop 179:97, 1983

33. Goel M: Vertebral osteotomy for correction of fixed flexion deformity of the spine. J Bone Joint Surg [Am] 50:287, 1968

34. Goldie IF, Althoff B: A simplified method for fixation in rheumatoid atlanto-axial dislocation. Reconstr Surg Traumatol 18:30, 1981

35. Guest M, Jacobson HG: Pelvic and extrapelvic

osteopathy in rheumatoid spondylitis. AJR 65:760, 1951

36. Hague T: Chronic rheumatoid polyarthritis and spondyloarthritis associated with neurological symptoms and signs occasionally simulating an intraspinal expansive process. Acta Chir Scand 120:395, 1961

37. Halla JT, Fallahi S: Cervical discovertebral destruction, subaxial subluxation and myelopathy in a patient with rheumatoid arthritis. Arthritis Rheum 24:944, 1981

38. Halla JT, Fallahi S, Hardin JG: Nonreducible rotational head tilt and lateral mass collapse: a prospective study of frequency, radiographic findings and clinical features in patients with rheumatoid arthritis. Arthritis Rheum 25:1316, 1982

39. Hehne H, Zielke K, Bohm H: Polysegmental lumbar osteotomies and transpedicled fixation for correction of long curved kyphotic deformities in ankylosing spondylitis. Clin Orthop 258:49, 1990

40. Heilman AE, Crockard HA, Stevens J: Progressive myelopathy secondary to dens fracture: radiological features and surgical treatment. Presented at the Cervical Spine Research Society, San Antonio, TX, 1990

41. Herbert J: Vertebral osteotomy. J Bone Joint Surg [Am] 30:680, 1948

42. Herbert J: Vertebral osteotomy for kyphosis, especially in Marie-Strumpell arthritis. J Bone Joint Surg [Am] 41:291, 1959

43. Hollinshead WH: Anatomy for Surgeons: The Head and Neck. 2nd Ed. Harper & Row, Hagerstown, MD, 1968

44. Itoh T, Tsuji H, Katoh Y et al: Occipito-cervical fusion reinforced by Luque's segmental spinal instrumentation for rheumatoid disease. Spine 13:1234, 1988

45. Kanefield DG, Mullins BP, Freehafer AA et al: Destructive lesions of the spine in rheumatoid ankylosing spondylitis. J Bone Joint Surg [Am] 51:1369, 1969

46. Kaufman RL, Glenn WV Jr: Rheumatoid cervical myelopathy: evaluation by computerized tomography with multiplanar reconstruction. J Rheumatol 10:42, 1983

47. Kauppi M, Sakaguchi M, Konttinen YT, Hamalainen M: A new method of screening for vertical atlanto-axial dislocation. J Rheumatol 17:167, 1990

48. Kawaida H, Sakou T, Morizino Y: Vertical settling in rheumatoid arthritis: diagnostic value of the Ranawat and Redlund-Johnell methods. Clin Orthop 239:128, 1989

49. King TT: Rheumatoid subluxations of the cervical spine. Ann Rheum Dis 44:807, 1985 (*editorial*)

50. Kornblum D, Clayton ML, Nash NH: Nontraumatic cervical dislocations in rheumatoid spondylitis. JAMA 149:431, 1952

51. Krodel A, Refior HJ, Westerman S: The importance of functional magnetic resonance imaging (MRI) in the planning of stabilizing operations on the cervical spine in rheumatoid patients. Arch Orthop Trauma Surg 109:30, 1989

52. LaChapelle E: Osteotomy of the lumbar spine for correction of kyphosis in a case of ankylosing spondyloarthritis. J Bone Joint Surg 28:851, 1946

53. Lachiewicz PF, Schoenfeldt R, Inglis A: Somatosensory-evoked potentials in the evaluation of the unstable rheumatoid cervical spine: a preliminary report. Spine 8:813, 1986

54. Law W: Lumbar spinal osteotomy. J Bone Joint Surg [Br] 41:270, 1959

55. Lesoin F, Duquesnoy A, Destee A et al: Cervical neurological complications of rheumatoid arthritis: surgical treatment techniques and indications. Acta Neurochir (Wien) 78:91, 1985

56. Lightfoot RW Jr: Clinical reasoning in the management of rheumatoid arthritis. J Musculoskel Med 7:19, 1990

57. Ligniere GC, Montagnani G, Panarace G, Gualdi I: Magnetic resonance imaging for the study of cervical myelopathy in rheumatoid arthritis. Clin Exp Rheumatol 6:343, 1988

58. Lipson SJ: Rheumatoid arthritis of the cervical spine. Clin Orthop 182:143, 1984

59. Lipson SJ: Rheumatoid arthritis in the cervical spine. Clin Orthop 239:121, 1989

60. Little H, Urowitz MB, Smythe HA: Asymptomatic spondylodiscitis: an unusual feature of ankylosing spondylitis. Arthritis Rheum 17:487, 1974

61. Lorber A, Pearson C, Rene R: Osteolytic vertebral lesions as a manifestation of rheumatoid arthritis and related disorders. Arthritis Rheum 4:514, 1961

62. Mate C, Taylor M: Cervical myelopathy in rheumatoid arthritis. Nurs Times 83:71, 1987

63. McAfee PC, Bohlman HH, Riley LH Jr et al: The anterior retropharyngeal approach to the upper part of the cervical spine. J Bone Joint Surg [Am] 69:1371, 1987

64. McGrath H Jr, McCormick C, Carey ME: Pyogenic cervical osteomyelitis presenting as a

massive prevertebral abscess in a patient with rheumatoid arthritis. Am J Med 84:363, 1988

65. McMaster P: Osteotomy of the spine for fixed flexion deformity. J Bone Joint Surg [Am] 44:1207, 1962

66. Meijers KAE, Cats A, Kremer HPH et al: Cervical myelopathy in rheumatoid arthritis. Clin Exp Rheumatol 2:239, 1984

67. Moncur C, Williams HJ: Cervical spine management in patients with rheumatoid arthritis: review of the literature. Phys Ther 68:509, 1988

68. Morris J, Lucas D, Bresler B: Role of the trunk in stability of the spine. J Bone Joint Surg [Am] 43:327, 1961

69. Ono K, Ebara S, Fuji T et al: Myelopathy hand: new clinical signs of cervical cord damage. J Bone Joint Surg [Br] 69:215, 1987

70. Ovassapian A, Land P, Schafer MF et al: Anesthetic management for surgical corrections of severe flexion deformity of the cervical spine. Anesthesiology 58:37, 1983

71. Parish DC, Clark JA, Liebowitz SM, Hicks WC: Sudden death in rheumatoid arthritis from vertical subluxation of the odontoid process. J Natl Med Assoc 82:297, 1990

72. Pellicci PM, Ranawat CS, Tsairis P, Bryan WJ: A prospective study of the progression of rheumatoid arthritis of the cervical spine. J Bone Joint Surg [Am] 63:342, 1981

73. Pettersson H, Larsson EM, Holtas S et al: MR imaging of the cervical spine in rheumatoid arthritis. AJNR 9:573, 1988

74. Pocock DG, Agnew JE, Wood EJ et al: Radionuclide imaging of the neck in rheumatoid arthritis. Rheumatol Rehabil 21:131, 1982

75. Ranawat CS, O'Leary P, Pallicci P et al: Cervical spine fusion in rheumatoid arthritis. J Bone Joint Surg [Am] 61:1003, 1979

76. Rathburn J, MacNab I: The microvascular pattern of the rotator cuff. J Bone Joint Surg [Br] 52:540, 1970

77. Redlund-Johnell I: Subaxial caudal dislocation of the cervical spine in rheumatoid arthritis. Neuroradiology 26:407, 1984

78. Rivelis M, Freiberger R: Vertebral destruction in unfused segments in late ankylosing spondylitis. Radiology 93:251, 1969

79. Rivelis M, Freiberger R: Vertebral destruction at unfused segments in late ankylosing spondylitis. Radiology 93:251, 1969

80. Rockswold GL, Bergman TA, Ford SE: Halo immobilization and surgical fusion: relative indications and effectiveness in the treatment of

140 cervical spine injuries. J Trauma 30:893, 1990

81. Romanus R, Yden S: Destructive and ossifying spondylitic changes in rheumatoid ankylosing spondylitis. Acta Orthop Scand 22:88, 1952

82. Santavirta S, Kankaanpaa U, Sandelin J et al: Evaluation of patients with rheumatoid cervical spine. Scand J Rheumatol 16:9, 1987

83. Santavirta S, Konttinen YT, Lindqvist C, Sandelin J: Occipital headache in rheumatoid cervical facet joint arthritis. Lancet 2:695, 1986 (*letter*)

84. Santavirta S, Konttinen YT, Sandelin J, Slatis P: Operations for the unstable cervical spine in rheumatoid arthritis. Acta Orthop Scand 61:106, 1990

85. Santavirta S, Slatis P, Kankaanpaa U et al: Treatment of the cervical spine in rheumatoid arthritis. J Bone Joint Surg [Am] 70:658, 1988

86. Schils JP, Resnick D, Haghighi PN et al: Pathogenesis of discovertebral and manubriosternal joint abnormalities in rheumatoid arthritis: a cadaveric study. J Rheumatol 16:291, 1989

87. Seaman W, Wells J: Destructive lesions of the vertebral bodies in rheumatoid disease. AJR 86:241, 1961

88. Semble EL, Elster AD, Loeser RF et al: Magnetic resonance imaging of the craniovertebral junction in rheumatoid arthritis. J Rheumatol 15:1367, 1988

89. Sigler JW, Bluhm GB, Duncan H, Ensign DC: Clinical features of ankylosing spondylitis. Clin Orthop 74:14, 1971

90. Sim FH, Svien HJ, Bickel WH, Janes JM: Swanneck deformity following extensive cervical laminectomy. J Bone Joint Surg [Am] 56:564, 1974

91. Sllatis P, Santavirta S, Sandelin J Konttinen YT: Cranial subluxation of the odontoid process in rheumatoid arthritis. J Bone Joint Surg [Am] 71:189, 1989

92. Simmons E: Kyphotic deformity of the spine in ankylosing spondylitis. Clin Orthop 128:65, 1977

93. Simmons E: Osteotomy of the cervical spine in ankylosing spondy-litis: a 15-year experience. J Bone Joint Surg [Br] 64:635, 1982

94. Simmons EH: Surgery of the spine in rheumatoid arthritis and ankylosing spondylitis. p. 93. In Cruess RL, Mitchell NS (eds): Surgery of Rheumatoid Arthritis. JB Lippincott, Philadelphia, 1971

95. Smith AS, Blaser SI: Infectious and inflammatory processes of the spine. Radiol Clin North Am 29:809, 1991

96. Smith HP, Challa VR, Alexander E Jr: Odontoid compression of the brain stem in a patient with rheumatoid arthritis: case report. J Neurosurg 53:841, 1980

97. Smith PH, Benn RI, Sharp J: Natural history of rheumatoid cervical subluxation. Ann Rheum Dis 31:431, 1972

98. Smith-Petersen M, Larson C, Aufranc O: Osteotomy of the spine for correction of flexion deformity in rheumatoid arthritis. J Bone Joint Surg 27:1, 1945

99. Steinbrocker O, Traeger CH, Batterman RC: Therapeutic criteria in rheumatoid arthritis. JAMA 140:659, 1949

100. Teigland J, Magnaes B: Rheumatoid backward dislocation of the atlas with compression of the spinal cord. Scand J Rheumatol 9:253, 1980

101. Toolanen G, Knibestol M, Larsson SE, Landman K: Somatosensory evoked potentials (SSEPs) in rheumatoid cervical subluxations. Scand J Rheumatol 16:17, 1987

102. Urist M: Osteotomy of the cervical spine. J Bone Joint Surg [Am] 40:833, 1958

103. Verhagen WIM, v. Rens TJG, Merx J, Slooff JL: Myelopathy due to cervical spine rheumatoid arthritis: a case report. J Neurosurg Sci 31:195, 1987

104. Weatherly D, Jaffray D, Terry A: Vascular complications associated with osteotomy in ankylosing spondylitis: a report of two cases. Spine 13:43, 1988

105. Weiner S, Bassett L, Spiegel T: Superior, posterior and lateral displacement of C1 in rheumatoid arthritis. Arthritis Rheum 25:1378, 1982

106. Weissman BNW, Aliabadi P, Weinfeld MS et al: Prognostic features of atlantoaxial subluxation in rheumatoid arthritis patients. Radiology 144:745, 1982

107. White AA, Panjabi MM, Posner I et al: Spinal stability: evaluation and treatment. AAOS Instruct Course Lect 30:457, 1981

108. Whitehill R, Richman JA, Glaser JA: Failure of immobilization of the cervical spine by the halo vest: a report of five cases. J Bone Joint Surg [Am] 68:326, 1986

109. Wholey M, Pugh D, Bicker W: Localized destructive lesions in rheumatoid spondylitis. Radiology 74:54, 1960

110. Wiesel SW, Rothman RH: Occipital atlantal hypermobility. Spine 4:187, 1979

111. Wilkinson M, Bywaters E: Clinical features of ankylosing spondylitis. Ann Rheum Dis 17:209, 1958

112. Wills DG: Anaesthetic management of posterior lumbar osteotomy. Can Anaesth Soc J 32:248, 1985

113. Winfield J, Cooke D, Brook AS, Corbett M: A prospective study of the radiological changes in the cervical spine in early rheumatoid disease. Ann Rheum Dis 40:109, 1981

114. Winfield J, Young A, Williams P, Corbett M: Prospective study of the radiological changes in hands, feet and cervical spine in adult rheumatoid disease. Ann Rheum Dis 42:613, 1983

115. Wolfe BK, O'Keefe DO, Mitchell DM, Tchang SPK: Rheumatoid arthritis of the cervical spine: early and progressive radiographic features. Radiology 165:145, 1987

116. Zygmunt S, Saveland H, Brattstrom H et al: Reduction of rheumatoid periodontoid pannus following posterior occipito-cervical fusion visualized by magnet resonance imaging. Br J Neurosurg 2:315, 1988

19

Management of Juvenile Rheumatoid Arthritis

Douglas A. Dennis
Mack L. Clayton

Juvenile rheumatoid arthritis (JRA) is usually defined as a persistent arthritis involving one or more joints in children less than 16 years of age. Numerous other titles have been used to describe this condition, including juvenile chronic arthritis, chronic arthritis of childhood, Still's disease, and others.

Since Still's[74] classic description in 1897, our understanding of the disease has grown continually, although the etiology remains obscure. Infection, trauma, heredity, autoimmunity, and psychological stress have been implicated.[20] Formulation of diagnostic criteria and a classification system of JRA have been difficult owing to the multitude of clinical presentations. The American Rheumatism Association formulated a set of diagnostic criteria in 1977.[11] Their general criteria include a persistent arthritis that lasts 6 weeks or longer for which multiple other conditions have been excluded. Some of the latter include other rheumatic diseases such as systemic lupus erythematosus, ankylosing spondylitis, infectious arthritis, inflammatory bowel disease, neoplastic conditions, and hematologic diseases.

Juvenile rheumatoid arthritis is further classified based on its mode of onset into pauciarticular, polyarticular, and systemic subtypes. The relative frequency of each subtype varies depending on the study. The polyarticular subgroup usually predominates, comprising 50 percent of the cases, followed by the pauciarticular (30 percent) and systemic (20 percent) varieties.

The pauciarticular subtype is defined as JRA occurring in four or fewer joints. Those patients with systemic symptoms are excluded from this category. In half of these cases, only a single joint may be involved.[21] The knee is the most commonly affected joint.

With the polyarticular type of juvenile arthritis, five or more joints are involved. As with the pauciarticular subtype, the knee is the most commonly affected joint. The ankles, wrists, and elbows are also commonly involved.[12] Essentially any synovial joint may be affected, however, including the spine and temporomandibular joints. Extra-articular manifestations (e.g., low grade fever, lymphadenopathy, and hepatosplenomegaly) may occur, although they are usually of lesser severity than with the systemic-onset subgroup.

Systemic-onset JRA, as classically described by Still,[74] is characterized by a spiking, intermittent fever[17] accompanied by a rheumatoid rash[12,16,18,38,66] and joint inflammation. Temperature elevations typically occur once or twice daily, reaching levels of 104° to 105°F. The fever usually falls rapidly with return of normal body temperature in between temperature elevations. The child often appears ill when fever is present, only to feel well when body temperature returns to a normal level. The rheumatoid rash that usually accompanies the fever is transient in nature and therefore is occasionally missed by the treating physician. The rash is erythematous and macular in nature and usually not pruritic. Lesions vary in size although usually are less than 5 to 6 mm in diameter. The trunk and proximal extremities are the most commonly involved locations. Joint involvement may be diffuse or limited to a few joints. It may occur concomitantly with the onset of the fever and rash or appear weeks to months later. The characteristic rash and fever should alert the physician to the high likelihood of JRA, even in the absence of joint involvement. Arthritis is required for final diagnosis, however.

A multitude of additional extra-articular manifestations may be present with systemic-onset JRA,[13,15,20,76] including lymphadenopathy, hepatosplenomegaly, renal glomerulitis,[3] myocarditis,[10,54] cardiac valvulitis,[76] pericarditis,[6,8,10,48] and serositis of other organs. Central nervous system involvement[41,47] and vasculitis[33,34] may be encountered, including pneumonitis, interstitial fibrosis, idiopathic hemosiderosis, arteritis, and pleuritis, with or without effusion.[14,43] Pulmonary rheumatoid nodules occur rarely.

Subcutaneous nodules occur in JRA, although less commonly than with the adult type. The incidence varies from 2 to 12 percent.[13]

A most serious extra-articular manifestation of JRA is an anterior nongranulomatous iridocyclitis that may result in blindness.[19,22,23,44,46,60,64,65,71,72] Multiple sequelae may result, including band keratopathy, posterior synechiae, cataracts, secondary glaucoma, and phthisis bulbi.[11] Bilateral involvement is not uncommon. Eye involvement occurs most commonly in the pauciarticular subtype of JRA with more than 20 percent affected.[22] Also, females afflicted with JRA early in life[72] and those with antinuclear antibody positivity[60,64] are at greater risk to develop ocular complications. Eye involvement is often insidious in onset and frequently asymptomatic. Frequent eye examinations are therefore imperative.

Growth disturbances are not unusual, especially with JRA of increased severity and chronicity.[2,7,9,51,62,75] Overgrowth predominates in unilateral pauciarticular disease owing to the enhanced vascularity and subsequent epiphyseal stimulation. Growth retardation may result from epiphyseal depression or premature physeal closure. In addition to extremity abnormalities, growth retardation may also occur in the jaw, resulting in micrognathia.[62]

Amyloidosis is an uncommon, yet potentially fatal complication of JRA, with an incidence of 4 to 6 percent reported in European patient populations.[5] It has been found much less commonly in patients living on the North American continent. Fatality most often results from renal failure and less often from infection. Improved survival rates have been reported with cytotoxic therapy utilizing chlorambucil.[67]

ORTHOPAEDIC MANAGEMENT

Management of the child with JRA is best administered by a team, consisting of a pediatrician, rheumatologist, orthopaedic surgeon, physical and occupational therapists, and social workers. The primary objective of the orthopaedic surgeon is to provide early management of mechanical problems, e.g., deformity or contracture. Physical therapy is used to maintain, as well as improve, range of motion and strength. Orthotics that maintain alignment and prevent contracture are also helpful.

Operative intervention is uncommon during the period of growth, with most operative treatment performed during adulthood to treat residual destruction of long-standing inflammatory disease. Operative intervention is often delayed longer in the juvenile with uncontrolled rheumatoid arthritis (12 to 18 months), in contrast to the adult with rheumatoid arthritis (6 months), owing to the increased chance of spontaneous remission with the juvenile type. Each child must be carefully evaluated preoperatively to assess his or her ability to perform and cooperate with the required postoperative rehabilitative regimen, which is so important to the success of the proposed operative procedure.

Surgical procedures commonly employed include soft tissue contracture release, synovectomy, osteotomy, arthrodesis, limb length equalization procedures, and total joint replacement.

The typical patterns of the disease of the commonly affected joints and their management are discussed next. The reader is encouraged to refer to other chapters in this text or operative texts for a more detailed description of the various surgical procedures.

HIP

The earliest manifestations of hip disease in the patient with JRA typically involve soft tissue contracture. Flexion contracture is most commonly seen, although adduction or abduction contracture as well as contracture of the iliotibial band may be noted. Early diagnosis of soft tissue contracture is the key to treatment, as most contractures can be relieved with appropriate stretching and splinting under the guidance of the physical therapist. Occasionally, traction followed by a short period of crutch ambulation is used in cases of severe, persistent spasm. We have infrequently used corticosteroid injections in recalcitrant cases.

Early flexion contracture of the hip may not be readily apparent owing to compensation by an increased lumbar lordosis. More severe cases are not uncommon in patients who are limited ambulators, particularly in wheelchair-bound patients. In cases of flexion contracture unrelieved by appropriate physiotherapy and splinting, operative tendon release is indicated, so long as adequate joint space of the contracted joint is present. It usually involves release of the sartorius, rectus femoris, and iliopsoas tendons. Anterior capsulotomy of the hip joint and anterior synovectomy are indicated in certain cases. Aggressive physiotherapy postoperatively is required to maintain operative correction. In patients with severe, fixed contractures and a destroyed joint space, extension osteotomy may be considered. One must be aware that this procedure may complicate conversion to total hip replacement if it is required at a later date.

Adduction contracture of the hip is seen less frequently but requires aggressive treatment. Early stretching and abduction splinting constitute the initial phase of treatment. If associated lateral subluxation of the hip is noted, adductor tenotomy should be considered to prevent accelerated joint destruction due to the subluxed posture of the hip. Again, aggressive postoperative physiotherapy is mandatory.

Contracture of the iliotibial band has been observed in severe cases. It may be associated with genu valgum and external tibial rotational deformities as well as abduction contracture of the hip. Initial treatment, as with other soft tissue contractures, involves appropriate stretching exercises. Rarely, iliotibial band release is required. We recommend the method described by Yount-Ober.[13,40]

The role of hip synovectomy in JRA patients is indefinite, and we have minimal experience with it. Jacobsen et al.[39] reported that there may be gradual loss of motion postoperatively with continued roentgenographic deterioration despite synovectomy. Mogenson et al.[55] reported relief of pain in 13 of 18 patients following hip synovectomy but continued progression of roentgenographic deterioration. A limited Smith-Petersen anterior approach is recommended without dislocation of the femoral head to lessen the risk of avascular necrosis as reported by Brewer et al.[13] Traction is used postoperatively until spasm is relieved. Continuous passive motion (CPM) may assist in regaining range of motion.

Total hip replacement has been reserved for patients with marked functional disability as well as severe roentgenographic destruction of the hip joint; ideally, the epiphyses should be closed or as near to full growth as possible. The indication for this procedure is significant stiffness (more often than disabling pain). The typical pattern of progressive hip deterioration in these patients involves acetabular protrusion, with eventual ankylosis in some cases. Flexion and adduction contractures are commonly encountered.

As these patients are often candidates for total hip replacement at a young age, one must attempt to optimize all conditions, such as obtaining ideal body weight and encouraging more sedentary occupations after operation to enhance the longevity of this procedure. These patients must be informed of the likelihood of subsequent revision of their total hip replacement during their lifetime in light of their young age.

The orthopaedist planning total hip replacement in a patient with JRA must be alert to certain anatomic variations characteristic of these patients. Because of more frequent contractures, more aggressive soft tissue release is usually needed, including release of the iliopsoas and rectus femoris muscles as well as a complete capsulectomy. Excessive coxa valga and increased femoral anteversion may be encountered. The femoral medullary canal is often small and narrow, such that custom-made prosthetic components may be required. Bone grafting of the medial acetabular wall in cases of protrusion is frequently needed.

Good results can be expected after total hip replacement in these patients, with excellent relief of pain and improvement in function (Fig. 19-1). Postoperative range of motion, although increased over preoperative values, is usually less than that in the adult with rheumatoid arthritis.

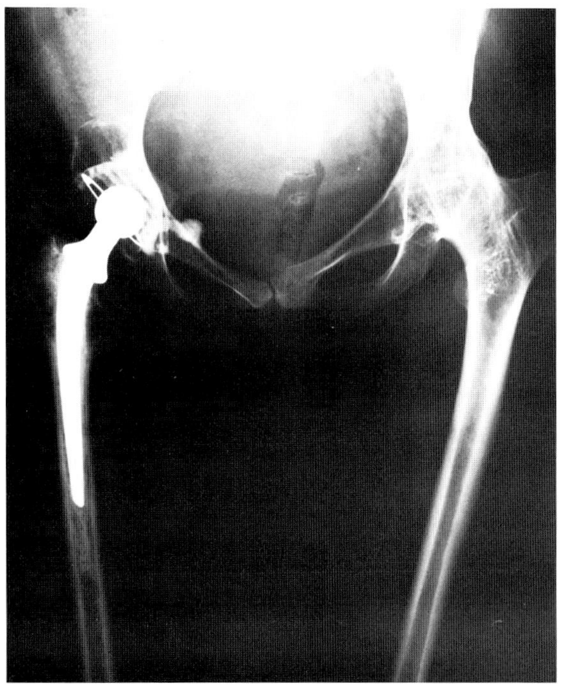

Fig. 19-1. Left hip shows autofusion in good position. Right total hip arthroplasty is a good example of the need for small or custom-made components. If patient develops later problems from her fused left hip, a total hip arthroplasty can be performed.

This difference can be attributed to the more severe soft tissue contractures found preoperatively in the juvenile group. The less substantial motion gains in the JRA patient undergoing total hip replacement have also been noted by Scott et al.[68]

We have found satisfactory results with the use of cementless biologic ingrowth prostheses over the short term. We presently recommend this mode of fixation in young patients if adequate bone stock is available. Longer follow-up is obviously needed to further address the appropriate mode of fixation in these patients.

In cases of severe bilateral hip disease in the young patient with no other major medical problems, we consider bilateral simultaneous total hip replacement. Generally, these patients can tolerate this procedure well, and it accelerates their rehabilitative process. In those with severe lower extremity involvement requiring multiple joint replacements of the hips and knees, we recommend ipsilateral total hip and total knee replacement at the same surgical setting, with the remaining total joint replacements performed after the patient is fully rehabilitated from the initial procedures. Again, these patients must be carefully selected for any bilateral procedures.

Hip arthrodesis is not recommended in the patient with JRA. These patients frequently have multiple joint involvement such that compensation by adjacent joints for the loss of hip motion is not adequate.

Accentuation of the physiologic valgus alignment of the knee is also often encountered. It may be aggravated by contracture of the iliotibial band. Initial management for mild deformity is close observation with appropriate medical management of the synovitis. Arthroscopic synovectomy is considered if synovitis persists with increasing deformity. McMaster[52] has shown resolution of knee angular deformity following this procedure. With progressive deformity in the earlier stages, we consider use of a long-leg three-point orthosis. In cases of more significant deformity, physeal stapling of the medial distal femoral or proximal tibial epiphyses or both is performed. Good correction of the valgus deformity has been obtained with this procedure. One must closely observe for overcorrection in these patients due to fluctuations in growth rates that may be related to corticosteroid use. As has been reported by Ansell et al.,[1] growth may rapidly increase after cessation of corticosteroids, leading to overcorrection and the need for staple removal. In the older child with limited or no growth remaining, the valgus deformity is corrected with osteotomy in the region of the deformity, usually the distal femur.[24] Jakobowski and Ruszcynska[40] reported correction of genu valgum after release of the iliotibial band just above the knee.

KNEE

One of the most frequent complaints presented to the orthopaedic surgeon is that of flexion contracture. It often occurs early in the disease process associated with chronic uncontrolled synovitis. It may also be caused or aggravated by ankle involvement with subsequent tightening of the heel cord and a crouch gait. Early cases are usually successfully managed with appropriate extension stretching exercises under the guidance of the physical therapist. For more severe cases, use of an extension orthosis may be of benefit. One must be aware of the potential of posterior tibial subluxation as well as cartilage pressure necrosis and resultant joint space narrowing with the use of this device. We rarely use serial extension casting, as we believe it can cause further joint stiffness secondary to immobilization of an already diseased joint.

In cases resistant to nonoperative measures but with adequate joint space, we recommend posterior soft tissue lengthening.[13,24] Extension distal femoral osteotomy can be considered in cases with severe joint space narrowing. Synovectomy of the knee has been helpful in selected patients, including those with a painful, persistent synovitis that has been resistant to appropriate medical management. As previously discussed, in contrast to the treatment of adults, synovectomy is frequently delayed for 12 to 18 months owing to the increased chance of remission in the juvenile patient, as recommended by Eyring et al.[32] During this time aggressive medical manage-

ment must be continued as well as continual evaluation of the knee joint to detect rapid deterioration of the joint space. In cases with progressive synovitis and significant flexion contracture, it is recommended to intercede with synovectomy earlier owing to the potential for pressure cartilage necrosis due to the flexion contracture.

Although many studies have reported favorable results of knee synovectomy in the short term,[4,32] as with synovectomy of other joints continued deterioration of the joint roentgenographically tends to occur.[39] This procedure provides good long-term pain relief and little change in range of motion postoperatively if an adequate rehabilitation program has been followed. It may be difficult in the young child, and we therefore prefer to perform synovectomy in children 6 to 7 years of age or older. Jani and Waigand[42] have reported their poorest results following synovectomy of the knee in children less than 5 years of age.

We have looked more favorably on knee synovectomy since beginning to perform the procedure arthroscopically, followed by postoperative CPM. Using this protocol, the morbidity is reduced and rehabilitation facilitated, with improved range of motion in most cases.

Total knee replacement has been reserved for the knee with severe destruction, and it has produced good results. It is often possible to delay this procedure many years after the onset of severe roentgenographic changes are noted, as pain in the juvenile-onset group is often less pronounced than in their adult counterparts. It is mandatory to delay total knee replacement until after physical closure, which is rarely a problem, as cases of severe and early involvement not infrequently have premature physeal closure.

In light of the marked valgus deformity and flexion contractures that may be encountered in these patients, aggressive soft tissue releases from the distal femur laterally and posteriorly, as described by Clayton et al.,[26] (See Chapter 14.) are often required. Occasionally, in cases of severe flexion contracture it is necessary to increase the amount of distal femoral resection to obtain adequate extension. Aggressive physiotherapy and occasionally extension casting are required postoperatively in these cases to pre-

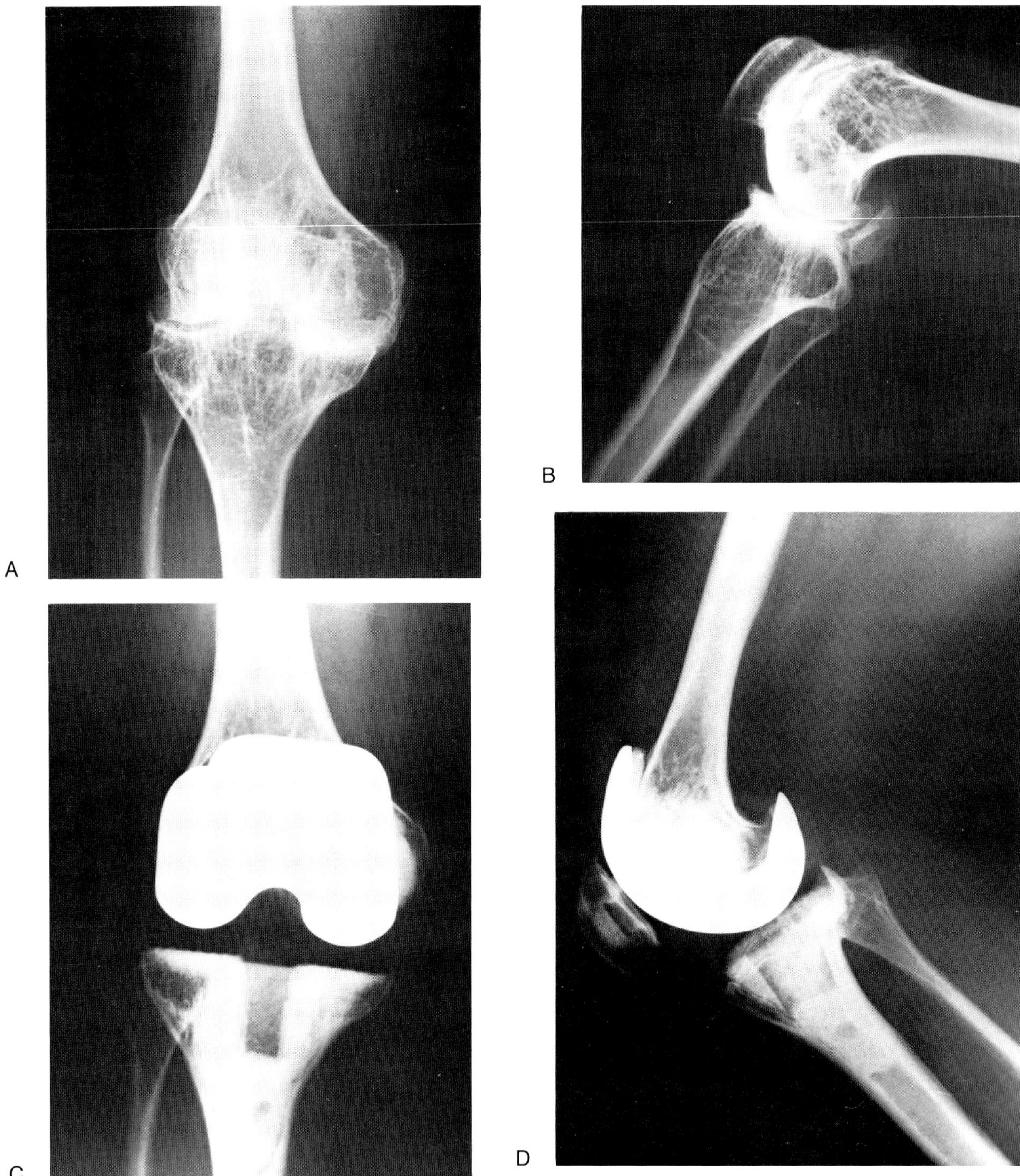

Fig. 19-2. (**A & B**) Preoperative anteroposterior and lateral roentgenograms of the involved knee before total knee arthroplasty. (**C**) Early total knee arthroplasty before extra small components were available. This knee is still functioning 12 years later. (**D**) Components are relatively oversized and thus lead to limited flexion (0 to 70 degrees).

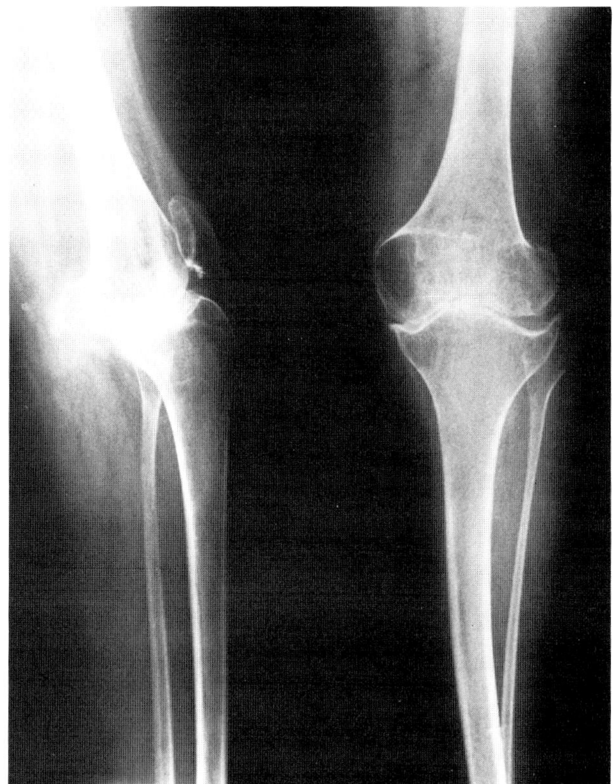

A

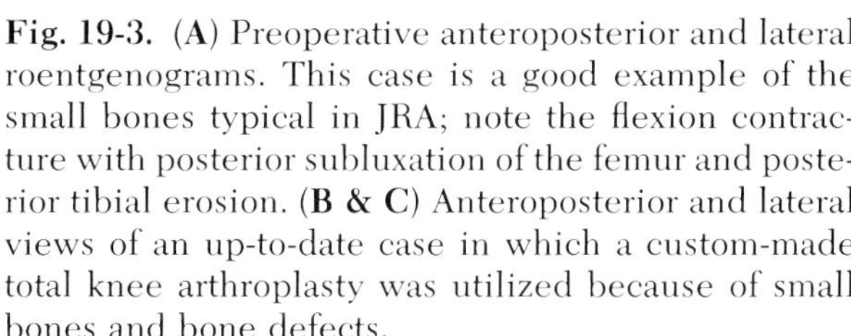

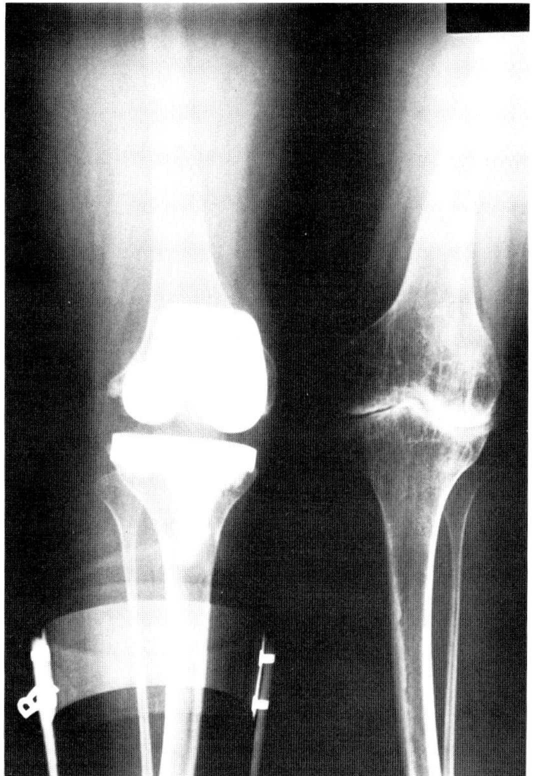

B

Fig. 19-3. (**A**) Preoperative anteroposterior and lateral roentgenograms. This case is a good example of the small bones typical in JRA; note the flexion contracture with posterior subluxation of the femur and posterior tibial erosion. (**B & C**) Anteroposterior and lateral views of an up-to-date case in which a custom-made total knee arthroplasty was utilized because of small bones and bone defects.

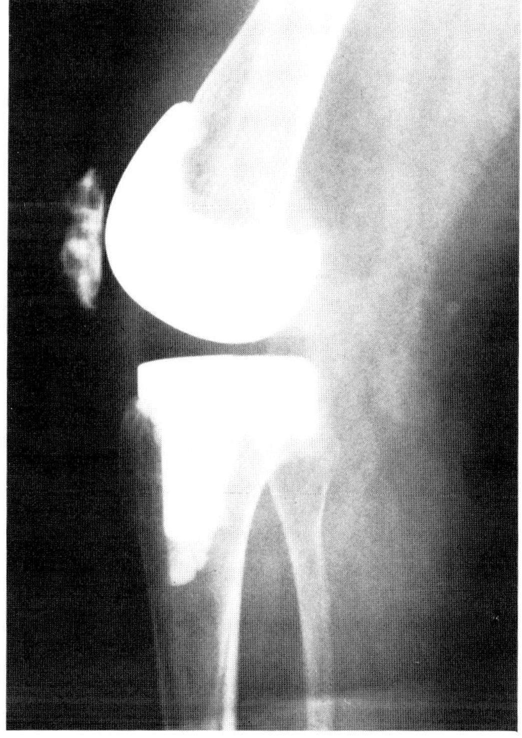

C

vent recurrence of flexion deformity. As with total hip replacement, bone architecture may be small, occasionally necessitating miniature custom components (Figs. 19-2 and 19-3).

After total knee replacement, one can expect excellent pain relief and improvement in function.[29] Final range of motion is generally less than that obtained in patients with adult rheumatoid arthritis owing to the more severe preoperative soft tissue contractures in the juvenile age group.[29] This difference has also been noted in other reports of total knee replacements in JRA patients by Sarokhan et al.[63] and Scott et al.,[68] who noted an average range of motion of 79 degrees, which was similar to that also found by Ranawat et al.[61]

We do not recommend arthrodesis as a primary procedure in the severely involved knee of the patient with JRA. As with the hip, if multiple joint involvement is present or occurs later, too much demand is placed on adjacent joints to compensate for the loss of knee motion. There is also no potential for later conversion to total knee replacement.

We have had no experience with interpositional arthroplasties about the knee in patients with JRA.

ANKLE

Whereas ankle involvement is not unusual in JRA, significant disability uncommonly occurs. Ankle synovitis is usually managed with appropriate medications and physiotherapy to maintain range of motion. Short periods of immobilization are occasionally required for control of the synovitis. Should synovitis become chronic, aggressive physiotherapy must be maintained to prevent equinus contracture. Brewer et al.[13] has reported the occurrence of dorsiflexion contracture in some cases. Corticosteroid injections may be required, although infrequently. We have little experience with ankle synovectomy, as it is rarely necessary, but successful results have been reported in limited reviews.[35,37,45]

For the patient with total loss of joint space and disabling pain, arthrodesis is recommended because of the poor long-term results of the total ankle arthroplasty.

FOOT

Any variety of foot deformities may be observed with JRA. Vaino[79] has compared maturation of the child's foot to modeling wax, guided in the right or wrong direction by rheumatoid inflammation and the load of weight-bearing. The goal of orthopaedic management is to maintain good foot alignment during this malleable period of childhood. It is usually accomplished with the use of orthotics, or occasionally serial casting, should deformity occur. With proper nonoperative care, few children require operative intervention (Fig. 19-4). Most surgery is usually deferred until skeletal maturation has been reached.

Either pes planovalgus (typical of adult rheumatoid arthritis) or cavovarus hindfoot deformities may be noted. They are often associated with intertarsal ankylosis (fibrous or osseous), which may occur early in cases of uncontrolled synovitis. Pes planovalgus deformity is initially managed with medial heel wedges and longitudinal arch supports in moderate cases. With more severe cases of hindfoot valgus, a double upright lower leg brace with corrective T strip is indicated. Cavovarus deformities, if recognized early, can be managed with stretching exercises and shoe modifications, including lateral heel and sole wedges and metatarsal pads if the cavus alignment precipitates metatarsalgia. For resistant cases, serial casting is used, as for the treatment of clubfoot. Surgical intervention (posterior tibial tendon lengthening, calcaneal osteotomies) has rarely been necessary in our experience. The key is early recognition. Infrequently, triple arthrodesis is necessary during the teenage years.

Forefoot problems are similar to those seen in the adult. They include hallux valgus with bunion, metatarsophalangeal (MTP) joint destruction with dorsal dislocation, metatarsal head prominence with metatarsalgia and plantar callosities, and hammertoe deformities. Custom-made shoes with extra-depth insoles, metatarsal pads or bars, and a wide accommodating toebox are used to manage most of these forefoot problems in the juvenile age group. If disabling residual deformity remains after skeletal maturity is obtained, a forefoot resectional arthroplasty is performed that includes MTP joint resections with plantar plate interpositional arthroplasties as described by Susman and Clayton.[77] Insertion of a silicone double-hinge implant in the first MTP joint is recommended only in an unusual case (see Ch. 16). Fusion of the first MTP is an alternative.

A patient with inactive arthritis and good cartilage who has isolated painful juvenile bunions

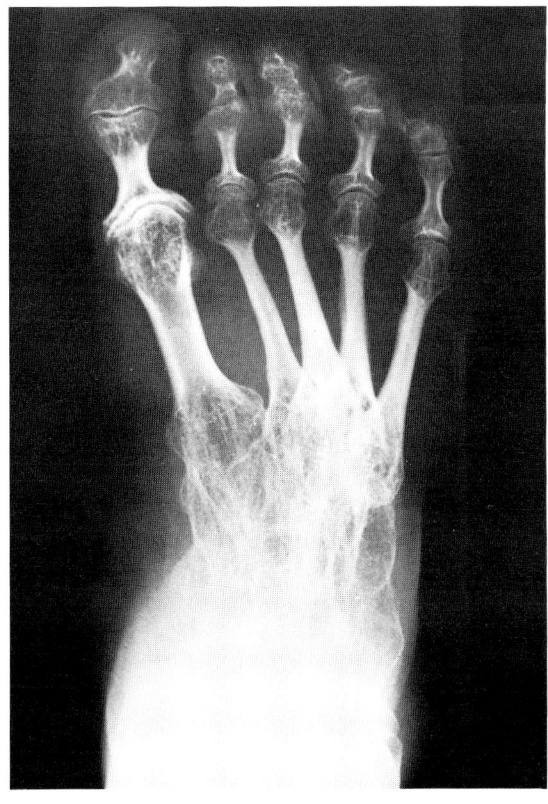

A

with hallux valgus can be treated effectively with a modified McBride bunionectomy including adductor halluces tendon transfer to the first metatarsal neck. Metatarsus primus varus of more than 15 degrees frequently coexists with the bunion in JRA. It is treated with corrective "dome" osteotomy of the first metatarsal base at the same time as bunionectomy is performed. One must carefully avoid an open physis when performing a basilar first metatarsal osteotomy.

LEG LENGTH DISCREPANCY

Children with JRA may demonstrate growth retardation or overgrowth. With the pauciarticular variety, overgrowth predominates, likely due to an increased metabolic rate of the physeal region, secondary to the inflammatory hyperemia. Because the physis at the knee accounts for most lower extremity growth, rheumatoid involvement in this region commonly leads to leg length discrepancy. Simon et al.,[70] in an evaluation of leg length discrepancy in JRA, found that the ma-

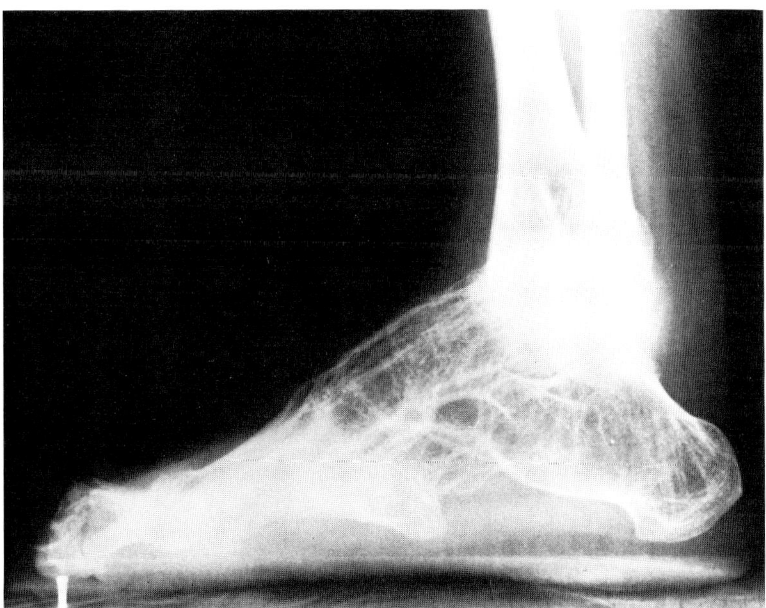

B

Fig. 19-4. Anteroposterior (A) and lateral (B) roentgenograms showing autofusion of the tarsal bones in a relatively neutral now painless position.

jor discrepancy developed within the first 4 years after onset of the disease and either increased slowly, remained unchanged, or decreased. Our experience has shown that the pattern of leg length inequality can be variable, affected by the disease duration, patient immobility and corticosteroid administration. It is therefore mandatory that leg length be frequently evaluated.

Most leg length discrepancies are observed if they are less than 0.5 inch. Shoe lifts are used for inequalities between 0.5 and 0.1 inch, with surgical procedures reserved for discrepancies greater than 1.0 inch. Epiphyseal stapling is preferred to epiphysiodesis because of the variability of growth rates in the patient with JRA. It allows for staple removal if growth of the nonstapled side is greater than predicted. Epiphyseal stapling also allows for immediate mobilization postoperatively, which is important when dealing with an inflammatory disease. In children with minimal growth potential remaining, closed femoral shortening is considered. Synovectomy should also be considered in cases of progressive overgrowth. McMaster[52] has shown that it halts overgrowth of the affected limb in some cases.

SHOULDER

The shoulder joint is involved less commonly than other joints in JRA. There is also usually less functional disability owing to the maintenance of scapulothoracic motion. The key to treatment is appropriate medical management as well as physiotherapy to maintain range of motion. Occasionally, corticosteroid injections are helpful in chronic cases. In cases of persistent, painful synovitis associated with progressive loss of motion nonresponsive to appropriate medical management, a closed manipulation under general anesthesia may be of benefit. In the past we have not been proponents of synovectomy because of the unpredictability of this procedure: A certain percentage of patients in the juvenile age group experience a significant loss of motion, and intensive physiotherapy after the operation is needed to prevent this loss. However, as with the knee, we are now looking more favorably on this proce-

dure because of the ability to perform it arthroscopically. We have seen good relief of pain with much less morbidity using this method.

Total shoulder replacement is reserved for the patient with disabling pain and severe roentgenographic destruction. It must be deferred, however, until after skeletal maturation. As with other total joint replacements in the patient with JRA, the bone architecture of the shoulder is often small such that custom-made components may be required.

ELBOW

The elbow joint is frequently involved in rheumatoid arthritis. One of the initial signs seen with elbow involvement is early loss of full extension, which may occur before the patient complains of pain or any palpable synovitis is noted. With more severe cases, total ankylosis may occur. As with the shoulder, medical therapy is the central focus of management along with physiotherapy to maintain range of motion. Night splinting and infrequent corticosteroid injections are used in persistent cases. Synovectomy is reserved for chronic, aggressive cases resistant to medical management. It is performed through a single posterolateral incision. The radial head is usually not excised in the skeletally immature patient so as to prevent postoperative deformity as growth continues.

In cases of total elbow destruction, total elbow arthroplasty is considered but again is deferred until later in adulthood.[28] Although we have had no experience with distraction arthroplasty of the elbow, Deland et al.[27] and Ewald[31] have reported success with it in patients with post-traumatic osteoarthritis. This form of treatment may lend itself well to the young patient with end-stage elbow destruction due to JRA.

WRIST

A classic early sign of wrist involvement is loss of wrist extension. In cases of progressive synovitis, fixed flexion contracture associated with an ulnar

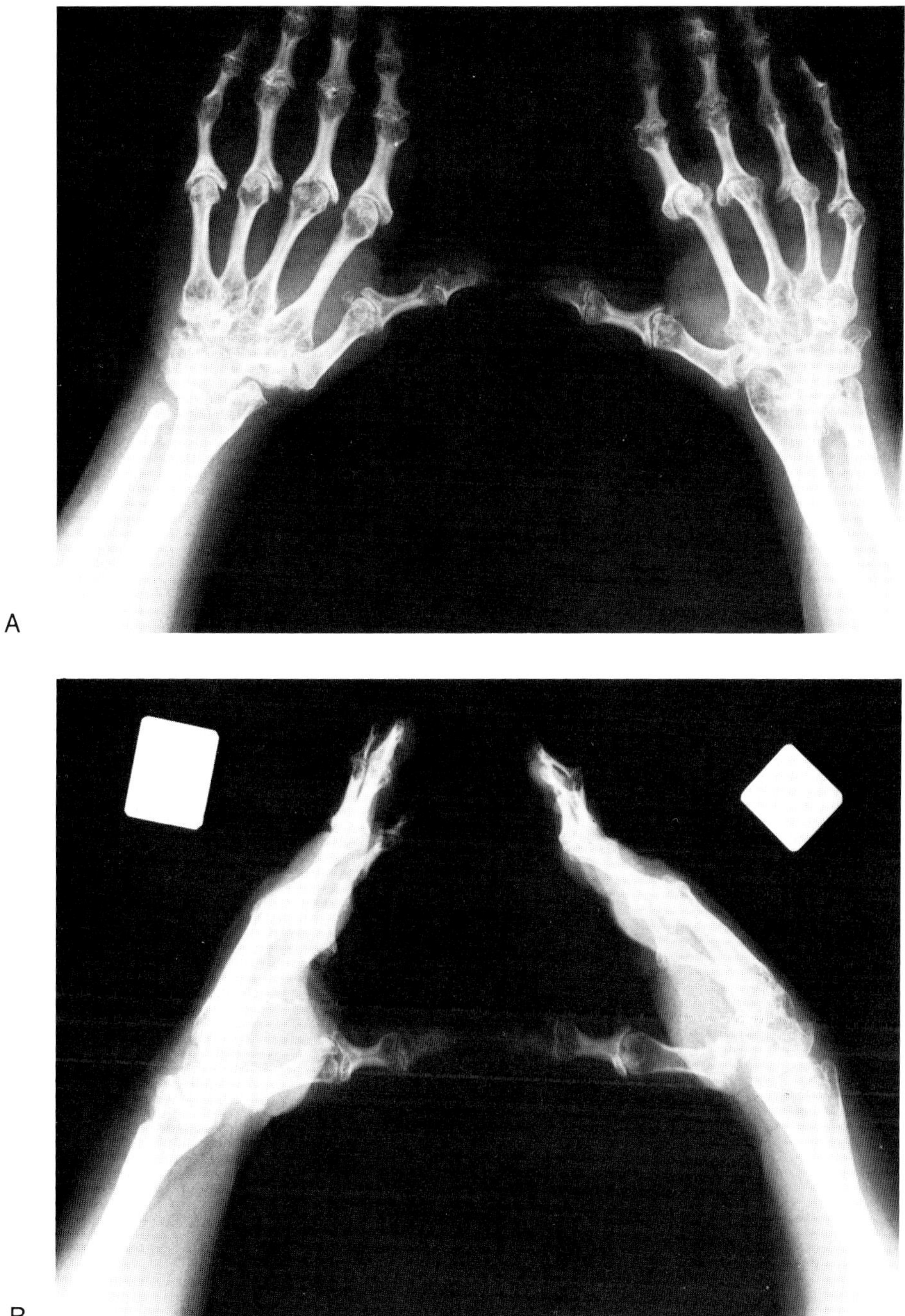

Fig. 19-5. Anteroposterior (**A**) and lateral (**B**) roentgenograms of a patient with small bone architecture and autofusion of carpal bones. The hands function well.

deviation deformity at the carpus may occur—in contrast to the typical radial carpal translocation seen in the adult with rheumatoid arthritis. The key to management of the wrist is maintenance of good wrist alignment. Wrist deformity may lead to finger deformities, as with the adult, due to imbalance of the intrinsic and extrinsic muscle forces on the digits.

As with other joints in the patient with JRA, intercarpal ankylosis—initially fibrous and later osseous—may occur (Fig. 19-5). It is important to maintain the wrist in a functional position with splinting in chronic, aggressive cases in which ankylosis is likely. The wrist is well suited for and responds well to splinting. We initially use the splint at night and during the day in more difficult cases. Splinting can maintain alignment as well as correct a deformity. Occasionally, serial casting is required. If wrist synovitis as well as tenosynovitis persist despite aggressive medical management and physiotherapy, tenosynovectomy with limited wrist synovectomy is considered. The distal ulna is not excised unless it is significantly destroyed with loss of growth potential associated with marked limitation of forearm rotation. Good pain relief as well as control of inflammation can be expected following this procedure. Tendon rupture, although less common in the JRA patient, can occur and is managed by the traditional tendon transfer techniques used in adults. The patient with disabling wrist pain, deformity, and severe roentgenographic deterioration of the carpus is best treated with an arthrodesis using intramedullary internal fixation as described by Clayton[25] (See Chapter 11) and modified by Mannerfelt and Malmsten[50] and Nalebuff.[57] We choose a neutral (0 degree flexion/extension) position for wrist arthrodesis to maintain a maximal global arc of motion, assuming maintenance of good forearm rotation. Although we have reported successful results with total wrist replacement in adults,[30] we do not recommend this procedure in the juvenile or young adult age group.

HAND

Hand involvement in JRA is characterized by progressive stiffness with associated loss of flexion of both the metacarpophalangeal (MCP) and proximal interphalangeal (IP) joints. In contrast to the adult, who typically demonstrates ulnar deviation of the MCP joints, children often develop mild radial deviation deformity at the MCP joint level. The ulnar deviation deformity seen at the wrist in the juvenile may contribute to the radial MCP joint deviation. It is uncommon to see significant volar subluxation or dislocation of the MCP joints in the child, as is commonly seen in the adult. In addition to the deformities at the MCP joint level, both boutonnière and swan-neck deformities can occur.

Treatment of MCP and proximal phalangeal joint involvement centers around physiotherapy, including both active and passive range of motion, hydrotherapy, and dynamic and static splinting. Occasionally, corticosteroid injections are of benefit. We have not found synovectomy of these joints to be overly successful owing to the propensity for loss of motion following operation.

Boutonnière deformities are initially managed with splinting to achieve a functional range of motion at both the proximal and distal IP joints. If deformity persists in the presence of a functional passive range of motion, consideration is given to distal extensor tendon release as described by Fowler[36] in cases of mild deformity. If more advanced deformity is present, distal tenotomy may need to be combined with central tendon and lateral band reconstruction, for which there are multiple methods (anatomic repair, substitution procedures, tendon transfers).[49,57,58] For the rigid boutonnière deformity with joint destruction unresponsive to appropriate splinting and physiotherapy, proximal IP joint fusion may be indicated, but it is delayed until after skeletal maturity. It is important to note that surgery on such deformities can be deferred permanently, as the children often learn to adapt well to the fixed deformities. Silicone arthroplasty of the proximal phalangeal joint is not indicated for either boutonnière or swan-neck deformities owing to the young age of the patient.

Treatment of swan-neck deformity varies with the stage of the deformity. It is important to realize that this deformity may be secondary to imbalance at the MCP joint, particularly volar subluxation with associated extensor lag. MCP joint imbalance, if present, must be corrected before addressing the swan-neck deformity.

Initial treatment consists in splinting, with an emphasis on stretching the intrinsic muscles, which are often contracted in this deformity. In cases of persistent deformity with passively supple joints, multiple treatment options are available, including flexor dermadesis,[59] flexor tenodesis using a single slip of the superficialis,[78] intrinsic muscle release (if tight), or a combination of these methods.

In moderate cases with a normal or near-normal joint roentgenographically but limited IP joint motion, lateral band mobilization with skin release is performed, as described by Nalebuff and Millender.[59] For severe cases with destruction of the proximal IP joint, options include (1) observation, if the deformity is well tolerated; (2) manipulation and pinning followed by intensive physiotherapy; or (3) arthrodesis.

Thumb deformities are usually better tolerated than those in the fingers. Loss of MCP motion of the thumb is less critical for good function. The primary goal of treatment should be to provide a stable "post" for articulation of the fingers. The most common thumb deformity encountered is a pseudoboutonnière deformity (Nalebuff type I[53]), with hyperflexion at the MCP joint and hyperextension at the IP joint secondary to attenuation of the dorsal soft tissues, including the capsule, extensor pollicis longus, and extensor pollicis brevis tendons. This deformity is initially managed with appropriate medication to control the synovitis and extension splinting of the MCP joint. If synovitis persists, corticosteroids are occasionally injected into the MCP joint. In cases with progressive deformity but adequate MCP joint space remaining that have not responded to nonoperative treatment, an extensor pollicis longus rerouting procedure[56] is performed in which the extensor pollicis longus tendon is brought through the dorsal MCP joint capsule and sutured back on itself, holding the MCP joint out of its hyperflexed posture. In cases of severe MCP joint destruction, arthrodesis of this joint is recommended after skeletal maturity. (See Chapter 12.)

We have rarely encountered a gamekeeper's thumb deformity in patients with JRA secondary to destruction of the ulnar collateral ligament by the inflammatory process. Treatment consists in surgical reconstruction, which usually requires tendon graft augmentation[73] or fusion.

SPINE

Involvement of the cervical spine in JRA patients differs from that of the adult variety in that there is a tendency for posterior ankylosis secondary to inflammatory disease of the facet joints. It typically begins proximally in the cervical spine and may extend distally to the midthoracic level. If untreated, an ankylosed spine, typically in a flexed posture, may result. The key to treatment of this problem is early recognition with appropriate physiotherapy to maintain range of motion and prevent fixed deformity. For acute cases with marked spasm and pain, rigid cervical collars are used until the acute episode subsides. In cases with severe involvement, ankylosis is often unavoidable. It is therefore critical to maintain the cervical spine in a functional position. We have not performed cervical spine osteotomy in cases of fixed deformity owing to the hazardous nature of this procedure.

Horizontal atlantoaxial subluxation secondary to inflammatory attenuation or rupture of the transverse ligament may occur and can lead to spinal cord compromise. Lateral roentgenograms of the cervical spine in full flexion and extension are imperative for diagnosis. The distance between the anterior aspect of the odontoid and the adjacent posterior border of C1 is measured to assess subluxation. If this distance measures more than 5 mm in a child, it is considered evidence of subluxation. It is critical to follow cases with subluxation carefully to assess progression and detect any neurologic compromise. Treatment of atlantoaxial subluxation must be individualized. Patients without neurologic compromise or severe pain often respond well to medication and the intermittent use of cervical collars. Patients with progressive subluxation, neurologic compromise, or severe and unrelenting pain are considered candidates for C1–C2 arthrodesis of the Gallie type recommended by Simmons.[69]

Infrequently, juvenile ankylosing spondylitis, similar to that seen in the adult, occurs. Early loss of lumbar flexibility with associated pain and involvement with the sacroiliac joints are common presenting signs. These children often test positive for the histocompatibility antigen HLA-B27. In progressive cases, sacroiliac joint fusion as well as ankylosis of the thoracolumbar spine in the typical "bamboo" fashion may occur. Treatment includes appropriate medications as well as physiotherapy, emphasizing extension of the spine. These patients are also instructed to avoid positioning themselves in a flexed posture for prolonged periods; it is recommended that they sleep on rigid surfaces and avoid pillows.

SUMMARY

Although it shares many characteristics with the adult counterpart, JRA represents a different pathologic entity with distinct clinical differences, as discussed. Medical management with intensive physiotherapy comprise the cornerstone of treatment. Surgical intervention, though not commonly required, can be helpful when indicated.

Individual procedures for juvenile rheumatoid arthritis have been discussed and illustrated in preceding chapters of this book. In general, however, prevention of permanent deformity is emphasized in the juvenile rheumatoid patient, and soft tissue surgery is the mainstay until the child is fully grown. After skeletal maturity, the procedures for adult rheumatoid arthritis apply, with the attention to details noted. Multiple joint replacements are often indicated for independent ambulation in young patients. Some young patients have expressed a desire "to have my 20 years between the ages of 20 and 40 rather than 40 and 60" (Ansell, personal communication).

REFERENCES

1. Ansell BM, Arden GP, McLennan I: Valgus knee deformities in children with juvenile chronic polyarthritis treated by epiphyseal stapling. Arch Dis Child 45:388, 1970
2. Ansell BM, Bywaters EGL: Growth in Still's disease. Ann Rheum Dis 15:295, 1956
3. Antilla R: Renal involvement in juvenile rheumatoid arthritis. Acta Paediatr Scand [Suppl] 227:3, 1972
4. Arden GP: Surgical treatment of Still's disease. Ann R Coll Surg Engl 53:288, 1973
5. Arden GP, Ansell BM: Surgical Management of Juvenile Chronic Arthritis. Academic Press, New York, 1978
6. Bernstein B: Pericarditis in juvenile rheumatoid arthritis. Arthritis Rheum 20:241, 1977
7. Bernstein BH, Stobie D, Singsen BH et al: Growth retardation in juvenile rheumatoid arthritis (JRA). Arthritis Rheum 20:212, 1977
8. Bernstein B, Takahashi M, Hanson V: Cardiac involvement in juvenile rheumatoid arthritis. J Pediatr 85:313, 1974
9. Brattstrom M, Sundberg J: Juvenile rheumatoid gonarthritis. Part I. Clinical and roentgenological study. Acta Rheumatol Scand 11:266, 1965
10. Brewer EJ Jr: Juvenile rheumatoid arthritis: cardiac involvement. Arthritis Rheum, suppl. 2, 20:231, 1977
11. Brewer EJ Jr, Bass J, Baum J et al: Current proposed revision of JRA criteria: JRA Criteria Subcommittee of the Diagnostic and Therapeutic Criteria Committee of the American Rheumatism Section of The Arthritis Foundation. Arthritis Rheum, suppl. 2, 20:195, 1977
12. Brewer EJ Jr, Giannini EH: A comparative study of the epidemiologic and clinical natural histories of rheumatoid arthritis subtypes. Arthritis Rheum 23:656, 1980
13. Brewer EJ Jr, Giannini EH, Person DA: Juvenile Rheumatoid Arthritis. 2nd Ed. WB Saunders, Philadelphia, 1982
14. Brinkman GL, Chaikof L: Rheumatoid lung disease; report of a case which developed in childhood. Am Rev Respir Dis 80:732, 1959
15. Calabro JJ: Other extra-articular manifestations of juvenile rheumatoid arthritis. Arthritis Rheum 20:237, 1977
16. Calabro JJ, Katz RM, Marchesano JM et al: Pruritus in juvenile rheumatoid arthritis. Pediatrics 46:322, 1970
17. Calabro JJ, Marchesano JM: Juvenile rheumatoid arthritis: observations on fever. N Engl J Med 276:11, 1967
18. Calabro JJ, Marchesano JM: Rash associated with juvenile rheumatoid arthritis. J Pediatr 72:611, 1968
19. Calabro JJ, Parrino GR, Atchoo PD et al: Chronic iridocyclitis in juvenile rheumatoid arthritis. Arthritis Rheum 13:406, 1970

20. Cassidy JT: Juvenile rheumatoid arthritis. p. 1289. In Kelley WN, Harris ED Jr, Ruddy S, Sledge CB: Textbook of Rheumatology. 3rd Ed. WB Saunders, Philadelphia, 1989
21. Cassidy JT, Brady GL, Martel W: Monarticular juvenile rheumatoid arthritis. J Pediatr 70:867, 1967
22. Cassidy JT, Sullivan DB, Petty RE: Clinical patterns of chronic iridocyclitis in children with juvenile rheumatoid arthritis. Arthritis Rheum 20:224, 1977
23. Chylack LT Jr, Bienfang DC, Bellows AR et al: Ocular manifestations of juvenile rheumatoid arthritis. Am J Ophthalmol 79:1026, 1975
24. Clayton ML: Surgery of the lower extremity in rheumatoid arthritis. J Bone Joint Surg [Am] 45:1517, 1963
25. Clayton ML: Surgical treatment at the wrist in rheumatoid arthritis. J Bone Joint Surg [Am] 47:741, 1965
26. Clayton ML, Thompson TR, Mack RP: Correction of alignment deformities during total knee arthroplasties; staged soft tissue releases. Clin Orthop 202:117, 1986
27. Deland JT, Walker PS, Sledge CB et al: Treatment of post-traumatic elbows with a new hinge-distractor. Orthopedics 6:732, 1983
28. Dennis DA, Clayton ML, Ferlic DC et al: Capitello-condylar total elbow arthroplasty for rheumatoid arthritis. J Arthroplasty 55:83, 1990
29. Dennis DA, Clayton ML, O'Donnell S et al: Posterior cruciate condylar total knee arthroplasty; average 11-year follow-up. Clin. Orthop (in press) 1992
30. Dennis DA, Ferlic DC, Clayton ML: Volz total wrist arthroplasty in rheumatoid arthritis; a long term review. J Hand Surg [Am] 11:483, 1986
31. Ewald F: Reconstruction of the elbow. Instr Course Lect 35:108, 1986
32. Eyring EJ, Longert A, Bass JC: Synovectomy in juvenile rheumatoid arthritis; indications and short term results. J Bone Joint Surg [Am] 53:638, 1971
33. Fauci AS, Haynes BF, Katz P: The spectrum of vasculitis, clinical pathologic, immunologic, and therapeutic considerations. Ann Intern Med 89:660, 1978
34. Fink CW: Polyarteritis and other diseases with necrotizing vasculitis in childhood. Arthritis Rheum 20:378, 1977
35. Fink CW, Baum J, Pardies LH et al: Synovectomy in juvenile rheumatoid arthritis. Ann Rheum Dis 28:612, 1969
36. Fowler SB: The management of tendon injuries. J Bone Joint Surg [Am] 41:579, 1959
37. Garrett AL, Campbell C: Synovectomy in children. p. 111. In Cruess RL, Mitchell NS (eds): Surgery of Rheumatoid Arthritis. JB Lippincott, Philadelphia, 1971
38. Isdale IC, Bywaters EGL: The rash of rheumatoid arthritis and Still's disease. Q J Med 99:377, 1956
39. Jacobsen ST, Levinson JE, Crawford AH: Late results of synovectomy in juvenile rheumatoid arthritis. J Bone Joint Surg [Am] 67:8, 1985
40. Jakobowski S, Ruszcynska J: The possibility of surgical treatment in cases of juvenile rheumatoid arthritis. Acta Rheumatol Scand 13:113, 1967
41. Jan JE, Hill RH, Low MD: Cerebral complications in juvenile rheumatoid arthritis. Can Med Assoc J 107:623, 1972
42. Jani L, Waigand D: Synovectomy of the knee in juvenile rheumatoid arthritis. Reconstr Surg Trauma 12:35, 1971
43. Jordan JD, Snyder CH: Rheumatoid disease of the lung and corpulmonale; observations in a child. Am J Dis Child 108:174, 1964
44. Jose DG, Good RA: Iridocyclitis pauciarticular juvenile rheumatoid arthritis. J Pediatr 78:910, 1971
45. Kampner SL, Ferguson AB Jr: Efficacy of synovectomy in juvenile rheumatoid arthritis. Clin Orthop 88:94, 1972
46. Key SN III, Kimura SJ: Iridocyclitis associated with juvenile rheumatoid arthritis. Am J Ophthalmol 80:425, 1975
47. Lang H, Antilla R, Svikus A et al: EEG findings in juvenile rheumatoid arthritis and other connective tissue diseases in children. Acta Paediatr Scand 63:373, 1974
48. Lietman PS, Bywaters EGL: Pericarditis in juvenile rheumatoid arthritis. Pediatrics 32:855, 1963
49. Littler JW, Eaton RG: Redistribution of forces in the correction of boutonnière deformity. J Bone Joint Surg [Am] 39:1267, 1959
50. Mannerfelt L, Malmsten M: Arthrodesis of the wrist in rheumatoid arthritis; a technique without external fixation. Scand J Plast Reconstr Surg 5:124, 1971
51. Martel W, Holt JF, Cassidy JT: Roentgenologic manifestations of juvenile rheumatoid arthritis. Am J Roentgenol Radium Ther Nucl Med 88:400, 1962
52. McMaster M: Synovectomy of the knee in juvenile rheumatoid arthritis. J Bone Joint Surg [Br] 54:263, 1972
53. Millender LH, Nalebuff EA: Reconstructive surgery in the rheumatoid hand. Orthop Clin North Am 6:709, 1975
54. Miller JJ III, French JW: Myocarditis in juvenile

rheumatoid arthritis. Am J Dis Child 131:205, 1977

55. Mogenson B, Brattstrom M, Ekelund L et al: Synovectomy of the hip in juvenile chronic arthritis. J Bone Joint Surg [Br] 64:295, 1982

56. Nalebuff EA: Restoration of balance in the rheumatoid thumb. p. 197. In Tubiana R (ed): La Main Rheumatoide. Expansion Scientifique Francaise, Paris, 1969

57. Nalebuff EA: Surgical treatment of finger deformities in the rheumatoid hand. Surg Clin North Am 49:833, 1969

58. Nalebuff EA, Millender LH: Surgical treatment of the boutonniere deformity in rheumatoid arthritis. Orthop Clin North Am 6:753, 1975

59. Nalebuff EA, Millender LH: Surgical treatment of the swan-neck deformity in rheumatoid arthritis. Orthop Clin North Am 6:733, 1975

60. Petty RE, Cassidy JT, Sullivan DB: Clinical correlates of antinuclear antibodies in juvenile rheumatoid arthritis. J Pediatrics 83:386, 1973

61. Ranawat CS, Bryan WJ, Inglis AE: Total knee arthroplasty in juvenile arthritis. Arthritis Rheum 26:1140, 1983

62. Sairanen E: On the etiology of growth disturbance of the mandible in juvenile rheumatoid arthritis. Acta Rheum Scand 16:136, 1970

63. Sarokhan AJ, Scott RD, Thomas WH: Total knee arthroplasty in juvenile rheumatoid arthritis. J Bone Joint Surg [Am] 65:1071, 1983

64. Schaller JG, Johnson GD, Holborow EJ et al: The association of antinuclear antibodies with the chronic iridocyclitis of juvenile rheumatoid arthritis (Still's disease). Arthritis Rheum 17:409, 1974

65. Schaller J, Kupfer C, Wedgwood RJ: Iridocyclitis in juvenile rheumatoid arthritis. Pediatrics 44:92, 1969

66. Schaller JG, Wedgwood RJ: Pruritis associated with the rash of juvenile rheumatoid arthritis. Pediatrics 45:296, 1970

67. Schnitzer TJ, Ansell BM: Amyloidosis in juvenile chronic polyarthritis. Arthritis Rheum, suppl. 2, 20:245, 1977

68. Scott RD, Sarokhan AJ, Dalziel R: Total hip and total knee arthroplasty in juvenile rheumatoid arthritis. Clin Orthop 182:90, 1984

69. Simmons EH: Surgery of the spine in rheumatoid arthritis and ankylosing spondylitis. In Cruess RL, Mitchell NS (eds): Surgery of Rheumatoid Arthritis. p. 93. Lippincott, Philadelphia, 1971

70. Simon S, Whiffen J, Shapiro F: Leg-length discrepancies in monoarticular and pauciarticular juvenile rheumatoid arthritis. J Bone Joint Surg [Am] 63:209, 1981

71. Smiley WK: Iridocyclitis in Still's disease; prognosis and steroid treatment. Trans Ophthalmol Soc UK 85:351, 1965

72. Smiley WK: The eye in juvenile rheumatoid arthritis. Trans Ophthalmol Soc UK 94:817, 1974

73. Smith RJ: Post-traumatic instability of the metacarpophalangeal joint of the thumb. J Bone Joint Surg [Am] 59:14, 1977

74. Still GF: On a form of chronic joint disease in children. Med Chir Trans 80:46, 1897

75. Sundberg J, Brattstrom M: Juvenile rheumatoid gonarthritis. II. Disturbance of ossification and growth. Acta Rheumatol Scand 11:279, 1965

76. Sury B, Vesterdal E: Extra-articular lesions in juvenile rheumatoid arthritis: a survey based upon a study of 151 cases. Acta Rheumatol Scand 14:309, 1968

77. Susman MH, Clayton ML: Surgery of the rheumatoid foot. Ann Acad Med (Singapore) 12:225, 1983

78. Swanson AB: Surgery of the hand in cerebral palsy and the swan-neck deformity. J Bone Joint Surg [Am] 42:951, 1960

79. Vainio K: The rheumatoid foot; a clinical study with pathological and roentgenological comments. Ann Chir Gynaecol [Suppl] 45:27, 1956

20

Case Report: Multiple Procedures in a Rheumatoid Arthritis Patient

Mack L. Clayton
Douglas A. Dennis

A 24-year-old woman presented with a 7-year history of rheumatoid arthritis in 1964. She complained of a swollen and painful right knee that began after an episode of strep throat 1.5 years before. She had been using crutches for 6 months. In the past she had tried cortisone and gold therapy; her current medication included only aspirin.

On examination she walked with crutches and protected her right knee. The right knee remained in flexion and valgus with attempted weight-bearing (Fig. 20-1A & B). Range of motion was 20 to 120 degrees. Marked tenderness was present with 2+ effusion and synovitis. Her left knee had a 1+ effusion without pain and with a free range of motion from 0 to 135 degrees. The feet and ankles rested in mild valgus. She had mild callus underneath the second metatarsal head on the right.

Both shoulders had forward flexion to 150 degrees without pain. The left elbow lacked 20 degrees of full extension but had free flexion; the right elbow had free motion. The right wrist was tender with pain on motion, and there was only a jog of motion. The joint, however, remained in a good position of 5 degrees dorsiflexion and mild ulnar deviation; pronation was 80 degrees and supination 30 degrees. There was a 2+ synovitis in various joints of her hand.

Weight-bearing roentgenograms of the knees revealed a marked loss of joint spacing on the right with valgus (stage IIIB); the left knee revealed normal joint spacing (stage I) (Fig. 20-1C). The standard procedure in 1964 for a knee with this amount of destructive change was an arthrodesis, but the patient preferred a movable joint, as it was explained to her that arthrodesis of a rheumatoid knee may lead to problem in other joints.

In June 1964 a custom-made Herman Young hinge[6] prosthesis was inserted in her right knee through a transverse incision with patellectomy. Screws served to stabilize each component to the knee. Postoperatively, the knee was immobilized in full extension for 2 weeks and then started on active motion. Three days later the patient had 25 degrees motion in her knee and was discharged. Eight weeks after surgery motion of the knee was only 5 to 30 degrees, and the patient was readmitted to the hospital and received manipulation; 8 weeks later the range of motion was 3 to 55 degrees.

About this time she experienced another episode of strep throat, coinciding with swelling and pain of the left knee with 2+ synovitis and synovial thickening; the left knee showed good joint spacing roentgenographically (stage I) (Fig. 20-2). The patient was concerned, as she realized what a disastrous course her opposite right knee had followed during the years before. Synovectomy of the left knee anterior compartments were performed in November 1964. The menisci were

389

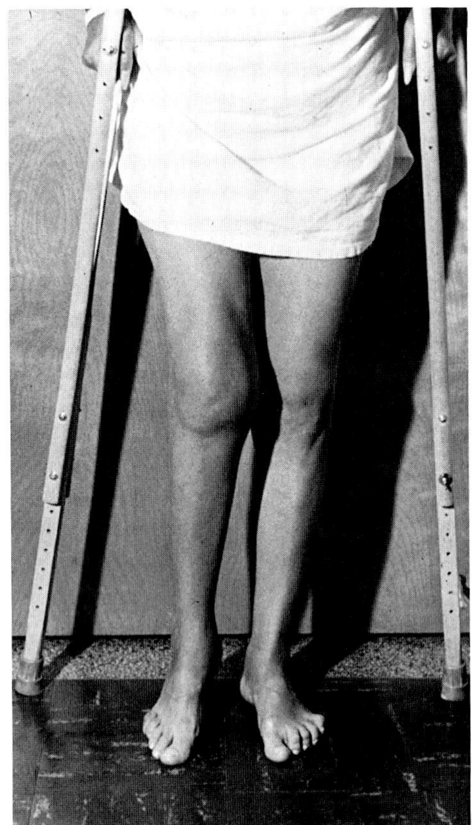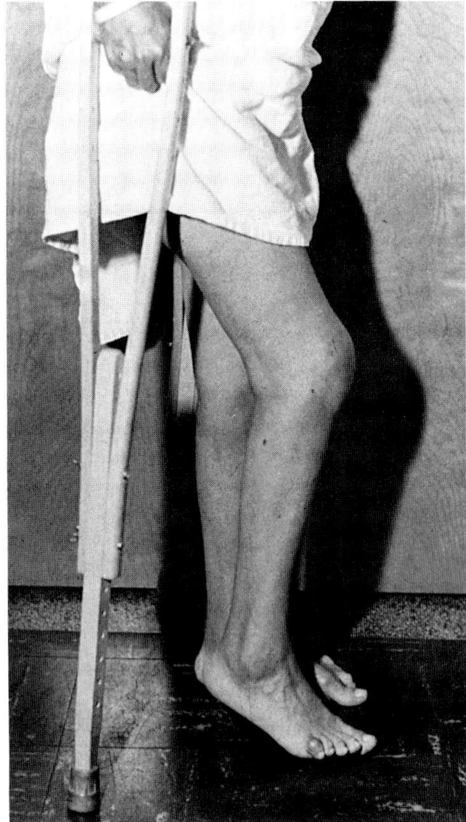

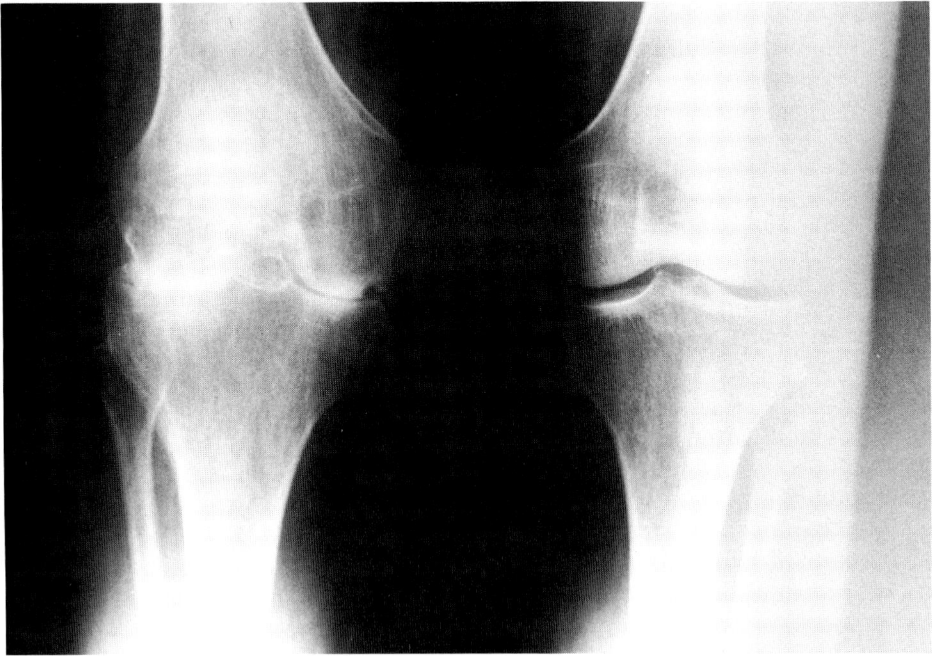

Fig. 20-1. Anteroposterior (**A**) and lateral (**B**) views in which swelling and deformity of the right knee are noted. (**C**) Standing roentgenogram (without crutches) shows complete narrowing of the right knee joint; there is normal joint spacing on the left.

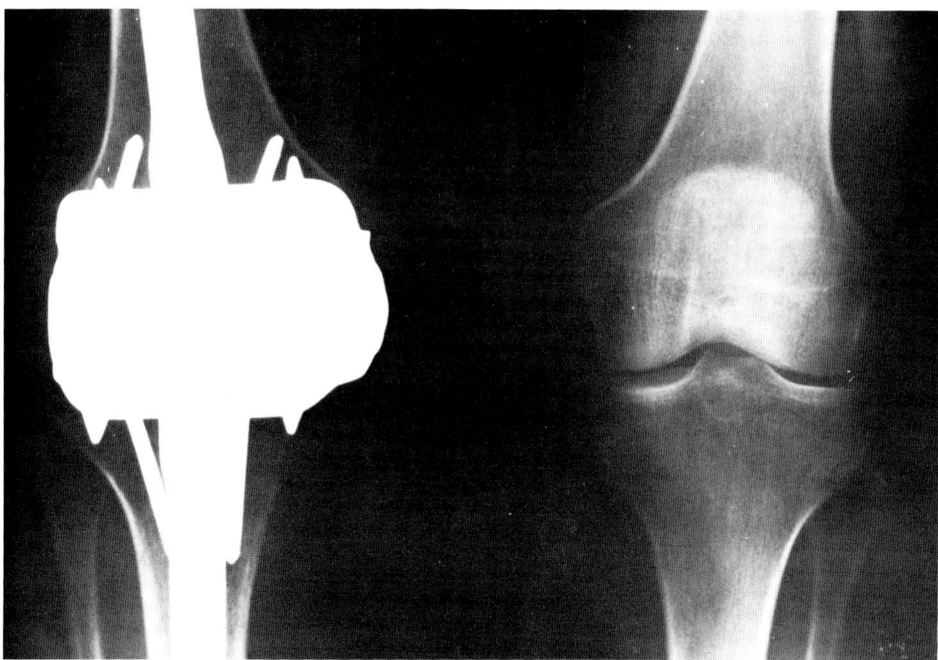

Fig. 20-2. Weight-bearing roentgenograms show the normal left knee joint (stage I) and the right knee with a Young hinge.

retained, as they appeared normal, and the posterior compartment appeared clear. The cartilage in the knee was well preserved (Fig. 20-3) as noted in the stage I roentgenograms. The knee was manipulated under anesthesia 1 week after surgery and essentially regained full range of motion. By June 1965 the patient was walking well without any support; the right knee motion was 0 to 80 degrees, and left knee motion was 0 to 135 degrees without effusion or pain.

The right wrist had become her next major complaint, again in 1965. She had pain, with dorsiflexion 10 degrees, volar flexion 5 degrees, and mild ulnar deviation, as well as pronation 60 degrees and supination 50 degrees. The right elbow moved freely from 0 to 150 degrees. Surgery consisted in tenosynovectomy of the extensor tendons and excision of the distal ulna on the right with local synovectomy of the wrist. She did well after this procedure and essentially regained full pronation and supination; there was no effusion in the wrist, the tendons were riding well, and her pain had been relieved.

The left wrist and elbow became her primary problem in 1966, with painful effusion and motion limited to 20 to 130 degrees in the elbow. The left wrist had 35 degrees dorsiflexion, 30 degrees palmar flexion, 60 degrees supination, and 80 degrees pronation, but with marked pain and crepitus about the radial head. In February 1966 synovectomy of the left wrist with excision of the distal ulna and tenosynovectomy were performed; left elbow synovectomy and radial head excision were done at the same time. She was started on early mobilization, as the postoperative care is essentially the same for these two procedures, and she did well.

By September 1966 she had no pain in her knees, but she did have marked pain and spasm in both of her feet, essentially in the area of the hindfoot. She had only a jog of motion in the subtalar joint, but it was painful. Ankle motion bilaterally was not painful with dorsiflexion to neutral and 35 to 40 degrees plantar flexion. The overall alignment of the foot was in satisfactory position on both the anteroposterior and lateral views. A

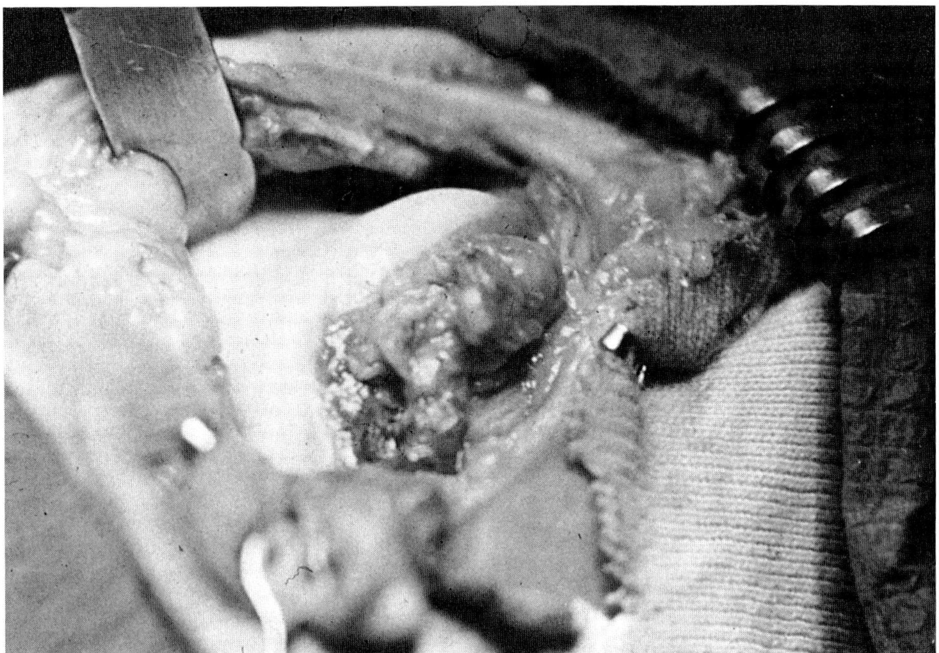

Fig. 20-3. Left knee at synovectomy. Note the normal appearance of the articular cartilage with proliferative synovium.

right triple arthrodesis was performed in October 1966, with plug grafts and a walking cast applied 2 weeks postoperatively (Fig. 16-26). She had a left triple arthrodesis 1 month later by the plug graft method. A walking cast again was utilized, and she was in the bilateral walking casts for 2½ months after operation. One month after cast removal she had no pain in the ankle or hindfoot and no swelling, and she had regained approximately 40 degrees of ankle motion. One year later she was walking well.

By 1968 her left elbow became increasingly painful, with motion from 30 to 120 degrees and full pronation and supination, but with tenderness and marked crepitus. In February 1968 a fascial arthroplasty was performed on the left elbow. Three months after surgery, she had no pain in the elbow, with motion from 35 to 105 degrees and full pronation and supination.

During late 1968 she developed increasing pain in her shoulders, particularly the right shoulder, with pain on motion and inability to sleep on the shoulder. The right shoulder had an active elevation of 160 degrees and external rotation of 60 degrees; synovial crepitation was present but no bone-to-bone crepitus. The left shoulder had a free range of motion without crepitus. A total acromionectomy of the right shoulder and synovectomy of the glenohumeral joint were performed in February 1969. She was started on early motion, and 6 weeks after surgery the shoulder was painless and was gaining free motion to 90 degrees forward elevation. Her shoulder exercises were continued, and she regained an excellent range of motion to 150 degrees of elevation without pain.

Considerable neck and shoulder pain was occurring because of the support necessary for her large breasts. Consultation was obtained with a plastic surgeon, and in October 1969 a bilateral reduction mammoplasty was performed. Routine pathologic sections revealed an early carcinoma in the left breast, which was treated with a modified radical mastectomy, and she has had no recurrence of the malignancy.

In August 1970 she began having increasing pain and swelling of the left knee. She had motion from 0 to 130 degrees with 3+ effusion and synovial thickening. It was now 6 years since the left knee synovectomy, and roentgenograms revealed mild narrowing of the joint spacing (Fig. 20-4A). Because of this recurrent effusion and pain, left knee synovectomy was repeated. Anterior and posterior compartment synovectomy was performed, with the synovium in the posterior compartment found to be more proliferative than that in the anterior compartment (Fig. 20-4B). A medial and lateral meniscectomy were done, and 2 weeks later she had manipulation of the left knee. She later regained full motion with no effusion or pain.

For more than 3 months in 1971–1972 she had been experiencing pain in her right elbow, with motion limited to 15 to 135 degrees, wrist dorsiflexion of 25 degrees, and palmar flexion of 5 degrees. Roentgenograms showed stage III elbow changes, and so in February 1972 a right elbow synovectomy and radial head excision were performed, including synovectomy of the metacarpophalangeal (MCP) joints and the proximal interphalangeal (PIP) joint on the index finger of the right hand. One year after surgery she had motion from 15 to 135 degrees in the right elbow with full pronation and supination and without synovitis. Her right shoulder at this time had 100 percent pain relief with full motion.

In 1974 she had bilateral foot pain in the forefoot with painful callus on the forefoot, particularly underneath the second metatarsals with cock-up toes. She had no pain in the hindfoot on either side. In June 1974 she had bilateral forefoot reconstructions with multiple metatarsophalangeal (MTP) joint resections and was relieved of pain. (See Chapter 16.)

By 1975–1976 her left shoulder had been causing her continuous pain for months, allowing elevation of only 80 degrees and external rotation of 20 degrees. Synovial crepitation was present. Roentgenograms showed an arthrogram of the left shoulder that demonstrated an intact rotator cuff and the extent of the synovitis. In March 1976 she underwent total acromionectomy and synovectomy on the right shoulder. Postoperatively, she recovered 75 percent of motion and was relieved of pain.

Her right elbow grew increasingly painful at this time, limiting range of motion to 40 to 90 degrees with full pronation and supination. Roentgenograms showed total loss of joint space in the right elbow. In August 1976 a right fascial

arthroplasty was performed, and motion was regained from 0 to 140 degrees.

Two years later the right hip had become painful, with limited motion and marked narrowing on the roentgenograms. In September 1978, a right total hip arthroplasty with a Turner-Aufranc component was performed. Three months later she had no pain in the hip and was walking with one crutch or a cane. She had 90 degrees free motion.

At this same time, her right shoulder again was a problem: She had marked pain with any attempt at motion. Roentgenograms revealed marked narrowing of the glenohumeral joint, and a right total shoulder replacement (Neer II) was performed in January 1979, including a glenoid replacement. Ten months later she was pain-free, could elevate her shoulder to 90 degrees, and could reach behind her head or behind her lower back.

Her next major complaint (late 1979) was a "giving out" of her painful left knee. On examination she had motion from 5 to 120 degrees. There was bone-to-bone crepitus laterally with marked tenderness medially and 3+ effusion. Therefore in January 1980 she had a left Miller multiradius condylar total knee replacement with cement injection to anchor the components. Postoperatively, she experienced peroneal nerve palsy; however, 5 months later the nerve had returned, and knee motion was 5 to 107 degrees.

In 1981 she developed increasing pain in her left shoulder, with loss of motion and an elevation of only 50 degrees. Roentgenograms showed progression with marked narrowing of the joint spacing. She received a left total shoulder replacement (Neer II) with glenoid replacement. She regained 90 degrees elevation in her shoulder and was relieved of pain. An osteotomy of the third metatarsal with tenotomy of extensor tendons two, three, and four was performed at the same time for recurrent problems with her left forefoot.

In March 1984, due to pain in the right thumb with subluxation of the MCP joint, she underwent an MCP joint fusion of the right thumb and a capsulotomy of the ring finger PIP joint to correct a flexion deformity. The thumb fusion produced excellent position of her thumb with the usual pain relief and optimum function. Finally,

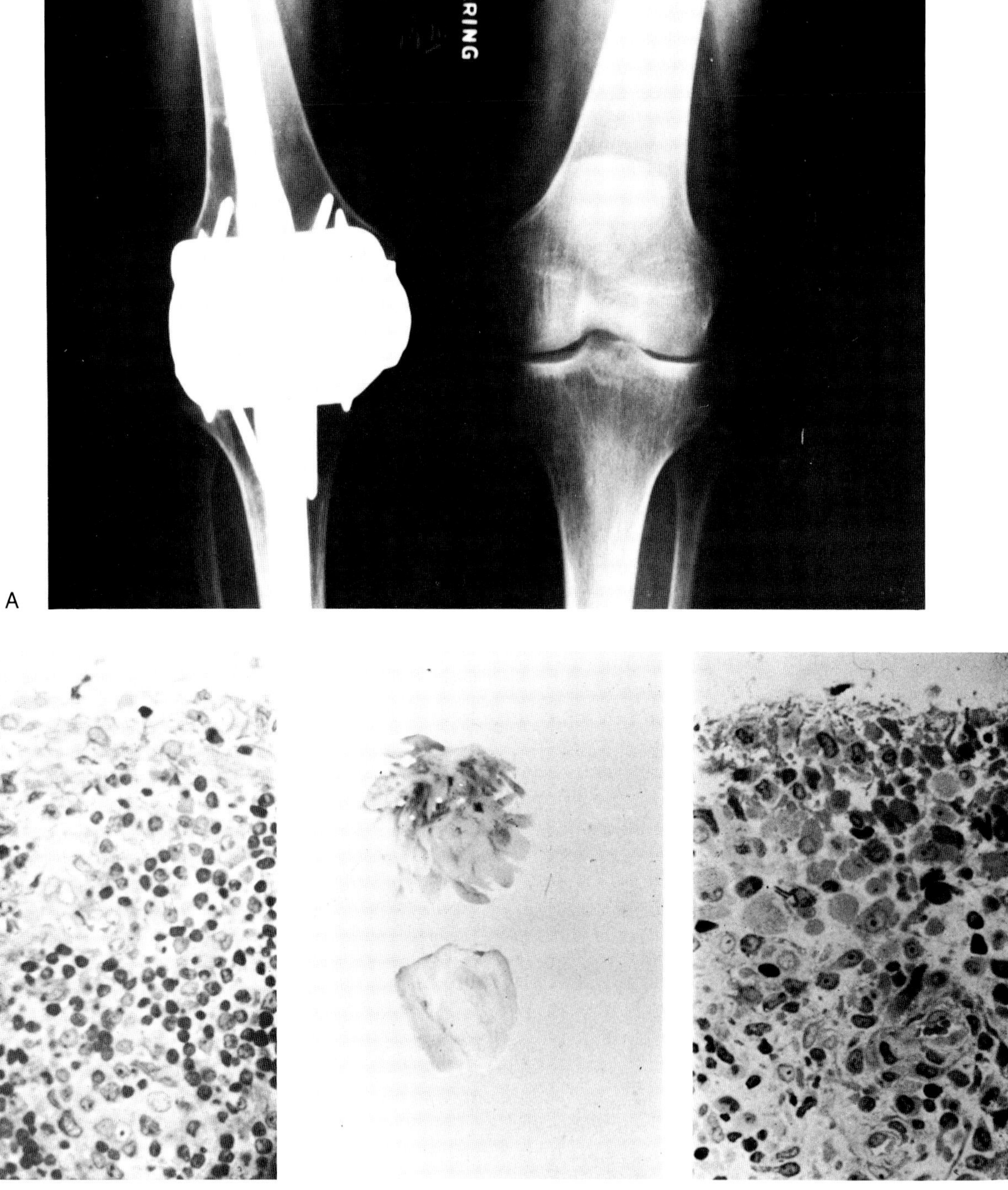

Fig. 20-4. (**A**) At 6 years after synovectomy of the left knee. Note the moderate narrowing of the joint spacing but no bone changes (early stage III). The hinge knee is in good position. (**B**) Center, top: Gross specimen of posterior compartment with villous proliferative synovium. Center, bottom: Gross specimen of anterior compartment with thickened but smooth synovium. Note the increased cellular activity in the posterior compartment (left) compared to that in the anterior compartment (right).

a left total hip replacement was performed in November 1988. A chronology of her surgeries is as follows.

6/1/64 Right Herman Young hinge total knee replacement (TKR)
8/3/64 Right knee manipulation
11/10/64 Left knee synovectomy
11/18/64 Left knee manipulation
6/21/65 Right wrist tenosynovectomy of extensor tendons, transposition of dorsal carpal ligament, excision of distal ulna
2/7/66 Left wrist synovectomy, tenosynovectomy of extensor tendons; left elbow arthrotomy with synovectomy and débridement and excision of radial head
10/14/66 Right foot triple arthrodesis with bone plug grafts
11/7/66 Left foot triple arthrodesis with bone plug grafts
2/13/68 Left elbow arthroplasty with fascia lata
2/3/69 Right shoulder synovectomy; right wrist partial synovectomy
10/15/69 Left radical mastectomy
11/23/70 Left knee synovectomy (repeat)
12/10/70 Left knee manipulation
2/14/72 Right elbow synovectomy with radial head excision; right hand synovectomy MCP 2–5, PIP 2
7/1/74 Bilateral forefoot reconstructions
3/9/76 Left shoulder synovectomy and tenodesis of biceps tendon
8/3/76 Right elbow fascial arthroplasty and excision of rheumatoid nodule (right leg)
9/8/78 Right total hip replacement (THR); tenotomy of both great toes
1/2/79 Right total shoulder replacement (TSR)
1/17/80 Left TKR
7/31/81 Left TSR; osteotomy of left metatarsal 3; left foot tenotomy of extensor tendons 2–4
4/12/84 Right thumb MCP fusion; finger capsulotomy
11/28/88 Left THR

DISCUSSION

The care of this patient illustrates much of the development and evolution of rheumatoid surgery since the 1960s. She has had more than 20 operative procedures, each of which was performed for her major complaint at the time with a specific objective in mind. The patient was kept ambulatory during these years and is still independent and ambulatory with a cane.

A discussion of her individual operations in a regional manner follows, beginning with the knee. *Note*: discussion of the knee is completely illustrated in this case report in order to demonstrate the evolution of surgery in the rheumatoid arthritic knee. Illustrations have been omitted for areas other than the knee to avoid duplicating illustrations from previous chapters.

Knee

6/1/64 Right Herman Young hinge TKR
8/3/64 Right knee manipulation
11/10/64 Left knee synovectomy
11/18/64 Left knee manipulation
11/23/70 Repeat left knee synovectomy
12/10/70 Left knee manipulation
1/17/80 Left TKR

When first seen in 1964, her major complaint was the right knee, which was destroyed with no remaining articular cartilage in the weight-bearing areas (Fig. 20-1). She exhibited the common changes—flexion, valgus, external rotation deformity with active synovitis and marked pain—and was unable to walk without crutches. It was too late for synovectomy. At that time there was no uniformly successful knee arthroplasty available, so the hinge knee was inserted to avoid an arthrodesis for an unknown length of time.

A few months after the hinge knee was inserted on the right, she experienced marked pain and swelling in the left knee (Fig. 20-2). Weight-bearing roentgenograms revealed normal joint spacing (stage I) (Fig. 20-3). Because of the destructive course followed in the right knee, an early synovectomy of the knee was indicated[3]; a disastrous course in the same patient in one knee is a prime indication for early synovectomy in the opposite knee.

As the posterior compartment did not seem to be involved at the time of synovectomy, no posterior synovectomy was performed, and the menisci appeared to be intact. She underwent manipulation of the knee 1 week after surgery, as this procedure was done almost routinely at that time in order to gain increased motion. Early in our series of knee synovectomies, we did not strive to gain motion beyond 90 degrees; later we realized that with more vigorous therapy and manipulation we could regain further flexion, which is important to rheumatoid patients, who usually have multiple joints involved. (Today, with continuous passive motion and supervised physical therapy, manipulation is rare.)

In 1970 she had recurrent pain and swelling in the left knee, but some joint spacing remained (early stage III) (Fig. 20-4A). A repeat synovectomy was performed, including anterior and posterior compartments. The posterior compartment seemed to show more proliferative synovitis than the anterior compartment, although both were involved (Fig. 20-4B). The menisci were involved and were removed at this time. Postoperatively, manipulation was again performed, and she regained essentially total motion in this knee. She remained free of pain for a number of years.

Today she most likely would have an arthroscopic synovectomy on the left knee. Her initial synovectomy produced excellent results for 6 years and the second one for 9 years. Neither procedure burned any bridges for later total knee replacement, and she gained 15 years of useful function. Synovectomy is the only procedure that maintains function in the patient's own joint, albeit for an unknown amount of time.

The left knee later became painful owing to loss of articular cartilage (Fig. 20-5), and in January 1980 she underwent a left total knee arthroplasty with a Miller multiradius knee anchored with cement by injection. It was basically a condylar type of resurfacing replacement for the knee; and the femur, tibia, and patella were all replaced (Fig. 20-6). Excellent alignment was obtained, and she regained motion of 110 degrees without manipulation (Fig. 20-7). Ten years later she was still active.

In 1990 she began having pain in the right hinge knee and right midtibial area. Pain increased, and motion decreased to 30 to 80 degrees. Roentgenograms showed that one screw in the proximal tibia had broken, and the distal tibial stem had eroded through the tibia posteriorly. A revision is necessary (Fig. 20-8).

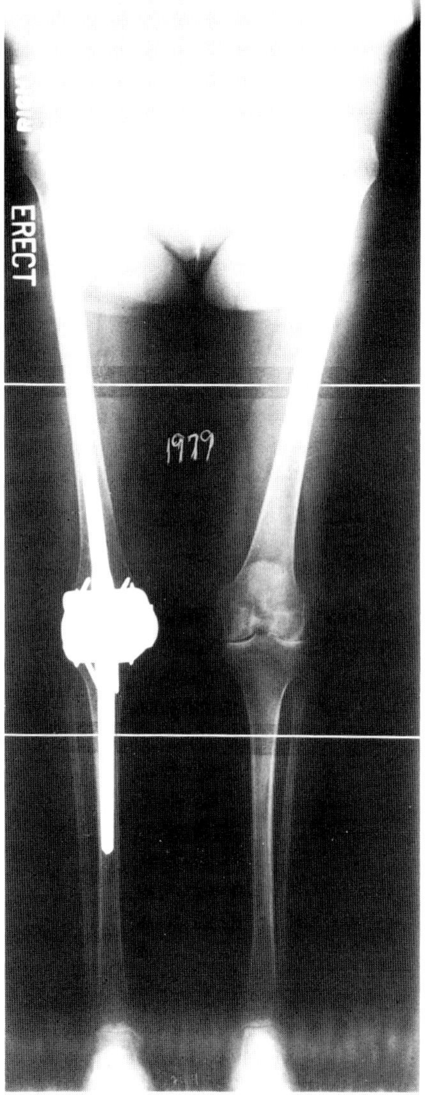

Fig. 20-5. Twelve years after right knee arthroplasty and 9 years after repeat synovectomy of the left knee. Note the marked joint narrowing (stage IIIb).

Currently, this case probably represents the longest known follow-up of a hinge-type knee arthroplasty. None of the arthroplasties of the knee available in 1964 is still used today. In 1968 we reported on the postmortem recovery of a Young hinge knee that had functioned for 2.5 years without a complication.[4] The wear was marked, although the knee continued to function. Small, black metallic fragments were found in the joint cavity and microscopically. At the present time,

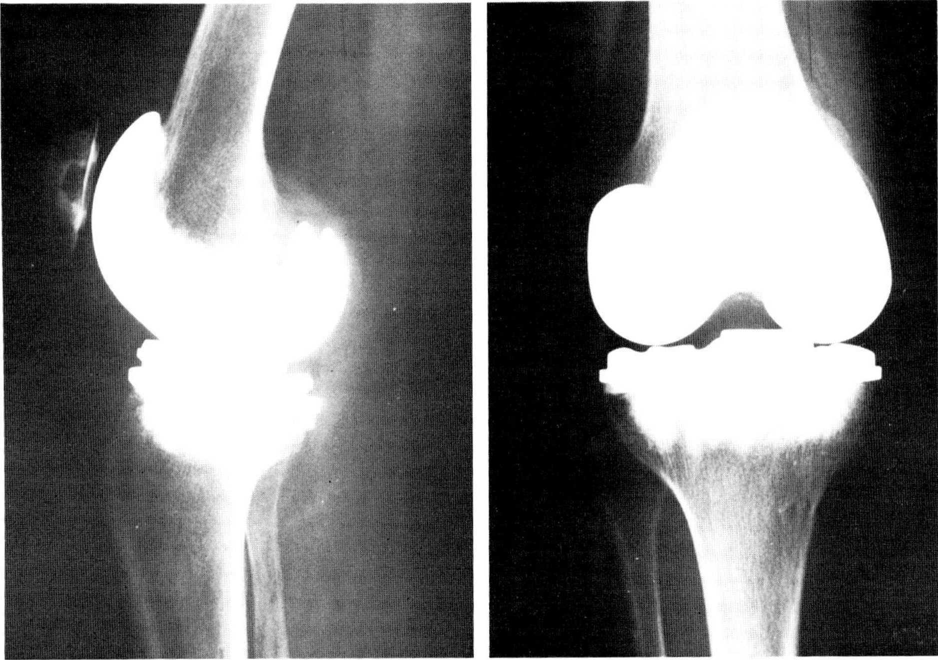

Fig. 20-6. Condylar-type left total knee arthroplasty (Miller multiradius) with cemented components.

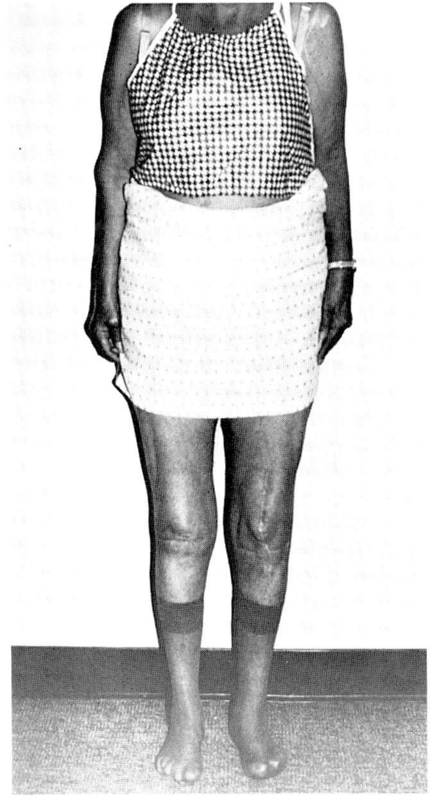

hinges are no longer used because they are constrained and caused too many problems. Actually, the more recent hinges used with cement have caused as many problems as the earlier, uncemented hinges. A number of hinges have had to be removed because of infection as well as loosening; arthrodesis has been necessary in some cases of infection. Rigid hinges have not been used since the early 1970s. The modern condylar posterior cruciate-sparing nonconstrained total knee replacement has provided more than 90 percent good to excellent results for more than 10 years in our experience.[5]

Foot

10/14/66 Right triple arthrodesis with iliac bone graft
11/7/66 Left triple arthrodesis with iliac bone graft

Fig. 20-7. Twenty years after right total knee hinge replacement and 4 years after left total knee replacement.

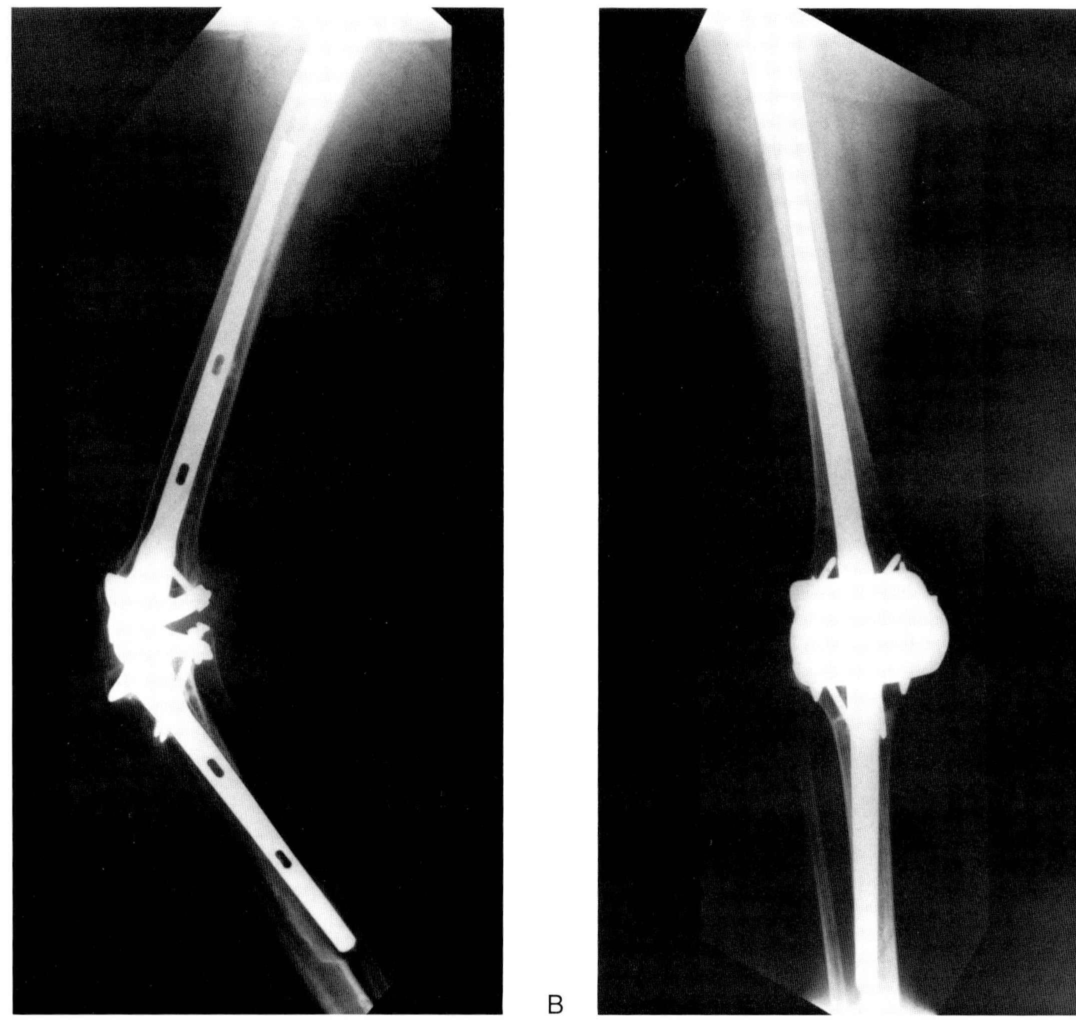

Fig. 20-8. Lateral (**A**) and anteroposterior (**B**) views of the Young hinge in place at 27 years. Note erosion of the posterior tibia and broken anchoring screws in the tibia. Revision is planned using a custom-made prosthesis.

7/1/74 Bilateral forefoot reconstructions
9/8/78 Tenotomy of both great toes
7/31/81 Left foot osteotomy of metatarsal 3 and extensor tenotomy of metatarsals 2–4

The patient had pain in the hindfoot, particularly in the subtalar joint, with tenderness. There was narrowing of the triple joints, but with good overall alignment of the foot on both the anteroposterior and lateral roentgenograms. She had good ankle motion (35 degrees without pain).

Triple arthrodesis was performed with iliac-type plug grafts, and she was immobilized in walking casts. During the healing period she was able to be ambulatory because the foot was in a stable position and there had been minimal dissection with the insertion of the plug grafts. If the foot either is in a good position or can be passively corrected, the triple arthrodesis is best performed with these types of plug graft, as there is less swelling and weight-bearing can often be attained. Weight-bearing must be deferred for a number of weeks if the foot is unstable and bone resection is necessary, even with staple fixation.

Bilateral forefoot reconstructions with MTP

joint resections were performed to relieve the forefoot pain. However, she did have minor operations at a later date with tenotomy of the extensor tendons to the great toe and osteotomy of the third metatarsal with extensor tenotomies on the left foot. (About 10 percent of all forefoot reconstructions require some type of later surgery.) This operation has been successful in our experience for more than 35 years, having a longer track record than any other lower extremity procedure today.

Hip

9/8/78 Right THR
11/28/88 Left THR

The patient had pain with destruction of the cartilage in the right hip, and a total hip arthroplasty was performed. Once a hip becomes involved, it almost inevitably progresses until intolerable pain indicates the need for surgery. The best single operation available for rheumatoid arthritis is the THR, and this patient has enjoyed an excellent result for 12 years.

Shoulder

2/3/69 Right shoulder synovectomy
3/9/76 Left shoulder synovectomy
1/12/79 Right TSR (Neer II)
7/31/81 Left TSR (Neer II)

Increasing pain in the patient's right shoulder caused synovial crepitus but allowed a functional range of motion. Roentgenograms revealed good joint spacing. Total acromionectomy was performed and provided excellent exposure. Two longitudinal incisions were made through the rotator cuff, and synovectomy was performed under vision with ronguers. The deltoid was carefully repaired following removal of the acromion, and she regained superb range of motion. The involved biceps tendon was tenodesed into the humerus. She underwent the same procedure in 1976 on the left shoulder. (When synovectomy is indicated today, it is usually performed arthroscopically. A partial rather than a total acromionectomy is utilized if indicated.) Her right

total shoulder was replaced in 1979 because of the progressive nature of the disease, but she had enjoyed good function for 10 years after synovectomy. The left shoulder was replaced 5 years after synovectomy. She is able to perform her activities of daily living without pain.

Elbow

2/7/66 Elbow synovectomy and radial head excision
2/13/68 Left elbow fascial arthroplasty with fascia lata
2/14/72 Right elbow synovectomy and radial head excision
8/3/76 Right elbow fascial arthroplasty

The patient's painful elbows were first treated by synovectomy with excision of the radial head, which provided considerable improvement for a number of years, but she subsequently had bilateral fascial arthroplasties. Although her elbows still function, there has been some bone absorption in the humerous, and she eventually may need total elbow replacements.

Fascial arthroplasty has produced good results in a number of patients, but if the patient has progressive bone absorption, fascial arthroplasty is not satisfactory. We have not done a fascial arthroplasty in a rheumatoid elbow since the early 1980s, and we prefer to use the non- or semiconstrained type of total elbow replacement when arthroplasty is necessary. We continue to use synovectomy and radial head excision as a primary operation, as it has provided good long-term results, with 78 percent of the patients still having improvement after 7.5 years.[2]

Wrist

6/21/65 Right wrist synovectomy, tenosynovectomy, excision of distal ulna
2/7/66 Left wrist synovectomy, tenosynovectomy, excision of distal ulna
2/14/72 Right hand MCP 2–5 synovectomy and index PIP joints
4/12/84 Right MCP fusion of thumb

The patient began to have problems with her right wrist in 1965, the wrist being the key joint to the hand. Synovectomy of the wrist with teno-synovectomy and excision of the distal ulna is still an excellent procedure. It helps restore pronation and supination, prevent tendon ruptures of the extensor tendons at the wrist, and relieve pain; it is the most successful procedure for the wrist. In the patient described, useful hand function has continued to be maintained.

In 1972 she had synovectomy of MCP joints two to five and index PIP joints at the time of elbow synovectomy. Twelve years later, pain and instability of the right thumb were treated by MCP fusion, the most successful procedure in the digits. Useful function in her hands has continued to be maintained.

CONCLUSIONS

The case of this patient outlines the evolution of surgery for rheumatoid arthritis over three decades. She was followed by rheumatologists and treated with the best available drug therapy, but her disease remained active in a slow, cyclic progression. Each operation has given some relief of pain as well as some gain in function to the area of the patient's major complaint at that time. "Early" procedures such as synovectomy did not "burn any bridges" for later procedures, and this patient has been able to lead an independent and useful life because of the team approach. (Details of described procedures are found in preceding chapters.)

REFERENCES

1. Clayton ML: Surgery of the lower extremity in rheumatoid arthritis. J Bone Joint Surg [Am] 45:1517, 1963
2. Ferlic DC, Patchett CE, Clayton ML, Freeman AC: Elbow synovectomy in rheumatoid arthritis: long term results. Clin Orthop 220:119, 1987
3. Geens S, Clayton ML, Leidholt JD et al: Synovectomy and débridement of the knee in rheumatoid arthritis. I. Historical review. II. Clinical and roentgenographic study of 31 cases. J Bone Joint Surg [Am] 51:626, 1969
4. Girzadas DV, Geens S, Clayton ML, Leidholt JD: Performance of a hinged metal knee prosthesis; a case report with a follow-up of three and one-half years and histologic and metallurgic data. J Bone Joint Surg [Am] 50:355, 1968
5. Papenfus K, Clayton ML, Dennis DA et al: The Clayton total hip arthroplasty: a ten-year follow-up. Clin Orthop (in press)
6. Young HH: Use of a hinged vitallium prosthesis for arthroplasty of the knee: a preliminary report. J Bone Joint Surg [Am] 45:1627, 1963

Appendix: Patient Letter

TO OUR TOTAL JOINT REPLACEMENT PATIENTS

It is important to remember that your new total joint replacement is not a "natural" joint, and special care must be taken. The following information should be kept for future reference.

1. ANTIBIOTICS AND INFECTION: Extremely important is the necessity of preventing blood-borne infections in your total joint. If you have any dental work done, even cleaning by the hygienist, you should receive protective antibiotics. You should inform your dentist. Our general recommendation is 2 grams of Penicillin VK oral one hour before the procedure and 1 grams six hours after the procedure.

If you have a bacterial infection anywhere in your body, including a sore throat, a urinary tract infection, or a respiratory system infection, you should always check with your family doctor so the appropriate antibiotics can be given.

2. RETURN OFFICE VISITS: It is vital that we follow your progress and that of your total joint annually *forever*. We cannot emphasize enough the importance of follow-up examinations. Total joint complications often first seen on x-ray films are easier to manage if detected early. A chronic problem can be much more difficult to resolve. If traveling to our office becomes a problem, please notify us as to who your local family physician or orthopaedist is, and we can keep in contact with him or her.

3. ADDRESS NOTIFICATION: Please include us in your address book and keep us notified if you move. We are in the midst of keeping current records on all our total joint replacement patients.

4. AIRPLANES: Enclosed is a wallet-sized card that we request you carry with you at all times. In the event that a metal detection device, such as those currently in use at airports, is activated by your total joint, this card provides ready explanation. This problem generally does not occur, as most implants used today are nonmagnetic. Our address is also included if you or your physician should need to reach us at any time.

Please feel free to call us should you or your doctor have any questions.

Index

Page numbers followed by f *indicate figures; those followed by* t *indicate tables.*

10 32√ √8

P15RX7

DATE DUE

	JUL 4 0 1992		